Surgical Management of Hepatobiliary and Pancreatic Disorders

Surgical Management of Hepatobiliary and Pancreatic Disorders

Edited by

Graeme J Poston MS, FRCS, FRCS(Ed)
Department of Surgery
The Royal Liverpool University Hospitals
Liverpool, UK

and

Leslie H Blumgart MD, FACS, FRCS, FRCPS
Hepatobiliary Service, Department of Surgery
Memorial Sloan–Kettering Cancer Center
New York, USA

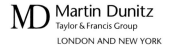
Martin Dunitz
Taylor & Francis Group
LONDON AND NEW YORK

© 2003 Martin Dunitz Ltd, a member of the Taylor & Francis group

First published in the United Kingdom in 2003
by Martin Dunitz Ltd, The Livery House, 7–9 Pratt Street, London NW1 0AE

Tel.:   +44 (0) 20 74822202
Fax.:   +44 (0) 20 72670159
E-mail: info@dunitz.co.uk
Website: http://www.dunitz.co.uk

A CIP record for this book is available from the British Library.

ISBN 1 899066 97 7

Distributed in the USA by
Taylor & Francis
10650 Tobben Drive
Independence, KY 41051, USA
Toll Free Tel.: +1 800 634 7064
E-mail: taylorandfrancis@thomsonlearning.com

Distributed in Canada by
Taylor & Francis
74 Rolark Drive
Scarborough, Ontario M1R 4G2, Canada
Toll Free Tel.: +1 877 226 2237
E-mail: tal_fran@istar.ca

Distributed in the rest of the world by
Thomson Publishing Services
Cheriton House
North Way
Andover, Hampshire SP10 5BE, UK
Tel.: +44 (0)1264 332424
E-mail: salesorder.tandf@thomsonpublishingservices.co.uk

Composition by Scribe Design, Gillingham, Kent
Printed and bound in Singapore by Imago

Contents

Contributors

Åke Andrén-Sandberg
Department of Surgery
Haukeland University Hospital
N–5021 Bergen, Norway

Philippe Bachellier
Centre de Chirurgie Viscérale et de Transplantation
Hôpital de Hautepierre
67200 Strasbourg, France

David L Bartlett
National Cancer Institute
National Institutes of Health
Building 10, Room 2B17
Bethesda, MD 20892, USA

Hans G Beger
Department of General Surgery
University Hospital of Surgery
Steinhovelstrasse 9
89075 Ulm, Germany

Thomas V Berne
Department of Surgery
University of Southern California Medical Center
1200 North State Street, Room 9900
Los Angeles, CA 90033, USA

Leslie H Blumgart
Hepatobiliary Service
Department of Surgery
Memorial Sloan–Kettering Cancer Center
1275 York Avenue
New York, NY 10021, USA

Giacomo Borgonovo
Dipartimento di Discipline Chirurgiche e
Metodologie Integrate
Università di Genova
Genova, Italy

Murray F Brennan
Department of Surgery
Memorial Sloan–Kettering Cancer Center
1275 York Avenue
New York, NY 10021, USA

Markus W Büchler
Department of General Surgery
University of Heidelberg
D–69120 Heidelberg, Germany

Kevin Conlon
Department of Surgery
Memorial Sloan–Kettering Cancer Center
1275 York Avenue
New York, NY 10021, USA

Margaret Finch-Jones
Department of Surgery
Bristol Royal Infirmary
Marlborough Street
Bristol BS2 8HW, UK

Ian Finlay
Department of Surgery
St George Hospital
Pitney Clinical Sciences Building
Kogarah
Sydney, NSW 2217, Australia

Yuman Fong
Hepatobiliary Service
Department of Surgery
Memorial Sloan–Kettering Cancer Center
1275 York Avenue
New York, NY 10021, USA

H Friess
Department of General Surgery
University of Heidelberg
D–69120 Heidelberg, Germany

Sivakumar Gananadha
Department of Surgery
St George Hospital
Pitney Clinical Sciences Building
Kogarah
Sydney, NSW 2217, Australia

Justin Geoghegan
Department of Surgery
St. Vincent's University Hospital
Elm Park
Dublin 4, Ireland

Hjörtur Gislason
Department of Surgery
Haukeland University Hospital
N–5021 Bergen, Norway

David Marcus Gore
Department of Surgery
Royal Liverpool University Hospital
5th Floor, Duncan Building
Daulby Street
Liverpool L69 3GA, UK

Lawrence E Harrison
New Jersey Medical School
University of Medicine and Dentistry of New Jersey
185 South Orange Avenue
Newark, NJ 07103, USA

Mark Hartley
Department of Surgery
Royal Liverpool University Hospital
Prescot Street
Liverpool L7 8XP, UK

Steven N Hochwald
University of Florida Medical School
Box 100286
Gainesville, FL 32610–0286, USA

Dag Hoem
Department of Surgery
Haukeland University Hospital
N–5021 Bergen, Norway

Arild Horn
Department of Surgery
Haukeland University Hospital
N–5021 Bergen, Norway

Clement W Imrie
Department of Surgery
Royal Infirmary
16 Alexandra Parade
Glasgow G31 2ER, UK

Daniel Jaeck
Centre de Chirurgie Viscérale et de Transplantation
Hôpital de Hautepierre
67200 Strasbourg, France

William R Jarnagin
Hepatobiliary Service
Department of Surgery
Memorial Sloan–Kettering Cancer Center
1275 York Avenue
New York, NY 10021, USA

Timothy G John
Department of Surgery
The North Hampshire Hospital NHS Trust
Aldermaston Road
Basingstoke RG24 9NA, UK

Alan G Johnson
Academic Surgical Unit
University of Sheffield
Department of Surgical and Anaesthetic Sciences
K-Floor
Royal Hallamshire Hospital
Sheffield S10 2JF, UK

Matthew Jones
Paediatric Surgery
Royal Liverpool Children's Hospital
Alder Hey
Eaton Road
Liverpool L12 2AP, UK

WY Lau
Department of Surgery
Prince of Wales Hospital
Shatin, New Territories, Hong Kong

Bernard Launois
formerly Centre de Chirurgie Digestive et
Hépatobiliaire
Hôpital Pontchaillou
Rue Henri Le Guilloux
35033 Rennes, France

CK Leow
Division of Hepatobiliary and Pancreatic Surgery
Department of Surgery
National University Hospital
5 Lower Kent Ridge Road
Singapore 119074

Michael PN Lewis
Department of Surgery
Norfolk and Norwich University Hospital
Colney Lane
Norwich NR4 7UZ, UK

Winston Liauw
Department of Surgery
St George Hospital
Pitney Clinical Sciences Building
Kogarah
Sydney, NSW 2217, Australia

David Lloyd
Paediatric Surgery
Royal Liverpool Children's Hospital
Alder Hey
Eaton Road
Liverpool L12 2AP, UK

J Peter A Lodge
Hepatobiliary and Transplant Unit
St. James's University Hospital
Beckett Street
Leeds LS9 7TF, UK

Ali W Majeed
Department of Surgical and Anaesthetic Sciences
K-Floor
Royal Hallamshire Hospital
Sheffield S10 2JF, UK

Dermot Malone
Diagnostic Imaging
St. Vincent's University Hospital
Elm Park
Dublin 4, Ireland

ME Martignoni
Department of General Surgery
University of Heidelberg
D–69120, Heidelberg, Germany

JC Meneu Diaz
Digestive Surgery Department
Hospital Universitario
12 de Octubre,
28041 Madrid, Spain

Olivier Monek
Centre de Chirurgie Viscérale et de Transplantation
Hôpital de Hautepierre
67200 Strasbourg, France

A Moreno
Digestive Surgery Department
Hospital Universitario
12 de Octubre,
28041 Madrid, Spain

Enrique Moreno Gonzalez
Digestive Surgery Department
Hospital Universitario
12 de Octubre,
28041 Madrid, Spain

David L Morris
Department of Surgery
St George Hospital
Pitney Clinical Sciences Building
Kogarah
Sydney, NSW 2217, Australia

James A Murray
Department of Surgery
University of Southern California Medical Center
1200 North State Street, Room 9900
Los Angeles, CA 90033, USA

Elie Oussoultzoglou
Centre de Chirurgie Viscérale et de Transplantation
Hôpital de Hautepierre
67200 Strasbourg, France

Ian Pope
Department of Surgery
The Royal Infirmary
Lauriston Place
Edinburgh EH3, UK

Graeme J Poston
Department of Surgery
The Royal Liverpool University Hospitals
Prescot Street
Liverpool L7 8XP, UK

Myrddin Rees
Department of Surgery
The North Hampshire Hospital NHS Trust
Aldermaston Lane
Basingstoke RG24 9NA, UK

Michael Rhodes
Department of Surgery
Norfolk and Norwich Hospital
Colney Lane
Norwich NR4 7UZ, UK

Pierre F Saldinger
Section of General Surgery
Danbury Hospital
24 Hospital Avenue
Danbury, CT 06810, USA

Wolfgang Schlosser
Department of General Surgery
University Hospital of Surgery
Steinhovelstrasse 9
89075 Ulm, Germany

Andreas Schwarz
Department of General Surgery
University Hospital of Surgery
Steinhovelstrasse 9
89075 Ulm, Germany

Marco Siech
Department of General Surgery
University Hospital of Surgery
Steinhovelstrasse 9
89075 Ulm, Germany

Claude Smadja
Digestive Surgery
University of Paris
Hôpital Antoine Béclère
157 rue de la Porte-de-Trivaux
92141 Clamart Cedex, France

Lygia Stewart
Department of Surgery
Department of Veterans Affairs
University of California
Surgical Service (112)
4150 Clement Street
San Francisco, CA 94121, USA

Francis Sutherland
Department of Surgery
Peter Lougheed Hospital
3500, 26th Ave, NE
Calgary
Alberta T2Y 6J4, Canada

Robert Sutton
Department of Surgery
Royal Liverpool University Hospital
5th Floor Duncan Building
Daulby Street
Liverpool L69 3GA, UK

Sandro Tagliacozzo
1st Institute of Surgical Clinic
Universita degli Studi di Roma 'La Sapienza'
Vaile del Policlinico
155–00161 Rome, Italy

Oscar Traynor
Department of Surgery
St. Vincent's University Hospital
Elm Park
Dublin 4, Ireland

Asgaut Viste
Department of Surgery
Haukeland University Hospital
N–5021 Bergen, Norway

Preface

Hepato-pancreato-biliary (HPB) surgery is now firmly established within the repertoire of modern general surgery. Indeed, in many major tertiary centres there are now specific teams for both pancreatic and liver surgery. However, in most hospitals outside these major centres the day-to-day management and decision-making for patients with these disorders remains the remit of the general surgeon.

The purpose of this book is therefore two-fold. Firstly, it is intended to cover the spectrum of common HPB diseases that will confront the general surgeon in his or her regular practice. The chapters are problem-based, rather than didactic descriptions of pathology and surgical technique. Secondly, we hope that this work will be sufficiently comprehensive to cover the broad spectrum of HPB surgery for candidates coming to examinations at the completion of surgical training.

We are indebted to the many international contributors for their perseverance and patience over the gestation of this project, which is greatly appreciated. Lastly, we are grateful to our publishers, Martin Dunitz, for their help during the preparation of this project.

Graeme J Poston
Liverpool

Leslie H Blumgart
New York

1 Surgical anatomy of the liver and bile ducts

Graeme J Poston and Leslie H Blumgart

The success of any surgical intervention on the liver and bile ducts is totally dependent on a thorough working knowledge of their anatomy. As more and more patients are now being considered for liver resection this anatomy should now be within the understanding of all surgeons with an interest in the gastrointestinal tract. Furthermore, a command of this anatomy is a prerequisite for any interpretation of radiological studies and other imaging of pathology within the liver and biliary system.

When operating on the liver, the surgeon has to obey three basic tenets. First, remove all pathologically involved tissue. Second, preserve the maximal amount of non-pathological liver tissue. Last, perform safe resection without excessive bleeding and impairment of vascularization of the remaining hepatic parenchyma. Similar principles apply to biliary surgery. First, achieve maximal effective drainage of the biliary tree. Second, resect all diseased tissue while protecting and maintaining the vascularity of the residual bile ducts thus allowing successful long term biliary enteric drainage.

Anatomy of the liver

Historically, the liver has been described according to its morphological appearance, but hepatic resection is wholly dependent on the functional and surgical anatomy of the liver.

Morphological anatomy

At laparotomy the liver is divided by the umbilical fissure and falciform ligament into a larger 'right' lobe and a smaller 'left' lobe (Figs 1.1 and 1.2). Situated on the inferior surface of this right lobe is

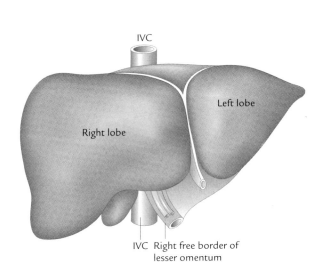

Figure 1.1 Morphological anatomy.

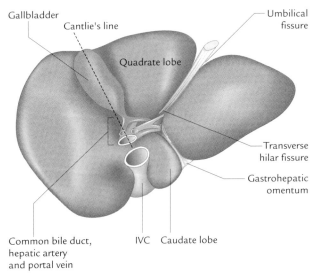

Figure 1.2 Anatomical features.

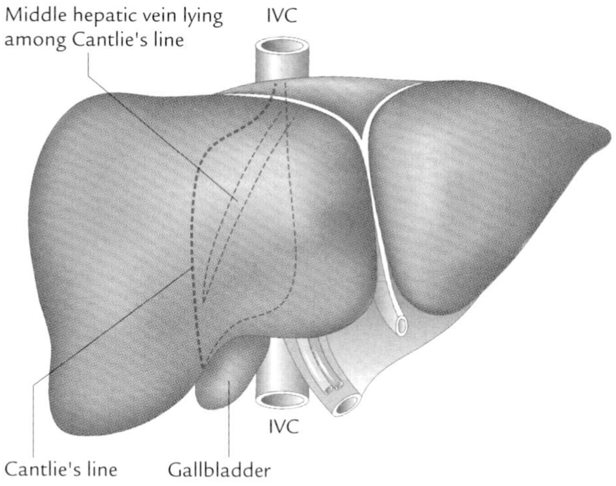

Middle hepatic vein lying among Cantlie's line

IVC

IVC

Cantlie's line   Gallbladder

Figure 1.3   Cantlie's line.

the transverse hilar fissure which constitutes the posterior limit of this lobe. That portion of the right lobe lying anterior to this fissure and to the right of the umbilical fissure is referred to as the quadrate lobe. The right side margin of the quadrate lobe is determined by the gallbladder fossa. Posterior to the hilum, lying between the portal vein and the inferior vena cava (IVC) is the caudate lobe, which is anatomically and functionally separate from the rest of the liver. This anatomical approach is only adequate for left lateral segmentectomy (see below) and is of no use in any other form of liver resection.

Functional anatomy

Francis Glisson of Cambridge first described the segmental anatomy of the liver in 1654,[1] but this work remained largely forgotten for nearly 300

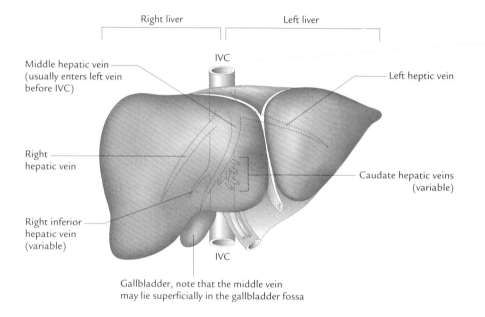

Right liver   Left liver

Middle hepatic vein (usually enters left vein before IVC)

IVC

Left heptic vein

Right hepatic vein

Caudate hepatic veins (variable)

Right inferior hepatic vein (variable)

IVC

Gallbladder, note that the middle vein may lie superficially in the gallbladder fossa

Figure 1.4   Venous drainage of the liver.

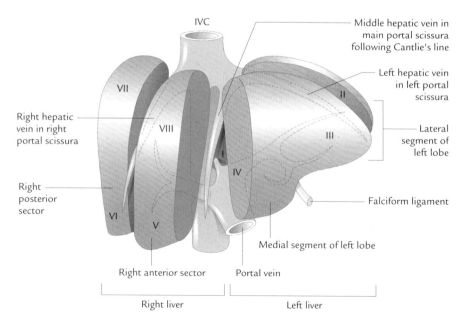

IVC

Middle hepatic vein in main portal scissura following Cantlie's line

Left hepatic vein in left portal scissura

Right hepatic vein in right portal scissura

Lateral segment of left lobe

Right posterior sector

Falciform ligament

Medial segment of left lobe

Right anterior sector   Portal vein

Right liver   Left liver

VII   VIII   II   III   IV   I   VI   V

Figure 1.5   Functional sectoral anatomy and relationship to hepatic scissurae.

years. In 1888, Rex reported a 'new' arrangement of the right and left lobes of the liver and further refined our understanding of lobar anatomy.[2] The modern first attempt to define the functional anatomy of the liver was made by Cantlie in 1898 while working as a pathologist in Hong Kong. Cantlie made a number of dissections of the livers of condemned prisoners following their execution in a Hong Kong jail.[3] He made vascular casts of the liver to demonstrate that the main lobar fissure is oblique and extends from right to left and from the visceral to the parietal surface at an angle of about 70°. From these studies, Cantlie demonstrated that the main division between the right and left lobe extends from approximately the bed of the gallbladder anteroinferiorly to the right side of the IVC posterosuperiorly (Figs 1.2 and 1.3).[4] Thirty years later, Cantlie's work was verified by McIndoe and Counsellor[5] and Hjorstjo.[6] In 1939, Ton That Tung described the role of the venous drainage of the liver in relationship to the functional lobar anatomy (Fig. 1.4),[7] and in 1953 Healey and Schroy, while constructing casts of the biliary tree, were able to show that the right lobe was further divided into an anterior and a posterior segment.[8] These studies also demonstrated that the left lobe was divided into a medial and lateral segment by the line of the falciform ligament (Fig. 1.5). From these descriptions, Goldsmith and Woodburne were able to recommend anatomical planes through the liver parenchyma for performing a right lobectomy (right hepatectomy), a left lobectomy (left hepatectomy) and a left lateral segmentectomy (Fig. 1.6).[9]

Early application of the functional anatomy

Although successful surgical treatments of isolated liver wounds had been described in the early seventeenth century by Hildanus and Berta,[10] and subsequent series of battlefield injuries described during the Napoleonic[11] and Franco-Prussian Wars,[12] The first attempt at resection of a liver tumour was not made until 1886 by Luis.[13] In November of that year, he excised a solid liver tumour by ligating and cutting through a pedunculated left lobe 'adenoma'. Attempts to suture the severed pedicle were unsuccessful, and the stump was returned to the peritoneal cavity. Not surprisingly, the patient succumbed some 6 hours later, after continuing haemorrhage from the stump.

The first successful elective liver resection is attributed to von Langenbuch, who excised a 370 g portion of the left lobe of the liver containing an adenoma in 1888.[14] Unfortunately, he had to reopen the abdomen several hours after the operation because of reactionary haemorrhage, but was able to ligate the bleeding vessels and return the oversewn

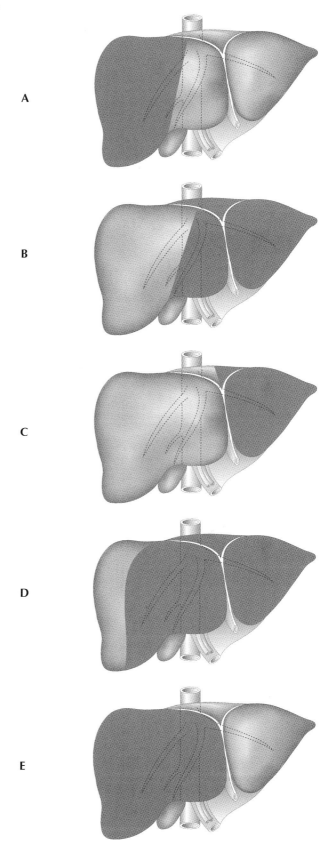

Figure 1.6 Formal hepatectomies: (A) right hepatectomy; (B) left hepatectomy; (C) left lateral segmentectomy; (D) extended left hepatectomy; (E) extended right hepatectomy.

liver to the abdomen. Two years later, the Baltimore surgeon McLane Tiffany reported the successful removal of a benign liver tumour,[15] and the following year Lucke described the successful resection of a cancerous growth of the liver.[16] In 1911, Wendel reported the first case of right lobectomy for a primary tumour,[17] and in 1940 Cattell was first to remove successfully a colorectal hepatic metastasis.[18] In 1943, Wangensteen performed a coincidental partial hepatectomy while performing a gastrectomy for a carcinoma with direct extension into the left lobe of the liver.[19]

The first left lateral segmentectomy was probably performed by Keen in 1899, but because of a lack of understanding of anatomical planes was described as a left hepatic lobectomy.[20] The first anatomically correct description of a left lateral segmentectomy was made by Raven in 1948 while resecting metastatic colon cancer.[21] An anatomical resection was performed in which the triangular and coronary ligaments were divided, and the left portal vein, left hepatic artery and left hepatic ducts were ligated within the hepatoduodenal ligament. The left hepatic vein was then isolated extrahepatically and then divided before the parenchyma was transected. Four years later, Lortat-Jacob and Robert described a similar approach to right hepatic lobectomy (Fig. 1.6).[22]

Appreciation of segmental anatomy

Probably the most important anatomical contribution to modern liver surgery comes from the work of Claude Couinaud, who in 1957 published the findings of a large number of vasculobiliary casts made by plastic injection followed by corrosion of the surrounding parenchyma.[23] These studies followed on 5 years after his demonstration of a right paramedian and latero-inferior sectors,[24] which paralleled the work of Healey and Schroy.[8] Couinaud was able to demonstrate that the liver consists of eight segments, each of which can potentially be separately resected. Couinaud redefined the caudate lobe as segment I and Goldsmith and Woodburne's left lobe as segments II and III. The quadrate lobe is now segment IV and more recently has been further subdivided by its portal blood supply into segments IVA lying superiorly and IVB inferiorly. The right liver consists of segments V (anteroinferiorly), VI (posteroinferiorly), VII (postero-superiorly) and VIII (anterosuperiorly) (Fig. 1.7). Couinaud later suggested a further clarification of the caudate lobe in which the part to the left of the IVC remains segment I and that to the right is redefined as segment IX.[25]

Resections based on these segments would minimize residual functional hepatic impairment. The

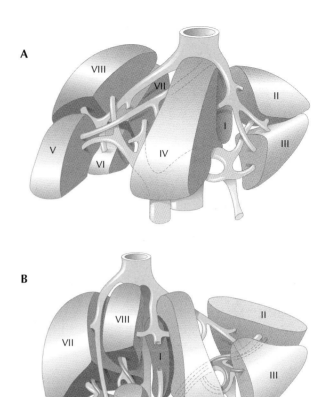

Figure 1.7 Functional division of the liver and of the liver segments according to Couinaud's nomenclature: (A) as seen in the patient and (B) in the ex vivo position.

description of Couinaud is the most complete and exact and also the most useful for the operating surgeon, and it is this description which will be used throughout this book.

Resection of segment I usually requires a preliminary left lobectomy to facilitate access and this procedure was first described by Ton That Tun, who was also the first to describe resection of segment VIII.[26] The first description of resection of segment IV was by Caprio in 1931, but in essence this was a resection of the inferior part of what was then the quadrate lobe.[27] Bismuth was first to report isolated resection of segment VI,[28] and in parallel with Ton That Tun described bisegmentectomy of segments VI and VII (right posterior sectorectomy).[26,28] Bi-segmentectomy of segments V and VI (right inferior hepatectomy) was described in 1955 by Mancuso and colleagues,[29] while in 1957 Couinaud was proposing en bloc resection with the gallbladder of segments IV, V and VI for carcinoma of the gall-bladder (Fig. 1.8).[23]

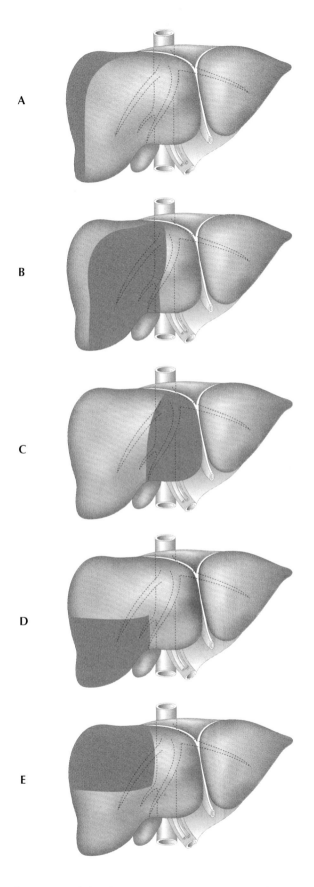

Figure 1.8 Other hepatic sectorectomies: (A) right posterior sectorectomy; (B) right anterior sectorectomy; (C) left medial sectorectomy (segment IVA and IVB); (D) right inferior hepatectomy; (E) right superior hepatectomy.

The study of the functional anatomy of the liver allows us to describe hepatic segments based upon the distribution of the portal pedicles and the location of the hepatic veins (Fig. 1.5). The three main hepatic veins (right, middle and left) divide the liver into four sectors, each of which receives a portal pedicle of hepatic artery, hepatic duct and portal vein, thus producing an alternation between hepatic veins and portal pedicles. These four sectors demarcated by the hepatic veins are the portal sectors, since each sector receives an independent portal supply. For the same reason, the scissurae containing the hepatic veins are called portal scissurae, while the scissurae containing portal pedicles are the hepatic scissurae (Fig. 1.5). Thus the liver is divided by the main portal scissura along the line of the middle hepatic vein into two discrete hemilivers, the line previously described by Cantlie.[3] We prefer to refer to these hemilivers as right and left livers, rather than right and left lobes, to avoid confusion with the anatomical lobes, particularly since there is no visible surface marking that permits individualization of a true lobe.

As described by Cantlie, the main portal scissura runs posteriorly from the middle of the gallbladder fossa to the right side of the IVC (Fig. 1.5). This scissura describes an angle of 75° with the horizontal plane opened to the left. Therefore, the right and left livers individualized by the main portal scissura are independent as regards their portal and arterial vascularization and biliary drainage.

These right and left livers are both further divided into two by the other two portal scissurae delineated by the right and left hepatic veins. Goldsmith and Woodburne refer to these further divisions as segments,[9] but we will use the more generally accepted nomenclature of Couinaud, which refers to these divisions as sectors.[23] The right liver is divided by the right portal scissura (right portal vein) into an anteromedial (or anterior) sector containing segments V inferiorly and VIII superiorly, and a posterolateral (or posterior) sector containing segments VI inferiorly and VII superiorly (Fig. 1.5). This right portal scissura is inclined 40° to the right (Fig. 1.5). However, when the liver lies in its normal unmobilized position within the upper abdominal cavity, the posterolateral sector lies directly behind the anteromedial sector and the scissura is almost in a coronal plane. Therefore in the clinical setting (particularly when imaging the liver) it is better to speak of the anterior and posterior sectors (Fig. 1.5). The exact location of the right portal scissura is imprecise because it has no external landmarks. According to Couinaud,[23] it extends from the anterior border of the liver at the middle of the distance between the right angle of the liver and the right side of the gallbladder bed to the confluence between the IVC and the right hepatic vein posteriorly. In Ton That Tung's description of 1939, this scissura follows a line that runs parallel to the right lateral edge of the liver, some three fingers' breadth anteriorly.[7]

The venous drainage of the right liver is variable in that in addition to the right and middle hepatic veins, there are often a number of smaller hepatic veins draining directly into the IVC from segments VI and VII. Not infrequently (63–68%) segment VI drains directly into the IVC through a large inferior right hepatic vein, which can be a significant bonus in the preservation of residual hepatic function in extended left hepatectomies (Fig. 1.4).[29,30]

The left portal scissura, along the left hepatic vein, divides the left liver into an anterior sector containing segments III laterally and IV medially, and a posterior sector containing segment II (Fig. 1.5). Note that the left portal scissura is not the umbilical fissure since this fissure is not a portal scissura; a portal scissura contains a hepatic vein and the umbilical fissure contains a portal pedicle. Therefore the left portal scissura lies posteriorly to the ligamentum teres inside the left lobe of the liver (Fig. 1.5). It is important to note that the middle hepatic vein (defining the main portal scissura) usually enters the left hepatic vein some 1–2 cm before the left hepatic vein joins the IVC (Fig. 1.4).[30] Occasionally the middle and left hepatic veins enter the IVC separately and in 2 of 34 of Couinaud's casts of the middle-left hepatic veins, the middle vein and left veins joined more than 2.5 cm from the IVC.[30] Such an anomaly must be detected and excluded during isolated resection of segment IV, since if not seen and the last 2 cm of the left vein is damaged, then segments II and III will be needlessly sacrificed.

The caudate lobe (segment I or segments I and IX) is the dorsal portion of the liver lying posteriorly and surrounding the retrohepatic IVC. As a result it lies directly between the portal vein lying anteriorly and the IVC posteriorly. The main bulk of the caudate lobe lies to the left of the IVC, with its left and inferior margins being free in the lesser omental bursa (Fig. 1.2). The gastrohepatic (lesser) omentum separates the left portion of the caudate from segments II and III of the left liver as it passes between them to be attached to the ligamentum venosum. The left portion of the caudate lobe thus traverses inferiorly to the right between the left portal vein and the IVC as the caudate process, which then fuses inferiorly with segment VI of the right liver. This portion of the caudate lobe that lies on the right side is variable but usually small. The anterior surface of the caudate lobe lies within the hepatic parenchyma against the posterior intrahepatic surface of segment IV, demarcated by an oblique plane slanting from the left portal vein to the left hepatic vein.

The caudate lobe must be considered from a functional viewpoint as an isolated autonomous segment, since its vascularization is independent of the portal division and of the three main hepatic veins. It receives both an arterial and a portal blood supply from both the right and left portal structures and this is variable, although the right caudate lobe receives an arterial supply consistently from the right posterior artery. Biliary drainage is likewise into both the right and left hepatic ducts. However, the left dorsal duct can also join the segment II duct. The small hepatic veins of the caudate lobe drain directly into the IVC. This independent isolation of the caudate lobe is clinically important in Budd–Chiari syndrome, if all three main hepatic veins are obliterated and the only hepatic venous drainage is through the caudate lobe, which then undergoes compensatory hyperplasia.

Anatomical classification of hepatectomies

We would classify these as 'typical' and 'atypical'. Typical hepatectomies (hepatectomies reglees) are defined by resection of a portion of liver parenchyma following one or several anatomical portal or hepatic scissurae. These resections are called left or right hepatectomies, sectorectomies and segmentectomies. Atypical hepatectomies involve resection of a portion of hepatic parenchyma not limited by anatomical scissurae. Such resections are usually inappropriate as they will leave behind devascularized residual liver and will probably also not adequately excise all the pathologically involved parenchyma.

The usual typical hepatectomies can be considered in two groups. First, right and left hepatectomies in which the line of transection is the main portal scissura separating the right and left livers along the middle hepatic vein (as proposed by Couinaud).[23] Second, right and left hepatectomies in which the line of transection commences in the umbilical fissure. For some time the latter definition, proposed by Goldsmith and Woodburne,[9] has been the accepted convention in the Anglo-Saxon literature. We prefer to use the definition of Couinaud, since segment IV (quadrate lobe) is anatomically part of the left liver (Fig. 1.9) and therefore right hepatectomy consists of the resection of segments V, VI, VII and VIII. Left hepatectomy is the removal of segments II, III and IV (Fig. 1.6). In certain pathologies (multiple liver metastases or large tumours transgressing the main portal scissura) hepatectomies can be extended

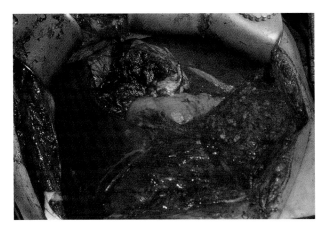

Figure 1.9 Completion of segment IV resection with portal bifurcation lying inferiorly in front of the inferior vena cava.

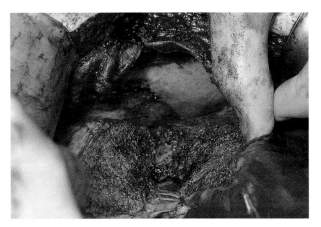

Figure 1.10 Left lateral segmentectomy immediately prior to division of the portal structure lying inferiorly and the left hepatic vein lying superiorly.

to include adjacent segments and sectors of the other liver. Therefore extended right hepatectomy will also include resection of segment IV, taking portal structures to the right of the falciform ligament (which Goldsmith and Woodburne describe as a right hepatic lobectomy)[9] (Fig. 1.6). Similarly, extended left hepatectomy would include resection of segments V and VIII en bloc with segments II, III and IV (Fig. 1.6).

Using this functional approach to liver anatomy, there are numerous other potential liver resections.[28] Individual segments can be resected in isolation or in adjacent pairs depending upon the distribution of pathology. This includes complete resection of segment IV, which leaves segments II and III in complete isolation from the right liver (Fig. 1.8). One area of confusion in the definitions of hepatectomies comes in the simultaneous resection of segments II and III (Fig. 1.10). Goldsmith and Woodburne describe this procedure as a left hepatic lobectomy.[9] However, left lateral segmentectomy is by technical definition wrong since the true left lateral segment (and sector) comprises no more than segment II. However, it is now accepted convention that resection of segments II and III is regarded as a left lateral segmentectomy.

Sectorectomies of the right liver are easier to define. Resection of segments V and VIII between the main portal scissura (middle hepatic vein) and right portal scissura (right portal vein) on their pedicle of the anterior division of the right portal vein is defined as a right anterior sectorectomy, while resection of segments VI and VII posterior to the right portal scissura (on the pedicle of the posterior division of the right portal vein) is a right posterior sectorectomy (Fig. 1.8). Similarly, segments V and VI can be resected en bloc (right inferior hepatectomy) and if there is a significant right inferior hepatic vein

draining segments V and VI, then segments VII and VIII can be resected with the right hepatic vein (right superior hepatectomy) (Fig. 1.8).

Surgical approach to the caudate lobe (dorsal sector)

This is initially achieved by dissection of the coronary ligament up to the right of the IVC, but avoiding the right hepatic vein. The falciform ligament is then dissected to the IVC and the lesser omentum incised close to the liver. Opening the left coronary ligament allows ligation of the inferior phrenic vein. The caudate veins to the IVC are now exposed and can be divided between ligatures as they run up the back of the caudate lobe. After the hilar plate is lowered to expose the right and left portal pedicles, the portal inflow to both the right and left caudate segments can be identified, ligated and divided. The caudate lobe is now isolated and the main portal fissure is divided to separate segments IV, VII and VIII. However, the caudate segment is not defined macroscopically from segment VI.

The biliary tract

Accurate biliary exposure and precise dissection are the two most important steps in any biliary operative procedure and are both totally dependent on a thorough anatomical understanding of these structures. Several authors have thoroughly described the anatomy of the biliary tract,[6,7,23] but unfortunately the surgical implications have been incompletely described and continue to be misunderstood by many surgeons.

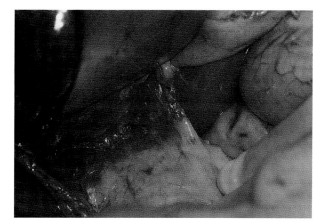

Figure 1.11 Exposing the hilar plate by raising the inferior surface of segment IVB, thus demonstrating the condensation of Glisson's capsule which will cover the extra hepatic confluence of the right and left hepatic ducts.

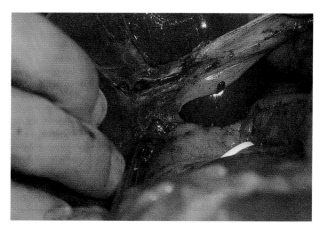

Figure 1.12 Exposing the recessus of Rex by distraction of the falciform ligament to demonstrate the bifurcation of segment III and segment IV bile ducts.

Intrahepatic bile duct anatomy

The right liver and left liver are respectively drained by the right and the left hepatic ducts, whereas the caudate lobe is drained by several ducts joining both the right and left hepatic ducts.[8] The intrahepatic ducts are tributaries of the corresponding hepatic ducts which form part of the major portal tracts invaginating Glisson's capsule at the hilus and penetrating the liver parenchyma (Fig. 1.11). There is variation in the anatomy of all three components of the portal triad structures, hepatic ducts, hepatic arteries and portal vein, but the latter of these shows the least anatomical variability. In particular, the left portal vein tends to be consistent in location.[23] Bile ducts are usually located above the portal vein whereas the corresponding artery will lie below. Each branch of the intrahepatic portal vein corresponds to one or two intrahepatic bile ducts which converge outside the liver to form the right and left hepatic ducts, in turn joining to form the common hepatic duct.

The left liver is divided between segments III and IV by the umbilical fissure, although this division may be bridged by a tongue of liver parenchyma of varying depth. The ligamentum teres passes through this umbilical fissure to join the left portal vein within the recessus of Rex (Figs 1.12 and 1.13). However, all these biliary and vascular elements are liable to anatomical variation. The left hepatic duct drains segments II, III and IV which constitute the left liver. The duct draining segment III is found a little behind the left horn of the umbilical recess, from where it passes directly posteriorly to join the segment II duct to the left of the main portal branch to segment II. At this point the left branch of the portal vein turns forward and caudally in the recessus of Rex[23] (Fig. 1.14). As the duct draining segment

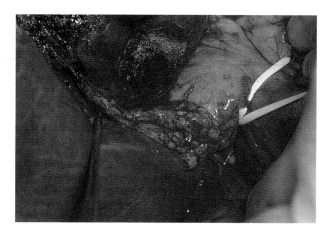

Figure 1.13 Demonstration of the right hepatic duct lying within the gallbladder fossa.

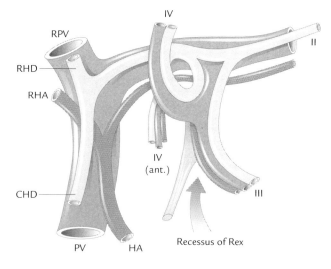

Figure 1.14 Biliary and vascular anatomy of the left liver. Note the position of segment III duct above the corresponding vein and its relationship to the recessus of Rex.

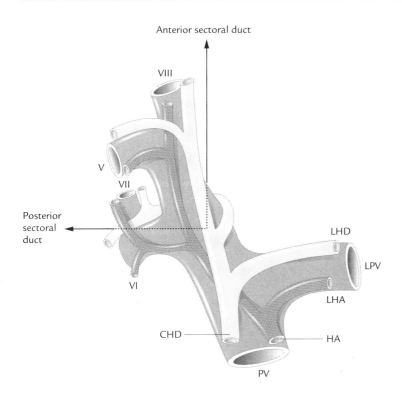

Anterior sectoral duct

VIII

V

VII

Posterior sectoral duct

VI

CHD

PV

LHD

LPV

LHA

HA

Figure 1.15 Biliary and vascular anatomy of the right liver. Note the horizontal course of the posterior sectoral duct and the vertical course of the anterior sectoral duct.

III begins its posterior course it lies superficially in the umbilical fissure, often immediately under Glisson's capsule. As such it is usually easily accessible at surgery to allow a biliary–enteric (segment III hepaticojejunostomy) anastomosis for biliary drainage if such access is not possible at the porta hepatis. The left hepatic duct then passes beneath the left liver at the posterior base of segment IV, lying just above and behind the left branch of the portal vein. After the left duct crosses the anterior edge of that vein it joins the right hepatic duct to form the common duct at the hepatic ductal confluence. In this transverse portion, where it lies below the liver parenchyma, it receives one to three small branches from segment IV.[23]

The right hepatic duct drains segments V, VI, VII and VIII and arises from the convergence of the two main sectoral (anterior V and VIII and posterior VI and VII) tributaries. The right posterior sectoral duct runs almost horizontally[26] and comprises the confluence of the ducts from segments VI and VII (Fig. 1.15). The posterior duct joins the anterior sectoral duct (formed by the confluence of the ducts from segments V and VIII) as it descends vertically.[26] This anterior sectoral duct lies to the left of the right anterior sectoral branch of the intrahepatic portal vein as it ascends within the parenchyma (Fig. 1.15). The junction of the two main right biliary ducts usually occurs immediately above the right branch of the portal vein.[23] The right hepatic duct is considerably shorter than its counterpart on the left, which it joins to form the common hepatic duct in front of the right portal vein (Fig. 1.15).

The caudate lobe (segment I) has its own separate biliary drainage. This segment comprises two anatomically and functionally distinct portions, a caudate lobe proper (which consists of a right and left part) located at the posterior aspect of the liver and a caudate process passing behind the portal structures to fuse with the right liver. In nearly half of individuals, three separate bile ducts drain these distinct parts, while in a quarter of individuals there is a common bile duct between the right portion of the caudate lobe proper and the caudate process, while the left part of the caudate lobe is drained by an independent duct. However, the site of drainage of these ducts is variable. In over three-quarters of individuals, the caudate lobe drains bile into both the right and left hepatic ducts, but in the rest, the caudate lobe drains exclusively into the left (15%) or right (7%) hepatic duct. Many authors now advocate en bloc resection of the caudate lobe during resection of hilar cholangiocarcinoma,[31] since the tumour usually infiltrates these ducts draining the caudate lobe. Certainly these authors have demonstrated that in 88% of cases of hilar cholangiocarcinoma coming to resection there is histological evidence of tumour infiltration of the caudate lobe along these ducts.

Extrahepatic biliary anatomy

The detail of this section will be confined to the upper part of the extrahepatic biliary tree, above the common bile duct, since the common bile duct is also covered in Chapter 2. The right and left hepatic ducts converge at the right of the hilum of the liver,

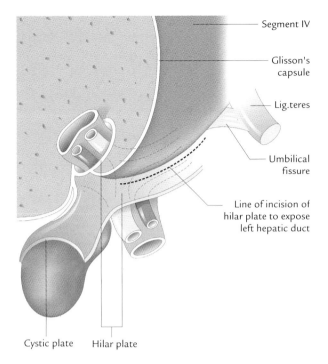

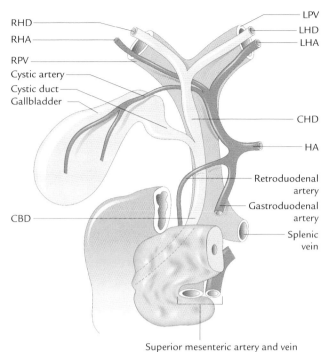

Figure 1.16 Demonstration of the relationship between the posterior aspect of the base of segment IV and the biliary confluence. Note the extension of Glisson's capsule to invest the portal structures at the hilum (hilar plate) and extending over the hepatic surface of the gallbladder (cystic plate). Exposure of the extrahepatic left hepatic duct is achieved by incising the hilar plate at the base of segment IV medially as far as the umbilical fissure.

Figure 1.17 Anterior aspect of biliary anatomy. Note the hepatic duct confluence anterior to the right hepatic artery and origin of the right portal vein. Note also the course of the cystic artery, arising from the right hepatic artery and passing posteriorly to the common hepatic duct.

anterior to the portal venous bifurcation and overlying the origin of the right portal vein. The biliary confluence is separated from the posterior aspect of the base of segment IV by a fusion of connective tissue investing from Glisson's capsule to form the fibrous hilar plate. This hilar plate has no vascular interposition and, when opened behind the posterior aspect of the base of segment IV, will display the extrahepatic confluence of the right and left hepatic ducts (Fig. 1.16).

The main bile duct is divided into its upper part, the common hepatic duct, and lower part, the common bile duct, by the entry of the cystic duct from the gallbladder. This point of entry is widely variable. The main bile duct normally has a diameter of 6 mm and passes downwards anterior to the portal vein in the right free border of the lesser omentum. The bile duct is closely related to the hepatic artery as it runs upwards on its left side before dividing into its left and right branches, the right hepatic artery usually passing posteriorly to the bile duct. The cystic artery which usually arises from the right hepatic artery crosses the common hepatic duct as frequently anteriorly as it does posteriorly (Figs 1.17 and 1.18).

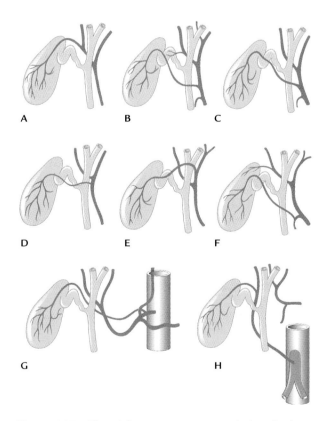

Figure 1.18 The eight most common variations in the anatomy of the arterial supply (cystic artery) to the gallbladder.

A

B

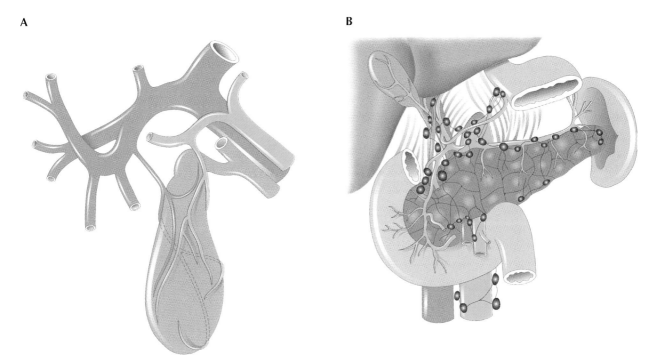

Figure 1.19 (A) Venous drainage of the gallbladder. (B) The lymphatic drainage of the gallbladder towards the coeliac axis.

Calot's triangle was originally defined by the common hepatic duct lying medially, inferiorly by the cystic duct and superiorly by the cystic artery.[32] However, the usually accepted surgical definition of Calot's triangle defines the upper border as the inferior surface of the liver.[33] The junction of the cystic duct and common hepatic duct varies widely and may even occur behind the pancreas. The retropancreatic portion of the bile duct approaches the duodenum obliquely, accompanied by the terminal part of the duct of Wirsung (see Chapter 2). These two ducts join to enter the duodenum through the sphincter of Oddi at the papilla of Vater.[34,35]

Gallbladder and cystic duct

The gallbladder lies within the cystic fossa on the underside of the liver in the main liver scissura at the junction between the right and left livers. It is separated from the hepatic parenchyma by the cystic plate, which is an extension of connective tissue from the hilar plate (described previously). The relationship of the gallbladder to the liver ranges from hanging by a loose peritoneal reflection to being deeply embedded within the liver substance. The gallbladder varies in size and consists of a neck, body and fundus which usually reaches the free edge of the liver, still closely applied to the cystic plate. Large gallstones impacting within the neck of the gallbladder may create a Hartmann's pouch,[33] and inflammation secondary to this can obscure the anatomical

plane between the gallbladder and the common hepatic duct leading to damage of the latter during cholecystectomy.[36] Other structures similarly threatened during this manoeuvre include the right hepatic artery and occasionally the right hepatic duct.

The cystic duct arises from the neck of the gallbladder and descends to join the common hepatic duct in its supraduodenal course in 80% of people. Its length varies widely but its lumen is usually between 1 and 3 mm. The mucosa of the cystic duct is arranged in spiral folds (valves of Heister).[33] In a small number of cases the cystic duct joins the right hepatic duct or a right hepatic sectoral duct.

The gallbladder receives its blood supply by the cystic artery, the anatomy of which varies widely (Fig. 1.18). The most common variant arises directly from the right hepatic artery and then divides into an anterior and posterior branch. The venous drainage of the gallbladder is directly through the gallbladder fossa to the portal vein in segment V (Fig. 1.19).

Biliary ductal anomalies

The biliary anatomy described above, comprising a right and left hepatic duct joining to form a common hepatic duct occurs in between 57%[23] and 72%[8] of cases. This variance may be because Couinaud[23] specifically identified a triple confluence of right posterior sectoral duct, right anterior sectoral duct and left hepatic duct in 12% of cases, which Healey and Schroy do not describe. Furthermore, Couinaud also describes a right sectoral duct joining the main bile duct in 20% of individuals (right anterior sectoral in 16%, right posterior sectoral in 4%). In addition, a right sectoral duct (posterior in 5%, anterior in 1%) may join the left hepatic duct in 6% of cases. In 3% of cases there is an absence of a defined hepatic duct confluence with all the sectoral ducts joining separately and in 2% the right posterior sectoral duct may join the neck of the gallbladder or be entered by the cystic duct[23] (Fig. 1.20).

Similarly, there are common variations of the intrahepatic biliary anatomy. Healey and Schroy[8]

describe the classical intrahepatic biliary arrangement (described above) in 67% of cases, with ectopic drainage of segment V in 9%, segment VI in

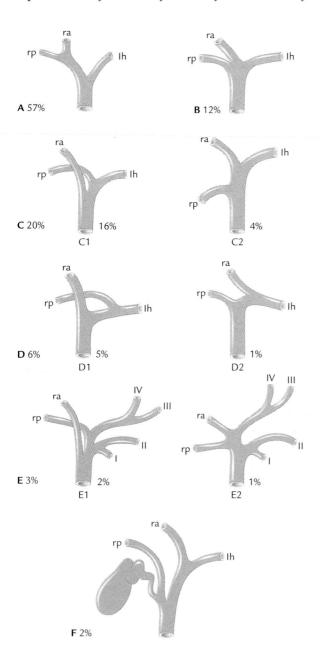

Figure 1.20 Main variations of the hepatic duct confluence.

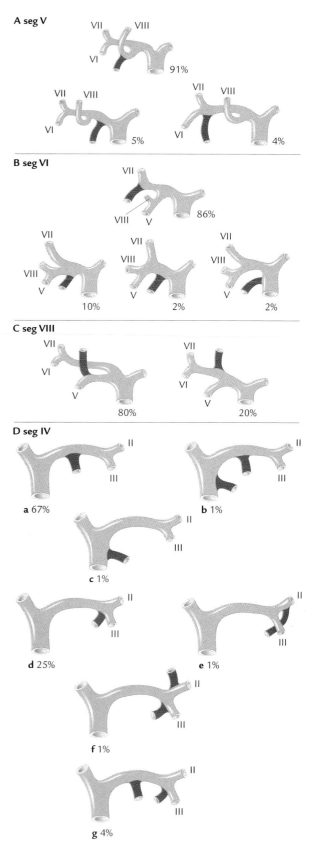

Figure 1.21 Variations of the intrahepatic biliary anatomy.

14% and segment VIII in 20% of cases. In addition, they describe a subvesical duct in 20–50% of cases.[8,37] This subvesical duct may lie deeply embedded in the cystic plate and can join either the common or right hepatic ducts. This duct does not drain any specific area of the liver and never communicates with the gallbladder, but may be damaged during cholecystectomy and therefore contribute to postoperative biliary leak. On the left side the commonest anomaly is a common union of segment III and IV ducts in 25% of cases, and in only 2% does the segment IV duct independently join the common hepatic duct (Fig. 1.21).

Anomalies of the accessory biliary apparatus

Gross described a number of anomalies of the accessory biliary apparatus in 1936.[38] These include bilobed and duplicated gallbladder,[39,40] septum and diverticulum of the gallbladder and variations in cystic duct anatomy including a double cystic duct.[41] More rare is agenesis of the gallbladder[42,43] (Fig. 1.22). Furthermore, the gallbladder may be abnormally positioned, either lying deep within the liver parenchyma or lying under the left liver.[44]

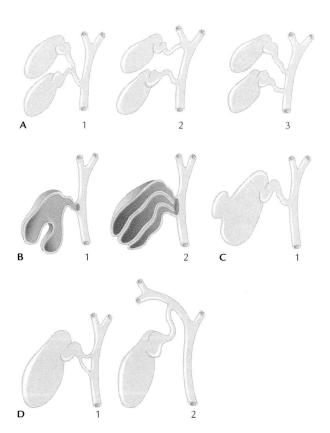

Figure 1.22 Main variations in gallbladder and cystic duct anatomy: (A) bilobed gallbladder; (B) septum of gallbladder; (C) diverticulum of gallbladder; (D) variations in cystic duct anatomy.

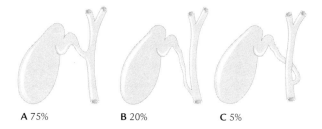

A 75%   B 20%   C 5%

Figure 1.23 Different types of union of the cystic duct and common hepatic duct: (A) angular (75%); (B) parallel (20%); (C) spiral (5%).

The union of the cystic duct with the common hepatic duct may be angular, parallel or spiral. The most frequent union is angular (75%),[45] while the cystic duct may run parallel with the hepatic duct in 20%, both encased in connective tissue. In 5% of cases the cystic duct may approach the hepatic duct in a spiral fashion, usually passing posteriorly to the common hepatic duct before entering on its left side (Fig. 1.23).

The arterial blood supply of the liver and bile ducts

The hepatic artery
The hepatic artery usually arises as one of the three named branches of the coeliac trunk along with the left gastric and splenic arteries (Fig. 1.24). The first named branch of the hepatic artery is the gastroduodenal artery and either of these arteries may then give rise to the right gastric and retroduodenal arteries (Fig. 1.24). The hepatic artery then divides into right (giving rise to the cystic artery) and left hepatic arteries. This arrangement holds true for 50% of cases.

In nearly 25% of cases the right hepatic artery arises separately from the superior mesenteric artery, indicative of the joint fore and midgut origin of the liver (Fig. 1.25), and in nearly another 25% of cases the left hepatic artery arises from the left gastric artery. In a small number of people other variations of these arrangements will occur (Fig. 1.25). However, these variations will be readily apparent to an experienced surgeon at operation and the authors do not advocate preoperative visceral angiography to delineate these anomalies before routine hepatectomy.

The blood supply of the extrahepatic biliary apparatus

The extrahepatic biliary system receives a rich arterial blood supply,[46] which is divided into three

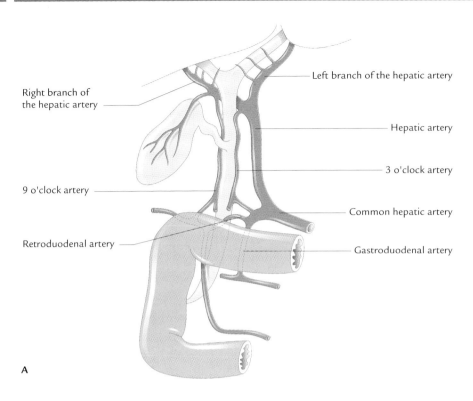

Right branch of the hepatic artery

9 o'clock artery

Retroduodenal artery

Left branch of the hepatic artery

Hepatic artery

3 o'clock artery

Common hepatic artery

Gastroduodenal artery

A

Figure 1.24 (A) The biliary duct blood supply; (B) conventional arterial anatomy of the liver (50%).

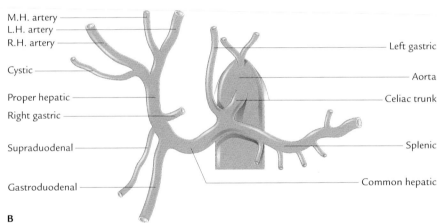

M.H. artery
L.H. artery
R.H. artery

Cystic

Proper hepatic

Right gastric

Supraduodenal

Gastroduodenal

Left gastric

Aorta

Celiac trunk

Splenic

Common hepatic

B

sections. The hilar section receive arterioles directly from their related hepatic arteries and these form a rich plexus with arterioles from the supraduodenal section. The blood supply of the supraduodenal section is predominantly axial, most vessels to this section arising from the retroduodenal artery, the right hepatic artery, the cystic artery, the gastroduodenal artery and the retroportal artery. Usually, eight small arteries, each 0.3 mm in diameter, supply the supraduodenal section. The most important of these vessels run along the lateral borders of the duct and are referred to as the 3 o'clock and 9 o'clock arteries. Of the arteries supplying the supraduodenal section, 60% run upwards from the major inferior vessels while 38% run downwards from the right hepatic artery. Only 2% are non-axial, arising

directly from the main trunk of the hepatic artery as it runs parallel to the bile duct. The retropancreatic section of the bile duct receives its blood supply from the retroduodenal artery.

The veins draining the bile duct mirror the arteries and also drain the gallbladder. This venous drainage does not enter the portal vein directly but seems to have its own portal venous pathway to the liver parenchyma.[47]

It has been proposed that arterial damage during cholecystectomy may result in ischaemia leading to postoperative stricture of the bile duct,[47] although it seems unlikely that ischaemia is the major mechanism in the causation of bile duct stricture after cholecystectomy.

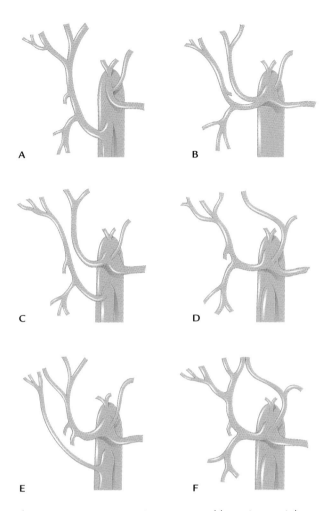

Figure 1.25 Variations in anatomy of hepatic arterial supply.

The anatomy of biliary exposure

Although intraoperative ultrasound has made easier the location of dilated intrahepatic biliary radicals, surgical exposure of the extrahepatic biliary confluence and the segment III duct demands knowledge of precise anatomical landmarks. Biliary–enteric anastomosis necessitates precise bile duct exposure to facilitate the construction of a mucosa to mucosa apposition.[36,48–50]

To expose the extrahepatic biliary confluence, the base of the quadrate lobe (segment IV) is lifted upwards and Glisson's capsule is incised at its base (see Fig. 1.16).[51] This technique is also sometimes referred to as lowering the hilar plate. In only 1% of cases is this made difficult by any vascular imposition between the hilar plate and the inferior aspect of the liver. This manoeuvre will expose considerably more of the left hepatic duct than the right, which runs a shorter extrahepatic course. Contraindications to this approach include patients with a very deep hilum which is displaced upwards and rotated laterally,[36] and those patients who have

undergone removal or atrophy of either the right or left livers resulting in hilar rotation. In this situation the bile duct may come to lie behind the portal vein.

When approaching the segment III duct (segment III hepaticojejunostomy), follow the round ligament (in which runs the remnant of the obliterated umbilical veins) through the umbilical fissure to the point where it connects with the left branch of the portal vein within the recessus of Rex. This junction may sometimes be deeply embedded within the parenchyma of the fissure. The bile ducts of the left liver are located above the left branch of the portal vein, whereas the corresponding arteries lie below the portal vein. Dissection of the round ligament on its left side allows exposure of either the pedicle or anterior branch of the duct from segment III. This is achieved by mobilizing the round ligament and pulling it downwards, thereby freeing it from the depths of the umbilical fissure. This procedure usually requires the preliminary division of the bridge of liver tissue which runs between the inferior parts of segments III and IV. The umbilical fissure is then opened and with downward traction of the ligamentum teres an anterior branch of the segment III duct is exposed on its left side.

Sometimes it may be necessary to perform a superficial liver split to gain access to this duct. In the usual situation of chronic biliary obstruction with dilatation of the intrahepatic bile ducts, the segment III duct is generally easily located above the left branch of the portal vein. However, in the situation of left liver hypertrophy, it may be necessary to perform a more extensive liver split to the left of the umbilical fissure in order to widen the fissure to achieve adequate access to the biliary system.

Access to the right liver system is less readily achieved than to the left as the anatomy is more imprecise. However, intraoperative ultrasonography greatly enhances the ability of the surgeon to locate these ducts at surgery. The ideal approach on the right side is to the segment V duct,[52] which runs on the left side of its corresponding portal vein.[23] The duct is exposed by splitting the liver over a short distance to the right of the gallbladder fossa, commencing at the right side of the porta hepatis. The segment V duct should lie relatively superficially on the left aspect of the portal vein to that segment.

Key points

- A full understanding of the lobar, sectoral and segmental anatomy of the liver and biliary system is an essential prerequisite for successful liver surgery.
- The surgeon must appreciate the wide variation in extrahepatic biliary anatomy.

REFERENCES

1. Glisson F. *Anatomia hepatis*. London: Typ. Du-Gardianis, 1654

2. Rex 1888. Cited in Hobsley M. The anatomical basis of partial hepatectomy. Proc R Soc Med Engl 1964; 57: 550–4

3. Cantlie J. On a new arrangement of the right and left lobes of the liver. J Anat Physiol (Lond) 1898; 32:4–9

4. Schwartz SI. Historical Background. In: McDermott WV Jr, ed. Surgery of the liver. Boston: Blackwell Scientific Publications, 1989: 3–12

5. McIndoe AH, Counsellor VX. A report on the bilaterality of the liver. Arch Surg 1927; 15: 589

6. Hjortsjo CH. The topography of the intrahepatic duct systems. Acta Anat 1951; 11: 599–615

7. Ton That Tung. La vascularisation veineuse du foie et ses applications aux resections hepatiques. These, Hanoi, 1939

8. Healey JE Jr, Schroy PC. Anatomy of the biliary ducts within the human liver. Arch Surg 1953; 66: 599–616

9. Goldsmith NA, Woodburne RT. Surgical anatomy pertaining to liver resection. Surg Gynaecol Obstet 1957; 195: 310–18

10. Lau WY. The history of liver surgery. J R Coll Surg Edin 1997; 42: 303–9

11. Mikesky WE, Howard JM, DeBakey ME. Injuries of the liver in three hundred consecutive cases. Int Abstr Surg 1956; 103: 323–4

12. Dalton HC. Gunshot wound of the stomach and liver treated by laparotomy and suture of the visceral wounds. Ann Surg 1888; 8: 81–100

13. Luis A. Di un adenoma del fegato. Centralblatt fur chirg 1887; 5: 99. Abstract from Ganzy, delle cliniche 1886, 23, No 15

14. Langenbuch C. Ein Fall von Resektion eines linksseitigen Schnurlappens der Leber. Berl Klin Wosch 1888; 25: 37–8

15. Tiffany L. The removal of a solid tumor from the liver by laparotomy. Maryland Med J 1890; 23: 531

16. Lucke F. Entfernung der linken Krebsiten Leber Lappens. Centrallbl Chir 1891: 6: 115

17. Wendel W. Beitrage zur Chirurgie der Leber. Arch Klin Chir Berlin 1911; 95: 887–94

18. Cattell RB. Successful removal of liver metastasis from carcinoma of the rectum. Lehey Clin Bull 1940; 2: 7–11

19. Wangensteen OH. The surgical resection of gastric cancer with special reference to: (1) the closed method of gastric resection; (2) coincidental hepatic resection; and (3) preoperative and postoperative management. Arch Surg 1943; 46: 879–906

20. Keen WW. Report of a case of resection of the liver for the removal of a neoplasm with a table of seventy six cases of resection of the liver for hepatic tumor. Ann Surg 1899; 30: 267–83

21. Raven RW. Partial hepatectomy. Br J Surg 1948; 36: 397–401

22. Lortat-Jacob JL, Robert HG. Hepatectomie droite regle. Presse Med 1952; 60: 549–50

23. Couinaud C. Le foie. Etudes anatomiques et chirurgicales. Paris: Masson, 1957

24. Couinaud C. Lobes et segments hepatiques. Note sur l'architecture anatomiques et chirurgicales du foie. Presse Med 1952; 62: 709–12

25. Couinaud C. Anatomy of the dorsal sector of the liver. In: Couinaud C, ed. New considerations on liver anatomy. Paris: Couinaud, 1998: 39–61

26. Ton That Tung. Les resections majeures et mineures du foie. Paris: Masson, 1979

27. Caprio G. Un caso de extirpacion die lobulo izquierdo die hegado. Bull Soc Cir Urag Montevideo 1931; 2: 159

28. Bismuth H, Houssin D, Castaing D. Major and minor segmentectomies 'reglees' in liver surgery. World J Surg 1982; 6: 10–24

29. Mancuso M, Nataline E, Del Grande G. Contributo alla conoscenza della struttura segmentaria del fegato in rapportto al problema della resezione epatica. Policlinico, Sez Chir 1955; 62: 259–93

30. Couinaud C. Surgical anatomy of the liver revisited. C Couinaud, 15 rue Spontini, Paris, 1989

31. Mizumoto R, Kawarada Y, Suzuki H. Surgical treatment of hilar carcinoma of the bile duct. Surg Gynecol Obstet 1986; 162: 153–8

32. Rocko JM, Swan KG, Di Gioia JM. Calot's triangle revisited. Surg Gynecol Obstet 1981; 153: 410–14

33. Wood D. Eponyms in biliary tract surgery. Am J Surg 1979; 138: 746–54

34. Byden EA. The anatomy of the choledochaoduodenal junction in man. Surg Gynecol Obstet 1957; 104: 641–52

35. Delmont J. Le sphincter d'Oddi: anatomie traditionelle et fonctionelle. Gastroenterol Clin Biol 1979; 3: 157–65

36. Bismuth H, Lazorthes F. Les traumatismes operatoires de la voie biliaire principale. Paris: Masson, Vol 1, 1981

37. Champetier J, Davin JL, Yver R, Vigneau B, Letoublon C. Aberrant biliary ducts (vasa aberrantia): surgical implications. Anatom Clin 1982; 4: 137–45

38. Gross RE. Congenital anomalies of the gallbladder. A review of a hundred and forty-eight cases with report of a double gallbladder. Arch Surg 1936; 32: 131–62

39. Hobby JAE. Bilobed gallbladder. Br J Surg 1979; 57: 870–2

40. Rachad-Mohassel MA, Baghieri F, Maghsoudi H, Nik Akhtar B. Duplication de la vesicule biliaire. Arch Francais des Maladies de l'Appareil Digestif 1973; 62: 679–83

41. Perelman H. Cystic duct duplication. J Am Med Assoc 1961; 175: 710–11

42. Boyden EA. The accessory gallbladder. An embryological and comparative study of aberrant biliary vesicles occurring in man and the domestic mammals. Am J Anat 1926; 38: 177–231

43. Rogers HI, Crews RD, Kalser MH. Congenital absence of the gallbladder with choledocholithiasis. Literature

review and discussion of mechanisms. Gastroenterology 1975; 48: 524–9

44. Newcombe JF, Henley FA. Left sided gallbladder. A review of the literature and a report of a case associated with hepatic duct carcinoma. Arch Surg 1964; 88: 494–7

45. Kune GA. The influence of structure and function in the surgery of the biliary tract. Ann R Coll Surg Engl 1970; 47: 78–91

46. Northover JMA, Terblanche J. A new look at the arterial blood supply of the bile duct in man and its surgical implications. Br J Surg 1979; 66: 379–84

47. Northover JMA, Terblanche J. Applied surgical anatomy of the biliary tree. In: Blumgart LH, ed. Biliary tract. Edinburgh: Churchill Livingstone, Vol 5, 1982

48. Bismuth H, Franco D, Corlette NB, Hepp J. Long term results of Roux-en-Y hepaticojejunostomy. Surg Gynecol Obstet 1978; 146: 161–7

49. Voyles CR, Blumgart LH. A technique for construction of high biliary enteric anastomoses. Surg Gynecol Obstet 1982p; 154: 885–7

50. Blumgart LH, Kelley CJ. Hepaticojejunostomy in benign and malignant bile duct stricture: approaches to the left hepatic ducts. Br J Surg 1984; 71: 257–61

51. Hepp J, Couinaud C, L'abord et L'utilisation du canal hepatique gauche dans le reparations de la voie biliaire principale. Presse Med 1956; 64: 947–8

52. Smadja C, Blumgart LH. The biliary tract and the anatomy of biliary exposure. In: Blumgart LH, ed. Surgery of the liver and biliary tract, 2nd edn. Edinburgh: Churchill Livingstone, 1994: 11–24

2 Surgical anatomy of the pancreas

Mark Hartley and Margaret Finch-Jones

Microanatomy

Exocrine

The acinus is the secretory unit for digestive enzymes. The glandular or acinar cells of the pancreas form the major part of the lining of the acini and are the most abundant cells within the exocrine lobule (Fig. 2.1).[1,2] The acinar cells are pyramidal in shape and contain prominent endoplasmic reticulum, golgi apparatus and zymogen granules which correspond to their main function of digestive enzyme secretion. These cells are interspersed with epithelial cells which are cuboidal or flat and are termed centroacinar cells. The epithelial cell lined ductules drain the acini and coalesce to form intralobular and interlobular ducts. The epithelial cells lining the centroacinar and interlobular ducts are flat and have interdigitating lateral basement membranes. This structure corresponds to their function of fluid and ion transport including the secretion of bicarbonate. The interlobular ducts are lined by pyramidal cells with microvilli and mucoprotein containing secretory granules. The main pancreatic duct is lined by columnar cells interspersed with goblet cells.

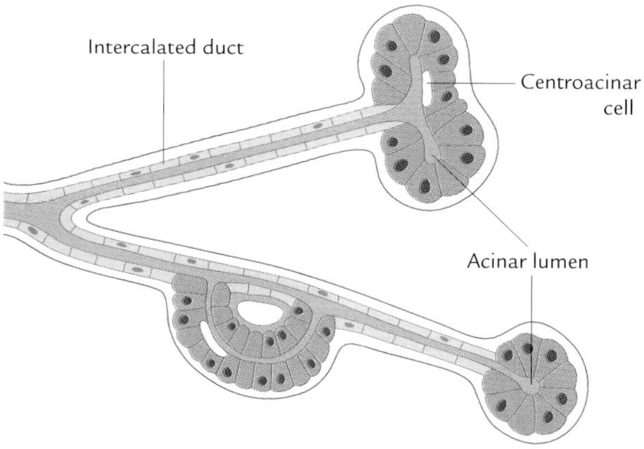

Endocrine

Pancreatic islet cells make up only 2% of the weight of the pancreas but receive 20% of its blood flow. The islets of Langerhans are essentially clumps of hormone secreting cells, including 25% α cells, 60–80% β cells and 15% δ cells. These proportions vary within the regions of the pancreas, for example the majority of β cells are located within the tail. Within each islet the β cells lie centrally, the δ cells surround these and the α cells lie at the perimeter. The portal drainage of the islets is arranged such that the acinar cells have greater contact with this draining blood than does any other cell in the body. Acinar cells in the peri-insular regions are larger and have more insulin receptors. This structure is thought to reflect an interaction between the endocrine and exocrine systems.

Ductal anatomy

A brief review of the embryology of the pancreas is required for an understanding of normal ductal anatomy and its variants. The pancreas begins as dorsal and ventral buds arising from the duodenum, each with its own duct. The ventral bud rotates posteriorly and to the left to become the uncinate process, while the dorsal bud becomes the head, body and tail (Fig. 2.2). The dorsal and ventral ducts carry the eponyms Santorini and Wirsung, respectively. In 70% of the cases these two ducts fuse and the connection of both ducts to the duodenum disappears (see Fig. 2.3A). In these cases the

Figure 2.1 Schematic representation of exocrine microanatomy of the pancreas.

Labels in figure: Intercalated duct; Centroacinar cell; Acinar lumen

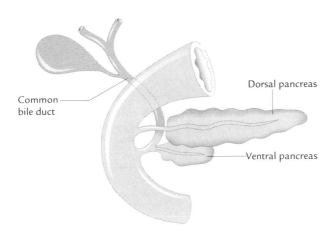

Figure 2.2 Embryology of the pancreas: position of pancreatic ducts before fusion and after rotation.

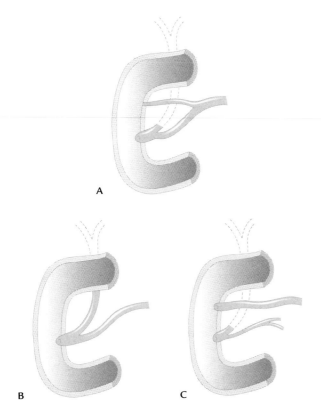

Figure 2.3 Variations in the pancreatic ducts: (A) Normal configuration (60% of population): major and minor ducts empty into duodenum through the major and minor papilla respectively—connection between ducts is maintained. (B) The accessory duct is suppressed and loses its connection to the duodenum (30% of population). (C) The main duct is suppressed and loses its connection to the accessory duct (pancreas divisum: 10% of population).

opening of the dorsal duct of Santorini into the duodenum is termed the minor papilla (Fig. 2.3A). When this is combined with failure of fusion of the two ducts, the situation is termed pancreas divisum (Fig. 2.3C). The other variations of ductal anatomy

include either the suppression or the absence of the accessory or dorsal duct. The exact incidence of these variants is unknown, but they are thought to be present in between 15% and 30% of the population. The incidence of pancreas divisum is higher in patients undergoing endoscopic retrograde cholangio-pancreatography (ERCP) for idiopathic pancreatitis, but whether pancreas divisum is aetiologic in this condition remains controversial.[3]

The relationship of the main pancreatic duct and common bile duct is also variable. The two join to form a common channel within the wall of the duodenum in the majority of normal subjects[4] (see Fig. 2.2). This is because the ventral pancreatic duct originates as a branch of the bile duct embryologically[4] (Fig. 2.4C). The common channel is termed the ampulla of Vater. This common channel has been shown to be longer (>5 mm) in patients who have had acute pancreatitis.[5] In these patients this anatomical situation is associated with reflux of bile from the bile duct into the pancreatic duct.[5] The pancreatic duct of such patients has also been found to sit at a wider angle in relation to the bile duct and tends to have a greater diameter, although this latter finding may well be secondary to the pathological process.[5] In a smaller percentage of patients the common channel is completely resorbed into the duodenal wall, resulting in separate openings of the pancreatic duct and bile duct into the duodenum. In each of these configurations both ducts or their common channel are surrounded in their most distal extent by a muscular sphincter termed the sphincter of Oddi. This circular smooth muscle is of a variable length of 6 to 30 mm and lies largely within the duodenal wall. It is, in fact, a sphincter complex made up of four different sphincters: the sphincter pancreaticus encircling the pancreatic duct, the superior and inferior choledochal sphincters around the bile duct and the sphincter ampullae around the ampulla.[4] It is this muscle which must be divided during endoscopic sphincterotomy or surgical sphincteroplasty. The bulge seen at the papilla is due to these fibres.

The relationship of the distal common bile duct to the head of the pancreas is also variable. It most commonly lies within the pancreatic tissue, but may also lie posteriorly within a groove in the pancreatic tissue.[6] There are multiple variations between these extremes, including cases where the duct is intra-pancreatic superiorly but lies extrapancreatic distally before joining the pancreatic duct and duodenum.[6,7]

The dimensions of the main pancreatic duct have been defined in ERCP studies by several authors. Its length varies from 175 to 275 mm. The diameter is greatest in the pancreatic head at 3 to 4 mm and

A

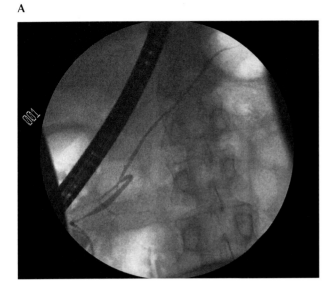

Figure 2.4A Normal pancreatic duct as seen at ERCP.

B

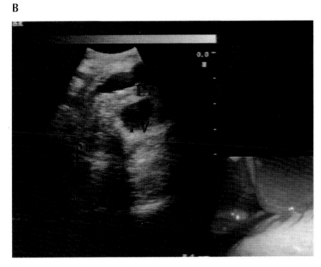

Figure 2.4B Conventional image of a tumour (T) in the head of the pancreas with adjacent portal vein (PV) and obstructed pancreatic duct (PD).

C

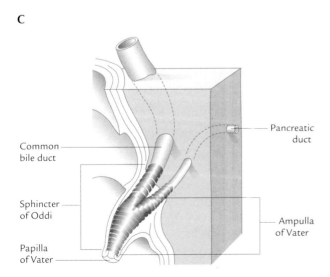

Common bile duct

Sphincter of Oddi

Papilla of Vater

Pancreatic duct

Ampulla of Vater

Figure 2.4C Anatomy of the ampulla of Vater and sphincter of Oddi.

decreases to 1 to 2 mm in the tail.[8] A gradual increase in ductal diameter occurs with age. A natural narrowing may be present at the point of fusion of the ventral and dorsal ducts.[9] Knowledge of normal ductal dimensions is helpful in identifying pathological states such as small tumours in the head of the gland, intraductal tumours and chronic pancreatitis. The normal pancreatic duct is smooth and tapered with side branches that are also smooth and tapered. Shortening, irregularity or dilatation of these ducts correlates with disease states such as chronic pancreatitis.[10,11] Evidence from endoscopic ultrasound studies indicates that changes in the ducts are preceded by morphological changes within the pancreatic parenchyma. The main ultrasonographic features of these parenchymal changes are alternating echo-poor and echo-rich areas and an irregular pancreatic margin rather than the usual uniform echogenicity and smooth margin.[12]

Vascular anatomy

Venous anatomy of the pancreas and duodenum

Attention to the portal venous system in and around the pancreas is the most important aspect in preventing blood loss during pancreatic surgery (Fig. 2.5). These high flow vessels are situated in awkward positions and if they are torn the application of proximal and distal vascular control is often neither advisable nor possible.

The portal vein itself can be further defined as the hepatic portal vein and the pancreatic portal vein. The latter runs behind the neck of the pancreas and

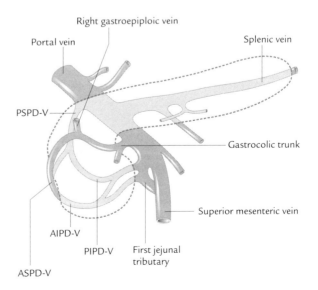

Right gastroepiploic vein

Portal vein

Splenic vein

PSPD-V

Gastrocolic trunk

Superior mesenteric vein

AIPD-V

PIPD-V

First jejunal tributary

ASPD-V

Figure 2.5 Venous anatomy of the head of the pancreas.

the former extends from the superior border of the pancreas to its bifurcation into the right and left portal vein branches. The pancreatic portal vein sits within a groove in the back of the gland. This groove may be further accentuated by the presence of a tumour within the head of the pancreas. It is formed from the confluence of the splenic and superior mesenteric veins. The inferior mesenteric vein may also contribute to this junction, although it classically joins the splenic vein and occasionally joins the superior mesenteric vein directly. Ligation of the inferior mesenteric vein is often a necessary step in mobilization of the body and tail of the pancreas. The venous drainage of the head of the pancreas and duodenum is via an anterior and a posterior arcade termed the anterior superior and inferior pancreaticoduodenal veins (ASPD-V and AIPD-V) and the posterior superior and inferior pancreaticoduodenal veins (PSPD-V and PIPD-V). It is important to recognize the common sites at which these vessels join the portal vein when performing a resection of the pancreatic head. The posterior superior vein commonly drains directly into the portal vein near the superior border of the pancreas after crossing anterior to the bile duct.[13] The anterior superior vein drains directly into the loop of Henle, or gastrocolic trunk. This latter vessel is both a common landmark and a source of trouble if not dealt with carefully. It is formed by the confluence of the right gastroepiploic vein and an unnamed middle colic vein. It joins the superior mesenteric vein just below the neck of the pancreas. Ligation of the gastroepiploic vein near this junction facilitates exposure of the superior mesenteric vein and pancreatic portal vein. Some studies seem to indicate that an anterior superior vein may not be present in all cases and that venous drainage in the corresponding region is directly into the gastrocolic trunk.[13] Both the anterior and posterior inferior veins drain directly into the first jejunal tributary to the SMV after it passes posterior to the SMV itself, although an anterior inferior vein is not always identified.[13]

Arterial anatomy

The arterial supply to the head of the pancreas is through an anterior and a posterior arcade. The anterior superior and posterior superior arteries arise from the gastroduodenal artery (GDA), the posterior being the last branch after the right gastroepiploic artery. The gastroduodenal in turn is a branch of the common hepatic artery and arises within the porta hepatis, where it marks the transition to the hepatic artery proper. It runs in the same general direction as the latter vessel, but when viewed from behind the mobilized and anteriorly retracted pylorus appears to run transversely. Ligation of the gastroduodenal artery is a necessary step for pancreaticoduodenectomy and can be helpful in controlling bleeding from difficult duodenal ulcers. The right gastric artery is the first branch of the hepatic artery proper, but often appears to arise at the same point as the GDA and runs in the same general direction as the GDA, and can therefore sometimes be confused with it. According to some authors, preservation of the right gastric artery is crucial during a pylorus preserving pancreatico-duodenectomy.[14] Some surgeons, however, do not preserve it on the basis that its preservation may not allow adequate lymph node clearance.

The anterior and posterior inferior pancreaticoduodenal arteries form the inferior blood supply to the head of the pancreas and duodenum. They arise either as a single trunk or separately directly from the superior mesenteric artery. The anterior arcade follows the course of the duodenal wall, passing posterior to the inferior pancreatic head as it overhangs the duodenum. The posterior arcade passes anterior to the common bile duct before it enters the pancreas and follows the margin of the head of pancreas posteriorly. It is relatively easy to detach from the pancreatic head.

The most frequent arterial anatomical variant related to the head of the pancreas is a replaced or accessory right hepatic artery arising from the superior mesenteric artery (25% of the population) (Fig. 2.6A). In 2–4.5% of cases, the main hepatic artery arises aberrantly from this position and its branches therefore arise behind the pancreas and pass to the liver posterior to the portal vein (Fig. 2.6B).[15–17] Much more rarely, an aberrant left hepatic can arise from the superior mesenteric artery (SMA) (Fig. 2.6C).[15] The presence of one of these variations, such as a left hepatic artery arising from the left gastric artery, makes the presence of another more likely. The pulse of an accessory or replaced right hepatic can normally be palpated in the porta hepatis posterior to the bile duct. Failure to identify such a vessel can result in ligation of part of the hepatic blood supply during pancreaticoduodenectomy.

With respect to the identification of vascular variants, some surgeons have advocated preoperative angiography. However, angiography can be misleading. Trede reports examples of its failure to demonstrate an accessory right hepatic artery and points out that when such an artery is identified its position anterior to, posterior to or within the head of the pancreas cannot be ascertained.[18] Angiography can also identify vascular abnormalities which may not be significant. One example is atherosclerotic stenosis of the coeliac axis. Very rarely this condition can be associated with collateral blood flow to the liver provided by the superior mesenteric artery through the pancreaticoduodenal

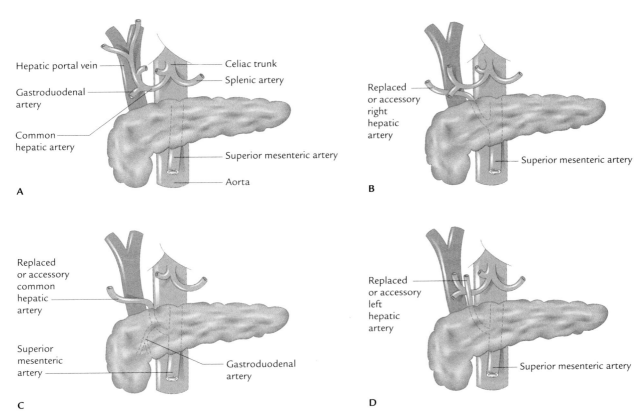

Figure 2.6 Variations in the hepatic arteries and the gastroduodenal artery. (A) Most common configuration: right and left hepatic arteries arise from hepatic artery proper; gastroduodenal artery arises from common hepatic artery. (B) Replaced or accessory right hepatic artery arising from superior mesenteric artery; gastroduodenal artery in normal position. Can be associated with left hepatic artery arising from left gastric artery. (C) Replaced or accessory common hepatic artery arising from superior mesenteric artery. Note posterior position of gastroduodenal artery. (D) Replaced or accessory left hepatic artery arising from superior mesenteric artery.

arcade, thus precluding pancreaticoduodenectomy. However, this rare situation can be identified intraoperatively when blood flow to the liver ceases upon temporary occlusion of the gastroduodenal artery.[18]

The blood supply to the body and tail of the pancreas is through a number of collateral branches running posteriorly to the pancreas arising principally from the dorsal pancreatic artery. The origin of this artery is variable, arising from the splenic artery in 38%, directly from the coeliac trunk in 22%, the common hepatic in 22%, the superior mesenteric artery in 12.7% and the gastroduodenal artery in 5%.[19] The splenic artery also gives rise separately to a caudal pancreatic artery.

Nerve supply to the pancreas

The pancreas receives both sympathetic and parasympathetic input. The parasympathetic input to the pancreas is by way of vagal fibres passing through the right and left coeliac ganglia which are situated adjacent to the coeliac axis. The sympathetic input is from the greater and lesser splanchnic nerves which are formed by branches from the T4 through T10 and T9 through L2 sympathetic ganglia, respectively. These then synapse in the coeliac plexus and ganglia. Sympathetic and parasympathetic fibres then enter the pancreas by several routes. The supply to the pancreatic head is by way of the plexus pancreaticus capitalis I, which runs directly from the right coeliac ganglion to the posterior pancreatic head,[20] the plexus pancreaticus capitalis II, which runs from both coeliac ganglia to the left margin of the uncinate process by way of the plexus surrounding the superior mesenteric artery,[21] and through the plexus surrounding the common hepatic artery and the gastroduodenal artery to the anterior region of the head of the pancreas. The supply to the body and tail is from the left coeliac ganglion via the plexus associated with the splenic artery and directly from the left ganglion and coeliac plexus to the posterior body.[22]

The significance of the nerve supply clinically is in the relationship to the control of endocrine and exocrine function, to the perineural spread of pancreatic malignancies and to strategies for the control of the pain of chronic pancreatitis and pancreatic malignancy. The parasympathetic nerves along the arteries enter the pancreatic parenchyma along with the arteries and end on intrinsic ganglia which lie near the parenchyma, in keeping with their role in stimulating secretion of pancreatic juice.[1] Parasympathetic afferents provide feedback through the same routes. The sympathetic fibres also enter the pancreas with the arterial branches. They are distributed to the vascular plexus and the islets.[1] With regard to pain control, the approach used has been the destruction of the splanchnic nerves, either within the thorax where they are formed from the sympathetic chain or by way of ablation within the abdomen as they enter through the hiatus and the horn of the semilunar ganglia.[23] The right and left semilunar ganglia are located in the retroperitoneum, the left lying caudal to the splenic artery and the renal vein with the aorta to the right and the left adrenal to the left, the right lying anterior to the aorta superior to the left renal vein.[23]

Anatomy in relation to surgical access

Relations and attachments of the pancreas and duodenum

The pancreas is a retroperitoneal structure (Fig. 2.7). The head of the pancreas is defined as that portion to the right of the left border of the superior mesenteric and portal vein. It sits within the loop of the

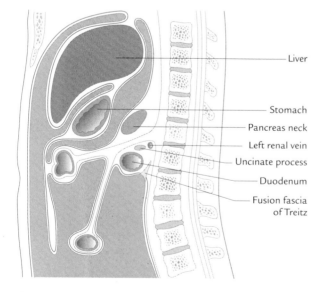

Figure 2.7 Cross-section of peritoneal and retroperitoneal attachments at the level of the pancreatic neck.

Liver

Stomach
Pancreas neck
Left renal vein
Uncinate process
Duodenum
Fusion fascia of Treitz

duodenum, by which it is partly covered anteriorly. The uncinate process is the extension of the head posterior to the portal vein and superior mesenteric artery and normally lies caudal to the pancreatic head. The pancreatic neck is that portion lying directly over the portal vein and superior mesenteric artery. It is covered anteriorly by the pylorus. The body and tail extend obliquely in a cranial direction toward the hilum of the spleen. The area anterior to the body and tail is termed the lesser sac and is bordered by the body of the stomach and gastrocolic ligament anteriorly and the transverse mesocolon and the transverse colon inferiorly. The pancreas is contained within the retroperitoneal space, which is bordered anteriorly by the visceral peritoneum and posteriorly by the transversalis fascia. The fusion of visceral peritoneum to the posterior parietal peritoneum fixes the pancreas in the retroperitoneum. This 'fusion fascia' is termed the fascia of Treitz in the region of the head and neck and the fascia of Toldt in the region of the body and tail.

Surgical access to the pancreatic head and duodenum

Mobilization or Kocherization of the duodenum and head of pancreas is a familiar manoeuvre used in many upper gastrointestinal procedures. The plane of dissection and the extent of mobilization will vary with the procedure. When mobility only is needed, the peritoneal fusion fascia can be separated from the duodenum using sharp dissection, leaving the fascial sheath overlying the inferior vena cava and aorta. For more extensive mobilization or more radical surgery, the fascia overlying the vena cava is divided and mobilized medially along with the duodenum and pancreatic head. This mobilization of the pancreatic head and neck may be carried to the left far enough to expose the anterior aorta. Such a manoeuvre is part of a radical pancreatico-duodenectomy as it is thought to provide more adequate posterior clearance of tumour and the opportunity for dissection of lymph nodes in the retropancreatic region. Further exposure of the head of pancreas and duodenum in the region of the uncinate process requires division of attachments between the third part of the duodenum and transverse mesocolon, thus exposing the right side of the root of the mesentery containing the portal vein. Careful dissection of the portal vein allows exposure of the posteriorly lying uncinate in some cases, but full exposure for resection usually requires transection of the proximal jejunum with division of its most proximal arterial and venous branches. Further exposure of the head of the pancreas in its anterior aspect is achieved by opening the lesser sac by separation of the omentum from the transverse mesocolon or by division of the gastrocolic ligament.

This dissection will reveal a right middle colic vein which leads to the gastrocolic trunk (loop of Henle), formed by its junction with the right gastroepiploic vein. Ligation of the right gastroepiploic vein will facilitate further dissection along the gastrocolic trunk, which then joins the superior mesenteric vein on its anterior aspect. This point in turn defines the neck of the pancreas and serves as a starting point for the dissection of a tunnel anterior to the portal vein during pancreaticoduodenectomy. To complete exposure of the anterior pancreatic head the pylorus and first part of the duodenum can be mobilized by division of small mesenteric vessels. This manoeuvre is used in pylorus preserving resections of the pancreatic head.

Surgical access for pancreatic necrosectomy

Several descriptions of the technique of necrosectomy have been published.[24–26] All include the exposure and debridement of the contents of the lesser sac. The group in Verona have consistently used a technique of more extensive mobilization and drainage, with excellent results.[27] Highlights of that technique will be described here. The aim of the technique is to expose the entire pancreas anteriorly and posteriorly as well as the entire upper abdominal retroperitoneum. An extended Kocher's manoeuvre is performed. The lesser sac is entered by opening the gastrocolic omentum. The anterior pancreatic capsule is removed. In the healthy state this capsule consists of a peritoneal layer overlying a layer of fatty tissue. In the diseased state it may

consist of necrotic or saponified peripancreatic fat. Posterior mobilization of the body and tail is achieved by finger dissection, beginning behind the pancreas and the splenic vessels at the ligament of Treitz and extending toward the pancreatic tail. Irrigation drains are then placed posterior to the head and the tail and in the lesser sac for continuous lavage.

Staging of pancreatic and periampullary tumours

The TNM staging of pancreatic and periampullary adenocarcinomas refers to the systems published by the International Union against Cancer (UICC) and to other similar systems such as the Japanese system.[28] The UICC TNM system was modified in 1997 for both tumour types (Table 2.1).[29]

T Staging

The T stage defines the primary tumour with respect to size and its relationship to pancreatic and peripancreatic structures. Pancreatic exocrine tumours are defined as those arising from the pancreatic ducts (although the cell of origin has been debated) and most commonly arise in the pancreatic head. Periampullary tumours are those arising from the ampulla or common channel of the pancreatic and main bile duct. In practice this is not always an easy differentiation to make. For

Table 2.1 1997 UICC pathological TNM staging of cancer of the exocrine pancreas: comparison with 1987 version

	1987	1997
T Stage		
< 2 cm	T1a	T1
> 2 cm	T1b	T2
Invasion of duodenum, bile duct or peripancreatic tissues	T2	T3
Invasion of major vessels, stomach, spleen or colon	T3	T4
N Stage		
Regional lymph node involvement	N1	N1
Single regional node	N1	N1a
Multiple regional nodes	N1	N1b
Stage grouping		
Stage I	T1-2N0M0	T1-2N0M0
Stage II	T3M0N0	T3M0N0
Stage III	T1-3N1M0	T1-3M0N0
Stage IV	T1-3N0-1M1	
IVA		T4N0-1M0
IVB		T1-4N0-1bM1

pancreatic tumours confined to the pancreas, those less than 2 cm are designated T1 (previously T1a) and those greater than 2 cm are designated T2 (previously T1b). T3 tumours are those extending into the duodenum, bile duct, retroperitoneal fat, mesenteric fat, mesocolon, omentum or peritoneum.

N Staging

The various staging systems for pancreatic cancer differ mostly in the classification of lymph node metastases. The UICC system is the simplest in this regard as only regional lymph nodes are included. For tumours of the pancreatic head these are classified as superior, inferior, anterior, posterior and coeliac. For body and tail tumours splenic hilum nodes are included as well. Within this system the only differentiation regarding the extent of lymph node involvement is between no involvement, single node involvement and multiple node involvement. The Japanese system is more detailed, giving specific numerical designations to specific lymph node stations (Fig. 2.8).[28] Such designations have been shown to be clinically important as some of

these sites harbour metastases in a high percentage of cases, whereas others rarely do so.[30]

The progression of nodal metastases from tumours of the head of the pancreas begins in the anterior and posterior pancreaticoduodenal nodes, areas 17 and 13, respectively. These regional nodes then drain into the inferior head nodes (areas 15b, c, d, v) and from there into the juxta-aortic nodes (areas 19, 14a) and the para-aortic group (area 16). The juxta-aortic nodes most commonly involved are those in area 16b which lie between the aorta and the inferior vena cava from the level of the coeliac axis to the superior mesenteric artery.[30] Because of the clinical utility of the Japanese system a recent European consensus conference on pancreatic resection has recommended definitions of standard, radical and extended resections based largely on this system (personal communication). Lymph nodes which are removed in a standard Whipple's resection according to this system are considered regional lymph nodes and those removed with a more radical lymphadenectomy are considered to be level 2 or 3 in the Japanese system and juxtaregional in the new European designation. The UICC system does not make such a differentiation, although there is an

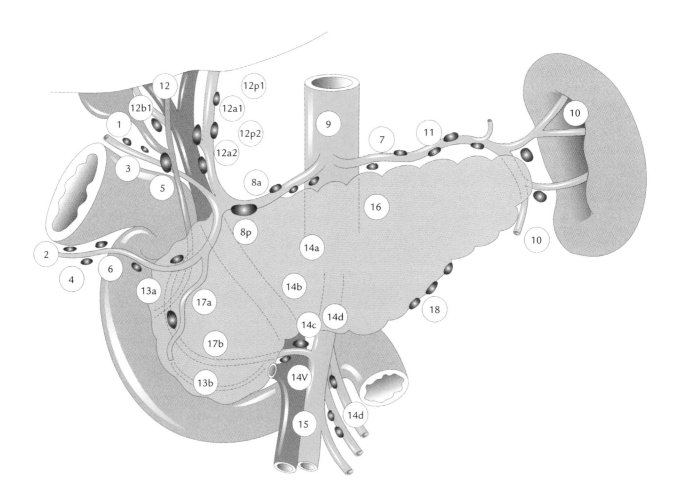

Figure 2.8 Regional lymph nodes of the pancreas according to the Japanese staging system.

option within that system of considering certain node sites as distant metastases.

M Staging

This aspect of staging is fairly straightforward as it relates to the presence of disseminated disease, most commonly in the form of peritoneal or liver deposits. There is some discussion over whether lymph node involvement at certain sites should be considered as distant metastases.

Staging modalities

The main aim of staging of pancreatic cancer currently focuses on the question of resectability. The emphasis is therefore on M stage and T stage. CT scanning has been the mainstay of such assessments in recent years and indeed some reports using techniques such as dual phase contrast injection and fine cut imaging intervals have shown excellent results.[31] Nevertheless, this type of experience with CT scanning is not universal. Even in specialist centres, pancreatic surgeons have seen both false positive and false negative predictions of resectability from this investigation.[32] For this reason other modalities for staging have been developed. Endoscopic ultrasound has been shown by some groups to provide excellent local tumour staging.[33,34] Nevertheless, the technique does not overcome one of the main shortcomings of CT which is the failure to detect small peritoneal and liver deposits. Laparoscopic staging has been used to address this problem.[35] The addition of laparoscopic ultrasound has been found by some groups to increase the sensitivity for detecting intraparenchymal liver deposits and to provide very accurate local tumour staging.[36] Despite some excellent reports of CT staging, comparative studies have so far shown laparoscopic ultrasound to provide more accurate overall staging.[32,37] The hallmark of such staging is a positive predictive value of 100% for predicting unresectable disease. This reflects the certainty of assessment which laparoscopic ultrasound provides, which so far has not been provided by other techniques. None of the techniques mentioned has so far demonstrated sufficient accuracy in lymph node staging to be of clinical value.

The examples (Fig. 2.2B) show the relationships between tumour, portal vein, pancreatic duct and common bile duct which can be demonstrated using laparoscopic ultrasonography and intraoperative ultrasonography. With the addition of the colour flow Doppler technique, disturbances of flow within the portal vein may help to determine whether a tumour is resectable.

Key points

- Attention to vascular anatomy is essential for low blood loss during pancreatic surgery.
- Most frequent arterial variant is the origin of the right hepatic artery from the superior mesenteric in 25% of cases.
- Staging modalities of pancreatic tumours include:
   Spiral CT
   ERCP and endoscopic ultrasound
   Laparoscopy with peritoneal cytology and laparoscopic ultrasound.

REFERENCES

1. Bockman DE. Histology and fine structure. In: Beger HG, Warshaw AL, Buchler MW et al., eds. The pancreas. Oxford: Blackwell Science, 1998: 19–26
2. Carter DC. In: Trede M, Carter DC, eds. Surgery of the pancreas. Edinburgh: Churchill Livingstone, 1993
3. Rosmurgy AS II, Carey LC. Pancreas divisum. In: Cameron JL, ed. Current surgical therapy. St Louis: Mosby, 1995: 419–23
4. Skandalakis JE, Gray SW, Rowe JS Jr et al. Anatomical complications of pancreatic surgery. Contemp Surg 1979; 15: 17–50
5. Armstrong CP, Taylor TV, Jeacock J, Lucas S. The biliary tract in patients with acute gallstone pancreatitis. Br J Surg 1985; 72: 551–5
6. Smanio T. Varying relations of the common bile duct with the posterior face of the pancreatic head in negroes and white persons. J Int Coll Surg 1954; 22: 150–72
7. Reyes GA, Fowler CL, Pokorny WJ. Pancreatic anatomy in children: emphasis on its importance in pancreatectomy. J Pediatr Surg 1993; 28: 712–5
8. Kausagi T, Nobuyoushi K, Kobayashi S, Kazuhiko H. Endoscopic pancreatocholangiography 1. The normal pancreatocholangiogram. Gastroenterology 1972; 63: 217–26
9. Parsons WG, Carr-Locke DL. Retrograde cholangiopancreatography. In: Beger HG, Warshaw AL, Buchler MW et al., eds. The pancreas. Oxford: Blackwell Science, 1998

10. Sarner M, Cotton PB. Classification of pancreatitis. Gut 1984; 25: 756–9

11. Axon ATR, Classen M, Cotton PB, Cremer M et al. Pancreatography in chronic pancreatitis: international definitions. Gut 1984; 25: 1107–12

12. Natterman C, Goldschmidt AJW, Dancygier H. Endosonography in chronic pancreatitis – a comparison between endoscopic retrograde pancreatography and endoscopic ultrasonography. Endoscopy 1993; 25: 565–70

13. Kimura W, Nagai H. Study of surgical anatomy of duodenum preserving resection of the head of the pancreas. Ann Surg 1995; 221: 359–63

14. Longmire WP, Traverso LW. The Whipple procedure and other standard operative approaches to pancreatic cancer. Cancer 1981; 47: 1706–17

15. Michels NA. The hepatic, cystic and retroduodenal arteries and their relations to the biliary ducts. Ann Surg 1951; 133: 503–4

16. Pansky B. Anatomy of the pancreas – emphasis on blood-supply and lymphatic drainage. Int J Pancreatol 1990; 7: 101–8

17. Woods MS, Taverso LW. Sparing a replaced common hepatic artery during pancreaticoduodenectomy. Am Surg 1993; 59: 719–26

18. Trede M. Vascular problems and techniques associated with pancreatectomy and regional pancreatectomy. In: Trede M, Carter DC, eds. Surgery of the pancreas. Edinburgh: Churchill Livingstone, 1993

19. Fiedor P, Kaminsky P, Rowinski W, Nowak M. Variability of the arterial system of the human pancreas. Clin Anat 1993; 6: 213–6

20. Donatini B, Hidden G. Routes of lymphatic drainage from the pancreas: a suggested segmentation. Surg Radiol Anat 1992; 14: 35–42

21. Yashioko H, Wakabayashi T. The pancreatic neurotomy on the head of the pancreas for relief of pain due to chronic pancreatitis: a new technical procedure and its results. Arch Surg 1958; 76: 546–54

22. Kuroda A, Nagai H. Surgical anatomy of the pancreas. In: Howard JM, ed. Surgical diseases of the pancreas. Baltimore: Williams and Wilkins, 1998

23. Hollander LF, Laugner B. Pain relieving procedures in chronic pancreatitis. In: Trede M, Carter DC, eds. Surgery of the pancreas. Edinburgh: Churchill Livingstone, 1993

24. Bradley III EL. Surgical indications and techniques in necrotising pancreatitis. In: Bradley III EL, ed. Acute pancreatitis: diagnosis and therapy. New York: Raven Press, 1994: 105–17

25. Warshaw AL, Jin G. Improved survival in 45 patients with pancreatic abscess. Ann Surg 1988; 202: 408–17

26. Beger HG, Krautzberger W, Bittner R et al. Results of surgical treatment of necrotizing pancreatitis. World J Surg 1984; 9: 972–9

27. Pederzoli P, Bassi C, Vesentini S et al. Retroperitoneal and peritoneal drainage and lavage in the treatment of severe necrotizing pancreatitis. Surg Gynecol Obstet 1990; 170: 197–203

28. Japan Research Society. Japanese classification of pancreatic carcinoma: first English edition. Tokyo: Kanehara, 1996

29. Sobin LH, Whittekind CH. TNM classification of malignant tumours, 5th edn. New York: Springer Wiley, 1997: 87–90

30. Nagakawa T, Kobayashi I, Ueno K et al. The pattern of lymph node involvement in carcinoma of the head of the pancreas. A histologic study of surgical findings in patients undergoing extensive surgical dissections. Int J Pancreatol 1993; 13: 15–22

31. Diehl SJ, Lehmann KJ, Sadick M et al. Pancreatic cancer: value of dual-phase helical CT in assessing resectability. Radiology 1998; 206: 373–8

32. John TG, Wright A, Allan PL et al. Laparoscopy with laparoscopic ultrasonography in the TNM staging of pancreatic carcinoma. World J Surg 1999; 23: 870–81

33. Tio TL, Tytgat GN, Cikot RJ et al. Ampullopancreatic carcinoma: preoperative TNM classification with endosonography. Radiology 1990; 175: 455–61

34. Rosch T, Braig C, Gain T et al. Staging of pancreatic and ampullary carcinoma by endoscopic ultrasonography. Gastroenterology 1992; 102: 188–99

35. Warshaw AL, Gu Z, Wittenberg J, Waltman AC. Preoperative staging and assessment of resectability of pancreatic cancer. Arch Surg 1990; 125: 230–3

36. John TG, Greig JD, Carter DC, Garden OJ. Carcinoma of the pancreatic head and periampullary region. Tumor staging with laparoscopy and laparoscopic ultrasonography. Ann Surg 1995; 221: 156–64

37. VanDelden OM, Phoa SS et al. Comparison of laparoscopic US and contrast-enhanced spiral CT in the staging of potentially resectable tumors of the pancreatic head region. Radiology 1997; 205 SS: 619

3 Caudate lobectomy

William R Jarnagin and Leslie H Blumgart

Introduction

The caudate lobe, deeply situated and surrounded by major vascular structures, is an area of the liver often seen as forbidding and dangerous. The pioneering work of Couinaud[1] provided a much clearer understanding of hepatic anatomy and allowed a safer, anatomically-based approach to hepatic resectional surgery. As hepatic surgery has advanced, surgeons have increasingly and successfully pursued resection of caudate lobe lesions. The caudate lobe is not infrequently involved in primary and secondary malignancies. While rarely performed as an isolated procedure, caudate lobectomy is most often included in conjunction with other hepatic resections to achieve complete tumor clearance. A thorough understanding of the caudate lobe anatomy is necessary for safe resection.

Anatomy

Landmarks

The caudate lobe (segment I) is that portion of hepatic parenchyma situated posterior to the hilum and anterior to the inferior vena cava (IVC)[2] (Fig. 3.1). In many respects, the caudate is an independent anatomical segment composed of three distinct parts.[3] The caudate lobe proper, or Spiegel lobe, lies

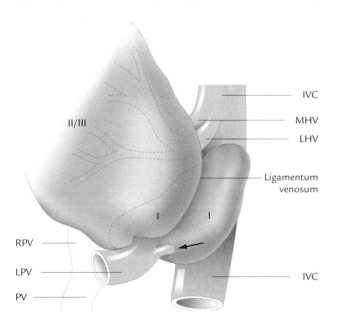

Figure 3.1 Schematic view of the caudate lobe (segment I, shaded), looking from above with the left lateral segment (segments II/III) retracted to the patient's right. The caudate is bounded anteriorly by the left portal vein (LPV) and posteriorly by the inferior vena cava (IVC). The principal portal venous supply, arising from the LPV, is indicated by the arrow. The ligamentum venosum runs along the anterior border of the caudate, from the LPV to the base of the left hepatic vein (LHV). PV, main portal vein; RPV, right portal vein; MHV, middle hepatic vein.

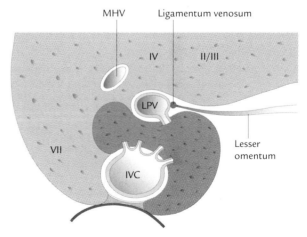

Figure 3.2 Cross-sectional view looking from below upwards. The caudate (segment I, shaded) is situated between the left portal vein (LPV) and the inferior vena cava (IVC). The main portal venous supply from the LPV and the caudate veins draining into the inferior vena cava are clearly shown. The lesser omentum separates the caudate from the left lateral segment (segments II/III). The posterior aspect of segment IV and the medial surface of segment VII mark the rightward extent of the caudate, which is in close proximity to the middle hepatic vein (MHV).

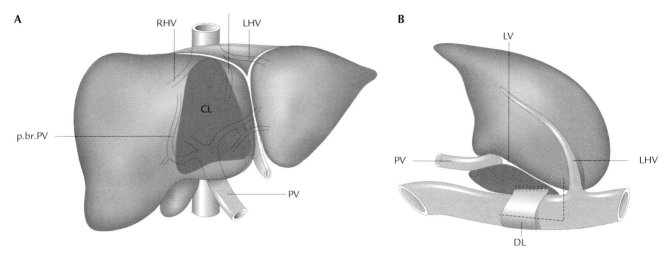

Figure 3.3 Two views of the caudate lobe, from above (A) and from the left with the left lateral segment retracted upwards and to the patient's right (B). The extent of the caudate from the hilum to the insertion of the hepatic veins is clearly shown. A plane from the origin of the right posterior sectoral portal vein (p.br.PV) to the confluence of the right hepatic vein (RHV) and inferior vena cava approximates the right border of the caudate (right). The ligamentous attachment, or dorsal ligament (DL), extending from the caudate to the IVC and segment VII is shown (left). CL, caudate lobe; PV, main portal vein; MHV, middle hepatic vein; LHV, left hepatic vein; LV, ligamentum venosum.

to the left of the vena cava and under the lesser omentum, which separates it from segments II and III. The paracaval portion of the caudate lies anterior to the IVC and extends cephalad to the roots of the major hepatic veins. The caudate process is located between the main right Glissonian pedicle and the IVC and fuses with segment VI of the right lobe[3–5] (Fig. 3.2).

The caudate lobe is bounded posteriorly, along its entire length, by the retrohepatic vena cava, and superiorly by the left and middle hepatic veins at their insertion. Its anterior border is formed by the left portal vein, the hilum and the base of segment IV (Figs 3.1–3.3). The ligamentum venosum, the obliterated ductus venosus, courses along the medial aspect of the caudate from the umbilical portion of the left portal vein to the inferior border of the left hepatic vein (Figs 3.1–3.3). The rightward extent of the caudate is variable, but is usually small and is indistinctly delimited by the posterior surface of segment IV and the medial surfaces of segment VI and VII[2,5–7] (Fig. 3.2). A plane passing from the origin of the right posterior sectoral portal vein to the confluence of the right hepatic vein (RHV) and IVC serves as a useful approximation of the right border[2] (Fig. 3.3). The middle hepatic vein is adjacent to the right portion of the caudate, and may be the source of significant hemorrhage if damaged during resection[6] (Figs 3.2 and 3.3). The posterior edge of the caudate on the left has a fibrous component that attaches to the crus of the diaphragm and extends posteriorly behind the vena cava to join segment VII (Fig. 3.4). In up to 50% of patients, this fibrous band

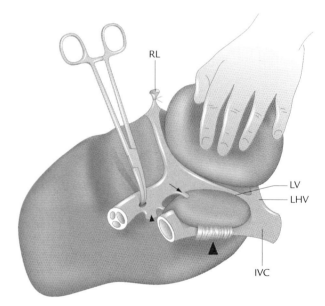

Figure 3.4 View of the caudate from the left. The left lateral segment is retracted upwards and to the patient's right. The ligamentous attachment extending from the caudate to the inferior vena cava (IVC) and segment VII is indicated (large arrowhead). The principal portal venous branch to the caudate arises from the left portal vein (small arrow), while a smaller branch arises from the right (small arrowhead). LV, ligamentum venosum; RL, round ligament; LHV, left hepatic vein; IVC, inferior vena cava.

may be replaced by hepatic parenchyma, so that the caudate lobe may completely embrace the vena cava at this level.[6]

Blood supply and biliary drainage

Both the left and right portal pedicles contribute to the blood supply and biliary drainage of the caudate.[2,5,6,8–10] Portal venous blood is supplied by 2–3 branches from the left portal vein and the main right or right posterior sectoral portal vein. From a practical standpoint, the left branch is much more constant and supplies a greater proportion of the lobe than the right branch(es)[2,9] (Figs 3.1 and 3.2). It is important that the left branch be identified and preserved during conventional left hepatectomy (i.e., without concomitant caudate resection).[6] The right posterior sectoral portal vein provides a branch to the right caudate in approximately 50% of patients.[9] The arterial anatomy is much more variable than the portal venous supply. The most common pattern is one branch from the main left hepatic artery and a second, smaller branch from the right posterior sectoral hepatic artery. Three branches may be seen in up to one-third of patients.[9] The principal biliary drainage of the caudate is through one or, less commonly, two branches that empty into the left main duct. A much smaller branch drains the right caudate and caudate process via the right posterior sectoral duct.[2,8,9] Failure to recognize and ligate these branches often results in troublesome biliary leak after caudate lobe resection.[6]

Hepatic venous drainage

The caudate lobe is the only hepatic segment that does not drain into one of the main hepatic veins. The hepatic venous drainage of the caudate is accomplished by a variable number of short venous branches that enter directly into the anterior and left aspect of the vena cava[2,6,9] (Fig. 3.2). Branches draining into the back of the vena cava may be encountered if there is a significant retrocaval caudate process.[6] Approximately 20% of patients have a solitary venous branch, but most patients have multiple branches and over one-third will have more than three.[9] This independent venous drainage allows continued decompression of the caudate in patients with complete hepatic venous outflow obstruction (Budd–Chiari), resulting in increased perfusion and compensatory hypertrophy.[2,7]

Embryogenesis

Many anatomical features of the caudate are thus unique relative to the other hepatic segments. Although often considered a left-sided structure, the caudate maintains physical attachments to the right liver, from which it derives some of its blood supply and biliary drainage. Consideration of its embryogenesis may

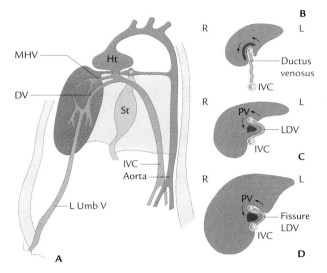

Figure 3.5 (A) Schematic representation of the ductus venosus and the fetal circulation. The left umbilical vein (L Umb V) carries placental blood to the left portal vein, which is shunted directly into the inferior vena cava (IVC) by the ductus venosus (DV). MHV, middle hepatic vein; Ht, heart; St, stomach. (B–D) The counterclockwise rotation of the liver as it enlarges, and the resulting insertion of the caudate lobe between the ductus venosus and IVC. PV, left portal vein; LDV, ligament of the ductus venosus.

provide a clearer understanding of the caudate lobe anatomy in the adult.[7] During the second trimester of fetal life, the persistent left umbilical vein enters the liver via the umbilical fissure and empties into the left portal vein (Fig. 3.5). The ductus venosus is suspended within the dorsal mesentery of the liver, shunting placental blood from the left portal vein directly into the vena cava. With hepatic enlargement and counterclockwise rotation, a small portion of the right liver inserts behind the ductus venosus mesentery, anterior to the IVC. The extrahepatic portion of the ductus venosus and its mesentery progressively shorten, and the future caudate lobe comes to rest between the IVC and the left portal triad. The ductus venosus obliterates shortly after birth and persists as the ligamentum venosum[7] (Fig. 3.5).

Surgical approaches

Surgical approaches to the caudate are critically dependent on the size and location of the tumor(s) and the type of associated resection. Caudate lobectomy may be undertaken as an isolated procedure or, more often, in conjunction with a right or left hepatic resection.[2,6] Bulky tumors, even though limited to the caudate, may be difficult to remove without associated left or right hepatectomy, as this may provide safer access without compromising the resection margin.[6,11] Other situations that require more extensive resection in addition to caudate lobectomy include: (1) tumors that arise from other segments and extend into the caudate, or vice versa; (2) primary or secondary tumors involving multiple segments, including the caudate; (3) hilar cholangiocarcinoma involving the caudate ducts.

General principles

The techniques of liver resection favored by the authors have been previously published and are described elsewhere in this book.[12] Full examination of the abdomen, pelvis, retroperitoneum and porta hepatis is performed to exclude the presence of extrahepatic disease. The lesser omentum is incised and the caudate is inspected and palpated. The liver is mobilized sufficiently to allow intraoperative ultrasound. The central venous pressure (CVP) is carefully controlled and not allowed to rise above 5 mmHg until the parenchymal transection is completed. Maintaining a low CVP greatly facilitates mobilization of the liver off the vena cava and control of the retrohepatic vena caval branches, and minimizes blood loss from small tears in hepatic venous branches. The possibility of air embolization is minimized by keeping the patient in a 15° Trendelenburg position. Parenchymal transection is accomplished with a Kelly clamp to expose ducts and vessels, which are then clipped or ligated. The authors make liberal use of vascular staplers for major pedicle and hepatic venous structures,[13] and favor intermittent rather than continuous portal triad clamping (Pringle maneuver).

Because of their location, tumors within the caudate often compress the IVC. Preoperative imaging often cannot distinguish tumor invasion from compression, and an attempt at resection should not be denied based solely on this radiographic finding.[6] Many tumors can be dissected free of the vena cava, and in selected cases vena caval resection can be performed. A short segment of resected vein may be amenable to primary repair or may require autogenous graft. On the other hand, a chronically occluded vena cava can often be resected without the need for reconstruction, since collateral flow has usually been established.[6]

Isolated caudate resection

Many of the critical maneuvers required for isolated caudate lobectomy apply also to combined resections. The caudate may be approached from the left or the right, depending on the size and location of the tumor. Often, dissection from both sides is

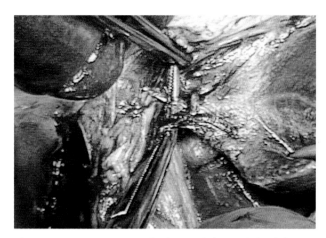

Figure 3.6 Dissection at the base of the umbilical fissure reveals the principal portal venous branch to the caudate (elevated on the clamp) arising from the left portal vein. The caudate lobe is being retracted to the patient's left and the right lobe upwards and to the patient's right.

necessary.[2,6,11,14] The essential elements of the procedure can be summarized in three steps.[6] First, control of the inflow blood supply is achieved by lowering the hilar plate and exposing the principal branches of the left and right hepatic artery and portal vein. As described above, the branches from the left are usually the most prominent. Second, the posteriorly draining caudate veins must be divided. A substantial tumor will often render the caudate stiff and difficult to manipulate, making exposure of these veins difficult. Third, after complete devascularization, the hepatic parenchyma between the base of segment IV and the left border of segment VII must be transected. During this phase of the dissection, one must always consider the close proximity of the middle hepatic vein and the possibility of major hemorrhage from inadvertent injury.[6]

Lowering the hilar plate is a necessary initial step for exposing the caudate blood supply and biliary drainage. Cholecystectomy may improve access to the base of segment IV and should be considered. The principal branches, arising from the left at the base of the umbilical fissure, are readily identified and divided (Fig. 3.6). The right sided branches must also be identified and controlled[2,6] (Fig. 3.7). The left lobe of the liver is mobilized and retracted upwards, exposing the ligamentous attachments to the IVC on the left (Fig. 3.8). If parenchyma is found to completely encircle the IVC, as discussed above, then complete mobilization from the left side may be difficult and an approach from the right should be considered.[6,11] When this ligament is divided, the caudate can be elevated and the hepatic venous branches safely controlled with clips or ligatures (Fig. 3.9).

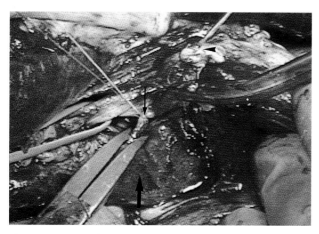

Figure 3.7 Portal venous branch to the right portion of the caudate and caudate process (large arrow), arising from the right portal vein (small arrow), is controlled and divided.

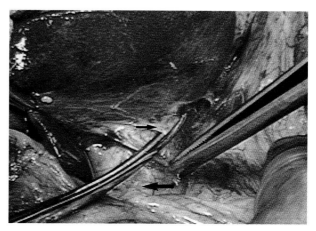

Figure 3.8 The ligamentous attachment extending from the caudate lobe to the inferior vena cava (IVC) is divided (small arrow). The caudate lobe is retracted upwards and to the patient's left. The IVC is indicated by the large arrow.

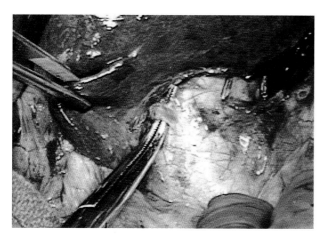

Figure 3.9 The caudate is retracted upwards and to the patient's left, exposing the inferior vena cava (IVC). A venous branch draining directly into the IVC is prepared for ligation and division.

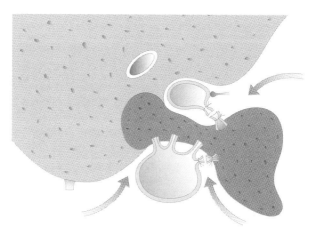

Figure 3.10 Cross-sectional view of the partially mobilized caudate lobe. The ligamentous attachments and the portal venous inflow have been divided. The posteriorly draining hepatic veins can be controlled and divided from the left or right.

Complete or nearly complete mobilization of the caudate can often be achieved in this manner, working from the left (Fig. 3.10). However, in the presence of a large, bulky tumor or retrocaval hepatic parenchyma extending from the caudate to segment VII, an initial approach from the right side is safer.[6,11,14] This requires complete mobilization of the right lobe from its diaphragmatic and retroperitoneal attachments, as well as from the right adrenal gland. The right lobe is rotated upwards and to the left, and the retrohepatic veins are serially divided, starting at the level of the caudate process and continuing upwards to the hepatic veins (Fig. 3.11). The ligamentous or parenchymal attachments to segment VII can also be divided working from the

right (Fig. 3.12). As the dissection progresses, it is usually a simple matter to continue across the anterior surface of the IVC and gain control of the caudate veins on the left.[6,11,14]

At this point, the caudate is devascularized, leaving only its parenchymal attachments to segment IV and segment VII to be divided (Fig. 3.10). The possibility of vigorous bleeding from a posterior tear in the middle hepatic vein makes this part of the procedure particularly hazardous.[6] This is especially true for a large tumor that extends anteriorly and to the right. When caudate resection is combined with right or left hepatectomy, this danger is reduced by controlling the vein prior to this portion of the procedure,

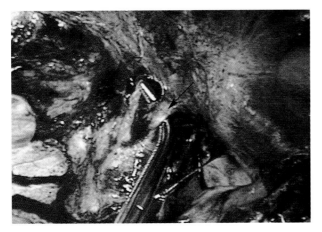

Figure 3.11 Mobilization of the right hepatic lobe off the vena cava. The diaphragmatic attachments have been divided, and the liver is retracted upwards and to the patient's left. A large retrohepatic vena caval branch is prepared for ligation and division (arrow).

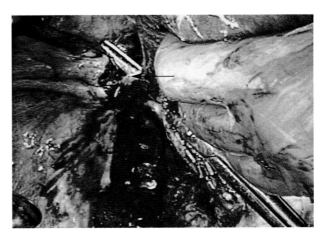

Figure 3.12 Division of the ligamentous attachment to segment VII. The liver has been mobilized and retracted upwards and to the patient's left. A clamp is passed between the inferior vena cava and the fibrous ligament (arrow), which in this case contains no hepatic parenchyma.

either extrahepatically or within the hepatic parenchyma. Likewise, for isolated caudate lobectomy, the authors have found it valuable to isolate the middle and left hepatic veins at their insertion into the suprahepatic IVC.[6] This allows temporary control with a vascular clamp during parenchymal transection. An alternative approach has been described, which entails partial occlusion of the vena cava at the confluence of all three hepatic veins.[5] Others have described splitting the hepatic parenchyma in the interlobar plane, separating the right and left hemilivers along the right border of segment IV[15] (Fig. 3.13). This transhepatic approach allows the transection of the remaining caudate parenchyma under direct vision of the middle hepatic vein, thereby minimizing the risk of injury. Total vascular isolation for caudate resection has also been described, but is usually unnecessary.[11]

Caudate resection with left hepatectomy

This technique is indicated for large caudate lesions where isolated resection is not safe, tumors that involve other segments of the left liver in addition to the caudate, and for cholangiocarcinoma of the hepatic duct confluence with extension into the left hepatic duct. In the latter case, tumor often extends into the principal caudate duct, arising from the left hepatic duct, and caudate resection is necessary to achieve tumor clearance.[2,6,16,17]

The left and right lobes should be mobilized completely. The falciform ligament is divided to the level of the suprahepatic vena cava. The hilar plate should be lowered and the left aspect of the caudate

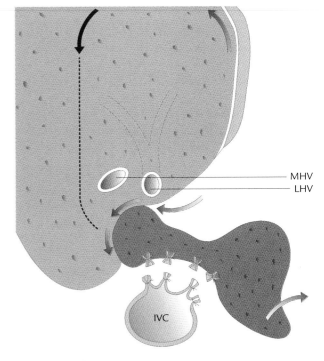

Figure 3.13 Cross-sectional view of the devascularized caudate lobe, which is attached only by its right border to segment VII medially and segment IV superiorly. As an alternative approach, the liver parenchyma may be split in the interlobar plane (black arrow), allowing the remaining caudate attachments to be divided under direct vision of the middle hepatic vein (MHV). LHV, left hepatic vein; IVC, inferior vena cava.

exposed as described above. The left portal vein and hepatic artery are exposed within the porta hepatis and divided at a point proximal to the principal caudate branches. Similarly, portal venous and hepatic arterial branches arising from the right should be sought and controlled.[2,6] It is the authors' practice to control and divide the hepatic venous outflow, if feasible, before starting parenchymal transection.[12] Dissecting from the left, the root of the left hepatic vein can be identified at the cephalad extent of the ligamentum venosum. Careful dissection in this area, anterior to the caudate, and above the liver along the anterior surface of the suprahepatic IVC, usually exposes the vein. Commonly, the left and middle hepatic veins enter the IVC as a common trunk, which can be exposed in a similar fashion. Once adequately exposed, the common trunk may be divided with a vascular stapler or oversewn.[6] Alternatively, the left and middle veins may be divided separately. If extrahepatic control of the hepatic veins is not feasible, this may be accomplished during the parenchymal transection phase. The posteriorly draining caudate veins are then exposed and divided. The retrohepatic veins coursing from the right lobe into the IVC should also be divided, as this makes transection of the right portion of the caudate easier. The liver tissue is then divided along the principal resection plane, encompassing the middle hepatic vein. The left hepatic vein may be divided during the hilar dissection or during parenchymal transection. It is essential to avoid narrowing the biliary confluence when the left hepatic duct stump is oversewn.[2]

The approach to the bile duct is much different when this procedure is performed for hilar cholangiocarcinoma. In this circumstance, the entire supraduodenal bile duct and lymphatic tissues are reflected upwards early in the procedure and included with the specimen. Also, the right hepatic duct should be divided at a point beyond the tumor and before dividing the liver. It may be necessary to divide the duct at the level of the right anterior and posterior sectoral hepatic ducts. The bile duct margins should be sent for frozen section histology to ensure complete tumor clearance.[2,16,18]

Extended left hepatectomy with caudate lobectomy is one of the more complex and technically challenging of all hepatic resections.[19] This procedure is indicated for multiple tumors that also involve the caudate or large central hepatic tumors of the left lobe that extend into the caudate and the right anterior sector. Tumors situated high in the liver, involving the left and middle hepatic veins and extending into segment VIII, may also involve the caudate and require this type of resection. Adding caudate lobectomy requires exposing and mobilizing the caudate, as described above for left hepatectomy. With the left liver and caudate completely prepared, the line of parenchymal transection is oblique from the right, anterior to the right hepatic vein and then carried posteriorly along the right border of the caudate.[19]

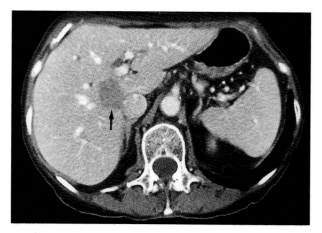

Figure 3.14 Computed tomographic scan showing a metastatic tumor within the right portion of the caudate lobe and extending into segment IV superiorly and segment VII medially (arrow). The tumor extended very near to the insertion of the middle and right hepatic veins. Complete removal required an extended right hepatectomy and caudate lobectomy en bloc.

Caudate resection with right hepatectomy

This procedure is typically indicated for solitary tumors of the right hepatic lobe that extend into the caudate (Fig. 3.14) or multiple tumors of the right lobe and caudate.[2,6] Occasionally, this procedure is necessary for cholangiocarcinoma of the hepatic duct confluence with extension into the right hepatic duct. Often, however, these tumors spare the principal caudate duct, and caudate resection is not necessary.[20] This is in contrast to cholangiocarcinomas of the left hepatic duct, which nearly always involve the orifice of the principal caudate duct and usually require caudate resection.

Caudate resection is somewhat easier to perform in conjunction with right hepatectomy, mainly because the potentially hazardous disconnection of the right portion of the caudate is avoided.[2] The right and left lobes should be fully mobilized. The gallbladder should be removed and the hilar plate lowered. The right hepatic artery and right portal vein are exposed within the porta hepatis. In situations where the extrahepatic bile duct is not sacrificed, exposing the right portal vein may be difficult. This is especially true when the bifurcation is high. It is usually helpful to first isolate and divide the right hepatic artery. Ligatures left on the divided cystic duct and right hepatic artery can be used to retract the common bile duct and hepatic artery upwards and to the left, allowing access to the portal vein from the right side[6] (Fig. 3.15). Continued cephalad dissection will usually reveal the portal venous bifurcation. A small posterolateral branch to the right portion of the caudate is usually encountered

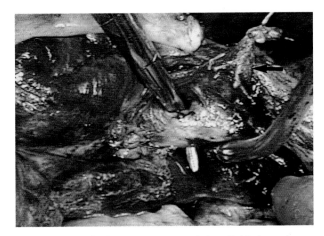

Figure 3.15 The hepatic artery and the divided cystic duct (arrow) are retracted upwards and to the patient's left, allowing access to the portal vein (right portal vein elevated on the clamp).

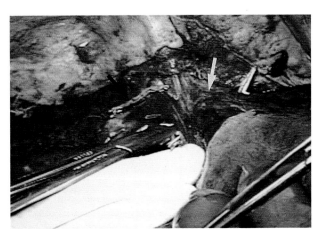

Figure 3.16 The staple line of the divided right hepatic vein is shown (black arrow). A clamp has been passed around the common trunk of the middle and left hepatic veins (white arrow).

(Fig. 3.7). This branch should be divided early in the dissection to avoid inadvertent injury and to allow better exposure of the right portal vein.[6] Not infrequently, the anterior and posterior portal vein branches arise separately, requiring that they be divided individually. With the inflow to the right lobe controlled, a clear line of demarcation should be evident along the principal resection plane. Dissection of the left portal vein at the base of the umbilical fissure exposes the principal caudate branch, which is divided (Fig. 3.6).

The liver is now fully mobilized off the vena cava by dividing the accessory hepatic veins. The right lobe must be liberated from all of its diaphragmatic and retroperitoneal attachments. The right adrenal may be adherent to the undersurface of the liver, just lateral to the vena cava, and may be the source of troublesome bleeding if dissection is not pursued in the proper tissue plane. The falciform ligament should be divided to the level of the suprahepatic vena cava, and the origin of the right hepatic vein identified. With the liver retracted upwards and to the left, ligation of the retrohepatic veins should commence from below and proceed to the level of the hepatic vein[2,6] (Fig. 3.11). It is often possible to extend this dissection across the anterior surface of the vena cava and control some or all of the caudate veins.[2,6] As the dissection proceeds cephalad, the ligamentous attachments along the lateral aspect of the vena cava are encountered and divided to allow access to the right hepatic vein. In approximately one half of patients, parenchymal tissue from the caudate will extend behind the vena cava and attach to segment VII.[6] This tissue, if present, must be carefully separated from the right hepatic vein and divided. Continued dissection from below and at the

level of the suprahepatic vena cava exposes the right hepatic vein, which may be divided at this point (Fig. 3.16).

The left liver is now retracted upwards and to the right, and mobilization of the caudate lobe is completed. Any remaining caudate veins are divided. The hepatic parenchyma may be divided just to the right of the middle hepatic vein.[6] As the dissection proceeds posteriorly, the surgeon's left hand is placed anterior to the vena cava, retracting the left portion of the caudate toward the right.[2] The remaining parenchyma can then be divided along the right lateral aspect of the middle hepatic vein. When necessary, the middle hepatic vein may be divided, either extrahepatically or from within the liver parenchyma. This can be done without fear of causing venous congestion of segment IV, since drainage will continue via the umbilical vein.

It should be noted that the right hepatic duct need not be divided during the hilar dissection. It is safer and easier to control the right duct by dividing and oversewing the main right portal pedicle, which is encountered early during parenchymal transection (Fig. 3.17). When this procedure is performed for hilar cholangiocarcinoma, the bile duct must be approached as discussed above.

It is usually a straightforward matter to extend this resection to include most or all of segment IV as an extended right hepatectomy. The procedure is carried out as described above, except that the segment IV pedicles are ligated at their origin within the umbilical fissure. Alternatively, these pedicles may be isolated and divided during the parenchymal transection phase. Likewise, the middle hepatic

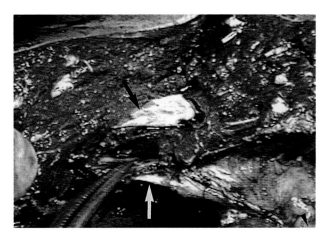

Figure 3.17 Hepatic parenchymal transection during right hepatectomy and caudate lobectomy. A sling has been placed around the portal triad. The main right pedicle is exposed (white arrow) and is prepared for ligation and division. Note the close proximity of the middle hepatic vein (black arrow).

vein may be divided extrahepatically or from within the parenchyma.[19]

Results of caudate lobectomy

Much of the published literature on caudate resection consists of case reports or small series (three or less).[5,14,15,21] These reports provided important insights into the technical aspects of caudate resection and documented its feasibility. Since 1990, however, many centers have reported their experience with an increasingly larger number of procedures (Table 3.1), allowing a more thorough analysis.[4,6,11,16,17,22,23]

It is readily apparent from these studies that caudate resection represents a small percentage of the total number of hepatic resections from any one center, generally 10% or less. In one of the largest series of partial hepatectomy for hepatocellular carcinoma, caudate lobectomy was performed in less than 1% of patients.[24] Moreover, isolated caudate resection is performed even less frequently. While some authors have reported a greater incidence of complications associated with caudate resection,[4] most series cite morbidity and mortality figures that are comparable to those of standard hepatic resection.[6,11,16,22,23] These results suggest that caudate resection, either alone or in conjunction with a larger resection, can be performed without excessive risk.

Some authors have suggested that isolated caudate resection for metastatic tumors or hepatocellular carcinoma may not provide adequate tumor clearance. Two studies have documented narrow resection margins and early recurrences in patients undergoing isolated caudate resection for hepatocellular carcinoma and metastatic tumors.[4,11] However,

Table 3.1 Selected series of caudate resections, diagnoses and procedures performed. The numbers in parentheses indicate the frequency of caudate resection as a percentage of all hepatic resections

Author	Number	Diagnoses	Procedures
Nimura et al.[16]	45	Cholangiocarcinoma (45)	En bloc complete caudate resection (42)
			Isolated complete caudate resection (3)
Elias et al.[11]	20 (9.4%)	Metastatic tumors (16)	En bloc complete caudate resection (4)
		Hepatocellular carcinoma (3)	Isolated complete caudate resection (3)
		Cholangiocarcinoma (1)	Partial caudate resection (13)
Nagasue et al.[22]	19 (4%)*	Hepatocellular carcinoma (19)	En bloc complete caudate resection (3)
			Isolated complete caudate resection (6)
			Partial caudate resection (10)
Yang et al.[23]	6	Hepatocellular carcinoma (6)	En bloc complete caudate resection (3)
			Partial caudate resection (3)
Shimada et al.[4]	9	Hepatocellular carcinoma (9)	Isolated complete caudate resection (2)
			Partial caudate resection (7)
Bartlett et al.[6]	21 (7.5%)	Metastatic tumors (9)	En bloc complete caudate resection (17)
		Other, not specified (12)	Isolated complete caudate resection (4)
Ogura et al.[17]	39	Cholangiocarcinoma (39)	En bloc complete caudate resection (34)
			Isolated complete caudate resection (5)

*2.2% of all patients with primary HCC had caudate involvement; of those resected, 4% of patients with primary HCC and 11% of patients with recurrent HCC underwent caudate resection.

many of these resections were partial or wedge excisions. Moreover, studies containing a greater number of complete resections also report adequate tumor clearance and acceptable recurrence rates.[6,22] Reasonable judgment must be exercised in selecting patients for isolated caudate lobectomy. The cumulated evidence supports the efficacy of isolated complete caudate lobectomy for small or medium sized tumors. Certainly, large tumors usually require a more extensive resection in order to achieve clear margins, and wedge resections, except for very small tumors, should be avoided.[6]

Several studies have documented the relatively frequent involvement of caudate lobe ducts in patients with hilar cholangiocarcinoma. Nimura et al. reported involvement of the caudate ducts in 44 of 46 patients in whom caudate resection was performed.[16] In a separate study by Ogura et al., microscopic tumor involvement of the caudate lobe was less common (9 of 21 patients).[17] It would seem clear that, in light of the predominant biliary drainage pattern of the caudate lobe,[9] tumors of the left hepatic duct almost always require caudate lobectomy. Tumors involving the right hepatic duct, by contrast, do not always require complete caudate resection.[20] Indeed, the ducts draining the caudate process will likely be involved, but this portion of the liver and the associated bile ducts are usually included with the resection. The results of several large series of resections for hilar cholangiocarcinoma, including a report from the authors, support this policy of selective caudate resection.[25–27]

Summary

Resection of the caudate lobe is occasionally necessary for primary or secondary hepatic tumors. While some lesions may be excised with an isolated caudate lobectomy, the majority will require right or left hepatectomy and caudate resection en bloc. The addition of caudate lobectomy does not significantly increase the morbidity above that expected for major hepatectomy. In properly selected patients, isolated caudate resection can achieve adequate tumor clearance without excessive morbidity. The surgical approach to caudate resection is critically dependent on the size and location of the tumor. The surgeon should be completely comfortable with the relevant anatomy and the common variations, as well as the standard techniques of hepatic resection.

Key points

- Caudate lobectomy is rarely performed as an isolated procedure.
- A thorough understanding of the anatomy of the caudate lobe is essential for safe resection.
- Tumors of the caudate lobe often involve the inferior vena cava.
- Caudate lobectomy is often performed in conjunction with other major liver resections.
- Resection margins of 1 cm may not be possible with caudate lobectomy in view of caval proximity.

REFERENCES

1. Couinaud, C. Etude anatomiques et chirugicales. Paris: Masson, 1957: 400–9
2. Mazziotti A, Cavallari A (eds). Techniques in liver surgery, 1st edn. London: Greenwich Medical Media, 1997: 101–15
3. Kumon M. Anatomy of the caudate lobe with special reference to portal vein and bile duct. Acta Hepatol Jpn 1985; 26: 1193–99
4. Shimada M, Matsumata T, Maieda T, Yanaga K, Taketomi A, Sugimachi K. Characteristics of hepatocellular carcinoma originating in the caudate lobe. Hepatology 1994; 19: 911–5
6. Bartlett D, Fong Y, Blumgart LH. Complete resection of the caudate lobe of the liver: technique and results [review]. Br J Surg 1996; 83: 1076–81
7. Dodds WJ, Erickson SJ, Taylor AJ, Lawson TL, Stewart ET. Caudate lobe of the liver: anatomy, embryology, and pathology [see comments]. AJR 1990; 154: 87–93
8. Furukawa H, Sano K, Kosuge T et al. Analysis of biliary drainage in the caudate lobe of the liver: comparison of three-dimensional CT cholangiography and rotating cine cholangiography. Radiology 1997; 204: 113–7
9. Mizumoto R, Suzuki H. Surgical anatomy of the hepatic hilum with special reference to the caudate lobe. World J Surg 1988; 12: 2–10
10. Stapleton GN, Hickman R, Terblanche J. Blood supply of the right and left hepatic ducts. Br J Surg 1998; 85: 202–7
11. Elias D, Lasser PH, Desruennes E, Mankarios H, Jiang Y. Surgical approach to segment I for malignant tumors of the liver. Surg Gynecol Obstet 1992; 175: 17–24
12. Cunningham JD, Fong Y, Shriver C, Melendez J, Marx

WL, Blumgart LH. One hundred consecutive hepatic resections: blood loss, transfusion, and operative technique. Arch Surg 1994; 129: 1050–6

13. Fong Y, Blumgart LH. Useful stapling techniques in liver surgery. J Am Coll Surg 1997; 185: 93–100

14. Lerut J, Gruwez JA, Blumgart LH. Resection of the caudate lobe of the liver. Surg Gynecol Obstet 1990; 171: 160–216

15. Yamamoto J, Takayama T, Kosuge T et al. An isolated caudate lobectomy by the transhepatic approach for hepatocellular carcinoma in cirrhotic liver. Surgery 1992; 111: 699–702

16. Nimura Y, Hayakawa N, Kamiya J, Kondo S, Shionoya S. Hepatic segmentectomy with caudate lobe resection for bile duct carcinoma of the hepatic hilus. World J Surg 1990; 14: 535–44

17. Ogura Y, Kawarada Y. Surgical strategies for carcinoma of the hepatic duct confluence. Br J Surg 1998; 85: 20–4

18. Blumgart LH, Hadjis NS, Benjamin IS, Beazley RM. Surgical approaches to cholangiocarcinoma at the confluence of the hepatic ducts. Lancet 1984; 1: 66

19. Blumgart LH. Liver resection – liver and biliary tumors. In: Blumgart LH, ed. Surgery of the liver and biliary tract, 2nd edn. Edinburgh: Churchill Livingstone, 1994: 1495–537

20. Blumgart LH, Benjamin IS. Cancer of the bile ducts. In: Blumgart LH, ed. Surgery of the liver and biliary tract, 2nd edn. Edinburgh: Churchill Livingstone, 1994: 967–95

21. Colonna JO, Shaked A, Gelabert HA, Busuttil RW. Resection of the caudate lobe through 'bloody gultch'. Surg Gynecol Obstet 1993; 176: 401–2

22. Nagasue N, Kohno H, Yamanoi A et al. Resection of the caudate lobe of the liver for primary and recurrent hepatocellular carcinomas [see comments]. J Am Coll Surg 1997; 184: 1–8

23. Yang MC, Lee PO, Sheu JC, Lai MY, Hu RH, Wei CK. Surgical treatment of hepatocellular carcinoma originating from the caudate lobe. World J Surg 1996; 20: 562–5

24. Tung TT, Bach TT. Bilan d'une experience de la chirurgie d'exerese hepatique pour cancer par la technique d'hepatectomie reglee par voie transparenchymateuse: a propos de 941 hepatectomies. Chirurgie 1983; 109: 27–30

25. Baer HU, Stain S, Dennison A, Eggers B, Blumgart LH. Improvements in survival by aggressive resections of hilar cholangiocarcinoma. Ann Surg 1993; 124: 248–52

26. Burke EC, Jarnagin WR, Hochwald SN, Pisters PWT, Fong Y, Blumgart LH. Hilar cholangiocarcinoma: patterns of spread, the importance of hepatic resection for curative operation, and a presurgical clinical staging system. Ann Surg 1998; 228(3): 385–94

27. Klempnauer J, Ridder GJ, von Wasielewski R, Werner M, Weimann A, Pichlmayr R. Resectional surgery of hilar cholangiocarcinoma: a multivariate analysis of prognostic factors. J Clin Oncol 1997; 15: 947–54

4 Ex-vivo resection for liver tumours

J Peter A Lodge

Introduction

These days it seems that virtually no liver tumour should be considered to be unresectable, even though the majority of patients continue to present at a late stage in their disease. Many experts have challenged the old dogma relating to hepatic resection and candidates with multiple and bilobar hepatic tumours as well as patients with limited extrahepatic tumour infiltration are now considered for resection. In addition, patients with metastases from tumours other than colorectal cancer are also regularly undergoing liver resection.

Improvements in anaesthesia have been integral to the success of hepatic surgery, primarily through the use of low central venous pressure techniques for liver resection. In this author's centre only 30% of cases require blood transfusion. This is despite the fact that 85% of our current resection practice is hemihepatectomy or more and the majority is trisectionectomy (extended hepatectomy) and bilateral resection work. In the majority of hepatobiliary centres, Pringle's manoeuvre and total vascular isolation (hepatic vascular exclusion) are used routinely,[1-16] and this short-term warm ischaemia is reported to be well tolerated. However, it has been our preference in recent years to avoid ischaemia whenever possible as we had noticed an increased postoperative morbidity and longer hospital stay in those patients in whom vascular isolation techniques had been used for prolonged periods.

In our experience, the use of hepatic ischaemia techniques and blood transfusion is more often necessary for the more complex resections. Whereas right and left hepatectomy and right hepatic trisectionectomy (right trisegmentectomy, extended right hepatectomy – resection of hepatic segments IV, V, VI, VII, VIII) should be regarded as routine and only rarely require transfusion, left hepatic trisectionectomy (left trisegmentectomy, extended left hepatectomy – resection of hepatic segments II, III, IV, V, VIII), for example, is more challenging. Recent internal audit of the first 22 left hepatic trisegmentectomies carried out by this author has shown that 11 required Pringle's manoeuvre and five needed a period of total vascular isolation. In 14 cases the caudate lobe (segment I) was also resected. Eleven of the 22 patients required blood transfusion, although the median requirement was only 1.5 units. This may partly be explained by a high proportion of cholangiocarcinoma cases (32%) in this series as resection of these tumours is associated with a greater degree of operative difficulty. In this group of 22 patients, six of the seven patients with major postoperative morbidity had required either Pringle's manoeuvre or total vascular isolation, confirming our previous observation. It is also true to say that increasing experience helps to reduce the use of ischaemia and blood transfusion, and there has been little morbidity in a further 15 left trisectionectomies carried out recently by this author.

Although orthoptic liver transplantation and cluster resection are the most radical forms of tumour clearance, results for otherwise unresectable tumours have been uniformly disappointing. Tumours account for only 3% of our liver transplant programme in terms of primary indication. However, transplantation remains a valuable option for patients with tumours as secondary indications: principally small hepatomas within cirrhosis. Our centre has been investigating cluster resection and multivisceral grafting as an alternative for extensive tumours and the neuroendocrine group lends itself neatly to this concept. These are most often tumours of midgut origin with foregut metastases and adequate lymphadenectomy involves both the coeliac and superior mesenteric arterial distributions, and if purely foregut (pancreatic tail) then a lesser cluster resection can also be appropriate.

These concepts will be discussed at the end of this chapter as they are helpful in defining the place of ex-vivo liver resection in the spectrum of hepatic surgical techniques. In addition there are many lessons to be learnt from the practice of liver transplantation, not least anaesthesia and the role of veno–venous bypass.

The short-term survival of untreated patients with both primary and secondary liver tumours, the unpredictability of chemotherapy response on an individual patient basis and the disappointing results of transplantation for cancer provide adequate impetus for attempts to extend the boundaries of liver resection as far as possible. Hilar involvement can be adequately dealt with by short periods of vascular isolation and warm ischaemia and this can often be done without caval or hepatic

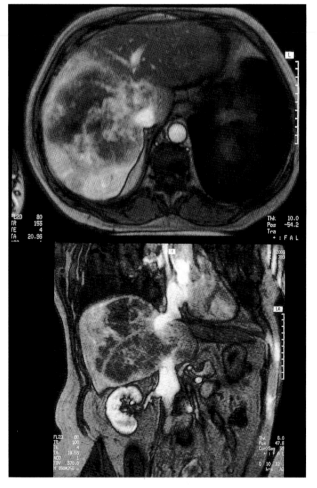

Figure 4.1 This MRI scan demonstrates a typical case for ex-vivo liver resection. The patient had liver metastases from colorectal cancer. The tumour is closely applied to the hepatocaval confluence, the IVC and the portal triad structures. At ex-vivo resection, a section of IVC was resected and replaced with a prosthetic graft. The patient survived for 12 months but died with bone metastases.

vein isolation.[17] Portal vein and hepatic artery resection and reanastomosis or replacement now accounts for 40% of this author's experience of primary hepatic resection for cholangiocarcinoma. Inferior vena cava (IVC) involvement can often be dealt with by simple venous side-clamping or in more extensive cases by total hepatic vascular isolation with IVC clamping and the selective use of veno–venous bypass. IVC resection accounts for 4% of this author's metastatic work, and replacement by graft has been necessary in most. This fraction is expected to increase as more advanced cases are being considered and it accounts for 6% of cases during the past 12 months in our centre. Tumours involving all of the major hepatic veins with or without IVC invasion, and particularly tumours involving the hepatocaval confluence and needing IVC replacement, continue to pose a surgical challenge, particularly if portal hilar structures are involved bilaterally (Fig. 4.1). Ex-vivo resection[18–20] offers a potential lifeline for this group of patients and this technique deserves discussion, although it accounts for less than 2% of this author's total hepatic resection experience. The processes of patient selection and operative assessment of operability by more conventional yet advanced techniques have meant that we have found ex-vivo resection to be necessary in only five of 28 cases (21%) considered during the past 7 years.

Patient selection

Cardiorespiratory assessment

Before considering a surgical procedure of this scale it is essential to be as sure as possible that the patient is fit enough to withstand the operation. It is important to take a detailed history of previous cardiovascular disease, including myocardial infarction, angina pectoris and hypertension. Clearly, a history of smoking or peripheral vascular disease should raise the clinical suspicion of coronary artery disease. Respiratory diseases, particularly emphysema and chronic bronchitis, are quite prevalent in the elderly population and clinical examination with chest radiology can be helpful.

Resting and exercise electrocardiography are the standard cardiological objective assessment tests in our centre. Failure to achieve an adequate heart rate for true stress testing can be a problem in the elderly population, most often due to osteoarthritis of the hips and knees. In this situation a great deal of useful information can be gained from echocardiography, with measurement of end diastolic and systolic volumes to calculate left ventricular ejection fraction, or by radioisotope assessment with dobutamine stress. Failure to complete these investigations or a significant depression of the S-T segment on the exercise ECG is a clear indication for coronary artery angiography. This procedure is carried out in 10% of major liver surgery candidates in our experience, ruling out surgery in 3% but providing reassuring information in the rest. Only five patients in our experience have been suitable for preoperative coronary artery angioplasty, stenting or bypass grafting prior to liver surgery, but these are clearly potential treatment options to consider.

Routine lung function tests including vital capacity and forced expiratory volume form part of our standard assessment as well as chest radiology. Useful information is also gained from the chest CT, which is done primarily to look for lung metastases and diaphragm involvement by the hepatic tumour. The CT appearances of emphysema in particular are characteristic. In our northern UK population, because of the high incidence of emphysema and chronic obstructive airways disease, we often consider blood gas sampling preoperatively. In cases where severe pulmonary hypertension is suspected a pulmonary artery wedge pressure line is placed at the commencement of anaesthesia before definitely deciding to proceed with the resection. If there is a very high index of suspicion then we prefer to check the pulmonary artery pressures as a day case procedure in advance of the planned surgical date so that the patient can be advised more accurately about operative risk.

Hepatic reserve

Preoperative blood tests necessary before proceeding to major resection include full blood count, urea and electrolytes, liver function tests, clotting screen and tumour marker studies. Prothrombin time, bilirubin and albumin give a fairly accurate indication of global hepatic function, but in some cases a liver biopsy of the residual tumour-free liver will also be necessary if there is a doubt about hepatic reserve, in particular in hepatoma. This is particularly important in the group of patients with a previous history of excess alcohol consumption or if there is serological evidence of hepatitis B or C. It is also useful when dealing with cholangiocarcinoma, as there may be underlying sclerosing cholangitis.

Some consideration needs to be given to the number of viable tumour-free hepatic segments that will be reimplanted, but this should not usually be less than two, unless there is considerable hypertrophy of the tumour-free liver (Fig. 4.2). Although it has not been our practice to use detailed CT-based volumetric analysis of the planned residual hepatic volume, careful review of preoperative imaging is clearly

important to make the decision for surgery. It is inevitable that a degree of temporary hepatic failure will be induced in some patients undergoing very major resection. More work needs to be done in this interesting area. If the tumour-free segments are affected by biliary obstruction, it is our current practice to attempt biliary decompression by endoscopic or percutaneous techniques a few days in advance of surgery as this may speed up the postoperative recovery.

Tumour type

It is reasonable to consider any malignant tumour of the liver, primary or secondary, for ex-vivo liver resection if there is an acceptable chance of clearance of all the disease. It is not our routine to biopsy the tumour unless there is a serious doubt about the diagnosis after radiological assessment. There is a potential for peritoneal tumour spread from the biopsy site and if a tumour biopsy is absolutely necessary then it is best done under ultrasound or CT guidance, traversing a section of normal liver as this may prevent tumour cell spillage. A biopsy can be useful if a benign tumour is suspected, for example hepatic adenoma occurring as a result of a glycogen storage disease, as liver transplantation may be more appropriate in that case.

Radiology assessment

Although MRI is the imaging method of choice for the liver in our centre, other groups routinely use CT arterioportography with similar results. Three-dimensional CT and MRI imaging technology continues to improve and may be of value in planning the surgical approach. Hepatic angiography with portal venography may also be useful. Small metastases or hepatomas not detected by other methods will rule out some candidates and variations in hepatic arterial anatomy can be helpful in some cases, particularly in cholangiocarcinoma. For example, an aberrant left hepatic artery from the left gastric artery can enable radical right hepatic trisectionectomy with bilateral portal vein resection and left portal vein reconstruction without interruption of the hepatic arterial supply to segments II and III at any stage of the operation. Venography to examine the inferior vena cava and hepatic veins is occasionally useful if all three major hepatic veins are involved with tumour as an adequate inferior or middle right hepatic vein (Fig. 4.3) may obviate the need for ex-vivo venous reconstruction.[21,22] It is our current practice to use CT scanning of chest, abdomen and pelvis to exclude extrahepatic disease for all tumour types. Screening for primary site recurrence (e.g. colonoscopy) is also clearly important. An isotope

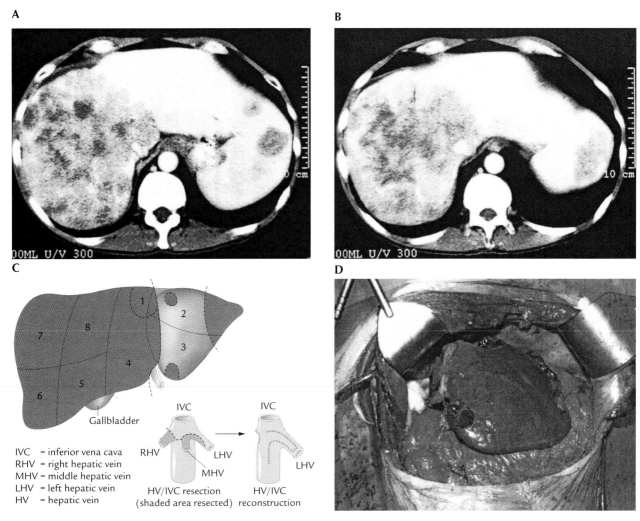

Figure 4.2 Considerable hypertrophy of the uninvolved hepatic segments can occur as demonstrated on this CT scan (A, B). In this case, in-situ hypothermic perfusion was used to preserve parts of segments II and III with left hepatic vein reconstruction using a flap from the IVC (C: schematic diagram of resection, D: operative photograph following reperfusion). The patient had undergone 6 months of preoperative chemotherapy. At the time of writing he was alive and disease-free at 4 months postoperatively.

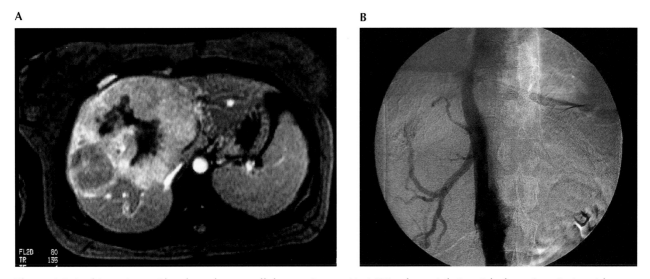

Figure 4.3 In this patient with a large hepatocellular carcinoma (A: MRI) a large inferior right hepatic vein is evident on venography (B) and in-situ resection was possible despite involvement of the three major hepatic veins.

bone scan may be useful in hepatoma, cholangiocarcinoma and some metastatic tumours, and we have recently found it to be of use in colorectal metastatic disease. This is at variance with our usual practice for patients with hepatic metastases from colorectal cancer and may reflect the late stage of presentation of the ex-vivo candidates.

Can it be avoided?

New surgical techniques such as resections that rely on the presence of an inferior or middle right hepatic vein and the possibility of hepatic venous reconstruction in situ will mean that ex-vivo liver resection will rarely be performed. In-situ hypothermic perfusion and the 'ante situm technique', which do not require hepatic arterial or biliary reconstruction, may be preferable in some cases where it is anticipated that the parenchymal dissection will be difficult. Careful thought must be given to these techniques both preoperatively and during the eventual operation as these methods are widely thought to have a greater applicability than the ex-vivo technique. However, the only disadvantage of the ex-vivo method is the number of necessary vascular anastomoses and the associated thrombotic risk and in this author's opinion this is outweighed by the advantages of superb exposure and adequate hypothermic protection in some cases.

In-situ hypothermic perfusion

The techniques involved in in-situ hypothermic perfusion (Fig. 4.4) are very similar to those employed in total vascular isolation. The aim is to provide a bloodless field combined with hypothermic cellular protection, allowing a prolonged and more precise dissection.[18,19–25] It is thought to be more straightforward than hepatic excision and reimplantation (ex-vivo method), but it should be noted that cooling may not be even and difficulties remain when considering access to the IVC and hepatic veins. It may be performed without portal or systemic venous bypass. Cooling can be achieved by portal vein or hepatic artery perfusion and a small dose of heparin is usually given before arterial and portal vein clamping. The IVC should be dissected enough to be clamped above and below the liver and the right suprarenal (adrenal) vein is slung as this will usually need to be clamped. The IVC is clamped above and below the liver (and also the right suprarenal vein if necessary) and the infrahepatic IVC is incised above the lower clamp. Perfusion is started with a cold hepatic preservation solution and the venous effluent is actively sucked from the IVC to prevent excessive body cooling. Liver cooling

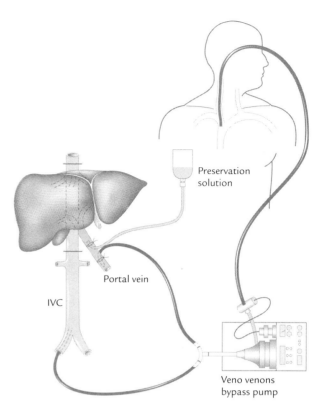

Figure 4.4 In-situ hepatic perfusion is summarized in this line drawing.

can be maintained by continuous slow perfusion during the resection or by repeated cooling by perfusion every 30 minutes. A practical point is to avoid rewarming by inadvertently allowing portal perfusion to continue: in a recent case we perfused and established veno–venous bypass through the cut end of the right portal vein and some blood flowed past the cannula from the main portal vein to the left liver.

The ante situm procedure

The ante situm procedure combines in-situ hypothermic perfusion with separation of the suprahepatic IVC to allow mobilization for dissection of the cranial and posterior parts of the liver under direct vision. It is usual to ligate and divide the right suprarenal vein in order to gain adequate rotation of the organ. In our experience, it has been necessary also to divide the infrahepatic IVC, with replacement by a prosthetic graft or by venous patches. This should allow the whole upper part of the liver to be moved onto the abdominal wall in order to allow access to the cranial and posterior aspects of the liver. Veno–venous bypass may be an advantage. Hepatic perfusion is as for the in-situ technique, although the liver can be placed on a heat exchange plate to help keep it cool during the resection.[18]

Patient preparation

Counselling

Preoperative counselling is one of the most important aspects of modern medical practice. When considering ex-vivo liver resection, the patient must be warned that worldwide experience is small. It is appropriate to explain the reasons behind this option and the risks and results of alternative operative and chemotherapeutic strategies. It is our unit's practice to give each patient being assessed for liver surgery a patient information booklet. This booklet details preoperative investigations, basic anatomy and pathophysiological aspects and the impact of hepatic surgery in broad terms. It includes a review of possible postoperative complications and a description of dietary recommendations and an integrated exercise programme to aid recovery. It is written in a reassuring but realistic fashion so that patient's expectations are not too high and so that they have stages in recovery to aim for. This booklet is given to each patient prior to assessment as it provides a useful basic knowledge for the patient before detailed discussion on an individual basis. The individual patient also requires a face-to-face discussion with the operating surgeon and anaesthetist to run over concerns including operative risk and it is our practice to overstate this aspect and to do this in the presence of the patient's next of kin. For ex-vivo liver resection candidates we suggest a potential inoperability rate of 20% and potential mortality risk of 20%, tending to exaggerate the risk when compared to standard liver resection or transplantation work. We suggest that our hope is that about 40% of survivors should expect to be cured by either conventional or ex-vivo liver surgery, but that it is difficult to make an accurate judgement before laparotomy. We explain that unfortunately statistics mean little to an individual and that if things go wrong then the outcome can result in a disadvantage in terms of survival. It is important that the patient is given an adequate amount of time to make his/her decision and also to discuss things with their family. Having made a decision to go ahead, the patient should clearly be supported in this decision by the medical and nursing team as a positive psychological approach to the surgery will influence the recovery time.

Preoperative preparation

Routine blood tests in our unit include full blood count, urea and electrolytes, liver function tests, coagulation screen and tumour marker studies (primarily carcinoembryonic antigen – CEA, CA19-9 and alpha feto protein) immediately before surgery as a baseline. A 10 unit blood cross match is our routine and 4 units of fresh frozen plasma are available at the start of surgery to prevent abnormalities in coagulation during the anhepatic phase. It is our routine to use some mechanical bowel preparation as this may help to reduce postoperative encephalopathy, but this is not excessive as it is important to avoid dehydration. A low molecular weight heparin is administered on the night before surgery to reduce the risk of deep vein thrombosis and pulmonary embolism. Broad spectrum antibiotics are given at the time of anaesthetic induction.

Setting up

Time factors

We have found that ex-vivo liver resection surgery can take up to 12 hours to perform. Consideration must be given to the time needed for each phase of the surgical procedure: anaesthesia, assessment of operability, veno–venous bypass, hepatectomy, liver cooling and preservation, bench resection and reconstruction, reimplantation and patient recovery. Clearly some surgical teams are quicker than others, but in comparison we would normally allow about 2 to 3 hours for a routine hemihepatectomy, 4 to 5 hours for a routine liver transplant and 9 hours for a more complex liver transplant in our centre.

Practice

For any new surgical procedure it is best to have a well-rehearsed team approach. Ex-vivo liver resection involves a combination of the techniques used in liver resection and transplantation, so a centre where these are routine should be able to proceed without special consideration. This is especially true in centres where cut-down and split liver transplantation is practised as there is no fundamental difference in the approach. Valuable lessons about the tolerance of cold ischaemia by the liver can be extrapolated from the data provided by these units, but it would be unusual for the ischaemic period to be longer than 4 hours as there is no requirement for organ transport.

Surgery with a liver available

For conditions where liver transplantation is a realistic and sensible option, it may be reasonable to consider listing the patient for major hepatic resection to be done as an emergency when a suitable donor becomes available. We have used this technique on occasion in our centre but have not applied it to the ex-vivo group. A back-up liver recipient is brought into hospital to receive the liver if the resection/transplant candidate is found to be resectable by conventional or ex-vivo means. The major drawback is the potential for a long cold ischaemia time for the donor liver if the decision for operability is difficult and it is our practice to begin the surgery whilst the donor team is at the donor site so that the delay is reduced to a minimum. Ideally, a second surgical team should be standing by to carry out the transplant on the second patient once the decision is taken. Patients assessed for ex-vivo surgery are probably not applicable to this situation at this time. If a tumour is not resectable by an ex-vivo technique it will not be a tumour that is treatable by transplantation. In our programme we have used this back-up technique for severe benign diseases, particularly intrahepatic biliary strictures, and it is mentioned here only for completeness.

Anaesthesia

A standard liver resection anaesthetic becomes a liver transplant anaesthetic if the ex-vivo dissection proceeds. It is our routine to place a central venous line, pulmonary artery wedge pressure catheter, arterial line, an oesophageal temperature probe and urinary catheter for careful monitoring. In the near future we plan to add to this by also using trans-oesophageal echocardiography. A warm air flow device covers the patient as well as a standard warming blanket underneath. We use an air–oxygen–desfurane-based anaesthesia which has been shown to minimize the derangement of postoperative liver function, with infusions of N-acetyl cysteine and antioxidants to confer hepatic protection.[26] Veno–venous bypass lines are inserted percutaneously into the internal jugular and femoral veins as the morbidity associated with this technique is lower than with the classical surgical method.

It is sensible to begin using accepted methodology for low central venous pressure anaesthesia as in most cases the surgery will proceed in situ. In our centre we use an epidural catheter for central venous pressure manipulation as well as postoperative analgesia, although vasodilators are sometimes necessary in addition. Inotropic support, primarily with adrenaline, is often necessary for the elderly patient in particular to maintain an adequate blood pressure during the low venous pressure phase.

If the ex-vivo operation proceeds then veno–venous bypass with high central venous pressure will be necessary. The bypass lines are heparin bonded so no additional anticoagulation should be used. The use of fresh frozen plasma early in the procedure is sensible to limit clotting abnormalities during the anhepatic phase, and cryoprecipitate and platelets should be given around about the time of reperfusion. Tranexamic acid or aprotinin is often necessary to prevent fibrinolysis and to maintain platelet function after reperfusion of the ischaemic liver. In our practice, the mean arterial blood pressure is maintained above 50 mmHg by the use of a phenylephrine infusion and after reperfusion of the liver dopexamine is infused to optimize hepatosplanchnic blood flow.[27] Despite these manoeuvres, it would be unwise to proceed without adequate availability of cross-matched red blood cells as sometimes transfusion will be necessary. It is not our practice to use a cell saver or other blood recycling device as there is a theoretical risk of tumour cell dissemination into the blood stream.

Assessment of operability

Surgical assessment

The initial phase of surgery is full laparotomy to determine operability. In this author's opinion, there seems little role for an initial laparoscopy except to exclude peritoneal disease and usually these cases have had major abdominal surgery in the past so adhesions may prevent a full assessment. It is our practice to use an incision that will give adequate access for assessment, whilst being fairly minimalist initially in case there are clear signs of inoperability. It is often possible to make use of an old incision site from previous surgery, but inevitably a variety of approaches are satisfactory and depend on surgeon preference and the availability of mechanical retractors. Transverse, midline, rooftop and Mercedes incisions are most usual. Adhesions should be divided to assess the primary tumour site and a careful examination of all peritoneal surfaces is carried out. Doubtful areas should be sampled for frozen section histopathological analysis and samples should also be taken from the coeliac nodes as this may suggest a more conservative approach for metastatic disease. The liver should be fully mobilized to allow adequate examination of the tumour and non-involved liver. It is usual to sling the portal triad structures individually and the inferior vena cava above and below the liver. In addition, one must decide whether to divide the right suprarenal vein or not and this will depend on the position of the tumour in relation to the inferior vena cava.

Intraoperative ultrasound

The use of intraoperative ultrasound can provide additional information about the relationship of the tumour to portal triad and hepatic venous structures, and may detect small metastases not seen on the preoperative CT or MRI.

Blood vessel and biliary involvement

Although much information will have been gained by preoperative radiology, careful dissection to examine the hepatic artery and portal vein in cholangiocarcinoma or the inferior vena cava in metastatic disease or hepatoma is sensible. This can normally be done without taking any irreversible steps, although we have found that final decisions about the degree of vessel invasion will need to be made once the liver has been removed. For example, we have found that in cases where only parts of segments II and III are to be reimplanted, close application of the tumour to the portal bifurcation may necessitate resection to the level of the segmental divisions of the left portal vein. In addition, involvement of the biliary tree by metastatic tumours can necessitate a cholangiocarcinoma style approach, with resection of the biliary tree to the segmental level in order to gain a margin of surgical clearance.

Conduits

Major blood vessel involvement should not prevent successful surgical resection as there are many strategies for vessel repair and conduit formation. Often an adequate repair can be created by a simple suture technique or end-to-end anastomosis. We have found that a satisfactory angioplasty/venoplasty patch can be created using vein remnants from the excised portion of the liver. Alternatively, the saphenous vein can be used to replace the hepatic artery, or opened out sections can be sutured together to create a wider vessel to repair the portal vein or inferior vena cava. The internal jugular vein, internal iliac vein or common iliac vein can be used to replace a section of portal vein without long-term detriment as collateral channels should open up. If a wide area of inferior vena cava must be excised then it is our preference to use a prosthetic graft. Some experience with vascular conduits made from vessels retrieved along with donor organs has also been reported but there is a theoretical risk of allograft rejection and stricture formation. It has been our practice to use a jejunal Roux loop for biliary diversion to reduce the chance of ischaemic stricture formation following biliary reanastomosis.

Surgical techniques for ex-vivo liver resection

Liver mobilization and excision

The liver needs to be completely separated from the posterior abdominal wall and any lumbar veins draining into the IVC between the diaphragm and the right renal vein must be ligated and divided so that the IVC can be encircled in slings in these two positions. In addition, in most cases it is necessary to ligate and divide the right suprarenal vein in order to gain adequate clearance of the tumour. The common bile duct is divided and ligated. The portal vein and hepatic artery should be mobilized so that they can be clamped individually, maximizing lengths for subsequent reanastomosis. The femoral (IVC) bypass is begun at this stage and heparin (5000 units intravenously) can be given before vascular clamps are applied to the portal vein, hepatic artery and the superior and inferior levels of the IVC to be excised. The liver is now ischaemic and it should be rapidly removed to the bench. The portal limb of the bypass is inserted and secured with a snugger technique, and once portal and systemic veno–venous bypass has been established the patient should remain stable for several hours.

Hepatic perfusion and preservation

Once the liver has been removed it must be flushed (down the portal vein for cooling then down the hepatic artery and biliary tree) with a suitable organ preservation solution and cooled to 0–4°C as in liver transplantation (Fig. 4.5). University of Wisconsin (UW) solution is the current 'gold standard' for liver preservation and is our choice for ex-vivo work, although it is certainly possible to preserve a whole liver adequately for a few hours with several other preservation fluids such as HTK solution.[28–31] It is not yet known how long a liver can be preserved during bench dissection, but in the accepted practice of cut-down and split liver transplantation most groups report bench times of 2–5 hours, with good results after reimplantation

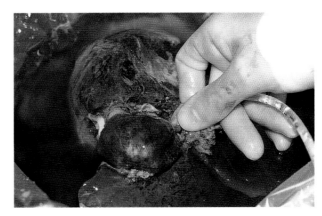

Figure 4.5 University of Wisconsin solution is flushed first through the portal vein for rapid cooling and then via the hepatic artery and biliary tree.

A

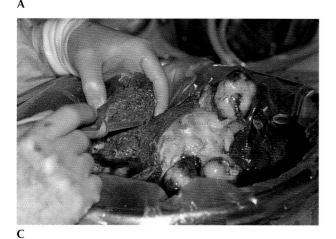

C

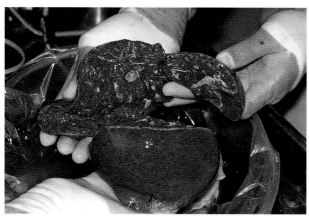

B

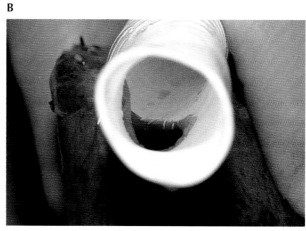

Figure 4.6 Bench dissection is performed without fear of blood loss. (A) Resection of all except parts of segments II and III; (B) reconstruction of IVC by anastomosis of left hepatic vein to 20 mm ringed PTFE graft; (C) resection of all except segments IVb, V and VI, with subsequent reanastomosis of right and middle hepatic vein stumps to a vascular graft.

following total cold ischaemic times of more than 12 hours. In our own practice, the median bench time for ex-vivo resection for tumour is 2 hours and the longest has been 4 hours, although the total ischaemic time was a little over 5 hours up to reperfusion.

Bench resection and reconstruction

Hepatic parenchymal fracture techniques or ultrasonic dissection may be used without the fear of blood loss, but great care must be taken to ligate or clip all visible vessels or ducts to avoid significant haemorrhage at reperfusion (Fig. 4.6). It is our practice to use a tissue sealant such as fibrin glue at the end of dissection. The most common reason for ex-vivo hepatic work will be extensive involvement of the IVC or hepatic veins by tumour. Although the major hepatic veins are quite thick walled near the IVC, more peripherally they are very friable and great care needs to be taken with the choice of suture material and technique. In our three most recent resections, where parts of hepatic segments II and III have been reimplanted, we anastomosed the left hepatic vein stump to a 20 mm ringed Gore-Tex graft with a 4-0 Gore-Tex suture.

Hepatic reimplantation and reperfusion

The reimplantation technique is identical to that used in orthoptic liver transplantation. After the upper IVC and 75% of the lower IVC have been sutured, the liver remnant should be flushed via the portal vein with a rinse solution (as UW solution contains a high concentration of potassium and adenosine). The lower IVC is then completed and the portal vein bypass is stopped and the portal vein reanastomosed. The IVC and portal vein clamps are removed for reperfusion. It is sensible to stay on systemic venous bypass via the femoral vein cannula until after reperfusion as this lowers the IVC pressure and may help to prevent rapid blood loss at this stage. Once haemostasis has been achieved, the bypass can be stopped and a further period aimed at control of haemorrhage follows. A direct hepatic artery to hepatic artery anastomosis will usually be possible, although a saphenous vein conduit may be needed, and if so this is most easily anastomosed first to the liver end on the bench. It is likely that a direct biliary anastomosis will be under some tension so it has been our choice to use a Roux loop to create an hepaticojejunostomy to the residual biliary tree, in our most recent cases to the segment II/III duct

A

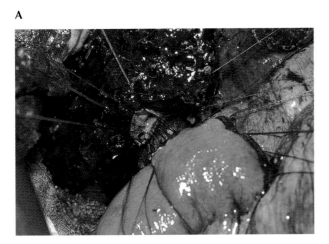

B

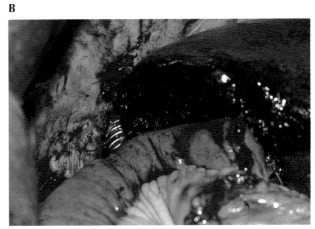

Figure 4.7 A Roux loop of jejunum for biliary anastomosis may prevent stricture formation. In this case the hepaticojejunostomy is to the segment II/III duct (A) following reimplantation of the liver remnant (B).

(Fig. 4.7). There is no need for a t-tube or other biliary stent. Other authors have used a duct-to-duct anastomosis but reported a high incidence of biliary stricturing.[20]

Finally, in our most recent cases we have used a 4 mm PTFE graft to create an arteriovenous fistula in the iliac vessels to increase the blood flow in the IVC graft. We have chosen 4 mm as this is unlikely to cause heart failure and we have used PTFE to prevent expansion of the fistula, which may occur with direct anastomosis or with venous conduits. It is our hope that the use of a small arteriovenous fistula may reduce the chance of IVC graft thrombosis and may obviate the requirement for long-term anticoagulation.

Postoperative care

The postoperative care of the ex-vivo liver resection patient should be similar to any major liver resection or liver transplant candidate. Nursing care should be initially on a high dependency ward or intensive care unit. Although inpatient care will usually be required for between 10 days and 3 weeks, our most recent case was fit for discharge at 6 days despite being 75 years old and having only parts of segments II and III reimplanted. Short stays can be anticipated in cases where there has been significant preresection hypertrophy because of the size of the tumour, as in this case where the major tumour was 17 cm diameter and the resected specimen weighed in excess of 2 kg. It is our practice to use intravenous antibiotics for the first 5 days whilst

assessments for liver failure are being made. A period of enteral supplementation may be useful in addition. Gastric acid secretion suppression with a proton pump inhibitor or H_2 antagonist is sensible as there is often an associated acute portal hypertension which may be additive to postoperative stress ulceration.

The prothrombin time seems to be most predictive of hepatic functional recovery. A daily requirement for fresh frozen plasma and 20% human albumin solution (200 ml/day) can be calculated from the blood results. The ALT is inevitably high (300–1000 IU/l) for the first few days and reflects the period of hepatic ischaemia. Our group uses N-acetyl cysteine by intravenous infusion for major hepatic resection cases as we have found it to be useful in our fulminant hepatic failure programme. In addition, there is usually a requirement for potassium, magnesium and phosphate supplementation intravenously following very radical resection. Low dose intravenous infusion heparin (40 unit/kg/24 hours) is used in our unit to help prevent hepatic arterial thrombosis in our liver transplant and ex-vivo resection programme and the haematocrit is kept low at 25–35%.

In the long term, we have chosen to anticoagulate all of our ex-vivo liver resection patients with warfarin, aiming for a prothrombin time of two to three times normal to prevent IVC thrombosis. The use of a small arteriovenous fistula, as described above, may obviate the need for long-term anticoagulation. However, if the warfarin is not causing any significant problems then it will provide an extra safeguard against thrombosis so it is likely that the majority of our patients will continue on this drug in the long term.

Complications of ex-vivo liver resection

Vascular thrombosis and stenosis

A sudden rise in ALT postoperatively should be an indication for Doppler analysis of the portal vein and hepatic artery, and if there is any doubt then arteriography should be performed. In our experience, if a thrombosis occurs more than 7 days postoperatively after major liver resection it can be managed conservatively. Anticoagulation with intravenous heparin and then by warfarin for 3 months should allow portal vein recanalization or arterial collateral formation. Dopexamine appears to increase splanchnic blood flow[27] and we have used this with both portal vein and hepatic artery thrombosis. This is at variance with experience in liver transplantation where regrafting is almost always required if early arterial thrombosis occurs. Unfortunately, in addition, significant stenosis can occur in any of the vascular anastomoses. They are usually detected by Doppler ultrasound in response to abnormalities in liver function tests, particularly a rise in ALT. Radiological intervention can solve most problems by balloon angioplasty or the use of endovascular stents.

Biliary strictures

There is a theoretical risk of biliary or biliary–enteric stricture formation. We have not experienced any difficulty in this regard and this may be because of our preference to hepaticojejunostomy. Strictures of the external biliary tree should be dealt with in standard fashion. Intrahepatic strictures as a result of preservation injury or arterial thrombosis are much more difficult to deal with and some consideration would have to be given to liver transplantation in order to correct this. We have used liver transplantation in one patient following a failed biliary reconstruction after the development of severe intrahepatic stricturing as a result of a right hepatectomy for colorectal metastases 18 months previously: at 5 years he is tumour free.

Long-term follow-up

Long-term follow-up after ex-vivo liver resection for tumour should be designed to examine the patients primarily for tumour recurrence, but also for complications related to the extensive hepatic resection and vascular replacement. Tumour marker studies (CEA, CA19-9, AFP) may indicate recurrent disease, although we have found CA19-9 to be often more related to biliary obstruction and it is more difficult to interpret than the other tumour markers. Regular CT of chest, abdomen and pelvis forms the basis of follow-up for complications and tumour recurrence at our centre, at 3, 6, 12, 18 and 24 months and then annually thereafter, but there are no clear cut guidelines. Isotope bone scans may also play a role in some tumour types. Regular blood tests for liver enzymes and bilirubin are helpful. A progressive rise in ALT may indicate a vascular stenosis impeding hepatic inflow or outflow. Doppler ultrasound should usually be diagnostic, with rapid recourse to arteriography and venography when necessary for consideration of endovascular correction. A rise in alkaline phosphatase or bilirubin may indicate an ischaemic biliary stricture or recurrent disease causing biliary obstruction.

Long-term results

There are very few series of ex-vivo liver resection in the world literature.[18,19] Published cases and small series have concentrated on surgical technique and even perioperative mortality is not well described and may be underreported. The perioperative mortality risk appears to be of the order of 10–40%, but these patients have been in the terminal phase of their illness at the time of surgery. Disease recurrence is inevitable for some of the surviving patients as the tumours have been so extensive at the time of presentation. Our experience does suggest, however, that a significant period of good quality palliation can be achieved by these elaborate techniques. In addition, as these techniques become more common place, the risk should reduce. This is exemplified by our most recent case where there was no requirement for blood transfusion and the patient was fit enough for discharge from hospital by day 6 despite being 75 years of age. At the time of writing this patient is alive with asymptomatic recurrent disease at 33 months from surgery.

Considering this author's direct experience to date with IVC resection and ex-vivo liver resection for malignant tumours, we have dealt with 12 cases to date of whom 10 had colorectal metastases. In five cases, ex-vivo resection was necessary and two of these patients died within 30 days from multiorgan failure. One of the other seven patients, in whom in-situ IVC resection was carried out, also died from multiorgan failure. This high mortality rate is comparable to that in other series and reflects the gravity of the surgery combined with the late stage of disease in these patients.

In the long term, disease recurrence has been a problem. Our longest surviving ex-vivo patient is alive at 33 months. A second patient lived for 30 months, and although the resection had been carried out for colorectal metastases, she died from complications relating to the development of a renal cell carcinoma. The other three ex-vivo patients have died with recurrent disease within 2 years. These data lend support to arguments for the use of adjuvant therapies despite the potential risk of systemic sepsis associated with the use of prosthetic graft material, and again relate to the late stage at presentation.

Prospects for transplantation

There is much experience in transplantation for hepatoma. There is no doubt that it is a suitable therapy for patients with small hepatomas in cirrhotic livers, where the cirrhosis is the primary indication for the transplant. Unfortunately, however, where the hepatoma is the primary indication for liver transplantation because of the enormity of the lesion, the results of transplantation have been almost universally poor.[32,33] Similar experience is reported for cholangiocarcinoma and for colorectal metastases. This is probably related to the necessary immunosuppression used following organ transplantation, and the development of more specific immunosuppressive agents may enable transplantation to be used in the future for these tumours.

Our group has been investigating the use of cluster resection and multivisceral grafting[34] as an alternative for neuroendocrine tumours. These are most often tumours of midgut origin with foregut metastases and adequate lymphadenectomy involves both the coeliac and superior mesenteric arterial distributions, so surgery involves excision of all organs supplied by these arteries: stomach, duodenum, liver, pancreas, spleen, jejunum, ileum and large bowel as far as the descending/sigmoid colon. This approach provides superb access to the para-aortic lymph nodes for adequate lymphadenectomy. This is followed by implantation of a multiorgan block of liver, pancreas, duodenum, jejunum and ileum. We have used a Roux loop (created from the transplanted jejunum) to the oesophagus, as gastric stasis can be a problem for several weeks following stomach transplantation. An ileostomy is used to provide access for regular endoscopic biopsies for careful monitoring for rejection and cytomegalovirus infection during the first few months, but it is our practice to reverse this at about 6 months if graft function is stable. We have found that the donor innominate artery forms an ideal conduit for anastomosis of the donor coeliac and superior mesenteric arteries to the recipient aorta.[35]

If purely a foregut neuroendocrine tumour (arising in the pancreatic tail), then a lesser cluster resection can also be appropriate to take the stomach, duodenum, liver, pancreas and spleen, with subsequent implantation of a liver–pancreas block. Our early results with neuroendocrine disease are more encouraging than with other tumours, but long-term analysis is necessary. This may be related to the more extensive resection or, more probably, to the tumour type.

We have also investigated the effect of liver transplantation and resection on the growth of a colorectal cancer cell line in an attempt to examine the links between cancer regrowth, hepatocyte growth factor (HGF) and immunosuppressed and non-immunosuppressed controls.[36] Serum samples were taken before and after operation (days 1, 4 and 30) from patients undergoing hepatic resection and liver transplantation, and from three control groups: major abdominal surgery, renal transplantation and normal volunteers. The human colonic cancer cell line LoVo was incubated for 4 days in a 5% concentration of the patient's serum in a medium. Tumour cell proliferation was measured by tritiated thymidine incorporation and an ELISA assay was used to measure hepatocyte growth factor (HGF). The immunosuppressed and non-immunosuppressed control groups showed no significant differences from normal. Serum from liver resection patients stimulated tumour cell growth throughout the experiment and this was associated with high levels of HGF. Serum from liver transplant recipients did not stimulate tumour cell line growth, but had high levels of HGF before and immediately after surgery, with rapid resolution after successful transplantation. This experiment, therefore, has not demonstrated a link between the HGF response of liver regeneration or recovery and cancer growth. An alternative growth factor may be active in the resection group both before and after resectional surgery. Our results supported the hypothesis that rapid tumour recurrence following liver transplantation is the result of the necessary immunosuppression. The development of more specific immunosuppressive agents may enable transplantation to be used in the future for more hepatic tumours, but for the moment the role of transplantation remains very limited.

Summary

Techniques for hepatic resection continue to advance and the involvement of liver transplant teams has aided the development of new types of resection and anaesthetic techniques. Short-term warm hepatic ischaemia is practised widely but there is often a necessity to hurry during this demanding surgery as prolonged warm ischaemia can result in irreversible liver failure. Transplant experience, particularly relating to cut-down and split liver techniques, has demonstrated that bench dissection and reimplantation after long periods of cold ischaemia can be successful in the majority of cases. Tumours involving all three major hepatic veins and IVC invasion continue to pose a surgical challenge and the combined techniques of hepatic resection and transplantation offer a potential lifeline for this unfortunate group of patients. Ex-vivo liver resection for tumour therefore deserves consideration.

Summary panel

The short-term survival of untreated patients with both primary and secondary liver tumours, the unpredictability of chemotherapy response on an individual patient basis and the disappointing results of transplantation for cancer provide adequate impetus for attempts to extend the boundaries of liver resection as far as possible. Major improvements in hepatic surgery have occurred during the past few years and improvements in anaesthesia have been integral to this success. Pringle's manoeuvre and total vascular isolation (hepatic vascular exclusion) are used widely, and this short-term warm ischaemia appears to be well tolerated. Tumours involving all of the major hepatic veins with or without IVC invasion, and

particularly tumours involving the hepatocaval confluence and needing IVC replacement, continue to pose a surgical challenge. Ex-vivo resection offers a potential lifeline for this group of patients.

Key points

- Hepatic resections involving IVC and portal structure reconstructions are occurring with increasing frequency.
- When considering patients for ex-vivo resection, a full cardiorespiratory work-up is mandatory.
- Careful consideration must be given to residual hepatic reserve.
- Patients and relatives must be counselled preoperatively with regard to the limited world experience and operative risk.

- Anaesthesia for ex-vivo liver resection:
  A standard liver resection anaesthetic becomes a liver transplant anaesthetic if the ex-vivo dissection proceeds.

- Phases of ex-vivo liver resection surgery:
  Liver mobilization and excision
  Hepatic perfusion and preservation
  Bench resection and reconstruction
  Hepatic reimplantation and reperfusion
  A Roux for biliary anastomoses may prevent stricture formation
  Consider a small a-v fistula if a prosthetic IVC graft has been used.

REFERENCES

1. Belghiti J, Noun R, Zante E et al. Portal triad clamping or hepatic vascular exclusion for major liver resection: a controlled study. Ann Surg 1996; 224: 155–61
2. Bismuth H, Houssin D, Ornowski J, Meriggi F. Liver resections in cirrhotic patients: a western experience. World J Surg 1986; 10: 311
3. Delva E, Camus Y, Nordlinger B et al. Vascular occlusions for liver resections – operative management and tolerance to hepatic ischemia: 142 cases. Ann Surg 1989; 209: 211–18
4. Elias D, Iasser P, Debaene B et al. Intermittent vascular exclusion of the liver (without vena cava clamping) during major hepatectomy. Br J Surg 1995; 82: 1535–9
5. Evans PM, Vogt DP, Mayes JT et al. Liver resection using total vascular exclusion. Surgery 1998; 124: 807–15
6. Ezaki T, Seo Y, Tomoda H et al. Partial hepatic resection under intermittent hepatic inflow occlusion in patients with chronic liver disease. Br J Surg 1992; 79: 224–6
7. Hannoun L, Borie D, Delva E et al. Liver resection with normothermic ischaemia exceeding 1 h. Br J Surg 1993; 80: 1161–6
8. Hewitt G, Halliday I, McCaigue M et al. Mortality, endotoxaemia and cytokine expression after intermittent and continuous hepatic ischaemia. Br J Surg 1995; 82: 1424–6
9. Huguet C, Gallot D, Offenstadt G. Normothermic complete hepatic vascular exclusion for extensive resection of the liver. N Engl J Med 1976; 294: 51–2
10. Huguet C, Gavelli A, Chieco A. Liver ischemia for hepatic resection: where is the limit? Surgery 1991; 111: 251–9
11. Kelly D, Emre S, Guy S et al. Resection of benign hepatic lesions with selective use of total vascular isolation. J Am Coll Surg 1996; 183: 113–16

12. Malassagne B, Cherqui D, Alon R et al. Safety of selective vascular clamping for major hepatectomies. J Am Coll Surg 1998; 187: 482–6

13. Pringle JH. Notes on the arrest of hepatic hemorrhage due to trauma. Ann Surg 1908; 48: 541–9

14. Starzl TE. Hepatic vascular exclusion and hepatic resection. Surgery 1984; 95: 376

15. Wu C-C, Hwang C-R, Liu T-J, P'Eng F-K. Effects and limitations of prolonged intermittent ischaemia for hepatic resection of the cirrhotic liver. Br J Surg 1996; 83: 121–4

16. Yamaoka Y, Ozawa K, Kumada K et al. Total vascular exclusion for hepatic resection in cirrhotic patients: application of venovenous bypass. Arch Surg 1992; 127: 276–80

17. Lygidakis NJ, van der Heyde MN, van Dongen RJAM et al. Surgical approaches for unresectable primary carcinoma of the hepatic hilus. Surg Gynecol Obstet 1988; 166: 107–14

18. Delrivière L, Hannoun L. In situ and ex situ in vivo procedure for complex major liver resections requiring prolonged hepatic vascular exclusion in normal and diseased livers. J Am Coll Surg 1995; 181: 272–6

19. Pichlmayr R, Grosse H, Hauss J et al. Technique and preliminary results of extracorporeal liver surgery (bench procedure) and of surgery on the in situ perfused liver. Br J Surg 1990; 77: 21–6

20. Yagyu T, Shimizu R, Nishida M et al. Reconstruction of the hepatic vein to the prosthetic inferior vena cava in right extended hemihepatectomy with ex situ procedure. Surgery 1994; 115: 740–4

21. Makuuchi M, Hasegawa H, Yamazaki S, Takayasu K. Four new hepatectomy procedures for resection of the right hepatic vein and preservation of the inferior right hepatic vein. Surg Gynecol Obstet 1987; 164: 69–72

22. Ozeki Y, Uchiyama T, Katayama M et al. Extended left hepatic trisegmentectomy with resection of main right hepatic vein and preservation of middle and inferior right hepatic veins. Surgery 1995; 117: 715–17

23. Fortner JG, Shiu MH, Kinne D et al. Major hepatic resection using vascular isolation and hypothermic perfusion. Ann Surg 1974; 180: 644–52

24. Hamazaki K, Yagi T, Tanaka N et al. Hepatectomy under extracorporeal circulation. Surgery 1995; 118: 98–102

25. Yang IK, Kobayashi M, Nakashima K et al. In situ and surface liver cooling with prolonged inflow occlusion during hepatectomy in patients with chronic liver disease. Arch Surg 1994; 19: 620–4

26. O'Beirne HA, Young Y, Thornton J, Bellamy MC. Desflurane versus isoflurane in liver transplantation: a comparison of outcomes. Br J Anaesth 1997; 79: 132

27. Smithies M, Tai HY, Jackson L et al. Protecting the gut and liver in the critically ill: effects of dopexamine. Crit Care Med 1994; 22: 789–95

28. Bretschneider HJ, Gebhard MM, Preu CJ. Reviewing the pros and cons of myocardial preservation within cardiac surgery. In: Longmire DB, ed. Towards safer cardiac surgery. Lancaster: MTP Press Limited, 1981: 21–53

29. Bretschneider HJ, Helmchen U, Kehrer G. Nieren protektion. Klin Wschr 1988; 66: 817–27

30. Jamieson NV, Sundberg R, Lindell S et al. Preservation of the canine liver for 24–48 hours using simple cold storage with UW solution. Transplantation 1989; 46: 517–22

31. Todo S, Nery J, Yanag K et al. Extended preservation of human liver grafts with UW solution. J Am Med Assoc 1989; 261: 711–14

32. Tan KC, Rela M, Ryder SD et al. Experience of orthoptic liver transplantation and hepatic resection for hepatocellular carcinoma of less than 8 cm in patients with cirrhosis. Br J Surg 1995; 82: 253–9

33. Bechstein WO, Kling N, Keck H et al. Hepatocellular carcinoma in cirrhosis: liver transplantation vs resection (abstract). Br J Surg 1994; 81(Suppl): 84

34. Starzl TE, Todo S, Tzakis A et al. Abdominal organ cluster transplantation for the treatment of upper abdominal malignancies. Ann Surg 1989; 210: 374–86

35. Lodge JPA, Pollard SG, Selvakumar S et al. Alternative techniques of arterialisation in multivisceral grafting. Transplant Proc 1997; 29: 1850

36. Corps C. An investigation of different mechanisms for tumour growth following liver resection and transplantation. MSc thesis, University of Manchester, UK, 1997

Further reading

Lodge JPA, Ammori BJ, Prasad KR, Bellamy MC. Ex-vivo and in situ resection of inferior vena cava with hepatectomy for colorectal metastases. Ann Surg 2000; 231: 471–9

5 Resection of small hepatocellular carcinoma in cirrhosis

Claude Smadja and Giacomo Borgonovo

Introduction

There is some discrepancy in the literature regarding the definition of small hepatocellular carcinoma (HCC). In surgical practice, 5 cm has emerged as the most suitable cut-off between small and large HCCs when a surgical approach is contemplated,[1,2] despite the fact that transplant surgeons consider 3 cm as the upper limit of small HCCs.[3] Although ablation by thermal injury and ethanol injection has gained a wide success, at present partial liver resection and liver transplantation still offer the best chance for cure. Neither adjuvant therapy with chemotherapy nor preoperative chemoembolization has been shown to be of any benefit in reducing the risk of recurrence or improving survival.[4] Despite the growing role and the encouraging results of liver transplantation in the treatment of HCC in cirrhosis, and in view of the shortage of organs, partial liver resection remains the therapy of choice. Over the last two decades, increased screening of patients with chronic liver disease has led to a rise in the number of resections of HCC in cirrhosis. In specialized centres, noteworthy progress in operative techniques and improvements in the surgical care of patients with liver cirrhosis have been achieved. However, while the risk of hepatic resection in cirrhosis has decreased dramatically during the last 15 years, the operation remains an arduous one in some cases. Nevertheless, it is imperative that we demystify this procedure, which can be relatively safe provided that some rules are respected. In other words, careful and precise preoperative evaluation is paramount in order to select those patients who might benefit from liver resection or liver transplantation.

Pathological classification of HCC

The recent increase in the number of resections performed for HCC in cirrhosis has allowed pathologists to establish prognostic factors, especially those indicating liver resection. In Western countries, indications for resection of HCC are less frequent than in the East. It is, however, essential to use a very simple classification that permits comparison of the results from different teams. In our centre, HCCs are divided into three groups: group I corresponds to an expanding tumour which is defined as a round, well-demarcated tumour, compressing the adjacent liver parenchyma and surrounded by a capsule which may be visible on gross examination (Fig. 5.1), and which is often

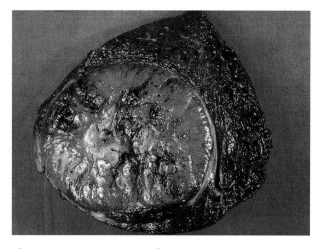

Figure 5.1 Group I HCC. The tumour is surrounded by a complete and thick capsule.

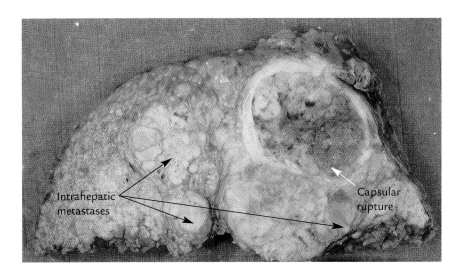

Figure 5.2 Group II HCC. The tumour is expanding, but the capsule is incomplete with a rupture (white arrow) and intrahepatic metastases (black arrows).

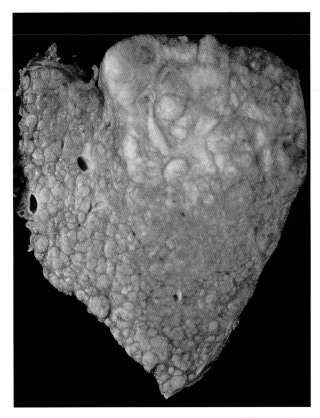

Figure 5.3 Group III HCC. The tumour is infiltrating the adjacent liver parenchyma, without capsular interposition.

normal parenchyma bordering the HCC is continuously replaced by neoplastic tissue. The prognosis of infiltrating tumour is poorer than expanding tumour.[6] This classification is simple and carries the major advantage over other classifications that HCC characteristics can be accurately detected by preoperative radiological imaging (Fig. 5.4).

Natural history of small HCC in cirrhosis

Precise knowledge of the natural history of the underlying disease is of major importance in the management of HCC, since more than 80% of patients suffering from HCC have associated cirrhosis.[7] Ginès et al.[8] studied the natural history of compensated cirrhosis, irrespective of its origin. They showed that 5 years after the diagnosis of cirrhosis the probability of developing decompensated cirrhosis was 35% and the survival rate probability was 70%. These data should be taken into account when adopting a therapeutic choice and in the analysis of the results of liver resection for small HCC in cirrhosis. Therefore, to evaluate the efficacy of surgical therapy, it is essential to know the natural history of small HCC in cirrhosis. There are limited data in the literature concerning this topic.[9–11] Ebara et al.[9] evaluated the outcome of 22 patients with untreated small HCCs (<3 cm). Patients were followed for 6 to 37 months without therapy. The mean 1-, 2-, and 3-year survival rates were 90.7%, 50.0% and 12.8%, respectively. In parallel, when taking into account also the severity of the liver disease, Barbara et al.[10] showed that cirrhotic patients with a good liver function (i.e. Child–Pugh's class A) and those with an impaired liver function (i.e. Child–Pugh's class B or C) had an estimated 3-year survival rate of 62% and 0%,

infiltrated by tumour cells but never ruptured; group II corresponds to an expanding HCC, but in which the capsule has been ruptured in some regions (Fig. 5.2). In our experience, tumour spreading to distal portal vein branches and satellite nodules was significantly less frequent in group I than in group II HCCs;[5] group III is an infiltrating tumour (Fig. 5.3), which is defined as a tumour with no precise landmarks, where the

Figure 5.4 CT scan aspect of the different anatomic types of HCCs. (A) Group I: expanding HCC, note the presence of a complete and thick capsule; (B) group II: expanding ruptured HCC, (1) rupture of the capsule (arrowhead) and thrombosis of the feeding portal branch (arrow), (2) rupture of the capsule (arrowhead) and intrahepatic metastases (arrow); (C) group III: infiltrating HCC, (1) portal venous phase study, (2) late phase study.

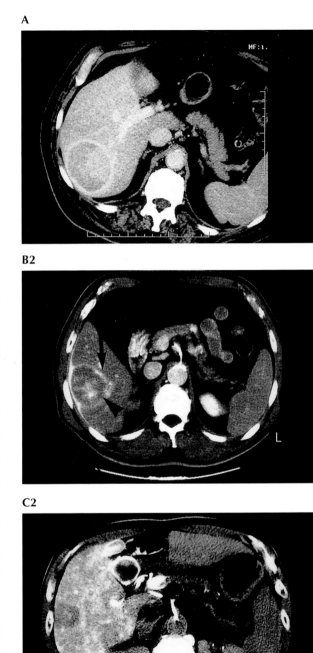

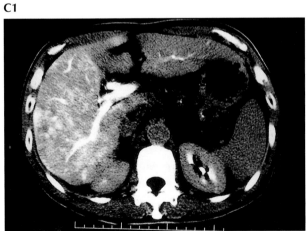

respectively. In this last series, the overall 3-year survival rate was 21%. Moreover, Llovet et al.[11] have shown that patients with HCC but without an extra-hepatic spread or a poor liver function had a sponta-neous survival at 1 and 3 years of 80% and 50% respectively. Given the results of these studies, the operative mortality of small HCCs treated by partial liver resection or liver transplantation should be less than 10% and the 3-year survival rate equal to or greater than 60% for the patients with good liver function.

Screening for HCC and preoperative radiological investigations

There is potential interest in screening cirrhotic patients, in order to detect symptomless HCCs of small size, which are more accessible to surgical therapy than symptomatic tumours.[12] Indeed, the annual risk of developing HCC in cirrhosis is estimated at 5%;[13] chronic hepatitis B and C are

A

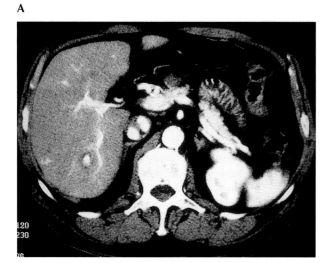

B

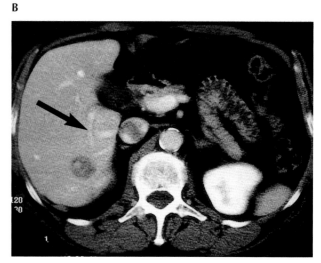

C

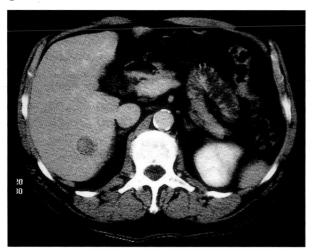

Figure 5.5 Helical CT scan assessment of a small HCC in cirrhosis located in segment VI. (A) Arterial phase study showing a hypervascular nodule, and the lack of intrahepatic metastases. (B) Portal vein phase study demonstrating the patency of the portal branch of segment VI (arrow). (C) Late phase study highlighting the presence of a thin capsule.

recognized as the major factors increasing the risk of HCC.[14,15] The most commonly used screening tests are serum α-fetoprotein and ultrasonography (US). Serum α-fetoprotein has low sensitivity and is not specific for small HCC, since it rises with flare-ups of active hepatitis.[16] However, a serum α-fetoprotein level >400 ng/ml is generally considered as diagnostic of HCC.[17] Ultrasonography is used as a first step in the diagnostic work-up of cirrhotic patients. Its accuracy has increased since the availability of broadband transducers and the introduction of new signal processing algorithms. The sensitivity of US in the detection of HCC in cirrhosis is 78% and the specificity 93%.[12] The use of ultrasound hepatospecific contrast medium seems to further ameliorate these percentages. On the other hand, US is relatively poor at identifying small multifocal lesions in cirrhotic patients. As a consequence, in order to confirm US findings and to assess the resectability of the tumour, other radiological investigations are used. Helical biphasic CT scans are the

most used technique of imaging for diagnosis and staging of HCC. This investigation must be performed by a very precise technique (Fig. 5.5),[18] in order to specify the characteristics of the tumour and to detect some prognostic factors, such as the presence of a capsule and its rupture,[19] satellite nodules, and vascular involvement,[20] which can be confirmed by a percutaneous biopsy of the thrombosed vessel.[21] The sensitivity of CT scanning in detecting nodules in the cirrhotic liver is proportional to the size of the lesion. Nodules larger than 3 cm are identified in 95% of cases, but this percentage drops to 80% for nodules of 1–3 cm.[22] Even less successful is the detection of small and hypovascular lesions whose identification is still very difficult. In these cases the place of magnetic resonance imaging in the diagnosis of HCC is still under discussion.[23]

Whenever the diagnosis is questionable a fine needle biopsy is mandatory. It can, nevertheless, be difficult to distinguish large cirrhotic nodules from well differentiated HCC or low-grade dysplastic nodules from HCC, using either needle or wedge biopsy.[24] Moreover, liver biopsy carries the risk of tumour spread,[25] although it is worth mentioning that one technique of tumour biopsy may obviate this risk.[26] In a recent prospective study, conducted by Maitre and undertaken at the Hôpital Antoine Béclère, comparing the preoperative radiological findings and the pathological data obtained from the resected liver, helical CT scanning turned out to be the most accurate investigation to determine the tumour characteristics and to assess correctly its resectability (unpublished data).

Factors influencing recurrence of HCC after partial liver resection

Following liver resection for HCC in cirrhosis, tumour recurrence is the main cause of poor prognosis. The risk of intrahepatic tumour recurrence after resection ranges from 70 to 100% at 5 years.[27-32] Most of these recurrences are the result of growth of HCCs, different to those of the resected tumour,[32] as documented by studies showing a different clonal origin between the initial and recurrent HCC.[33,34] Thus initial tumours that relapsed exhibited more profound genomic abnormalities than tumours followed by de novo neoplasms.[35] Precise knowledge of the preoperative factors that influence recurrence after resection and, in turn, postoperative survival, is of paramount importance, since it helps surgeons to select patients with the best prognosis after liver resection. Also, scores based on the histopathological examination of the resected specimen, such as the invasiveness scoring system based on pathological criteria,[31] may be useful for the selection of the potential candidates for adjuvant therapy studies. The risk of postoperative recurrence depends on tumour characteristics and decreases in the presence of a small, single and encapsulated HCC, in the absence of capsule rupture, portal vein invasion or intrahepatic metastases.[32,36-38] Hepatitis status has also been incriminated as a significant risk factor for tumour recurrence,[39] as well as the severity of liver fibrosis.[15] The underlying liver disease seems to have a greater influence on 5-year and long-term survival after liver resection than the characteristics of the initial tumour.[40]

Therapeutic options for HCC in cirrhosis

Partial liver resection and liver transplantation seem to offer the best chances of cure for small HCCs.

However, the lack of controlled data for most therapeutic modalities, including chemoembolization and percutaneous ethanol injection, thermal ablation by radiofrequency and cryotherapy, makes it difficult to assess whether any of these therapies is associated with a significantly improved survival. The development of surveillance programmes has allowed the detection of small asymptomatic HCCs which are amenable to surgical therapy. Nevertheless, it must be stressed that the prognosis of HCC is largely dependent on the underlying liver cirrhosis. This suggests that liver transplantation and non-surgical treatments should be included in the therapeutic armamentarium. Percutaneous ethanol injection and radiofrequency ablation have gained wide popularity.[41] Both techniques are highly effective and safe in the treatment of single small (<3 cm), encapsulated tumour, but their palliative role is confirmed by the high rate of local and distant recurrence.[42] Moreover, in patients with subcapsular tumour and poor degree of differentiation the risk of tumour seeding after percutaneous radiofrequency is augmented.[43] As far as transplantation is concerned, even if indications based on tumour size and the number of nodules seem to be slightly expandable,[44] only a fraction of patients with small HCCs have the opportunity to receive a transplant, since demand exceeds the number of donor organs and, as a consequence, in the centres where the therapy is available the waiting lists grow longer. All efforts must therefore be made to evaluate fully the possibilities of partial liver resection.

Partial liver resection in cirrhosis

Surgical anatomy

Modern hepatic surgery is based upon functional liver anatomy, according to the vascular architecture of the organ. The liver is schematically divided into three major portions: the right liver, the left liver and the dorsal sector (Figs 5.6 and 5.7). According to Couinaud,[45] the three hepatic veins (i.e. right, middle and left) divide the right and left livers in four sectors called portal sectors, each of which receives a portal pedicle. The limit between the right and left livers is represented by the main portal scissura (Cantlie's line) in which the middle hepatic vein runs. Each hemiliver includes two portal sectors. The left liver (Fig. 5.6) is divided by the left portal scissura containing the left hepatic vein into an anterior sector which includes two segments, III and IV, and a posterior sector represented by segment II. The quadrate lobe (segment IVB), located in front of the hilum, corresponds to the anterior part of segment IV, the posterior part corresponding

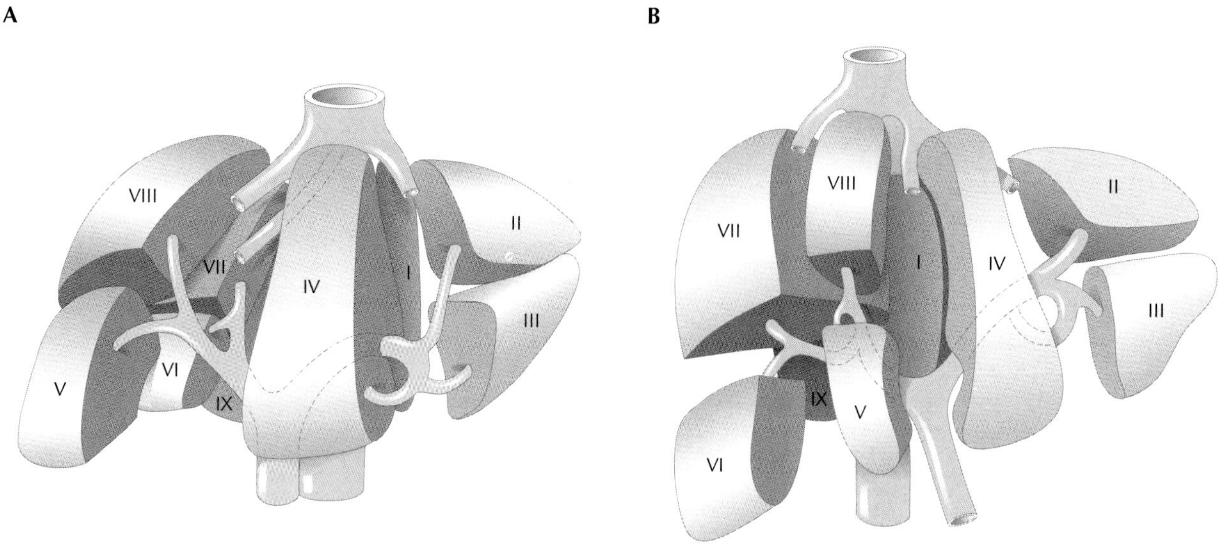

A

B

Figure 5.6 The functional division of the liver and the liver segments according to the nomenclature of Couinaud: (A) in the in vivo position; (B) in the ex vivo position. Note the recurrent direction of the feeding vessels of segment IV, the location of segments I and IX and the posterior situation of segments VI and VII in the in vivo position.

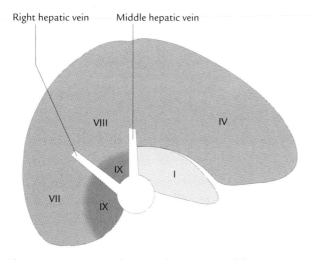

Figure 5.7 Diagram showing the anatomical location of the dorsal sector and its relationships with the hepatic veins. Note that the middle hepatic vein represents the boundary between segment I and segment IX and that there is no precise landmark between segment IX and the right liver.

to segment IVA. The anatomy of the right liver should be described with the liver in its normal place in the abdominal cavity (see Fig. 5.6). Indeed, the classic lateral right sector (i.e. segments VI and VII) is posterior and lies behind the median sector (i.e. segments V and VIII) which is in fact anterior. This in vivo anatomic description is clearly demonstrated by an analysis of the morphological appearance of the liver on CT scanning (Fig. 5.8).

This information is of paramount importance for the practice of liver resection in cirrhotic patients for

several reasons. First, atrophy or hypertrophy of the right liver currently observed in cirrhotic patients may alter the normal anatomy and should be taken into consideration for the type of resection to be performed: for example, major atrophy of the right liver should warrant formal right hepatectomy for HCC located in this hemiliver rather than segmentectomy or sectorectomy. Second, the difficulty of fully mobilizing the right liver in cirrhosis because of the presence of a right liver hypertrophy should be taken into account when resection is to be performed for HCC located into the right posterior sector. Third, the major anatomical alterations sometimes encountered in cirrhosis render the location of the surgical limit of a segment or a sector difficult to delineate. Each sector of the right liver (Fig. 5.6) is finally divided by the plane of the portal bifurcation into segments. The superior portion of the anterior sector is called segment VIII and the inferior portion segment V. For the posterior sector, the superior portion corresponds to segment VII and the inferior portion to segment VI. The dorsal sector is made up of two segments separated by the middle hepatic vein, left (segment I or caudate lobe) and right (segment IX), incorporated in the posterior portion of the right liver[46] (Fig. 5.7). This segment IX is a separate entity located behind the hilum and covering the inferior vena cava. The dorsal sector is tightly connected with the right liver without precise anatomic landmarks. It receives its own vessels from the right and left branches of the portal vein and hepatic artery. Its hepatic veins drain directly into the inferior vena cava and represent an important pathway of venous drainage into the inferior vena cava. Finally, it should be mentioned that, following Couinaud's study, Makuuchi et al.[47]

A

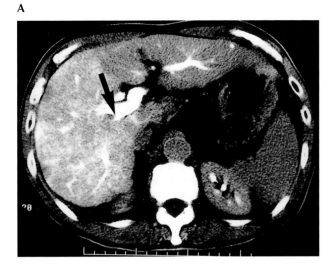

B

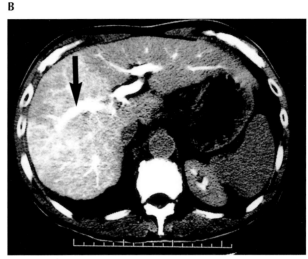

C

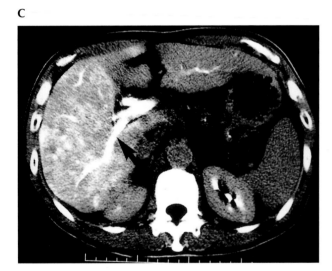

Figure 5.8 Radiological anatomy of the sectoral portal branches of the right liver on CT scan. (A) Right branch of the portal vein (arrow); (B) anterior sectoral portal branch (arrow); (C) posterior sectoral portal branch (arrow).

confirmed the ultrasonic presence of a significant inferior right hepatic vein in about 10 to 20% of cases, the existence of which offers new surgical possibilities. Indeed, tumours located in the superior portion of the posterior sector (i.e. segment VII) may lead to the performance of a bisegmentectomy VII–VIII and those encasing the right hepatic vein distally.

Specific risks linked to partial liver resection in cirrhosis

Liver resection is sometimes poorly tolerated by cirrhotic patients, with the potential risk of death by liver failure jeopardizing the overall clinical picture. The presence of portal hypertension may initiate postoperative complications such as variceal rupture and the development of ascites. Finally, non-specific postoperative surgical complications such as abdominal infection may also precipitate liver failure.

Postoperative liver failure

Liver regeneration is altered in cirrhosis.[48,49] Therefore, in patients with good preoperative liver function, postoperative liver failure is mainly related to the volume of non-neoplastic liver parenchyma removed during the resection.[50] Liver failure may be induced by intraoperative bleeding. Indeed, there is a direct relationship between intraoperative bleeding and supervening liver failure.[51,52] Noteworthy are findings that, despite selection of only Child's A patients for hepatic resection, the presence of a significant portal hypertension was the best predictive factor of unresolved postoperative liver decompensation.[53]

Complications of portal hypertension

Although there are no controlled data, and no clear relationship has been established,[54] the risk of variceal rupture after liver resection is obviously increased. It seems logical to postulate that the extent of parenchymal resection might influence the occurrence of this serious complication, which is related primarily to the diminution of the liver vascular bed after hepatic resection, which leads to an increase in portal pressure. In our experience, intractable ascites occurred in 6% of cirrhotic patients undergoing liver resection for HCC.[6] It has been shown that the presence of significant portal hypertension was the best predictor of postoperative ascites following hepatic resection for a small HCC.[53] Ascites occurred in 55% of cases and had a severe influence on prognosis.[53] Ascites formation has serious adverse effects, distends the abdominal cavity, has repercussions on the ventilatory function and may jeopardize the abdominal incision with wound dehiscence, resulting in ascitic leak and subsequent infection. Leakage of ascites through drains may result in major fluid loss and electrolyte imbalance.

Preoperative nutritional status, postoperative complications and infection

The prevalence of malnutrition in hospitalized cirrhotic patients varies from 30 to 70%.[55] Factors associated with an increased risk of postoperative complications are weight loss >10% of current weight and a serum albumin level <30 g/l. Whether patients undergoing hepatic resection benefit from preoperative artificial nutrition is a matter of debate. Some insight into the issue comes from the prospective randomized study of Fan et al.[56] who showed that perioperative total parenteral nutrition reduced postoperative morbidity, weight loss and liver failure. Cabre et al.[57] have shown that in selected malnourished patients a short course of enteral nutrition is able to ameliorate malnutrition or a hypercatabolic state. It often occurs that in our clinical practice these patients are unfit for hepatic surgery. In most cases, in our opinion, a short work-up readily allows prompt surgery without any form of preoperative nutrition.

The risk of septic complications is high in cirrhotic patients, due to defects in cellular and humoral immunity, and a deficiency in the non-immune acute infectious mechanism.[58] Moreover, total and prolonged hepatic pedicle clamping during hepatic resection might facilitate bacterial translocation from the gut to the blood.[59] Prevention of intraoperative bleeding and contamination of the peritoneal cavity by drains, and the use of perioperative short-term antibiotic prophylaxis in patients at risk should improve the results.

Selection of patients

Indications of partial liver resection in cirrhotic patients are dictated by the characteristics of the tumour and the hepatic reserve status. Patients with a single and small encapsulated nodule are the best candidates for liver resection. In any case, if doubts exist about the nature of an associated portal vein branch thrombosis, there is an indication to perform a fine needle guided biopsy.[21] When two nodules are present, great care should be taken to determine whether localized portal spreading has occurred. In such a case, resection is still possible, but should be extended to the territory supplied by the feeding portal branch.[60] It is a matter of debate, in view of the very poor prognosis and the significant risk of surgery, whether infiltrating tumours deeply located in the parenchyma should be removed. In our experience, even extensive removal of non-neoplastic liver parenchyma around the tumour did not reduce recurrence, and no patient lived more than 2 years after radical resection.[6]

Liver function status is crucial to the prognosis of cirrhotic patients undergoing liver resection. There is no single biochemical value that is predictive of postoperative liver failure, even if serum bilirubin of greater than 34 μmol/l (twice the normal value) is generally considered as an ominous sign and excludes the patient from surgery.[61,62] Pugh's modification of Child's classification is a simple, reproducible and reliable method to determine preoperatively the hepatic functional reserve. There is consensus that only patients with a score under 7 (i.e. Child–Pugh's class A) should be resected. The use of this criterion showed prospectively that the risk of hepatic resection was extremely low in patients with a good liver function (i.e. Child–Pugh's A patients; mortality 3.7%) and significant in cases of moderate liver failure or poor liver function (i.e. Child–Pugh's B and C patients; mortality 16.7%).[6] In no case are patients with ascites candidates for partial liver resection. It is our opinion that young cirrhotic patients with ascites and a small HCC should always be considered for liver transplantation.

Many sophisticated tests have been proposed for improved measurement of residual hepatic function, the most validated of them being indocyanine green clearance at 15 minutes.[3,62–64] When the retention rate is less than 10%, any type of resection is possible; for values between 10 and 20% a bisegmentectomy is well tolerated, while for values between 20 and 29% only a unisegmentectomy is indicated. The use of a combination of indocyanine green clearance, serum bilirubin level and the presence or absence of ascites has enabled Japanese surgeons to reduce operative morbidity to 1%.[65] Later, the assessment of wedged hepatic pressure was suggested as a means to improve the selection of patients for liver resection.[53] This last study suggests that hepatic resection should be proposed only in patients with a hepatic venous gradient below 10 mmHg. Information on the volume of the hepatic remnant measured by CT scanning may enhance the accuracy of assessment. The formation of monoethylglycinexylidide, the main lidocaine metabolite, might also provide an additional tool to assess preoperative liver function.[66] The potential usefulness of this test seems to be confirmed by the fact that formation of the metabolite decreases as liver disease evolves, probably because of a reduction in the cellular mass.[67] A further simplification in the preoperative assessment of liver function comes from the use of the C13-aminopyrine breath test that reproduces the results obtained by the monoethylglycinexylidide (MEGX) test.[68] Important signs of portal hypertension or previous haemorrhage from variceal rupture should be viewed as a relative contraindication to liver resection, although preoperative variceal eradication has been suggested to reduce the risk of bleeding.

Finally, given the current epidemiology of hepatitis C virus infection in Western countries, we should expect that most of the patients with HCC who are candidates for surgery will, in the future, be aged over 70 years. This implies that age should also be taken into account in the selection of patients for surgery, even though it has been shown that the treatment policy for HCC in the aged patient should be identical to that adopted in the young subject.[69,70]

General guidelines for liver resection of HCC in cirrhosis

Resection is more difficult in patients with cirrhosis than in those with a normal liver parenchyma. Perioperative bleeding is frequent. Difficulties are mainly related to the presence of portal hypertension and to the distortion of anatomy induced by the process of atrophy-hypertrophy and fibrosis. Haemorrhage and lymphatic spillage occur mainly during severance of the liver ligaments and the posterior peritoneum. These are usually thickened and contain dilated lymphatic and venous vessels; therefore, the simple dissection and mobilization requires careful haemostasis to avoid insidious perioperative bleeding and postoperative collection or ascites. The intense fibrosis that occurs in cirrhosis makes it difficult to identify intraparenchymal vascular structures and is, in association with portal hypertension and fragility of hepatic veins, the main cause of haemorrhage during parenchymal transection. In recent years, liver resections have been performed using minimally invasive techniques.[71] In cirrhotic patients, this approach may be used only for small tumours located anteriorly (i.e. segments III, IVB + V), or for HCCs requiring a bisegmentectomy II–III.[72]

Anatomical resection

As a consequence, the treatment of choice for small HCC in cirrhosis is limited resection which has the following advantages: (1) removal of a small amount of functioning parenchyma, but a free margin of 10 mm should be respected;[29] (2) since HCC spreads through the regional portal system, anatomical resection allows for the complete removal of the tumour-related domain, including possible microscopic daughter nodules around the mass; (3) dissection through the known anatomical planes prevents accidental injury to vascular structures and, consequently, potential major bleeding. By contrast, although proven feasible and safe in cirrhotic patients with large tumours,[73] major hepatic resections should be avoided in the case of small HCC, because of the risk of postoperative hepatic failure and portal hypertension complications. Nevertheless, it should be mentioned that it has been reported recently that preoperative portal vein embolization in cirrhotic patients might allow atrophy of the liver to be resected with compensatory hypertrophy of the remaining liver, thus increasing the safety of liver resection.[74]

Non-anatomical resection (atypical resection)

This is indicated only in cases of tumours confined at the boundaries of two or three adjacent segments when an anatomical resection is not feasible, mainly because of atrophy of the liver to be left after liver resection. Transection through non-anatomical planes exposes the patient to continuous haemorrhage during parenchymal transection, and prolonged total blood inflow clamping (with its attendant risk to parenchymal function) is often required to control major blood loss.

Liver exposure

Position of the patient

The patient is positioned supine, turned 30° to the left on his sagittal axis with the right arm along the body. Tilting the table will give an adequate view, even for posteriorly located tumours. When a bisegmentectomy of segments II–III has been planned, the patient is left supine. A crossbar or special device should be fitted at the head of the table for two self-retaining retractors in order to widen the laparotomy, by elevating the costal margin.

Incision

For most hepatic resections a right S-shaped subcostal incision extending from the midaxillary line to the external margin of left rectal muscle enables good liver exposure. Also the incision popularized by Hasegawa et al.[75] might be used. For tumours located in the left lateral segments (i.e. segments II and III), the right portion of the incision should be reduced or the subcostal incision replaced by an upper midline laparotomy. Once the peritoneum is entered, the round ligament (ligamentum teres) is not systematically divided in order to avoid suppression of possible collateral circulation through a recanalized umbilical vein that might augment portal hypertension.

Exploration and liver mobilization

Most of the information concerning morphology and location of the tumour is obtained from preoperative imaging; rarely does manual exploration add further information, in particular for deeply located tumours. Variations of arterial anatomy (which are detectable by CT scan) are preliminarily sought out in order to avoid accidental ligation and consequent ischaemia during liberation of the liver. The most common findings are a right hepatic artery originating from a superior mesenteric artery, and a left hepatic artery from a left gastric artery. The former runs on the right border of the hepato–duodenal ligament, the latter in the lesser omentum. Mobilization should be as minimal as possible, to avoid fluid spillage and haemorrhage. For anteriorly located tumours (segments III, IVB, V) sectioning of the falciform ligament (while preserving the ligamentum teres) usually suffices. In the other locations, division of the triangular and coronary ligaments on the side of the lesion is mandatory. For right-sided nodules the posterior peritoneum is divided as well. This manoeuvre, associated with division of the triangular ligament, allows the liver to be turned to the left, with initial exposure of the inferior vena cava that is fixed in its upper portion to the liver by the suspensor caval vein ligament. This ligament is particularly thickened in cirrhotic livers and its division should only be performed after having meticulously secured haemostasis. The retrohepatic vena cava is only completely free after careful ligation and division of all short accessory hepatic veins. This manoeuvre is mandatory for tumours located in the right posterior (i.e. segments VI–VII) and dorsal (i.e. segments I–IX) sectors. For tumours arising in the left segments of the liver and the dorsal sector, the lesser omentum is opened and the falciform, left triangular and coronary ligaments are divided. The round ligament is divided in the case of left hepatectomy (i.e. segments II–III–IV), but can be preserved in case of bisegmentectomy II–III.

Intraoperative ultrasonography

Although preoperative work-up provides most of the information needed for a correct surgical strategy, intraoperative US still plays an important role in defining intrahepatic anatomy and, in some cases, serves as a complement to diagnosis. In cirrhosis, the difficulty of finding the usual superficial landmarks makes US an indispensable tool for segmental resection.[76] Through systematic examination of the liver, the surgeon can easily identify segmental distribution of portal pedicles that are recognized because they are enveloped in a hyperechogenic fibrous sheath. The hepatic veins and their branches are also readily identified because of their thin wall, which is much less echogenic than that of the portal vessels. Hepatic veins are studied from their confluence with the inferior vena cava to their peripheral branches in order to detect their relationships to the territory to be removed. Therefore, the exact location of the lesion and its relationship with the vascular distribution make it easier to perform anatomically and oncologically correct, segmental resections. When re-resection is performed, US is mandatory for detection of the modified anatomy created by the previous surgery. This prevents both vascular injury and excessive parenchymal removal. Finally, US is a great aid for the surgeon who performs anatomic resection either under the guidance of tattooing, after injection of the dye into the segmental portal branch, or under selective segmental vascular occlusion through the introduction of a balloon into the segmental portal branch.[60]

The role of US in the diagnosis of a liver mass in cirrhosis is limited. Nevertheless, US may in some instances detect small additional nodules in the liver substance, resulting in major modifications of the surgical strategy.

Liver blood flow control, parenchymal transection and hepatic stump

Liver blood flow control

Because of associated portal hypertension and the characteristics of liver parenchyma, the risk of bleeding is generally considered to be higher in cirrhosis than in normal liver, although, we have not been able to confirm these data in a univariate analysis.[77] Many procedures have been suggested to prevent this complication.

Temporary total hepatic blood inflow occlusion
The Pringle's manoeuvre is the commonest of these procedures. It entails encircling the hepatic pedicle at the foramen of Winslow with a vascular tape, and then occluding the entire hepatic pedicle with a vascular clamp. This results in a critical reduction in bleeding, and if bleeding is persistent, it must originate from the hepatic veins. The tolerance of prolonged normothermic ischaemia in cirrhotic patients is good,[78] and this allows the performance

of complex liver resections in cirrhotic patients. Clamping of the portal triad can be continuous or intermittent. At present, most surgeons are used to performing intermittent clamping (alternating 15 minutes of occlusion with 5 minutes of re-circulation in order to reduce the period of liver ischaemia). It has been shown that continuous occlusion of the hepatic inflow is also well tolerated.[79]

Selective clamping

In order to avoid prolonged liver ischaemia due to total inflow occlusion, selective clamping has been proposed. This can be achieved at either the hilar or suprahilar level. In the former, main portal and arterial branches are dissected and occlusion is obtained by bulldogs, vascular clamps or special balloon catheters. In the latter, occlusion of sectoral portal branches is more difficult because dissection must be pursued deep within the liver substance, which may be the source of bleeding. In order to obviate this risk, selective occlusion of a segmental portal branch by a specially devised balloon catheter introduced into the vessel under ultrasonic guidance has been proposed.[60,80] The dissection and clamping of the ipsilateral hepatic artery better delineates the limits of dissection and further reduces bleeding during parenchymal transection. While the duration of portal occlusion is indefinite, arterial clamping should last no longer than that needed during Pringle's manoeuvre. This procedure, however, should be reserved only for experienced teams, as it is expensive, time-consuming and demands skill in intraoperative interventional US.

Total hepatic vascular exclusion

This procedure entails the concomitant occlusion of the inferior vena cava below and above the liver together with the hepatic pedicle.[81] Tolerance to continuous normothermic ischaemia is poor in cirrhosis, and despite attempts to reduce the risk of postoperative liver failure by inserting a veno-venous bypass and reducing total time of clamping,[82] this technique should be used with extreme caution in cirrhotic patients.[83]

Parenchymal transection and hepatic stump

The line of resection is marked on the liver surface by electric cautery, without penetrating too deeply into the hepatic parenchyma. The hepatic pedicle is then clamped and transection begins. Division of fibrous tissue in cirrhotic livers is made by progressive crushing of the liver parenchyma, using Kelly forceps, allowing skeletonization of the bilio-vascular structures. Intrahepatic vessels and bile ducts are progressively exposed and occluded by bipolar coagulation if the calibre is less than 1 mm. Larger structures are controlled by resorbable clips (author's technique)[84] or ligated. No clips are used

on the side to be removed. When major branches of the hepatic veins are encountered in the field, great care must be taken to encircle them without tearing their thin wall. The risk of brisk bleeding is high and not controlled by Pringle's manoeuvre. Every effort has to be made not to place forceps blindly to arrest the haemorrhage; it is preferable to use gentle compression by applying a damp gauze on the site of bleeding. Division of the hepatic vein is carried out after securing the haemostasis with two forceps, taking care to leave a long stump on the caval side. The vein is then closed by a running vascular suture with a monofilament 5/0. The main portal pedicle of the resected liver is then divided on two forceps and ligated by stout suture.

Parenchymatous division can be also accomplished by an ultrasonic surgical aspirator or by a high velocity water jet dissector. It is our opinion that in cirrhotic livers, transection is better achieved by Kelly crushing. Moreover, an ultrasonic dissector is very useful in the isolation of portal branches, but is potentially harmful when used in the proximity of hepatic veins. A device known as the harmonic scalpel (Ultracision) has been introduced on the market. According to the authors' experience it is reliable for both haemostasis and bilistasis. The slowness during dissection, poor ergonomy and its cost have so far limited the use of this tool. At the end of liver transection, if this has been carefully conducted, oozing from the liver remnant is minimal. Sources of bleeding are identified, and haemostasis is achieved by absorbable mattress sutures on the raw surface. It is equally important to identify bile leaks. Careful inspection with a clean swab usually facilitates location of the origin of bile leakage. Closure of a bilious leak is achieved by absorbable stitches. To improve further the haemostasis of the cut surface, fibrinogen sealant, microcrystalline collagen powder and argon beam coagulation have all been proposed. However, in our view careful haemostasis and securing of bile ducts during parenchymal transection is the best guarantee against postoperative collection and bile leakage.

Abdominal drainage

There is now strong evidence that abdominal drainage can be avoided even after hepatic resection.[85] This would imply that, in cirrhotic patients, prolonged ascitic fluid leakage and exogenous contamination of the abdominal cavity, which result in higher morbidity and prolonged hospital stay, could be prevented.[86] In the very few patients who have symptomatic postoperative collection, we rely on interventional radiological percutaneous drainage.

Current resections for small HCCs in cirrhosis

Although resection of each segment has been described, there are procedures that, because of their complexity, should be proposed with caution in cirrhotic patients. This is the case in bisegmentectomy VII + VIII with resection of the right hepatic vein, and venous graft reconstruction.[87] Three segmental resections are routinely performed: segmentectomy IV, V and VIII. Segmentectomy VII is technically feasible, but the posterosuperior location of this segment makes this procedure difficult. The presence of a large right inferior hepatic vein may allow the sacrifice of the right hepatic vein[47,60] or the performance of a bisegmentectomy VII–VIII, which is technically easier to perform. We seldom perform resection of segment VI, because we have found bisegmentectomy V–VI to be safer and quicker. Likewise, for tumours located in segment II or III, bisegmentectomy II–III, which removes a minor amount of functional liver, is a much simpler operation. Partial or complete resection of the dorsal sector, which some years ago was considered a hazardous operation, is technically feasible. Finally, small tumours located at the junction of segments II, III and IV or segments IV, V and VIII are a good indication for a left hepatectomy or a central hepatectomy (i.e. trisegmentectomy IV–V–VIII),[75] respectively. It is worth mentioning that parenchymal transection during segmental resection causes more bleeding than during conventional hepatectomy, since there is no previous control of the portal pedicles and the raw surface following sectioning is large.[88]

Segmentectomy IV

This segmental resection should remove the quantity of liver parenchyma situated between the umbilical fissure and the main portal scissura, up to the union of the middle and left hepatic veins. The initial step of this procedure entails division of the bridge of parenchyma which joins segments III and IV at the base of the umbilical fissure. Cholecystectomy is performed. Mobilization of the anterior part of segment IV (segment IVB) is then achieved by lowering the hilar plate (Fig. 5.9). This technique has been described in detail elsewhere.[89] Glisson's capsule is opened just above the fibrous tissue of the hilar plate to separate it from liver tissue. There is an almost avascular plane, with the exception of one artery directed upwards to the liver that has to be ligated. The main portal scissura is opened. Parenchymal division is shifted slightly to the left, thus preserving the middle hepatic vein. Resection is pursued until the level of the hilus. The liver is then divided slightly to the right side of the umbilical fissure. Arterial and biliary branches to segment IVA and segment IVB are ligated and

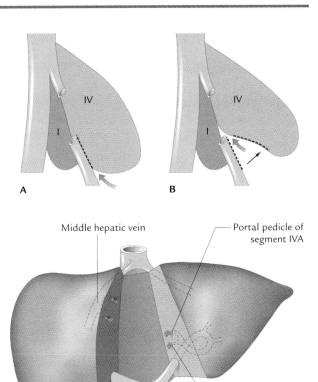

C

Figure 5.9 Complete resection of segment IV. (A) Sketch showing the relationship between the posterior aspect of segment IVB and the hepatic pedicle; the hilar plate (arrow) is formed by the fusion of the connective tissue enclosing the bilio-vascular elements with Glisson's capsule. (B) Diagram showing the anterior mobilization of the posterior aspect of segment IVB and the parenchymatous split between segment IV and segment I (arrow). (C) Complete segmentectomy IV. Note the site of division of the portal pedicles of segments IVA and IVB, and the relationships with the hepatic pedicle and the middle hepatic vein.

severed. The latter is found to come from the left, some 2 or 3 cm from the falciform ligament, immediately upwards of the left hepatic duct. It is easily recognized because of its horizontal direction and its consistency. The latter is located higher in the parenchyma and should not be searched for at the hilus because of its depth. Once both portal pedicles of segment IV have been divided, transection is begun on the right side following a plane 1 cm from the left side of the right hepatic vein. Portal branches are then divided in a slightly more posterior direction. Liver resection is pursued up to the inferior vena cava or the junction of the middle and left hepatic veins; during this step, collateral branches of these veins draining segment IV are divided. The procedure ends by the separation of

A

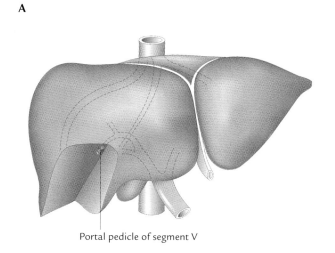

Portal pedicle of segment V

B

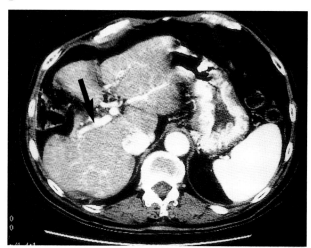

Figure 5.10 (A) Diagram showing a segmentectomy V. Note the location of the portal pedicle of segment V and the proximity of the tip of the right liver from the right area of resection. (B) Postoperative CT scan showing the resected area and the stump of the portal pedicle of segment V (arrow).

segment IV from the dorsal sector (Fig. 5.9). It is worth pointing out that there are no clear guiding landmarks for dividing between these two territories.

Segmentectomy V

The limits of segment V are as follows: the main portal scissura on the left and the right portal scissura on the right, which is in the vicinity of the anterior tip of the right liver and the plane of the hilus posteriorly. After cholecystectomy, the main portal scissura is first opened up to the hilum, avoiding injury to the middle hepatic vein. The right portal scissura is then opened. Liver division is slightly displaced to the left in order to preserve the right hepatic vein. This manoeuvre facilitates the division of the posterior boundary of segment V, which has a transverse direction and is located at the level of the plane of the hilum. The main biliovascular pedicle of segment V is divided at the left superior corner of the resected specimen (Fig. 5.10). This step of the procedure should be performed very cautiously, in order to avoid damage to the vascularization of segment VIII.

Segmentectomy VI

Segment VI, which is located in the posterior portion of the right liver, is limited on the left by the right portal scissura, which ends posteriorly near the inferior vena cava at the junction of the dorsal sector and the right hepatic vein. The superior limit is the plane of the hilum. After complete mobilization of the right liver, parenchymatous division is performed posteriorly and transversely at the level of the hilum without damaging the right hepatic

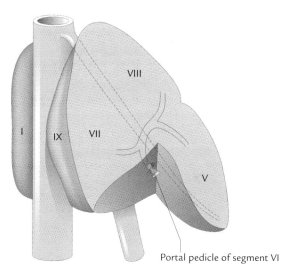

Portal pedicle of segment VI

Figure 5.11 Diagram showing a segmentectomy VI. Note the relationships with the right hepatic vein, segment IX and the site of ligation of the portal pedicle of segment VI.

vein. The right portal scissura is opened on the right side of the right hepatic vein, which marks the anterior limit of the resection. The liver is then divided in the direction of the inferior vena cava. The biliovascular pedicle of segment VI is divided at the junction of both parenchymatous divisions (Fig. 5.11). During this manoeuvre, great care is taken not to damage the blood supply of segment VII.

Segmentectomy VII

Removal of segment VII is a difficult procedure because of the posterior and superior location of this

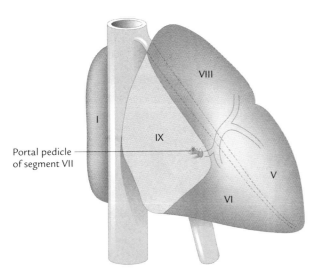

Figure 5.12 Diagram showing a segmentectomy VII. Note the site of ligation of the portal pedicle of segment VII and the relationship with segment IX and the right hepatic vein.

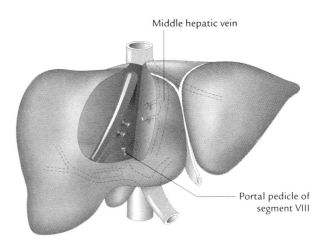

Figure 5.13 Diagram showing a segmentectomy VIII. Note the large raw liver surface, the vicinity of the middle and right hepatic veins, the site of ligation of the portal pedicle of segment VIII and the size of the resected area.

segment near the end of the right hepatic vein. Complete mobilization of the right liver up to the inferior vena cava and the distal portion of the right hepatic vein is paramount. The liver is first divided transversely at the level of the hilum. The right portal scissura is then opened and divided in the direction of the inferior vena cava. The right hepatic vein is left intact. The bilio-vascular pedicle of segment VII is divided at the junction of the parenchymal incisions (Fig. 5.12).

Segmentectomy VIII

Medial and lateral limits are the main and right portal scissurae. The boundary between segments V and VIII is given by the projection on the liver surface of the hilar fissure. Division of the right liver and falciform ligaments up to the confluence of the hepatic veins into the inferior vena cava allows exposure of segment VIII. Parenchymatous division is carried out, 1 cm to the right of the main portal scissura, taking care to ligate a large branch of the middle hepatic vein in the cranial portion of the liver division. On the right, the hepatic vein should not be exposed. Only its branches are ligated or, preferably, occluded by clips. The main pitfalls of this resection are injuries to the hepatic veins on the borders of the segment. Resection should be conducted by surrounding the segment on each side. The final shape of the removed liver is that of a truncated pyramid.[90] The natural tendency of coning surgery – the dissection into the axilla of right and middle veins – has to be avoided, as it entails the risk of non-oncological removal of the tumour. The portal pedicle is ligated intraparenchymally, taking care to avoid the accidental injury to the adjacent

pedicles of segment V when dividing the pedicle of segment VIII (Fig. 5.13).

Dorsal sectorectomy (segments I and IX)

This is one of the most challenging operations in cirrhosis. Removal of small tumours located in the left portion of the dorsal sector (segment I) is relatively easy to accomplish after liberation of segment I posteriorly from its connections to the vena cava, by sectioning the accessory veins and, anteriorly, by dividing the arterial and portal vein branches (Fig. 5.14). Much more difficult is the resection of tumours located in the cranial or in the right portion (segment IX) of this sector. In patients with a good liver function, the ablation of the dorsal sector is usually associated with a left hepatectomy or a bisegmentectomy II–III to simplify the procedure. However, similar to what has been suggested in a normal liver,[91,92] procedures of isolated dorsal sectorectomy have been described also in cirrhosis.[93,94] Two techniques are available for a complete dorsal sectorectomy. In the first, the liver is completely mobilized on both sides up to the insertion of the three main hepatic veins into the inferior vena cava by sectioning the right and left liver ligaments and dividing the accessory hepatic veins (Fig. 5.15). The dorsal sector is freed from the inferior vena cava posteriorly and from the hilum anteriorly. The posterior branches of the portal vein directed to the dorsal sector are ligated and divided. Because of uncertainty as to the right border of the sector, Japanese authors have suggested injecting dye into the posterior portal branches.[95] The limits of unstained liver posteriorly are traced on the surface by electric cautery. Parenchymatous transection is carried out with the liver turned medially. The resection starts from the

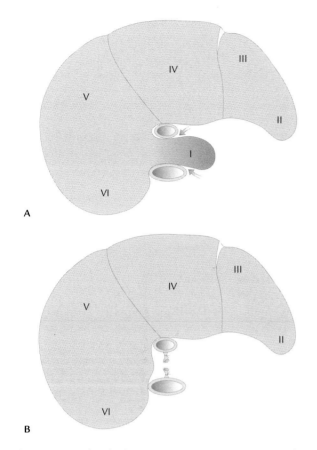

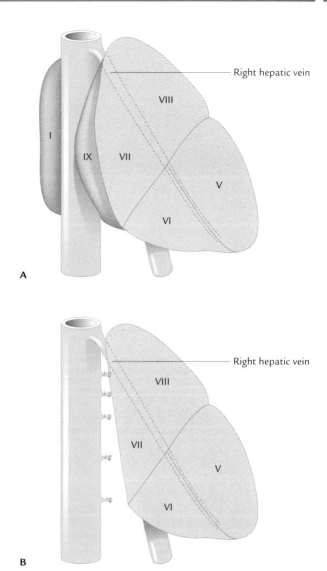

Figure 5.14 Sketch showing a segmentectomy I (caudate lobe). Note (A) the planes of dissection behind the portal vein and in front of the inferior vena cava and (B) the site of ligation of the accessory hepatic veins and posterior portal vein branches.

Figure 5.15 Diagram showing a complete resection of the dorsal sector (i.e. segments I–IX). (A) Note the relationships with the inferior vena cava and the right hepatic vein and the tight connections with the right posterior sector (i.e. segments VI–VII). (B) At the end of the procedure note the numerous ligations of accessory hepatic veins and that the anterior limit of the resection is represented by the segments of the right posterior sector.

right limit and advances beneath the hepatic veins up to Arantius' sulcus on the left, taking care to avoid injury to the main hepatic veins cranially and to the second-order portal branches, anteriorly (Fig. 5.15). In the second technique, dorsal sectorectomy can be performed by using a transhepatic approach, as described by Yamamoto et al.[93] for tumours that displace the middle hepatic vein. The liver is completely freed and transection is carried out along the main portal scissura, thus exposing the middle hepatic vein on most of its length. Two planes of transection are followed on each side of the vein: on the left, following the direction of Arantius' sulcus, and on the right, behind the middle hepatic vein towards the right side of the inferior vena cava (Fig. 5.16). Once Arantius' sulcus is joined, the left portion of the dorsal sector is separated from segments II and III. Pulling the resected dorsal sector forwards through the main portal scissura, the resection is ended by division of the portal branches directed towards the dorsal sector.

Central hepatectomy (segments IV–V–VIII)

Indications are tumours located at the confluence of the three segments deep within the liver

substance of patients with a very good hepatic reserve. The volume of non-tumourous liver removed is conspicuous (about 30%) and, therefore, the risks of hepatic failure and worsening portal hypertension are high. Moreover, the raw cut surface is the largest of the different hepatic resections and, as a consequence, postoperative fluid collection is not uncommon. Falciform and coronary ligaments are divided up to the inferior vena cava, whose anterior surface is exposed in order to locate the confluence of the hepatic veins, particularly the middle one, into the vena cava. The limits of the resection are the falciform

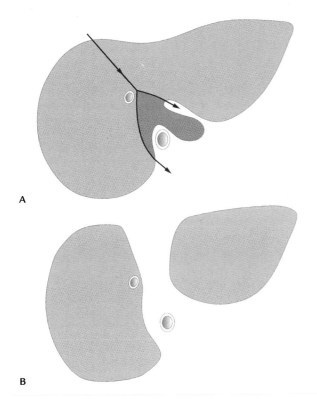

Figure 5.16 Sketch showing a representation of complete dorsal sectorectomy according to Yamamoto et al.[93] (A) The liver has been divided through the main portal scissura (arrow). Note the planes of liver division to the left in the direction of Arantius' sulcus (arrow) and to the right on the right side of the inferior vena cava (arrow), behind the middle hepatic vein. (B) The resected area at the end of the procedure.

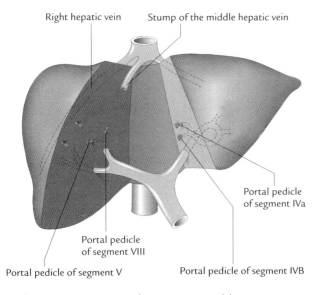

Right hepatic vein   Stump of the middle hepatic vein

Portal pedicle of segment IVa

Portal pedicle of segment VIII

Portal pedicle of segment V   Portal pedicle of segment IVB

Figure 5.17 Diagram showing a central hepatectomy. Note the size of the raw liver surface, the vicinity of the right hepatic vein and the site of ligation of the portal pedicles of segment IVA and IVB and segment V and VIII. The middle hepatic vein has been divided and occluded by a running suture.

ligament on the left and the right hepatic vein, whose direction has been traced on the surface of the right liver by US. The inferior limit is the hilar plate. The hilar plate is lowered as if for a segmentectomy IV, from the insertion of the ligamentum teres up to the gallbladder fossa. While extending the dissection into the liver substance, although difficult in cirrhosis, it is sometimes possible to identify, isolate and clamp the anterior sectoral portal pedicle for segments V and VIII. It is actually harmful, in most cases, to encircle the pedicle: it is easier and safer to ligate it intraparenchymally during transection. On the left side, there are two portal pedicles, one for segment IVB and one for IVA, that are divided as for a segmentectomy IV. If, for any reason, the right hepatic vein is encountered, the plane of section should be shifted medially. The pedicles of segments V and VIII are separately ligated into the liver parenchyma. In front of the inferior vena cava, the trunk of the middle hepatic vein is easily identified and ligated on a vascular clamp by a running suture. An adequate thickness of liver tissue should be kept posteriorly (i.e. the dorsal sector) (Fig. 5.17).

Perioperative treatment

Antibiotics

Although some authors argue for the use of antibiotic therapy in cirrhotic patients undergoing liver resection, we do not routinely use this approach. It is worth mentioning that there are no controlled data on the topic. Septic complications seem to be no higher in our patients compared to other series. In at-risk patients, third generation cephalosporins or quinolones are used. In patients in whom a prolonged total portal clamping is foreseen, a preoperative selective intestinal decontamination may be proposed to prevent bacterial translocation.

Blood transfusion

The risks entailed in allogeneic blood transfusion are manifest in cirrhotic patients undergoing liver resection, and include worsening of hepatic function, increase in postoperative complications and a higher recurrence rate. Therefore all attempts should be made to identify patients at risk of bleeding in order to minimize the risk of transfusion. As shown in a multivariate study,[77] patients undergoing extended resections or with abnormal coagulation should be specially considered for other procedures, such as autologous blood predeposit, isovolemic haemodilution or intraoperative autotransfusion.

To be effective, autologous blood transfusion requires painstaking organizational efforts prior to the patient's hospitalization. While the procedure is mandatory in patients with benign tumours, its use in patients with malignant disease is debatable in view of the very high cost/benefit ratio. The best candidates for this procedure are those patients with haemoglobin concentrations >13 g/dl. Two or three blood units are drawn and stored. Liver resection should be delayed for a period of 2 weeks. When haemoglobin is <11 g/dl, human recombinant erythropoietin and iron may also be effective in cirrhotic patients to accelerate erythrogenesis.[96] However, there is evidence that the use of the human recombinant erythropoietin in cirrhosis can hasten hypophosphataemia and worsening of hepatic function.

Isovolemic haemodilution represents a very inexpensive and reliable method to substitute allogeneic transfusion in cirrhotic patients,[97] provided that contraindications such as major coagulation defects, cardiac disease or anaemia do not co-exist. Haemodilution is probably the best alternative method to allogeneic blood transfusion.

The cell-saver for intraoperative blood recovery is practically unused in elective hepatic resection for malignant tumours because of its costs and the potential risk of tumoural cell dissemination, despite experimental evidence showing that this latter risk is absent.[98]

We have shown that the use of the antifibrinolytic aprotinin during surgery is effective in reducing both perioperative blood loss and the need for blood transfusions in patients undergoing hepatic resection for tumour.[99] Major limitations to its more widespread use are its high cost and the likelihood of allergic reaction.

A policy of fluid and sodium restriction in cirrhotic patients is the best method for preventing ascites formation in the postoperative period.[61] The daily amount of fluid given should not exceed 20 ml/kg and should be based on urinary osmolarity and excretion of sodium. In the case of ascites formation, the intravenous administration of albumin or macromolecules associated with furosemide usually induces a diuresis and a reduction in intraperitoneal fluid accumulation. Paracentesis is mandatory in patients with massive ascites, in order to avoid prolonged leakage of fluid through the abdominal incision. The loss of fluid via abdominal drains must also be compensated.

Postoperative nutritional support is not a common practice after hepatectomy in our experience. Provided that a good selection of patients has been made preoperatively on the basis of residual hepatic function, the appearance of encephalopathy is nearly always exceptional. As a consequence, the use of special formulations, such as branched-chain amino acid enriched solution, does not lead to any clinical advantage over other standard formulations. An early resumption of oral intake in patients without complications is, in our current view, the best way to manage cirrhotic patients.

Results of partial liver resection for small HCC in cirrhosis

The results of partial liver resection for small HCCs (<5 cm) in cirrhosis are summarized in Tables 5.1 and 5.2. The average operative mortality is 5.7 ± 4.9% (range 0–14.6%). When data from a number of series are collected, the mean 3- and 5-year survivals are 59.2 ± 15.2% (range 39–79%) and 48.5 ± 13.2% (range 37–63.8%), respectively. In a large series of 1000 patients treated by hepatectomy

Table 5.1 **Operative mortality following liver resection for small hepatocellular carcinoma in patients with cirrhosis**

Study	No of patients	Operative mortality (%)
Ohnishi et al.[100]	34	11.8
Tang et al.[36]	132	2.3
Bismuth et al.[3]	46	10
Castells et al.[101]	33	9.1
Kawasaki et al.[38]	93	0.9
Livraghi et al.[102]	82[a]	2.5
Fuster et al.[103]	48	4.2
Lee et al.[104]	48	0
Nagashima et al.[29]	41	14.6
Zhou et al.[105]	474	1.7
Llovet et al.[106]	77	4

[a] Child's A patients.

for small HCC, 10-year survival has been reported to be 46.3%.[2] Discrepancies between series are probably related to variations in the selection of patients regarding preoperative liver function and tumour invasiveness. Finally, the mean 3-year recurrence rate is 52.2 ± 7.9% (range 43–65%). The high recurrence rate is most likely linked to a small surgical margin, residual neoplastic foci of HCC and the ongoing carcinogenic process.

Table 5.2 **Long-term survival and recurrence rates following liver resection of small hepatocellular carcinoma in patients with cirrhosis**

Study	No of patients	Survival rate (%)		3-year recurrence rate (%)
		3-year	5-year	
Ohnishi et al.[100]	34	55[a]	28[b]	—
Tang et al.[36]	132	76.3	63.2	—
Franco et al.[6]	43	42	—	65
Bismuth et al.[3]	46	39[c]	—	49
Castells et al.[101]	33	44	—	52
Kawasaki et al.[38]	93	40[d]	—	—
Livraghi et al.[102]	82[e]	79	—	—
Fuster et al.[103]	48	64[f]	—	47
Lee et al.[104]	48	70	50	—
Nagashima et al.[29]	41	75[g]	53[h]	—
Nakajima et al.[107]	52[i]	48[e]	37[e]	57
Zhou et al.[105]	474	75.4	63.8	—
Poon et al.[108]	244	61.6	44.5	43

[a]65% in Child's A patients.
[b]38% in Child's A patients.
[c]HCC <3 cm; 17% in disease-free patients.
[d]Disease-free patients.
[e]Child's A patients.
[f]37% in disease-free patients.
[g]53% in disease-free patients.
[h]30% in disease-free patients.
[i]HCC <3 cm.

Liver transplantation for small HCC in cirrhosis

General considerations

Liver transplantation has the advantage over partial liver resection of curing the tumour and the underlying liver disease with its potential carcinogenic process which plays a major role in the outcome of patients. Nevertheless, it must be mentioned that reinfection of the transplanted liver by hepatitis B or hepatitis C virus is the rule in cases of viral infection prior to transplantation, which might interfere with the risk of tumour recurrence. Historically, total hepatectomy and liver transplantation have been considered the therapy of choice for HCCs that could not be removed by partial liver resection. The high tumour recurrence rate after liver transplantation in this indication has prompted surgeons progressively to abandon liver transplantation for huge tumours.[109] A 5-year survival rate for small HCCs not exceeding 25% at 5 years[110] has led to the proposal of liver transplantation for small HCCs.[3,111] However, the shortage in organ donors has hindered the widespread development of such a policy. As regards the operative protocol, a thorough examination of the peritoneal cavity should be carried out before transplantation, and specific operative measures should be respected during the procedure.[3] Very strict selection criteria are essential for the identification of patients who have the best chance of cure following liver transplantation. HCC recurrence following transplantation is largely dependent on the tumour stage, made according to the TNM classification[112,113] and vascular invasion.[3,112,114]

Indications for liver transplantation

At present, liver transplanation should ideally be proposed in patients with small HCCs without vascular invasion (i.e. stage I of the TNM classification) and which are not accessible to a limited curative resection. It is typically the case that HCC centrally embedded in the right liver, at the junction of segments V, VI, VII and VIII, requires a right hepatectomy for a small tumour. In such a situation, despite the presence of a good hepatic function, it seems advisable not to perform a major hepatic resection for a small HCC which could be poorly tolerated, or an atypical resection which might not be curative. However, an alternative therapeutic approach which reduces the operative risk is right hepatectomy, preceded by an embolization of the right branch of the portal vein, provided that a compensatory hypertrophy of the left liver with an atrophy of the right liver has been achieved.[74,115] The precise staging of HCC, based on the number and size of lesions that predicts recurrence after transplantation, has not yet been defined. However, the indications for transplantation may be expanded. Thus, patients with two or three nodules of HCC, each not exceeding 3 cm in diameter,[111] or patients with their largest nodule ≤4.5 cm and total tumour diameter not exceeding 8 cm,[44] could also be proposed for liver transplantation. Because of the shortage of organs, Majno et al.[116] have studied in selected patients the results of a primary liver resection and salvage transplantation, in patients with single, small HCC and preserved liver function, as against liver transplantation. They showed that life expectancy was similar in both groups. Finally, liver transplantation is strongly indicated in patients with a small asymptomatic HCC and a poor liver function.

Results of liver transplantation for small HCCs in cirrhosis

The results of liver transplantation for small HCCs are summarized in Tables 5.3 and 5.4. The operative mortality is quite high, with a mean of 15.6 ± 9.1% (range 5–30%). Three-year survival is 70.1 ± 12.0% (range 54–85%), superior to the results obtained after conventional resection. This last result is most likely related to a more stringent selection of patients for liver transplantation. The recurrence rate is low when compared to liver resection. Finally, recurrence rate is high, especially in patients with vascular invasion.[121]

Key points

- Precise knowledge of the natural history of HCC in cirrhosis.
- CT scanning assessment:
  Tumour characteristics
  Tumour resectability
  Type of hepatic resection.
- Partial liver resection in cirrhotic patients:
  Good liver function
  Economic parenchymal resection
  Free margin of 10 mm
  Specific postoperative complications.

Table 5.3 **Operative mortality following liver transplantation for small hepatocellular carcinoma in patients with cirrhosis**

Study	No of patients	Operative mortality (%)
Bismuth et al.[3]	45	5
Romani et al.[117]	27	11
Schwartz et al.[118]	40	30
Mazzaferro et al.[111]	48	17
Collella et al.[119]	69	25[a]
Otto et al.[120]	40	8
Hemming et al.[121]	112	13

[a]Within 3 months following liver transplantation.

Table 5.4 **Long-term survival and recurrence rates following liver transplantation for small hepatocellular carcinoma in patients with cirrhosis**

Study	No of patients	3-year survival rate %	Recurrence rate (%)
Bismuth et al.[3]	45	60[a]	0[b]
Romani et al.[117]	27	71	—
Schwartz et al.[118]	40	66	—
Mazzaferro et al.[111]	48	85	10[c]
Collella et al.[119]	69	85[d]	15.1[e]
Otto et al.[120]	40	54	30[b]
Figueras et al.[122]	84	77	4[f]
Hemming et al.[121]	112	63	65[g]

[a]HCC <3 cm.
[b]At 3 years.
[c]Median follow-up of 26 months.
[d]Disease-free patients.
[e]Median follow-up of 57 months.
[f]During follow-up.
[g]5-year actuarial tumour recurrence.

- Tumour recurrence after resection:
  Main cause of poor prognosis
  In most cases intrahepatic recurrence
  Anatomic prognostic factors.

- Liver transplantation:
  Better results than partial liver resection
  Highly selected patients.

REFERENCES

1. Hsu HC, Wu TT, Wu MZ, Sheu JC, Lee CS, Chen DS. Tumor invasiveness and prognosis in resected hepatocellular carcinoma. Clinical and pathogenetic implications. Cancer 1988; 61: 2095–9

2. Zhou XD, Tang ZY, Yang BH et al. Experience of 1000 patients who underwent hepatectomy for small hepatocellular carcinoma. Cancer 2001; 91: 1479–85

3. Bismuth H, Chiche L, Adam R, Castaing D, Diamond T, Dennison A. Liver resection versus transplantation for hepatocellular carcinoma in cirrhotic patients. Ann Surg 1993; 218: 145–51

4. Nagasue N, Galizia G, Kohno H et al. Adverse effects of preoperative hepatic artery chemoembolization for resectable hepatocellular carcinoma: a retrospective comparison of 138 liver resections. Surgery 1989; 106: 81–6

5. Kemeny F, Vadrot J, Wu A, Smadja C, Meakins JL, Franco D. Morphological and histological features of resected hepatocellular carcinoma in cirrhotic patients in the west. Hepatology 1989; 9: 253–7

6. Franco D, Capussotti L, Smadja C et al. Resection of hepatocellular carcinomas. Results in 72 European patients with cirrhosis. Gastroenterology 1990; 98: 733–8

7. Tiribelli C, Melato M, Croce LS, Giarelli L, Okuda K, Ohnishi K. Prevalence of hepatocellular carcinoma and relation to cirrhosis: comparison of two different cities of the world – Trieste, Italy, and Chiba, Japan. Hepatology 1989; 10: 998–1002.

8. Ginès P, Quintero E, Arroyo V et al. Compensated cirrhosis: natural history and prognostic factors. Hepatology 1987; 7: 122–8

9. Ebara M, Ohto M, Shinagawa T et al. Natural history of minute hepatocellular carcinoma smaller than three centimeters complicating cirrhosis. A study in 22 patients. Gastroenterology 1986; 90: 289–98

10. Barbara L, Benzi G, Gaiani S et al. Natural history of small untreated hepatocellular carcinoma in cirrhosis: a multivariate analysis of prognostic factors of tumor growth rate and patient survival. Hepatology 1992; 16: 132–7

11. Llovet JM, Bustamante J, Castells A et al. Natural history of untreated non-surgical hepatocellular carcinoma: rationale for the design and evaluation of therapeutic trials. Hepatology 1999; 29: 62–7

12. Pateron D, Ganne N, Trinchet JC et al. Prospective study of screening for hepatocellular carcinoma in caucasian patients with cirrhosis. J Hepatol 1994; 20: 65–71

13. Ikeda K, Saitoh S, Koida et al. A multivariate analysis of risk factors for hepatocellular carcinogenesis: a prospective observation of 795 patients with viral and alcoholic cirrhosis. Hepatology 1993; 18: 47–53

14. Benvegnu L, Fattovich G, Noventa F et al. Concurrent hepatitis B and C virus infection and risk of hepatocellular carcinoma in cirrhosis. A prospective study. Cancer 1994; 74: 2442–8

15. Koike Y, Shiratori Y, Sato S et al. Risk factors for recurring hepatocellular carcinoma differ according to infected hepatitis virus. An analysis of 236 consecutive patients with a single lesion. Hepatology 2000; 32: 1216–23

16. Di Biscegly AM, Hoofnagle JH. Elevations in serum alpha-fetoprotein levels in patients with chronic hepatitis B. Cancer 1989; 64: 2117–20

17. Heyward WL, Lanier AP, McMahon BJ, Fitzgerald MA, Kilkenny S, Paprocki TR. Early detection of primary hepatocellular carcinoma. Screening for primary hepatocellular carcinoma among persons infected with hepatitis B virus. JAMA 1985; 254: 3052–4

18. Frederick MG, McElaney BL, Singer A et al. Timing of parenchymal enhancement on dual-phase dynamic helical CT of the liver: how long does the hepatic arterial phase predominate? AJR 1996; 166: 1305–10

19. Freeny PC, Baron RL, Teefey SA. Hepatocellular carcinoma: reduced frequency of typical findings with dynamic contrast-enhanced CT in a non-Asian population. Radiology 1992; 182: 143–8

20. Baron RL, Oliver III JH, Dodd III GD, Nalesnik M, Holbert BL, Carr B. Hepatocellular carcinoma: evaluation with biphasic, contrast-enhanced, helical CT. Radiology 1996; 199: 505–11

21. Vilana R, Bru C, Bruix J, Castells A, Sole M, Rodes J. Fine-needle aspiration biopsy of portal vein thrombus: value in detecting malignant thrombosis. AJR 1992; 160: 1285–7

22. Solbiati L, Cora L, Ierace T et al. Liver cancer imaging: the need for accurate detection of intrahepatic disease spread. J Computed Assisted Tomogr 1999; 23: S29–S37

23. Livraghi T, Makuuchi M, Buscovini L. Guidelines. In: Livraghi T, Makuuchi M, Buscarini L, eds. Diagnosis and treatment of hepatocellular carcinoma. London: Greenwich Medical Media, 1997

24. International working party. Terminology of nodular hepatocellular lesions. Hepatology 1995; 22: 983–93

25. John TG, Garden OJ. Needle track seeding of primary and secondary liver carcinoma after percutaneous liver biopsy. HPB Surg 1993; 6: 199–203

26. Azoulay D, Johann M, Raccuia JS, Castaing D, Bismuth H. 'Protected' double needle biopsy technique for hepatic tumors. J Am Coll Surg 1996; 183: 160–3

27. Belghiti J, Panis Y, Farges O, Benhamou JP, Fékété F. Intrahepatic recurrence after resection of hepatocellular carcinoma complicating cirrhosis. Ann Surg 1991; 214: 114–7

28. Balsells J, Charco R, Lazaro JL et al. Resection of hepatocellular carcinoma in patients with cirrhosis. Br J Surg 1996; 83: 758–61

29. Nagashima I, Hamada C, Naruse K et al. Surgical resection for small hepatocellular carcinoma. Surgery 1996; 119: 40–5

30. Takenaka K, Kawahara N, Yamamoto K et al. Results of 280 liver resections for hepatocellular carcinoma. Arch Surg 1996; 131: 71–6

31. El-Assal ON, Yamanoi A, Soda Y, Yamaguchi M, Yu L, Nagasue N. Proposal of invasiveness score to predict recurrence and survival after curative hepatic resection for hepatocellular carcinoma. Surgery 1997; 122: 571–7

32. Kumada T, Nakano S, Takeda I et al. Patterns of recurrence after initial treatment in patients with small hepatocellular carcinoma. Hepatology 1997; 25: 87–92

33. Chen PJ, Chen DS, Lai MY et al. Clonal origin of recurrent hepatocellular carcinomas. Gastroenterology 1989; 96: 527–9

34. Nagasue N, Kohno H, Chang YC et al. DNA ploidy pattern in synchronous and metachronous hepatocellular carcinomas. Hepatology 1992; 16: 208–214

35. Chen YJ, Yeh SH, Chen JT et al. Chromosomal changes and clonality relationship between primary and recurrent hepatocellular carcinomas. Gastroenterology 2000; 119: 431–40

36. Tang ZY, Yu YQ, Zhou XD et al. Surgery of small hepatocellular carcinoma. Analysis of 144 cases. Cancer 1989; 64: 536–41

37. Nagasue N, Uchida M, Makino Y et al. Incidence and factors associated with intrahepatic recurrence following resection of hepatocellular carcinoma. Gastroenterology 1993; 105: 488–94

38. Kawasaki S, Makuuchi M, Miyagawa S et al. Results of hepatic resection for hepatocellular carcinoma. World J Surg 1995; 19: 31–4

39. Shirabe K, Takenaka K, Taketomi A et al. Postoperative hepatitis status as a significant risk factor for recurrence in cirrhotic patients with small hepatocellular carcinoma. Cancer 1996; 77: 1050–5

40. Bilimoria MM, Lauwers GY, Doherty DA et al. Underlying liver disease, not tumor factors, predicts long-term survival after resection of hepatocellular carcinoma. Arch Surg 2001; 136: 528–35

41. Livraghi T, Goldberg SN, Lazzaroni S et al. Hepatocellular carcinoma: radiofrequency ablation of medium and large lesions. Radiology 2000; 214: 761–8

42. Orlando A, D'Antoni A, Camma C et al. Treatment of small hepatocellular carcinoma with percutaneous ethanol injection: a validated prognostic model. Am J Gastroenterol 2000; 95: 2921–7

43. Llovet JM, Vilana N, Bru C et al. Increased risk of tumor seeding after percutaneous radiofrequency ablation for single hepatocellular carcinoma. Hepatology 2001; 33: 1124–9

44. Yao FY, Ferrel L, Bass NM. Liver transplantation for hepatocellular carcinoma: expansion of the tumor size limits does not adversely impact survival. Hepatology 2001; 33: 1394–403

45. Couinaud C. Le foie: etudes anatomiques et chirurgicales. Paris: Masson, 1957

46. Couinaud C. Secteur dorsal du foie. Chirurgie 1998; 123: 8–15

47. Makuuchi M, Hasegawa H, Yamazaki S, Bandai Y, Watanabe G, Ito R. The inferior right hepatic vein: ultrasonic demonstration. Radiology 1985; 148: 213–7

48. Nagasue N, Yukaya H, Ogawa Y, Kohno H, Nakamura T. Human liver regeneration after major hepatic resection. A study of normal liver and livers with chronic hepatitis and cirrhosis. Ann Surg 1987; 206: 30–6

49. Chen MF, Hwang TL, Hung CF. Human liver regeneration after major hepatectomy. A study of liver volume by computed tomography. Ann Surg 1991; 213: 227–9

50. Bismuth H, Houssin D, Mazmanian G. Postoperative liver insufficiency: prevention and management. World J Surg 1983; 7: 505–10

51. Makuuchi M, Takayama T, Gunven P, Kosuge T, Yamazaki S, Hasegawa H. Restrictive versus liberal blood transfusion policy for hepatectomies in cirrhotic patients. World J Surg 1989; 13: 644–8

52. Takenaka K, Kanematsu T, Fukuzawa K, Sugimachi K. Can hepatic failure after surgery for hepatocellular carcinoma in cirrhotic patients be prevented? World J Surg 1990; 14: 123–7

53. Bruix J, Castells A, Bosch J et al. Surgical resection of hepatocellular carcinoma in cirrhotic patients: prognostic value of preoperative portal pressure. Gastroenterology 1996; 111: 1018–22

54. Nagasue N, Yukaya H, Kohno H, Chang YC, Nakamura T. Morbidity and mortality after major hepatic resection in cirrhotic patients with hepatocellular carcinoma. HPB Surg 1988; 1: 45–56

55. Merli M, Romiti A, Riggio D, Capoccia L. Optimal nutritional indexes in chronic liver disease. J Parent Ent Nutr 1987; 11: S130–4

56. Fan ST, Lo CM, Lai ECS, Chu KM, Lu CI, Wong J. Perioperative nutritional support in patients undergoing hepatectomy for hepatocellular carcinoma. N Engl J Med 1994; 331: 1547–52

57. Cabre E, Gonzales-Huix F, Abad Lacruz A et al. Effect of enteral nutrition on the short outcome of severely malnourished cirrhotics. A randomized controlled trial. Gastroenterology 1990; 98: 715–20

58. Rimola A, Arroyo V, Rodes J. Infective complications in acute and chronic liver failure: basis and control. In:

Williams R, ed. Liver failure. Clinics in critical care medicine. London: Churchill Livingstone, 1986; 93–111

59. Ferri M, Gabriel S, Gavelli A, Franconeri P, Huguet C. Bacterial translocation during portal clamping for liver resection. A clinical study. Arch Surg 1997; 132: 162–5

60. Makuuchi M, Hasegawa H, Yamazaki S. Ultrasonically guided subsegmentectomy. Surg Gynecol Obstet 1985; 161: 346–50

61. Hasegawa H, Yamazaki S, Makuuchi M, Elias D. Hépatectomies pour hépatocarcinome sur foie cirrhotique: schémas décisionnels et principes de réanimation péri-opératoire. Expérience de 204 cas. J Chir (Paris) 1987; 124: 425–31

62. Makuuchi M, Kosuge T, Takayama T et al. Surgery for small liver cancers. Semin Surg Oncol 1993; 9: 298–304

63. Izumi R, Shimizu K, Li T et al. Prognostic factors of hepatocellular carcinoma in patients undergoing hepatic resection. Gastroenterology 1994; 106: 720–7

64. Wu CC, Ho WI, Yeh DC, Huang CR, Liu TJ, Peng FK. Hepatic resection of hepatocellular carcinoma in cirrhotic liver: is it unjustified in impaired liver function? Surgery 1996; 120: 34–9

65. Miyagawa S, Makuuchi M, Kawasaki S, Kakasu T. Criteria for safe hepatic resection. Am J Surg 1995; 169: 589–94

66. Oellerich M, Hartmann H, Ringe B, Burdelski M, Lautz HU, Pichlmayr R. Assessment of prognosis in transplant candidates by use of the Pugh-MEGX score. Transplant Proc 1993; 25: 1116–9

67. Testa R, Caglieris S, Risso D et al. Monoethylglycinexylidide formation measurement as a hepatic function test to assess severity of chronic liver disease. Am J Gastroenterol 1997; 92: 2268–73

68. Fasoli A, Giannini E, Botta F et al. $13CO_2$ excretion in breath of normal subjects and cirrhotic patients after 13C-aminopyrine oral load. Comparison with MEGX test in functional differentiation between chronic hepatitis and liver cirrhosis. Hepatogastroenterology 2000; 47: 234–8

69. Nagasue N, Chang YC, Takemoto Y, Taniura H, Kohno H, Nakamura T. Liver resection in the aged (seventy years or older) with hepatocellular carcinoma. Surgery 1993; 113: 148–54

70. Poon RTP, Fan ST, Lo CH et al. Hepatocellular carcinoma in the elderly: results of surgical and non-surgical management. Am J Gastroenterol 1999; 94: 2460–6

71. Huscher CG, Lirici MM, Chiodini S, Recher A. Current position of advanced laparoscopic surgery of the liver. J R Coll Surg Edin 1997; 42: 219–25

72. Cherqui D, Hussou E, Hammound R et al. Laparoscopic liver resections: a feasibility of 30 patients. Ann Surg 2000; 232: 753–62

73. Capussotti L, Borgonovo G, Bouzari H, Smadja C, Grange D, Franco D. Results of major liver resection for large hepatocellular carcinoma in patients with cirrhosis. Br J Surg 1994; 81: 427–31

74. Azoulay D, Castaing D, Krissat J et al. Percutaneous portal vein embolization increases the feasibility and safety of major liver resection for hepatocellular carcinoma in the injured liver. Ann Surg 2000; 232: 665–72

75. Hasegawa H, Makuuchi M, Yamazaki S, Gunven P. Central bisegmentectomy of the liver: experience in 16 patients. World J Surg 1989; 13: 786–90

76. Castaing D, Kunstlinger F, Habib N, Bismuth H. Intraoperative ultrasound study of the liver: methodology and anatomical results. Am J Surg 1985; 169: 676–82

77. Mariette D, Smadja C, Naveau S, Borgonovo G, Vons C, Franco D. Preoperative predictors of blood transfusion in liver resection for tumor. Am J Surg 1997; 173: 275–9

78. Kim YI, Nakashima K, Tada I, Kawano K, Kobayashi M. Prolonged normothermic ischaemia of human cirrhotic liver during hepatectomy: a preliminary report. Br J Surg 1993; 80: 1566–70

79. Capussotti L, Nuzzo G, Polastri R et al. Continuous vs. intermittent portal clamping during hepatectomy in cirrhotic liver. A prospective randomized clinical trial. Hepatogastroenterology 1998; 45 (Suppl 2): 13 (abstract)

80. Castaing D, Garden OJ, Bismuth H. Segmental liver resection using ultrasound-guided selective portal venous occlusion. Ann Surg 1989; 210: 20–3

81. Huguet C, Addario-Chieco P, Gavelli A, Arrigo E, Harb J, Clement R. Technique of hepatic vascular exclusion for extensive liver resection. Am J Surg 1992; 163: 602–5

82. Yamakoa Y, Ozawa K, Kumada K et al. Total vascular exclusion for hepatic resection in cirrhotic patients. Application of venous bypass. Arch Surg 1992; 127: 276–80

83. Bismuth H, Castaing D, Garden OJ. Major hepatic resection under total vascular exclusion. Ann Surg 1989; 210: 13–9

84. Franco D, Smadja C, Meakins JL, Wu WL, Berthoux L, Grange D. Improved early results of elective hepatic resection for liver tumours. One hundred consecutive hepatectomies in cirrhotic and non-cirrhotic patients. Arch Surg 1989; 124: 1033–7

85. Franco D, Karaa A, Meakins JL, Borgonovo G, Smadja C, Grange D. Hepatectomy without abdominal drainage. Ann Surg 1989 210: 748–50

86. Smadja C, Berthoux L, Meakins JL, Franco D. Patterns of improvement in resection of hepatocellular carcinoma in cirrhotic patients. HPB Surg 1989; 1: 141–7

87. Nakamura S, Sakaguchi S, Kitazawa T, Suzuki S, Koyano K, Mura H. Hepatic vein reconstruction for preserving remnant liver function. Arch Surg 1990; 125: 1455–9

88. Franco D, Smadja C, Kahwaji F, Grange D, Kemeny F, Traynor O. Segmentectomies in the management of liver tumors. Arch Surg 1988; 123: 519–22

89. Smadja C, Blumgart LH. The biliary tract and the anatomy of biliary exposure. In: Blumgart LH, ed. Surgery of the liver and biliary tract, Vol 1. Edinburgh: Churchill Livingstone, 1988; 11–22

90. Franco D, Bonnet P, Smadja C, Grange D. Surgical resection of segment VIII (antero-superior subsegment of the right lobe) in patients with liver cirrhosis and hepatocellular carcinoma. Surgery 1985; 98: 949–53

91. Lerut J, Gruwez JA, Blumgart LH. Resection of the caudate lobe of the liver. Surg Gynecol Obstet 1990; 171: 160–2

92. Elias D, Lasser PH, Desruennes E, Mankarios H, Jiang Y. Surgical approach to segment I for malignant tumors of the liver. Surg Gynecol Obstet 1992; 175: 17–24

93. Yamamoto J, Takayama T, Kosuge T et al. An isolated caudate lobectomy by the transhepatic approach for hepatocellular carcinoma in cirrhotic liver. Surgery 1992; 111: 699–702

94. Takayama T, Tanaka T, Higaki T, Katou K, Teshima Y, Makuuchi M. High dorsal resection of the liver. J Am Coll Surg 1994; 179: 73–5

95. Kosuge T, Yamamoto J, Takayama T et al. An isolated, complete resection of the caudate lobe, including the paracaval portion, for hepatocellular carcinoma. Arch Surg 1994; 129: 280–4

96. Kaikawa M, Nonami T, Kurokaw T et al. Autologous blood transfusion for hepatectomy in patients with cirrhosis and hepatocellular carcinoma: use of recombinant human erythropoietin. Surgery 1994; 115: 727–34

97. Séjourné, P, Poirier A, Meakins JL, Smadja C, Grange D, Franco D. Effect of haemodilution on transfusion requirements in liver resection. Lancet 1989; ii: 1380–2

98. Torre GC, Ferrari M, Favre A, Razzetta F, Borgonovo G. A new technique for intraoperative blood recovery in cancer patients. Eur J Oncol 1994; 20: 565–70

99. Lentschener C, Benhamou D, Mercier FJ et al. Aprotinin reduces blood loss in patients undergoing elective liver resection. Anesthaesiol Analg 1997; 84: 875–81

100. Ohnishi K, Tanabe Y, Ryu M et al. Prognosis of hepatocellular carcinoma smaller than 5 cm in relation to treatment: study of 100 patients, Hepatology 1987; 7: 1285–90

101. Castells A, Bruix J, Bru C et al. Treatment of small hepatocellular carcinoma in cirrhotic patients: a cohort study comparing surgical resection and percutaneous ethanol injection. Hepatology 1993; 18: 1121–6

102. Livraghi T, Bolondi L, Buscarini L et al. No treatment, resection and ethanol injection in hepatocellular carcinoma: a retrospective analysis of survival in 391 patients with cirrhosis. J Hepatol 1995; 22: 522–6

103. Fuster J, Garcia-Valdecasas JC, Grande L et al. Hepatocellular carcinoma and cirrhosis. Results of surgical treatment in a European series, Ann Surg 1996; 223: 297–302

104. Lee CS, Sheu JC, Wang M, Hsu HC. Long-term outcome after surgery for asymptomatic small hepatocellular carcinoma. Br J Surg 1996; 83: 330–3

105. Zhou XD, Tang ZY, Yu YQ et al. Long-term results of surgery for small primary liver cancer in 514 adults. J Cancerol Res Clin Oncol 1996; 122: 59–62

106. Llovet JM, Fuster J, Bruix J. Intention-to-treat analysis of surgical treatment for early hepatocellular carcinoma: resection versus transplantation. Hepatology 1999; 30: 1434–40

107. Nakajima Y, Shimamura T, Kamiyama T et al. Evaluation of surgical resection for small hepatocellular carcinomas. Am J Surg 1996; 171: 360–3

108. Poon RTP, Fan ST, Lo CM, Liu CL, Wong J. Intrahepatic recurrence after curative resection of hepatocellular carcinoma. Long-term results of treatment and prognostic factors. Ann Surg 1999; 229: 216–22

109. Pichlmayr R, Weimann A, Ringe B. Indications for liver transplantation in hepatobiliary malignancy. Hepatology 1994; 20: 33S–40S

110. Nagasue N, Kohno H, Chang YC et al. Liver resection for hepatocellular carcinoma: results of 229 consecutive patients during 11 years. Ann Surg 1993; 217: 375–84

111. Mazzaferro V, Regalia E, Doci R et al. Liver transplantation for the treatment of small hepatocellular carcinomas in patients with cirrhosis. N Engl J Med 1996; 334: 693–9

112. Mazzaferro V, Rondinara GF, Rossi G et al. Milan multicenter experience in liver transplantation for hepatocellular carcinoma, Transplant Proc 1994; 26: 3557–60

113. Regalia E, Sansalone C, Mazzaferro V et al. Pattern of recurrence of hepatocellular carcinoma after liver transplantation: Milan multicenter experience. Transplant Proc 1994; 26: 3579–80

114. Marsh JW, Dvorchik I, Subotin M et al. The prediction of risk of recurrence and time to recurrence of hepato-cellular carcinoma after orthotopic liver transplantation: a pilot study. Hepatology 1997; 26: 444–50

115. Elias D, Debaere T, Roche A, Bonvallot S, Lasser P. Preoperative selective portal vein embolizations are an effective means of extending the indications of major hepatectomy in the normal and injured liver. Hepatogastroenterology 1998; 45: 170–7

116. Majno PE, Sarasin FP, Mentha G, Hadengue A. Primary liver resection and salvage transplantation or primary liver transplantation in patients with single, small hepatocellular carcinoma and preserved liver function: an outcome-orientated decision analysis. Hepatology 2000; 31: 899–906

117. Romani F, Belli LS, Rondinara GF et al. The role of transplantation in small hepatocellular carcinoma complicating cirrhosis of the liver. J Am Coll Surg 1994; 178: 379–84

118. Schwartz ME, Sung M, Mor E et al. A multidisciplinary approach to hepatocellular carcinoma in patients with cirrhosis. J Am Coll Surg 1995; 180: 596–603

119. Colella G, De Carlis L, Rondinara GF et al. Is hepatocellular carcinoma in cirrhosis an actual indication for liver transplantation? Transplant Proc 1997; 29: 492–4

120. Otto G, Heuschen U, Hofmann WJ, Krumm HG, Hinz U, Herfarth C. Is transplantation really superior to resection in the treatment of small hepatocellular carcinoma? Transplant Proc 1997; 29: 489–91

121. Hemming AW, Cattral MS, Reed AI et al. Liver transplantation for hepatocellular carcinoma. Ann Surg 2001; 233: 652–9

122. Figueras J, Garcia-Valdecasas JC, Rafecas A et al. Prognosis of hepatocarcinoma in liver transplantation in cirrhotic patients. Transplant Proc 1997; 29: 495

6 Small solitary hepatic metastases: when and how?

David L Bartlett and Yuman Fong

Introduction

The management of patients with small hepatic metastases from colorectal cancer and other histologies requires the consideration of many diverse patient and tumor related factors. These factors include the natural history of the tumor type, the expected cure rate after surgical treatment, effectiveness of alternative treatments, and the morbidity of surgical resection. In general, the indications for any major surgical procedure include the potential for cure, prolongation of survival and palliation of symptoms. For metastatic tumors to the liver in selected cases the cure rate may be over 50% for colorectal cancer,[1] but will be exceedingly rare for other histologies such as gastric cases, and melanoma and sarcoma. Small metastases to the liver generally do not cause symptoms (except for hormone secreting neuroendocrine tumors) and, therefore, palliation of symptoms is not a common indication for management of these lesions. Nevertheless, many issues remain unresolved. Does resection of a small solitary hepatic metastasis prolong survival in cases where the patient is likely to develop widespread metastases in the future? Is there any harm in allowing a tumor to go untreated for a period of time, knowing that with close follow-up the resection option may still be possible in the future? Do metastases metastasize such that a delay in management may obviate the curative option? Unfortunately, all of these difficult issues are only addressed by sparse data in the literature.

The risk and extent of the surgical procedure plays a significant role in the decision making for management of small hepatic metastases. It is more reasonable to excise an enlarged subcutaneous lymph node for metastatic cancer than it is to perform a hepatic lobectomy when the chance of benefit is low in both cases. As other less invasive ablative options become routine therapy, it may be reasonable to consider these options in cases where surgical resection is unreasonable. These alternative options include percutaneous approaches at ablation such as radiofrequency ablation and percutaneous alcohol injection.[2] Laparoscopic procedures may also be an alternative for the management of small hepatic metastases, including laparoscopic resection of tumors and laparoscopically directed ablation such as cryotherapy. If the risks, discomfort, and hospital stay are truly minimal, then it becomes reasonable to consider local treatment of these lesions, even with a small chance of overall benefit to the patient.

This chapter will provide an overview of the data on survival benefit after resection of hepatic metastases and the techniques of surgical management. A brief discussion of minimally invasive and percutaneous procedures for management of small solitary hepatic metastases will follow. In addition, a discussion of the role for adjuvant therapy after resection or ablation of the hepatic metastases will be included.

Survival results for hepatic metastasectomy

While the purpose of this chapter is not to provide an in-depth review of the results of hepatic metastasectomy, a general sense of expected cure rate and prolongation of survival after hepatic metastasectomy for various histologies is required in order to make an informed decision regarding resection of small hepatic metastases.

Colorectal metastases

Colorectal cancer, compared to other histologies, is more likely to present as disease isolated to the liver. The natural history of unresected solitary hepatic

Table 6.1 Survival after hepatic resection for a solitary colorectal metastasis

Author	Date	N	Actuarial 5-year survival (%)	Median survival (months)
Hughes et al.[6]	1988	509	37	—
Rosen et al.[7]	1992	185	30	—
Scheele et al.[8]	1995	180	36[a]	45
Taylor et al.[9]	1997	77	47	54
Fong et al.[10]	1997	240	47	—

[a]Actual 5-year survival.

metastases from colorectal cancer was described by Wagner et al. where 39 patients with solitary metastases did not undergo therapy and the median survival was 24 months.[3] Wood et al. described 15 patients with solitary hepatic metastases left untreated with a mean survival of 17 months.[4]

There is a considerable body of literature on the results of hepatic metastasectomy for colorectal cancer. The overall 5-year survival ranges from 22% to 39%.[5] In many studies, low number and small size are associated with improved prognosis such that a small solitary metastasis from colorectal cancer has a greater than 50% 5-year survival. Nuzzo et al. report 56% actuarial 5-year survival in patients with solitary metachronous hepatic metastases from colorectal cancer less than 4 cm in size.[1] Table 6.1 reviews the results of the largest series for solitary metastasectomy. After resection of solitary metastases from colorectal cancer, 5-year survival ranges from 30% to 47%.[6–10] These reports do not consider the small solitary metastases separately from the entire group of solitary metastases. The size of the lesion is expected to affect prognosis and, therefore, the actual results for small solitary hepatic metastases may be even better than the numbers reported in Table 6.1. Liver resection for hepatic colorectal metastases is, therefore, safe and effective, and may be curative.

Neuroendocrine metastases

For cancers of other than colorectal origin, patients with hepatic metastases from neuroendocrine tumors have been thought to be the most likely to benefit from surgical resection. Certainly, if the tumor were symptomatic for either hormonal or physical reasons, resection should be considered even though cure is unlikely. Because of the indolent nature of these tumors, durable palliation can be achieved with cytoreduction. Five-year survival rates for untreated hepatic metastases from neuroendocrine tumors have ranged from 13 to 54%.[11–15]

In patients with no symptoms, the case for surgical resection, or any treatment for that matter, is less clear. We and others[16] have adopted a very aggressive approach even for asymptomatic tumors based only on retrospective data. Chen et al. compared liver resection for neuroendocrine tumors with a retrospectively matched cohort who did not undergo resection, demonstrating improved survival after resection.[17] The general recommendation is for aggressive surgical management of neuroendocrine metastasis.[18] We acknowledge that the variable growth rate and sometimes indolent nature of these tumors make firm conclusions based on retrospective data without a non-treated control group suspect. The rarity of these tumors, however, does not allow for random assignment trials. Certainly for small hepatic metastases, aggressive surgical resection is indicated, while it is acknowledged that definitive proof of its benefit may never be achieved.

Non-colorectal, non-neuroendocrine metastases

For histologies other than colorectal or neuroendocrine cancer, the utility of hepatic metastasectomy is not as obvious. For these tumors the liver is rarely the sole site of disease; liver metastases are rarely the ultimate cause of death, nor does it contribute significantly to symptoms prior to death. Nevertheless, selected cases of disease isolated to the liver after a long disease-free interval raise the possibility of a single site of metastatic disease that could be cured with surgical therapy. Table 6.2 reviews the largest series for hepatic metastasectomy with a variety of histologies.

Breast cancer
Many reviews have been published on hepatic metastasectomy for breast cancer. Due to the high incidence of breast cancer and the frequency of liver metastases for this histology, the first site of metastases is frequently observed to be hepatic. In highly selected patients, favorable results of section of such liver metastases have been reported. Raab et al. reported a 5-year survival of 18.4% in 34 patients after hepatic metastasectomy for breast cancer.[19] Elias et al reported 9% 5-year survival after resection in 21 patients.[20] The relatively few patients in these reports compared to the total number of breast cancer patients in each institution during the study period reflect the degree of patient selection for surgery. The survival rates reported are actuarial survival rates and the actual cure rate is much lower. At most, hepatic metastasectomy for breast cancer should be

Table 6.2 **Survival following hepatic metastasectomy for non-colorectal histologies**

Author	Histology	N	Actuarial 5-year survival (%)	Median survival (months)
Chen et al.[17]	Neuroendocrine	15	73	NR
Que et al.[57]	Neuroendocrine	74	73[a]	NR
Harrison et al.[26]	Genitourinary[b]	34	60	NR
Jaques et al.[21]	Sarcoma	14	0	30
Harrison et al.[26]	Breast/melanoma/sarcoma	41	26	32
Elias et al.[20]	Breast	21	9	26
Raab et al.[19]	Breast	34	18	27
Ochiai et al.[24]	Gastric	21	19[c]	18
Bines et al.[25]	Gastric	7	14[d]	15
Harrison et al.[26]	Gastrointestinal[e]	7	0	25

[a]4-year survival.
[b]Includes renal (5), testicular (9), adrenal (7), ovary (7), uterine (4), cervix (2).
[c]4 of 21 actual 5-year survivors.
[d]1 of 7 actual 5-year survivors.
[e]Includes gastric (5), pancreatic (2).
NR: not reached.

considered cytoreductive. It may delay the development of symptoms and prolong survival, but it has very little chance of curing the disease.

Sarcoma

Similarly, hepatic resection for sarcoma metastases may be associated with long-term survival in highly selected patients, but it is unlikely to result in cure. In a series of 14 hepatic resections for metastatic sarcoma, recurrence was found in all patients during follow-up, and 11 of 14 failed in the liver.[21] The median survival in that series was 30 months.

Melanoma

Metastatic cutaneous melanoma to the liver has been resected with long-term survival, but these tumors also ultimately recur.[22] The erratic behavior of melanoma makes conclusions regarding the benefit of hepatic metastasectomy difficult. Only in highly selected cases is it appropriate to consider resection of cutaneous melanoma. Ocular melanoma, on the other hand, has a unique natural history. Ocular melanoma preferentially metastasizes to the liver and the majority of patients die of liver failure as a direct result of tumor progression. Anecdotal reports exist of long-term survival after metastasectomy for ocular melanoma,[23] although these tumors are also almost always multifocal and resection of what appears to be a solitary metastasis is most often associated with liver recurrence. These hepatic metastases may show up many years after the treatment of the primary tumor. A long

disease-free interval reflects a slow tumor doubling time, and suggests resection may achieve durable palliation. Usually in this disease, however, the appearance of a solitary liver metastasis is merely a precursor of the later appearance of multiple metastases.

Other gastrointestinal cancers

In general, hepatic metastasectomy for gastrointestinal primaries other than colorectal is not associated with prolonged survival. For tumors such as esophageal, gastric, small bowel, and pancreatic cancer the pattern of spread includes regional lymph nodes, the peritoneal cavity, and lung metastases in addition to liver metastases. It is unlikely that these patients will die of liver failure as a result of progression of hepatic metastases, but instead, suffer other gastrointestinal sequelae from extrahepatic tumor progression. A major operative procedure can be of significant detriment to these patients with aggressive cancers where survival is expected to be of the order of weeks to months. Nevertheless, even for these tumors selected cases exist where one might consider resection, and the literature contains anecdotal reports of long-term survivors after liver resection.[24,25]

Genitourinary tumors

For non-colorectal, non-neuroendocrine tumors, metastases from genitourinary primaries seem to have the best prognosis following hepatic metastasectomy. In a recent review by Harrison et al.,

34 patients underwent hepatic resections for genitourinary primaries (including testicular, adrenal, ovary, renal, uterine, and cervix) with a 5-year actuarial survival of 60%.[26] Other investigators have reported prolonged survival after resection for renal cell cancer[27] and adrenal cancer.[28] While the natural history of genitourinary tumors contributes to these remarkable results, it does suggest a survival benefit to resection in selective cases.

Do metastases metastasize?

For small solitary hepatic metastases, where many months of growth would still not preclude resection, the question is whether a waiting period would allow for further spread of the tumor from the metastatic deposit itself. If metastatic tumors were unable to further metastasize, waiting for the first sign of progression prior to initiating treatment and allowing other metastatic disease to declare itself would seem a reasonable approach. If, however, metastases are able to spread during that waiting period, then the chance of potential cure may be adversely affected by the delay in definitive treatment. Unfortunately, it is clear that metastatic tumors do have the potential to metastasize themselves, and this must be considered when recommending observation alone.

Experimental evidence suggests that cells from spontaneous metastases are more likely to metastasize than cells populating the parent neoplasm.[29] Clinically, the most obvious examples of metastases from metastatic colorectal cancer deposits are in the cases of perihepatic lymph node metastases,[30] and satellite-tumor formation.[31]

Published data would indicate that metastases to periportal lymph nodes occur in 10–20% of cases of hepatic colorectal metastases.[30] The presence of lymph node metastases portends a poor prognosis. Therefore, excision of liver tumors before they spread to regional lymph nodes would be advantageous.

A recent paper examined the incidence of satellite micrometastasis in colorectal liver metastases by careful histologic examination of resection specimens and found that 56% of specimens had micrometastases as far as 3.8 cm away from the tumor being resected.[31] In some cases, these satellites could be traced to the original metastasis by a trail of cells, suggesting spread from the original metastasis. As discussed previously, the presence of satellitosis is an important independent poor prognostic factor. It may be that a delay in resection allows for the development of satellitosis, which negatively impacts on prognosis. On the other hand,

the presence of satellitosis may be an indicator of biologic aggressiveness which portends a poor prognosis regardless of when the tumor is resected.

Patient selection

Colorectal metastases

In order to decide when surgical resection is reasonable for small solitary hepatic metastases, it is important to review prognostic factors which are independent of size and number that may influence the decision regarding management of these tumors. Many studies have examined data on prognostic factors for outcome after hepatic resection for colorectal metastases. The time to development of liver tumor after resection of the primary, pathologic margin, stage of the primary tumor, tumor number, carcinoembryonic antigen levels, satellitosis, extrahepatic disease, and positive surgical margin have all been shown to predict survival after hepatic resection for colorectal metastases independent of size.[7,8,10,32]

Extrahepatic disease is considered a contraindication to hepatic resection. Even the presence of perihepatic lymph nodes portends a poor prognosis and generally is felt to be a contraindication to resection. Particularly in the cases of small solitary hepatic metastases with extrahepatic disease, there would be no advantage to resection or ablation of the liver tumor because systemic disease will likely be the ultimate cause of death regardless of what is done with the liver metastases. Of the other various factors that are prognostic for outcome, surgical margin, and satellitosis are the least useful in patient selection. No one would subject a patient to surgical resection expecting a positive margin. Satellitosis cannot be easily assessed preoperatively and therefore is a poor selection criterion for surgery.

We analyzed our recent data on factors prognostic for outcome after resection of hepatic metastases from colorectal cancer.[33] In data derived from our last 1001 liver resections for this disease, the seven factors found to be independent predictors of poor long-term outcome were:

(1) node positive outcome,
(2) presentation of liver disease within 12 months of the primary cancer,
(3) CEA >200 ng/dl,
(4) number of liver tumors >1,
(5) size >5 cm,
(6) positive margin, and
(7) extrahepatic disease.

From this we formulated a clinical risk score (CRS) based on the first five of these factors for use in

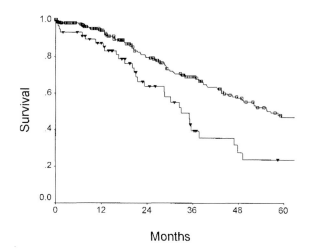

Figure 6.1 Prediction of long-term outcome for small (<3 cm) (N = 293) metastatic deposits based on clinical risk score (CRS). CRS is based on the following five criteria: (1) node positive primary cancer, (2) disease-free interval <12 months, (3) number of liver tumors >1, (4) size of liver tumor >5 cm and (5) CEA >200 ng/dl. For score = 0–2 (N = 236) (open box), the median survival was 56 months and the 5-year survival 47%. For score = 3–4 (N = 57) (filled triangles), the median survival was 32 months and the 5-year survival 24%.

patient selection for surgery and for stratification of patients for clinical studies. Using one point for each criterion, a summed score of 0–2 puts patients in a low risk group and is a strong indication for hepatectomy. In the patients with small tumors, a maximum score of 4 is possible. The 5-year survival of patients with small tumors and 0–2 points on the CRS is 47% and the median survival is 56 months.[33] Patients with a score of 3–4 are in a high risk group, with a median survival of 32 months and 5-year survival of 24% (Fig. 6.1). In these high risk patients, a period of observation with no therapy or systemic chemotherapy allowing for the extent of metastases to declare themselves is reasonable. Improved imaging techniques such as fluorodeoxyglucose positron emission tomography (FDG PET) scanning should be considered and may help discover extrahepatic disease non-invasively in these patients at high risk for additional cancer.[34] Finally, these patients should be considered for clinical studies of aggressive adjuvant chemotherapy after liver resection.

Neuroendocrine tumors

Patients with symptomatic neuroendocrine tumors should be considered for resection or ablation. For the small tumor, symptoms are most likely derived from hormonal secretion by the tumors, and such hormone levels will also provide a marker for effectiveness of the ablation or resection. For asymptomatic tumors, a

period of observation to allow assessment of the pace and aggressiveness of the tumors is reasonable when the tumors are small. At the first signs of progression, resection or ablation should be considered.

Non-colorectal, non-neuroendocrine tumors

Harrison et al. defined prognostic factors involved in the resection of non-colorectal, non-neuroendocrine hepatic metastases.[26] In this study, 96 patients underwent liver resection. The prognostic factors of significance on multivariate analysis included the disease-free interval (>36 months), curative resection (versus palliative incomplete resection) and primary tumor type. Their conclusions would suggest that regardless of histology, with a long disease-free interval patients may benefit from surgical resection.

Resection techniques

For small solitary metastases to the liver, the goal of resection is to completely excise the tumor while preserving the maximum normal hepatic parenchyma. Preserving parenchyma facilitates postoperative recovery and also provides flexibility for further resections should intrahepatic recurrences occur.[35] Small surface oriented metastases can be excised using a non-anatomic wedge resection, whereas deeper lesions require formal segmentectomies or sectorectomies. A goal of at least a 1 cm margin is reasonable.[36] The use of intraoperative ultrasound is important to rule out other small hepatic metastases which may not be evident on preoperative scans and in defining the intersegmental planes for designing the approach to segmentectomy. Even for wedge resections, ultrasound is beneficial in defining the vascular anatomy around the lesion, which may help minimize blood loss.

Wedge resections

Wedge resections must be performed meticulously to avoid inadvertently leaving a positive margin. Large chromic liver sutures can be placed and used for retraction during dissection. The parenchymal dissection should be performed along the lines used for other forms of liver resection. We prefer the Kelly clamp technique where the clamp is used to crush the normal parenchyma, exposing vessels that are then clipped, tied, suture ligated or stapled using a vascular stapling device.[37] The Pringle maneuver is used intermittently for 5 minutes at a time followed by reperfusion of the parenchyma, during which time the argon beam coagulator is used to coagulate small bleeding vessels on the surface. This technique is superior to the simple use of electrocautery for the dissection which is often attempted for what seems to be routine wedge resections. The char effect of the electrocautery prevents adequate visualization of the anatomy, making it quite easy to stray into large vessels or into the tumor.

The most difficult margin in performing a wedge resection is the deep margin of dissection. Using intraoperative ultrasound, the depth of dissection should be measured prior to the initiation of parenchymal dissection, including at least a 1 cm margin deep to the tumor. The dissection should be carried down perpendicular to the liver surface to the predetermined depth. At this point the tumor can be lifted up and dissection can proceed horizontally across the base of the wedge. The tendency to resect with a 'V-shaped approach' is more likely to be complicated by a positive deep margin. At the end of the dissection the Pringle maneuver is removed and the argon beam coagulator is used to control bleeding vessels. Careful examination is made for any evidence of a bile leak, which is controlled with suture ligature.

For larger lesions where it is especially difficult to achieve the deep margin safely, a cryoassisted wedge resection can be performed.[38] The cryotherapy probe is inserted into the tumor and freezing is begun with real time ultrasound imaging. When the zone of freezing is confirmed by ultrasound to be at least 1 cm beyond the tumor, wedge resection is performed using the freeze margin as the margin of resection. The cryotherapy probe makes a ready retracting device and the parenchyma is usually easy to dissect at the margin of the ice-ball. Freezing must continue intermittently during dissection to ensure that the ice-ball does not retract and expose the tumor.

Segmental resections

For all but the most superficial lesions, we prefer a segmental approach for the resection of tumor.[39] Segmental resections have a significantly lower rate of pathologic positive margins, and this translates into improved long-term survival.[40] Small, deep solitary metastases and surface lesions adjacent to major vascular structures lend themselves particularly well to segmentectomies or sectorectomies. The intersegmental planes can be identified intraoperatively using vascular landmarks with the aid of intraoperative ultrasound. Using these planes for parenchymal dissection will minimize blood loss and help ensure a safe margin.

Inflow occlusion for the segment can almost always be performed first, thereby producing demarcation of the segmental planes to further enhance the dissection. The portal triad to segments II, III and IV can be identified and controlled within the umbilical fissure with little parenchymal dissection.[37] The right posterior sectoral pedicle can be found by dividing the parenchyma along a horizontal cleft (fissure of Gans) present on the inferior surface of the right lobe of the liver. The pedicle can be traced to its bifurcation to segments VI and VII for control of the individual segmental portal triads. The anterior sectoral pedicle can be dissected from an inferior or anterior approach.

The major hepatic veins lie within the intersegmental planes, and can be a source of significant blood loss during the parenchymal transection phase of a segmentectomy. The use of low central venous pressure (0–5 mmHg) during parenchymal dissection can decrease back bleeding in these veins.[41] Extrahepatic control of the left, middle and right hepatic veins can also be achieved and the vein of concern temporarily clamped at its junction with the vena cava during parenchymal transection to further minimize blood loss.

When the solitary metastases lies near an intersegmental plane, two segments can be removed. This is most easily done as a formal sector such as the left lateral sectorectomy (segments II and III) and right posterior sectorectomy (segments VI and VII). The caudate lobe (segment I) can be resected as an isolated segmentectomy when the tumor is confined to this lobe.[42] This requires a more extensive dissection, including complete division of all the perforating caudate veins draining directly into the vena cava as well as the numerous small portal triads extending off the main left pedicle at the base of the umbilical fissure.

Figure 6.2 demonstrates a case of a small, solitary segment of hepatic metastasis for colorectal cancer which was detected on an MRI scan used for screening because of a rising CEA. Although this was a surface lesion, intraoperative ultrasound revealed the segment VI triad immediately adjacent to the tumor. The segment VI triad was located by ultrasound and ligated at its origin with minimal parenchymal dissection. The intersegmental planes were then marked by electrocautery and a formal segmentectomy was performed with negative margins. While an aggressive resection was indicated and performed, the patient can still undergo a formal left or right hepatic lobectomy in the future if indicated. No dissection of the vena cava or porta hepatis was required.

Morbidity and mortality

The mortality rates for major hepatic resection have decreased significantly over time to a common

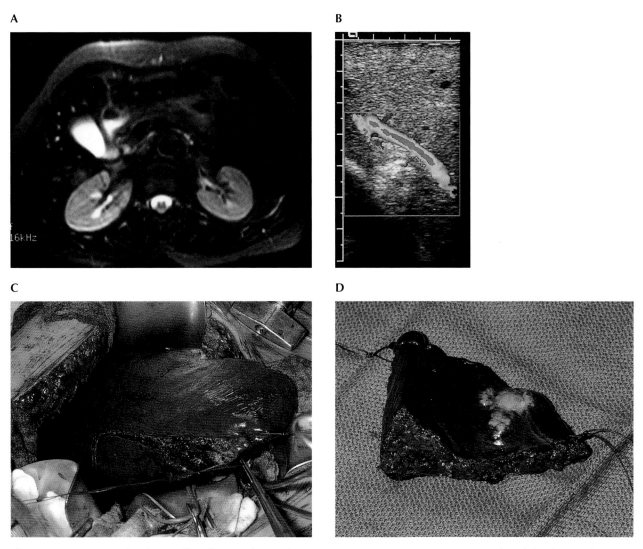

Figure 6.2 An example of a small, solitary colorectal metastasis to segment VI. (A) MRI reveals subtle abnormality not seen on CT scan. (B) Intraoperative ultrasound reveals the tumor and adjacent segment VI portal vein. (C) Intersegmental planes have been marked on the liver capsule with electrocautery and parenchymal dissection begun. (D) Resected segment with tumor (microscopic negative margins). (Special thanks to Dr Peter Choyke for MRI scan.)

reporting of mortality in the 1–4% range.[43] These values are even lower for wedge resections and segmentectomies. In a recent report of 270 wedge or segmental resections, the operative mortality was 0.5%.[40] This low mortality is not surprising considering that the main cause of death in studies of liver resection is liver failure secondary to inadequate residual normal parenchyma, an unlikely event for resection of small solitary hepatic metastases where minimal normal parenchyma is sacrificed.

While mortality rates are low, the complication rate for major hepatic resection is still relatively high, ranging from 20% to 50%.[5] Bile leaks, perihepatic abscess, hemorrhage, cardiopulmonary complications, pleural effusions, pneumonia, and pulmonary embolism are among the most common complications.[43] Many of these could be expected after segmentectomy and wedge resections as well as major hepatic resections. Even though these complications do not translate into a high mortality rate, they may affect recovery time and quality of life. While this is not a significant issue for patients expected to undergo a long-term disease-free interval or cure, it may be significant for patients whose survival is expected to be of the order of months. For those patients with aggressive tumors who are likely to fail outside the liver in the near future, less invasive techniques which are associated with a lower complication rate and quicker recovery time are more appealing.

Ablative techniques

Other minimally invasive techniques include local ablative therapies such as laparoscopically directed

A

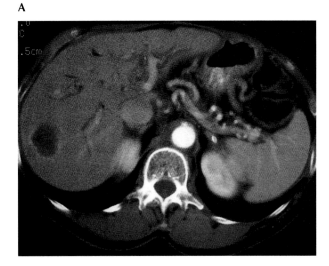

C

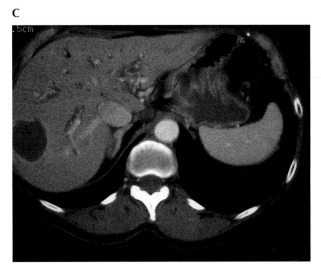

B

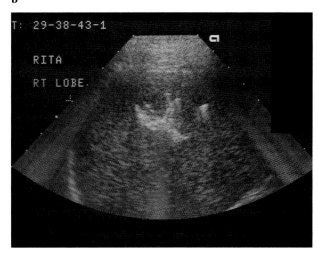

Figure 6.3 An example of a small, solitary pancreatic cancer metastasis treated with percutaneous radiofrequency ablation. (A) Pretreatment CT scan reveals hypodense 3 cm right lobe liver metastasis. (B) Ultrasound photo with radiofrequency probe inserted into tumor. (C) Post-treatment scan (3 weeks) reveals large zone of necrosis replacing prior tumor. (Special thanks to Dr Thomas Shawker for ultrasound photo.)

cryotherapy[44] or radiofrequency ablation.[45] These techniques will be discussed further in Chapter 8. They provide ideal alternatives to laparotomy and major liver resection for the treatment of small solitary hepatic metastases, since the small tumor is the most likely to be completely treated by ablation techniques. Furthermore, treatment by ablative techniques does not preclude future resection.

Percutaneous approaches to tumor ablation are even more attractive than laparoscopic procedures. Local injection of toxic agents such as ethanol has been shown to be effective for hepatocellular cancers, however these agents have not been proven for other histologies and are known to be poorly effective for colorectal cancer.[2] Radiofrequency ablation can be performed percutaneously under ultrasound guidance with local anesthesia. Figure 6.3 demonstrates a case of a metastatic pancreatic cancer 2 years after a dramatic primary response to gemcitabine and radiation therapy. Because the patient will likely begin to fail in multiple sites in the near future with limited survival potential, a

laparotomy and hepatic resection was not considered reasonable. She was treated with percutaneous radiofrequency ablation, achieving a good zone of necrosis encompassing the mass, and she spent only one day in the hospital with very minimal discomfort. How such procedures, which have low morbidity and which maintain quality of life, will factor in the treatment of patients with small hepatic metastases must be addressed by studies with sufficient follow-up to define the local recurrence rate.

Adjuvant chemotherapy

The role for adjuvant systemic chemotherapy after the removal of small solitary hepatic metastases is not well defined. Even for hepatic colorectal metastases, which are commonly treated with surgery, data on adjuvant chemotherapy after liver resection is sparse. Two retrospective studies have suggested a benefit of adjuvant systemic chemotherapy after

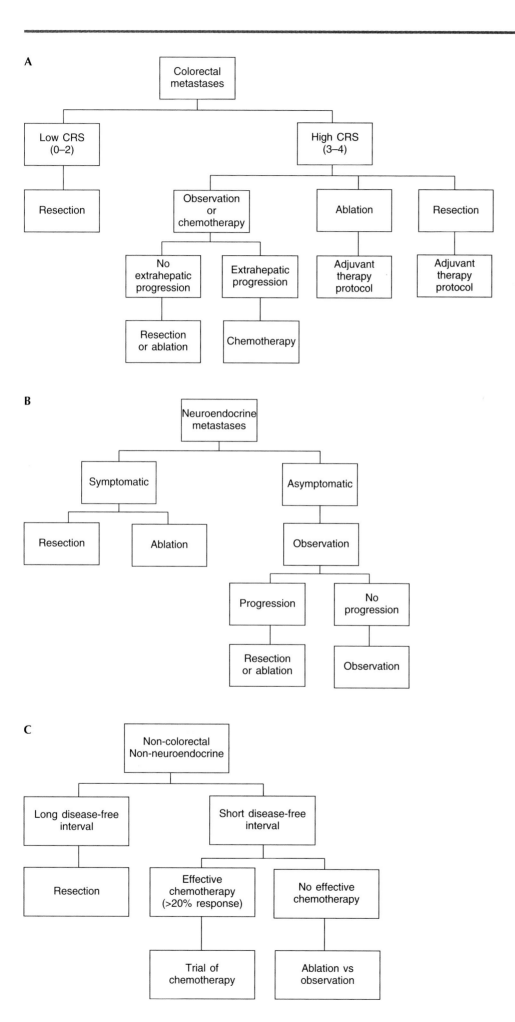

Figure 6.4 Algorithms for the management of small hepatic metastases. (A) Algorithm for colorectal metastases (CRS, clinical risk score). (B) Algorithm for neuroendocrine metastases. (C) Algorithm for non-colorectal, non-neuroendocrine metastases.

metastasectomy, but others have not supported this.[6,46–48] Use of systemic chemotherapy after resection of hepatic colorectal metastases is based mainly on data demonstrating adjuvant 5-fluorouracil (5-FU) and levamisol or 5-FU and leucovorin to decrease recurrence rate and improve survival when used after resection of the primary tumor.[49] It is hoped that a similar benefit will be seen when 5-FU-based chemotherapy is used after metastasectomy. Current practice is to offer adjuvant 5-FU-based chemotherapy after hepatic resection to patients who have had no previous chemotherapy. There are currently no data to support the use of irinotecan and oxaliplatin in an adjuvant setting, although studies are in progress.

For patients with hepatic colorectal metastases, the most common site of tumor recurrence after liver resection is the remnant liver.[50] In the treatment of patients with small hepatic metastases, there is particular concern that even smaller undetected metastases may subsequently present as a liver tumor recurrence. Regional chemotherapy to treat the liver site is therefore a theoretically attractive option for adjuvant care. Data addressing the utility for such hepatic arterial infusional (HAI) chemotherapy had been sparse, consisting only of four small single arm studies[51–53] and a single, small, randomized trial consisting of 36 patients.[54] These preliminary studies demonstrated safety of such an approach, but efficacy data were insufficient to support the routine use of adjuvant intra-arterial chemotherapy. Two large randomized trials examining adjuvant HAI have been completed. In the first trial,[55] 224 patients from 25 centers were randomized to either no adjuvant therapy, or adjuvant HAI 5-FU + systemic folinic acid. Although no difference was found between the groups, technical factors compromised this study such that only 34 of the 114 patients randomized to chemotherapy completed the adjuvant treatments. In another study, Kemeny et al. randomized 156 patients to either systemic 5-FU + leucovorin or HAI floxuridine (FUDR) + systemic 5-FU after complete resection of tumor.[56] There was a significant survival advantage to HAI that is most likely related to local liver tumor control. We believe HAI chemotherapy is effective and should be considered as an adjuvant to resection of hepatic colorectal metastases.

For non-colorectal, non-neuroendocrine histologies metastatic to the liver the most likely cause of death will be related to the disease outside the liver, regardless of how the liver is managed. For patients who are likely to develop systemic metastases in the near future it may be reasonable to offer chemotherapy prior to resection. If the tumor responds then a resection will be performed with confidence that other micrometastatic disease may be effectively treated with chemotherapy. If the tumor does not respond and the liver remains the only site of metastatic disease, resection is performed with increased confidence conferred by the longer period of observation. If the patient advances systemically during chemotherapy then it is very unlikely that a resection would have been of benefit and the patient will have avoided the potential morbidity, pain, discomfort and recovery time of an hepatic resection. That patient can go on to obtain second-line chemotherapy, investigational chemotherapy, or have no additional treatment.

Conclusions

Algorithms for the management of small solitary hepatic metastases are shown in Figure 6.4. Both patient and tumor characteristics must be considered in making management decisions. The most important tumor related characteristic is histology. For patients with colorectal cancer (Fig. 6.4A), the prognostic factors for tumor recurrence after resection are well defined. Using the clinical risk score (CRS) as selection criterion, patients with CRS = 0–2 are ideal candidates for resection. Those with CRS = 3–4 should consider observation or chemotherapy prior to a definitive hepatic procedure. Immediate ablation or resection should be performed in the setting of a clinical trial, and most appropriately a trial examining adjuvant therapy.

For neuroendocrine cancers (Fig. 6.4B), symptomatic tumors should be treated with resection and/or ablation when possible. When the cancer is found in an asymptomatic patient, a period of observation is not unreasonable because of the often indolent nature of these tumors. At resection, the principle should be to leave as much normal liver behind in order to minimize the risk of liver failure and in order to allow for repeat anatomic liver resections in the future for recurrent disease. Enucleation with positive margins is acceptable for treatment of this histology because resection is almost never curative, and such cytoreduction can provide significant and durable palliation with minimum risk.

For patients with small, solitary, non-colorectal non-neuroendocrine tumors the most significant factor in terms of prognosis seems to be the disease-free interval (Fig. 6.4C). For patients with a long disease-free interval from primary resection a curative surgical resection is indicated as the most effective means of therapy. While it may be still unlikely that these patients can be cured, they must be given the benefit of the doubt and the most optimal procedure performed. The definition of 'long' has been arbitrarily set at 36 months by Harrison et al.,[26] but in reality it must vary according to histology. For gastric cancer, 12–24 months would be considered long, whereas for ocular melanoma, 3–5 years would be more reasonable.

Patients with a short disease-free interval from a tumor with a poor prognosis should undergo a trial of chemotherapy if there is a known effective agent. If no effective agent exists (as is the case for most solid malignancies), then these patients are ideal for an experimental, minimally invasive, local ablative therapy. This provides an advantage to observation alone, given the low but definite risk of the metastases spreading during the observation period. It will be psychologically more comforting to the patient to know that the lesion has been ablated, and risk, pain and recovery duration are minimal. Observation alone is also quite reasonable, but it is often not accepted by patients. Patient related factors must also be taken into consideration. Patients who have concomitant illnesses which make them poor operative candidates may be better served with a minimally invasive or percutaneous technique, even in the case of potentially curable metastases from colorectal cancer.

Because of improvements in diagnostic techniques and the routine use of serum tumor markers, the detection of small solitary hepatic metastases from various tumors will likely increase in the future. A uniform approach to these patients such as that which is outlined in the treatment algorithm should be considered.

Key points

Factors that determine management

- Natural history of tumor type
- Expected cure rate after surgical treatment
- Effectiveness of alternative treatment strategies
- Morbidity of surgical resection.

Survival rates following hepatic resection

- Good evidence for long-term survival
  Colorectal metastases
  Neuroendocrine metastases.
- Survival possible in highly selected cases
  Breast cancer
  Sarcoma (especially gastrointestinal stromal tumors)
  Melanoma.

Patient selection factors in colorectal metastases

- Contraindications
  Extrahepatic disease (except solitary pulmonary metastases)
  Positive hilar lymph nodes.
- Relative contraindications
  Presentation within 12 months of resection of primary tumor
  CEA >200 ng/dl
  >1 liver tumor
  Tumor >5 cm in size
  Positive resection margin.

REFERENCES

1. Nuzzo G, Giuliante F, Giovannini I, Tebala GD, Clemente G, Vellone M. Resection of hepatic metastases from colorectal cancer. Hepato-gastroenterology 1997; 44: 751–9
2. Alexander HR, Bartlett DL, Fraker DL, Libutti SK. Regional treatment strategies for unresectable primary or metastatic cancer confined to the liver. In: DeVita VT Jr, Hellman S, Rosenberg SA, eds. Cancer: principles and practice of oncology. Philadelphia: JB Lippincott, 1996: 1–19
3. Wagner JS, Adson MA, van Heerden JA, Adson MD, Ilstrup DM. The natural history of hepatic metastases from colorectal cancer. A comparison with resective treatment. Ann Surg 1984; 199: 502–8
4. Wood CB, Gillis CR, Blumgart LH. A retrospective study of the natural history of patients with liver metastases from colorectal cancer. Clin Oncol 1976; 2: 285–8
5. Fong Y, Blumgart LH, Cohen AM. Surgical treatment of colorectal metastases to the liver. CA Cancer J Clin 1995; 45: 50–62
6. Hughes KS, Simon R, Songhorabodi S. Resection of the liver for colorectal carcinoma metastases: a multi-institutional study of indications for resection. Surgery 1988; 103: 278–88
7. Rosen CB, Nagorney DM, Taswell HF et al. Perioperative blood transfusion and determinants of survival after liver resection for metastatic colorectal carcinoma. Ann Surg 1992; 216: 493–505
8. Scheele J, Stang R, Altendort-Hofmann A, Paul M. Resection of colorectal liver metastases. World J Surg 1995; 19: 59–71
9. Taylor M, Forster J, Langer B, Taylor BR, Greig PD, Mahut C. A study of prognostic factors for hepatic resection for colorectal metastases. Am J Surg 1997; 173: 467–71

10. Fong Y, Cohen AM, Fortner JG et al. Liver resection for colorectal metastases. J Clin Oncol 1997; 15: 938–46

11. Moertel CG. An odyssey in the land of small tumors. J Clin Oncol 1987; 5: 1503–22

12. Thompson GB, van Heerden JA, Grant CS, Carney JA, Ilstrup DM. Islet cell carcinomas of the pancreas: a twenty-year experience. Surgery 1988; 104: 1011–7

13. Declore R, Friesen SR. Gastrointestinal neuroendocrine tumors. J Am Coll Surg 1994; 178: 188–211

14. Godwin JD. Carcinoid tumors: an analysis of 2837 cases. Cancer 1975; 36: 560–9

15. Sjoblom SM. Clinical presentation and prognosis of gastrointestinal carcinoid tumours. Scand J Gastroenterol 1988; 23: 779–87

16. McEntee GP, Nagourney DMN, Kvols LK, Moertel CG, Grant CS. Cytoreductive hepatic surgery for neuroendocrine tumors. Surgery 1990; 108: 1091

17. Chen H, Hardacre JM, Uzra A, Cameron JL, Choti MA. Isolated liver metastases from neuroendocrine tumors: does resection prolong survival? J Am Coll Surg 1998; 187: 88–92

18. Ihse I, Persson B, Tibblin S. Neuroendocrine metastases of the liver. World J Surg 1995; 19: 76–82

19. Raab R, Nussbaum KT, Behrend M, Weimann A. Liver metastases of breast cancer: results of liver resection. Anticancer Res 1998; 18: 2231–3

20. Elias D, Lasser PH, Montrucolli D, Bonvallot S, Spielmann M. Hepatectomy for liver metastases from breast cancer. Eur J Surg Oncol 1995; 21: 510–3

21. Jaques DP, Coit DG, Casper ES, Brennan MF. Hepatic metastases from soft-tissue sarcoma. Ann Surg 1995; 221: 392–7

22. Schwartz SI. Hepatic resection for noncolorectal nonneuroendocrine metastases. World J Surg 1995; 19: 72–5

23. Salmon RJ, Levy C, Plancer C, et al. Treatment of liver metastases from uveal melanoma by combined surgery-chemotherapy. Eur J Surg Oncol 1998; 24: 127–30

24. Ochiai T, Sasako M, Mizuno S. Hepatic resection for metastatic tumours from gastric cancer: analysis of prognostic factors. Br J Surg 1994; 81: 1175–8

25. Bines SD, England G, Deziel DJ, Witt TR, Doolas A, Roseman DL. Synchronous, metachronous and multiple hepatic resections of liver tumors originating from primary gastric tumors. Surgery 1993; 114: 799–805

26. Harrison LE, Brennan MF, Newman E et al. Hepatic resection for noncolorectal, nonneuroendocrine metastases: a fifteen-year experience with ninety-six patients. Surgery 1997; 121: 625–32

27. Fujisaki S, Takayama T, Shimada K, et al. Hepatectomy for metastatic renal cell carcinoma. Hepato-gastroenterology 1997; 44: 817–9

28. Iwatsuki S, Shaw BW, Starzl TE. Experience with 150 liver resections. Ann Surg 1983; 197: 247

29. Talmadge JE, Fidler IJ. Enhanced metastatic potential of tumor cells harvested from spontaneous metastases of heterogeneous murine tumors. J Natl Cancer Inst 1982; 69: 975–80

30. Elias D, Saric J, Jaeck D et al. Prospective study of microscopic lymph node involvement of the hepatic

pedicle during curative hepatectomy for colorectal metastases. Br J Surg 1996; 83: 942–5

31. Nanko M, Shimada H, Yamaoka H et al. Micrometastatic colorectal cancer lesions in the liver. Jpn J Surg 1998; 28: 707–13

32. Hughes KS, Simon R, Songhorabodi S, Adson MA. Resection of the liver for colorectal carcinoma metastases: a multi-institutional study of patterns of recurrence. Surgery 1986; 100: 278–84

33. Fong Y, Fortner J, Sun RL, Brennan MF, Blumgart LH. Clinical score for predicting recurrence after hepatic resection for metastatic colorectal cancer: analysis of 1001 consecutive cases. Ann Surg 1999; 230(3): 309–18

34. Delbeke D, Vitola JV, Sandler MP et al. Staging recurrent metastatic colorectal carcinoma with PET. J Nucl Med 1997; 38: 1196–201

35. Fernández-Trigo V, Shamsa F, Sugarbaker PH. Repeat liver resections from colorectal metastasis. Surgery 1995; 117: 296–304

36. Shirabe K, Takenaka K, Gion T et al. Analysis of prognostic risk factors in hepatic resection for metastatic colorectal carcinoma with special reference to the surgical margin. Br J Surg 1997; 84: 1077–80

37. Blumgart LH. Liver resection – liver and biliary tumours. In: Blumgart, LH ed. Surgery of the liver and biliary tract. New York: Churchill Livingstone, 1994: 1495–538

38. Polk W, Fong Y, Karpeh M, Blumgart LH. A technique for the use of cryosurgery to assist hepatic resection. J Am Coll Surg 1995; 180: 171–6

39. Billingsley KG, Jarnagin WR, Fong Y, Blumgart LH. Segment-oriented hepatic resection in the management of malignant neoplasms of the liver. J Am Coll Surg 1999; 187: 471–81

40. DeMatteo RP, Palese C, Jarnagin WJ, Sun RL, Blumgart LH, Fong Y. Anatomic segmental hepatic resection is superior to wedge resection as an oncologic operation for colorectal liver metastases. J Gastrointest Surg 2000; 4(2): 178–84

41. Cunningham JD, Fong Y, Shriver C. One hundred consecutive hepatic resections: blood loss, transfusion and operative technique. Arch Surg 1994; 129: 1050–6

42. Bartlett D, Fong Y, Blumgart LH. Complete resection of the caudate lobe of the liver: technique and results. Br J Surg 1996; 83: 1076–81

43. Fong Y, Blumgart LH. Hepatic colorectal metastasis: current status of surgical therapy. Oncology 1998; 12: 1489–94

44. Lezoche E, Paganini AM, Feliciotti F, Guerrieri M, Lugnani F, Tamburini A. Ultrasound-guided laparoscopic cryoablation of hepatic tumors: preliminary report. World J Surg 1998; 22: 829–36

45. Siperstein AE, Rogers SJ, Hansen PD, Gitomersky A. Laparoscopic thermal ablation of hepatic neuroendocrine tumor metastases. Surgery 1997; 122: 1147–55

46. Fortner JG, Silva JS, Golbey RB. Multivariate analysis of a personal series of 247 consecutive patients with liver metastases from colorectal cancer: I. Treatment by hepatic resection. Ann Surg 1984; 196: 306–16

47. Butler J, Attiyeh FF, Daly JM. Hepatic resection for metastases of the colon and rectum. Surg Gynecol Obstet 1986; 162: 109–13

48. Pagana TJ. A new technique for hepatic infusional chemotherapy. Semin Surg Oncol 1986; 2: 99–102

49. Moertel CG, Fleming TR, Macdonald JS et al. Levamisole and fluorouracil for adjuvant therapy of resected colon carcinoma. N Engl J Med 1990; 322: 352–8

50. Blumbart LH, Fong Y. Surgical management of colorectal metastases to the liver. Curr Prob Surg 1995; 5: 333–428

51. Goodie DB, Horton MD, Morris RW, Nagy LS, Morris DL. Anaesthetic experience with cryotherapy for treatment of hepatic malignancy. Anaes Int Care 1992; 20: 491–6

52. Moriya Y, Sugihara K, Hojo K, Makuuchi M. Adjuvant hepatic intra-arterial chemotherapy after potentially curative hepatectomy for liver metastases from colorectal cancer: a pilot study. Eur J Surg Oncol 1991; 17: 519–25

53. Curley SA, Roh MS, Chase JL, Hohn DC. Adjuvant hepatic artery infusion chemotherapy after curative resection of colorectal liver metastases. Am J Surg 1993; 166: 743–8

54. Kemeny MM, Goldberg D, Beatty D et al. Results of a prospective randomized trial of continuous regional chemotherapy and hepatic resection as treatment of hepatic metastases from colorectal primaries. Cancer 1986; 57: 492–8

55. Lorenz M, Muller HH, Schramm H et al. Randomized trial of surgery versus surgery followed by adjuvant hepatic arterial infusion with 5-fluorouracil and folinic acid for liver metastases of colorectal cancer. Ann Surg 1998; 228: 756–62

56. Kemeny N, Huang Y, Cohen AM et al. Hepatic arterial infusion of chemotherapy after resection of hepatic metastases from colorectal cancer. N Engl Med 1999; 341(27): 2039–48

57. Que FG, Nagorney DM, Batts KP, Linz LJ, Kvols LK. Hepatic resection for metastatic neuroendocrine carcinomas. Am J Surg 1995; 169: 36–43

7 Bilobar metastatic colon cancer

Daniel Jaeck, Olivier Monek, Elie Oussoultzoglou and Philippe Bachellier

At present, in the West, the main indication for hepatic resection is the treatment of colorectal liver metastases. Among these patients, those with bilobar metastatic disease represent the biggest challenge for the surgeon. In the multicentric retrospective study of the French Association of Surgery,[1] the largest series of liver resections for colorectal metastases to date, of the 1818 patients treated with a curative resection 20% of the cases were bilobar. (Figure 7.1).

We shall try to answer the following questions:
(1) Is it therefore justifiable to resect bilobar colorectal liver metastases?
(2) How should diagnostic procedures and the preoperative evaluation be managed? (With special reference to the hepatic functional reserve.)
(3) How should bilobar metastases be resected? (Intraoperative evaluation, contraindications and various types of resections.)

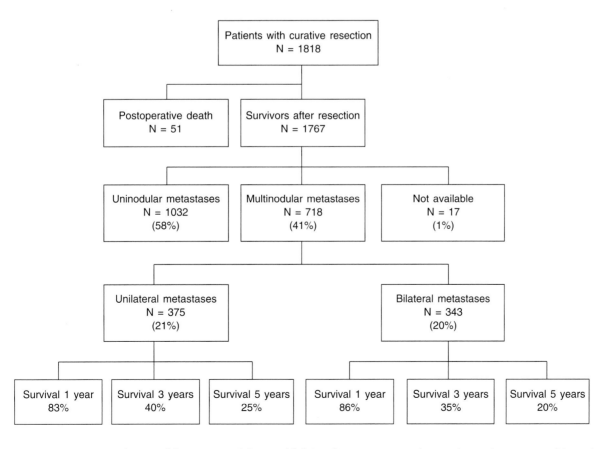

Figure 7.1 Comparison of survival between unilobar and bilobar liver metastases from colorectal cancer (multicentric retrospective study by the French Association of Surgery[1]).

(4) Which other local treatments can be used?

(5) What results can be expected after surgery?

(6) What strategies are available in certain conditions, especially with a small left lobe?

(7) Is there a place for adjuvant or neo-adjuvant chemotherapy?

(8) The follow-up: is repeat hepatectomy worthwhile?

Is it justifiable to resect bilobar colorectal liver metastases?

Surgical resection is currently accepted as a safe, and also the only potentially curative treatment available for patients with colorectal liver metastases, offering a chance of long-term survival with rates ranging from 25% to 50% at 5 years.[1-6] During the last decade, significative technical advances have been accomplished in liver surgery. They allow bilobar resections with very low mortality (around 1%) and low morbidity. However, it has been estimated[7,8] that a curative resection (RO resection), i.e. with complete excision of the metastatic deposits, can only be achieved in about 10% to 15% of all patients who develop colorectal liver metastases. Furthermore, there is still a lack of enthusiasm among many physicians regarding surgical resection of liver metastases when they are multiple; many of them are clearly reluctant in the case of bilobar disease.

Nevertheless, most studies in the literature show clearly that there is no difference in 5-year survival rate between patients with solitary or fewer than four metastases, whether the location is unilobar or bilobar.[3-5,9,10] The multicentric retrospective study that we performed with the French Association of Surgery[1] collected 1818 patients in whom the resection was considered to be curative. The data showed, on multivariate analysis, that the following factors were associated with a significantly better prognosis: presence of fewer than four metastases, diameter of less than 5 cm (Tables 7.1 and 7.2), no extra-hepatic disease, carcinoembryonic antigen (CEA) level below 30 ng/l and detection 2 years or more after resection of a primary tumor which had not involved the serosa or the pericolic lymph nodes. In contrast, unilobar versus bilobar location had no influence on survival in this group (Figure 7.1) of candidates for resection, provided that the deposits could be completely removed (RO resection) with a free resection margin of at least 1 cm. Similar results were reported by Elias[9] and Minagawa.[10] Giving one point to each factor, including the age of the patient, the population could be divided into three risk groups with different 2-year

Table 7.1 **Survival according to the size of the metastases (<5 cm, ⩾5 cm) (multicentric retrospective study by the French Association of Surgery[1])**

Size of metastases	No of patients	Survival (%)*		
		1 year	3 years	5 years
<5 cm	857	90	47	29
⩾5 cm	818	83	35	24
Not available	92			

*P<0.0001

Table 7.2 **Survival according to the number of the metastases (1–3, 4 or more) (multicentric retrospective study by the French Association of Surgery[1])**

Size of metastases	No of patients	Survival (%)*		
		1 year	3 years	5 years
1–3	1510	88	43	28
4 or more	214	79	28	13
Not available	43			

*P<0.0001

Table 7.3 **Prognostic scoring system[11]**

Number of risk factors[a]	2-year survival (%)
0–2	79
3–4	60
5–7	43

[a]Risk factors:
- age (>60 years)
- size of largest metastases (⩾5 cm)
- CEA (>30 ng/ml)
- stage of primary tumor extension to serosa lymphatic spread
- disease-free interval <2 years
- number of liver nodules (⩾4)
- resection margin (<1 cm).

survival rates: 0–2 (79%), (3–4 (60%) and 5–7 (43%) (Table 7.3).[11]

In contrast to some reports where bilobar liver involvement was found to be associated with lower

A

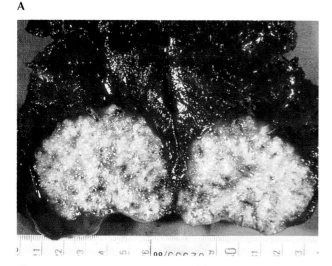

B

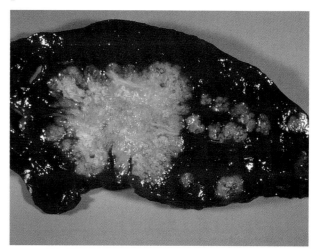

Figure 7.2 Macroscopic aspects of liver metastases from colorectal cancer. Uninodular type (A) compared to multinodular metastasis with satellite nodules (B).

survival and higher postoperative mortality and morbidity rates,[12–17] our study confirmed that the prognosis is not influenced by the location of the tumor deposits on one or both lobes of the liver or by the extent of the liver resection, provided the tumor was totally removed. Moreover, the postoperative complication rate is similar in subjects with unilobar or bilobar involvement. This means that surgical excision of two or three metastases, for example, should be undertaken if technically feasible, whether they are located on one half of the liver and require a lobectomy or in both lobes and demand two separate resections. It also means that if complete resection of the secondary tumors can be achieved with a wedge resection there is no need to perform a larger hepatectomy, provided a 1 cm clearance of normal parenchyma is resected with the tumor.

Several studies[18–20] have evaluated the prognostic impact of the surgical margin when, under certain circumstances, it has to be less than 1 cm (for example in the case of metastases located near a main vessel: vena cava, porta hepatis). It was concluded that if complete resection of the tumor is mandatory, a margin less than 1 cm should not be considered as an absolute contraindication to surgery. In these situations, cryotherapy has been recommended to improve the proportion of negative resection margins;[18] however, the proximity of a metastasis to a large blood vessel compromises an adequate freezing margin.

Finally, there is a strong argument in favor of segmentectomies or minor resections rather than extended resections if they can be undertaken safely. This approach contributes to preservation of the residual liver. Indeed, recurrences will

unfortunately occur in the majority of patients after the first liver resection. A clinical score predicting recurrences after hepatic resection for metastatic colorectal cancer has been established by Fong et al.[21] We demonstrated in our multicentric series that there is a clear survival benefit for repeat liver resections in some selected patients with long-term survival rates after the second resection similar to that obtained after the first resection.[22] These findings have been confirmed by others,[23–25] and they emphasize the need not only for a careful follow-up after hepatectomy in order to detect resectable recurrences, but also for a policy of economical but complete resections of the liver metastases rather than routine major hepatic resections when the size and/or the number of the tumors do not require it. Other studies tried to identify parameters that could help to select subpopulations of patients with recurrent liver metastases who have a better prognosis after repeat resections. Bozzetti[26] showed that patients with a disease-free interval greater than 1 year between the first and second liver resections had a greater disease-free survival after the second resection. However, in the largest series no parameter significantly related to outcome could be identified,[27] even for bilobar liver involvement. Several authors recommended an aggressive approach for patients with recurrent or multiple bilobar liver metastases from colorectal primaries.[1,9,10,28–31]

Pathophysiology of bilobar distribution

Many studies have attempted to explain (1) the ability of some primary tumors to develop metastases,[32] and (2) the lobar distribution of these metastases in the liver.[33] Several factors are involved,

A

B

C

D

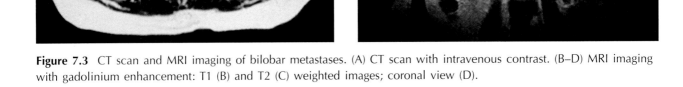

Figure 7.3 CT scan and MRI imaging of bilobar metastases. (A) CT scan with intravenous contrast. (B–D) MRI imaging with gadolinium enhancement: T1 (B) and T2 (C) weighted images; coronal view (D).

linked to the biology of the tumor and of the target organ. It has been suggested that right-sided colon cancers involve the right hepatic lobe more selectively while left-sided tumors involve the entire liver, according to streaming of flow in the portal vein.[33] These hypotheses need further investigations but should not influence the specific therapeutic strategy. Obviously, metastatic potential of the primary tumor correlates with several factors, including angiogenesis, or genetically coded disorders which will have a strong effect on the prognosis of the disease. Other prognostic factors have been studied including the macroscopic morphology of the metastases: simple nodular or confluent nodular, according to the characteristics of the cut surface of the tumor.[34] The presence of satellite nodules around the metastases predicts a poorer prognosis;[35] in this situation an extended hepatectomy seems to be a better option in order to reduce the risk of local recurrence (Fig. 7.2).

How should diagnostic procedures and the preoperative evaluation be managed?

Diagnostic procedures

Preoperative liver imaging and also intraoperative ultrasound are routinely used to detect hepatic metastases. The two main difficulties are distinguishing metastases from incidental benign focal liver lesions (particularly hemangioma) and being able to detect small metastases less than 2 cm in diameter. At the preoperative stage, some cases of bilobar invasion may not be recognized if the deposits on one side are too small.

Percutaneous ultrasound (US) is the most widely used imaging technique. For lesions greater than

A

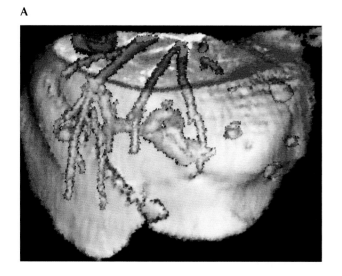

B

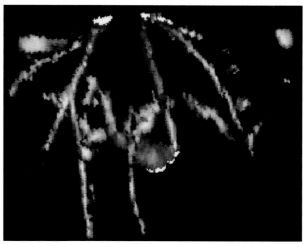

C

Figure 7.4 (A–C) Image reconstruction techniques in three dimensions showing connections between the vessels and the tumors.

2 cm the sensitivity exceeds 94%, but this falls to less than 56% for lesions below this size.[36] Ultrasound should always employ color Doppler, which may show more clearly displacement, interruption or thrombosis of the hepatic and portal vein or of the IVC.

The use of CT scanning with intravenous contrast (enhanced CT scanning), bolus dynamic CT, delayed scanning, and dynamic CT scanning during arterial portography has led to increased sensitivity in detection of liver metastases (68% of the nodules less than 1 cm diameter were detected and 99% of those larger than 1 cm)[37,38] (Fig. 7.3A). The portoscanner (dynamic CT during arterial portography CTAP) involves selective catheterization of the superior mesenteric artery followed by bolus contrast injection and CT scanning during the portal phase. This method is particularly helpful to detect lesions less than 5 mm in diameter; it has been proven to be significantly better than US, contrast CT or hepatic angiography in detecting metastases

less than 10 mm in diameter.[39] However, this investigation is invasive and the second major limitation is the number of false positive findings caused by perfusion defects from flow artefacts. Moreover, all focal intrahepatic abnormalities (biliary cyst, angiomas, benign tumors) appear as lucent areas with this imaging technique; if smaller than 5 mm they cannot be compared to other preoperative examinations and possible guided needle biopsy.

The development of MRI, including the use of gadolinium ferumoxide (Endorem),[40] and other enhancement methods, raised the possibility that this technique could be even better and more efficient in detecting small lesions (Fig. 7.3B,C). The T1-weighted MRI appears to have the lowest false positive rate (11%).[41] Staging laparoscopy with laparoscopic ultrasonography has also been reported.[42,43] This method allows accurate preoperative hepatic staging, needle biopsy and also assessment of peritoneal involvement. However, it is an invasive procedure which carries a potential risk for

A

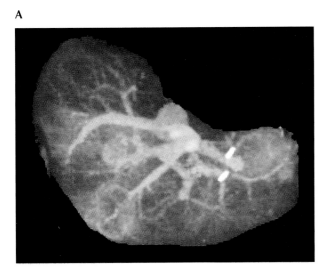

B

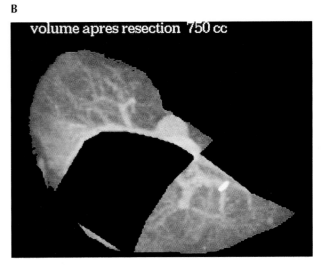

Figure 7.5 Preoperative measurement of the respective volumes of (A) hepatic resection (1310 ml) and (B) remnant liver (750 ml) according to simulation of central hepatectomy.

metastatic seeding of the port sites. In the near future, the PET (positron emission tomography) scan might be more sensitive and specific for detection of metastatic deposits in the liver, as well as for detection of local recurrences, carcinomatosis and metastatic lymph nodes.[44,45] Finally, a chest CT scan is used routinely to establish the presence or absence of pulmonary metastases. CT of the brain and isotope bone scans are usually only performed in the presence of clinical symptoms.

Evaluation of hepatic functional reserve and measurement of liver volume

The development of image reconstruction techniques in three dimensions is very helpful to evaluate the total volume of the tumors and the volume of healthy liver. It also shows very clearly the relationship between vessels and the tumors (Fig. 7.4). It enables the surgeon to determine an exact strategy of resection and to draw it on the computer screen.

Patients with bilobar metastases often require either extended hepatectomies or multiple resections and are therefore at risk of developing liver failure after hepatectomy. Although the normal liver is reported to tolerate removal of up to 70% of its volume,[46] the extent to which the liver parenchyma may be resected in patients with steatosis (after chemotherapy) or with chronic liver disease has not yet been completely elucidated. The hepatic functional reserve may be evaluated by measurement of the respective volumes of hepatic tumors together with the resection margin and of the remnant liver, or by evaluation of preoperative liver function as a guide before making decisions with regard to the extent of liver resection.

Measurement of liver volume

This has been performed by several imaging techniques (Fig. 7.5). However, CT has been shown to be the most adequate procedure both in liver resection[47–49] and liver transplantation, especially in assessing graft sizes for living-related liver transplantation.[50] It is currently accepted that in patients with normal hepatic function, resection of up to 60% of the non-cancerous parenchyma is well tolerated.[48] After excluding the tumor volume, the ratio of the non-cancerous parenchymal volume of the resected liver to that of the whole liver is the crucial value to estimate. Actually, when the volume of the future remnant liver estimated by CT-scan volumetry is less than 40%, right portal vein embolization has been recommended in order to improve the safety of the right hepatic lobectomy. This procedure efficiently reduces the size of the liver volume to be resected (right lobe) and induces hypertrophy of the contralateral liver (left lobe).[51–54]

Evaluation of preoperative liver function

Standard liver biochemistry tests have not been shown to be of any predictive value.[55] Other methods have included measurement of uptake of organic anions (such as bromsulphalein, rose bengal and indocyanine green (ICG),[55,56] the arterial ketone body ratio,[57] redox tolerance test,[58] aminopyralene breath test and the amino acid clearance test.[59] The ICG clearance test appears to be the best discriminating investigation.[56,59] Before a decision is made to undertake a major hepatectomy, ICG retention should be less than 20% at 15 minutes. Hepatectomy involving resection of up to 60% of the non-tumorous parenchyma can be justified in patients with normal liver function and with ICG 15 values >20%. Minor hepatectomies can be accomplished even if ICG retention at 15 minutes reaches

23 to 25%.[56,59] The lidocaine test (MEGX) can also be used to evaluate the hepatic function. Lidocaine is metabolized almost exclusively (97%) in hepatocytes by the P-450 cytochrome. Fifteen minutes after an IV bolus injection of 1 mg/kg of lidocaine, a venous blood sample is taken and the MEGX rate is assessed: values over 50 ng/ml are considered as normal, between 25 and 50 ng/ml intermediately reduced and below 25 ng/ml greatly reduced.

How should bilobar metastases be resected? (Intraoperative evaluation and contraindications and various types of resections)

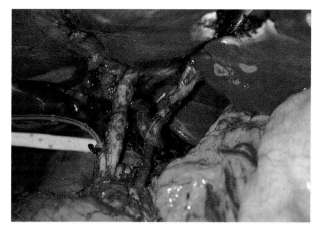

Figure 7.6 Operative view of extensive lymphadenectomy of the hepatic pedicle.

Surgical resection should only be undertaken if all the liver metastases can be removed (RO resection).[60] In the case of associated extrahepatic disease, resection is not justified except in cases where all the tumoral tissue—intrahepatic and extrahepatic—can be completely removed. The surgical strategy has to achieve two contradictory goals: (1) perform an oncological resection with clear free resection margins, and (2) save most of the non-cancerous parenchyma in order to avoid liver failure and to allow further repeat resection in case of possible recurrence.

Involvement of lymph nodes in the hepatic pedicle

Extensive lymph node dissection of the hepatic pedicle was undertaken prospectively in 100 consecutive patients undergoing curative hepatectomy for colorectal liver metastases in whom lymph node involvement of the hepatic pedicle was not macroscopically detectable.[61] Microscopic lymph node involvement was found in 14 patients, and the presence of microscopic disease related to the number of metastases, extent of liver involvement and CEA level. Colorectal tumors that spread to the lymph nodes of the hepatic pedicle or coeliac region are generally considered to be metastases derived from liver metastases.[62] The incidence of macroscopic involvement of these lymph nodes varied from 1 to 10% in a major series of liver resections for colorectal metastases.[1,3,62,63] One series showed up to 28% tumor infiltration of the hepatoduodenal ligament lymph nodes.[64] Low 5-year survival rates have been reported for these patients, despite complete resection of the macroscopically involved lymph nodes.[3,64] However, the 5-year survival rate of this group of patients was up to 12% in the study by the French Association of Surgery,[1] compared to the expected 0 to 2% without resection.[65] Therefore, our recommendation would be to perform hepatectomy even in the case of hepatic pedicle lymph node involvement, but to complete the procedure with an extensive lymphadenectomy from the liver hilum (Fig. 7.6) to the origin of the hepatic artery (coeliac axis). The prognostic and therapeutic value of such a lymphadenectomy is currently unknown;[66] the answer could only be found by a prospective randomized study comparing groups with and without lymphadenectomy.

Other extrahepatic involvement

Liver resection should only be undertaken when curative resection is possible, which clearly means complete resection of intrahepatic and extrahepatic deposits.[60] In the case of extrahepatic involvement, the probability for curative resectability is less: 5.9% compared to 27.1% without extrahepatic involvement in synchronous metastases and 5.4% compared to 37.4% in metachronous metastases.[5]

Intraoperative ultrasound (IOUS)

The importance of detecting all metastatic nodules present in the liver and also the need for a negative margin with adequate liver function after resection emphasize the role of intraoperative ultrasonography combined with Doppler examination. Assessment of the hepatic vasculature and the localization of the tumors with regard to any adjacent vessels is essential in order to provide an overall assessment of the extent of the lesions and also to determine the limits of the resection. The information obtained at the beginning of the operation will avoid unnecessary tissue dissection or traumatic surgical maneuvers. Small linear probes are most commonly used for hepatic surgery. Ultrasound frequency ranges from 5 to 10 MHz. The 5 MHz probe offers a reasonable compromise between optimal resolution and maximum depth of exploration.[67] The examination may be repeated during the operation, for instance in assessing the resection margins or in identifying the relations between the tumor and the main intrahepatic vessels. The concept of ultrasound-guided segment-orientated procedures has been developed and is particularly useful in resection of multiple metastases.[68–72] IOUS is able to detect lesions as small as 4 or 5 mm and to find metastases which were not diagnosed preoperatively: detection of 5–10% of unsuspected liver lesions has been reported by employing this technique.[73,74] One prospective study designed to compare diagnostic accuracy of preoperative ultrasonography, surgical examination and IOUS showed a higher sensitivity and specificity for IOUS.[67] During liver resection, IOUS is repeated to ensure a sufficient safety margin and to follow an adequate plane of parenchymal division with respect to the limit of the tumor.

How to choose the type and the number of hepatic resections in bilobar metastases

Complete knowledge of the segmental structure of the liver is essential for the performance of this type of surgery. The description by Couinaud[75,76] was originally adopted in France and then throughout the world (see Chapter 1). It divides the liver into eight segments (or even nine),[77,78] based on the portal and hepatic veins distribution (Fig. 7.7). A new terminology, accepted by the scientific committee of the International Hepato-Pancreato-Biliary Association (IHPBA), has also been reported.[79]

In the case of bilobar metastases it seems convenient and realistic to consider schematically five types of situations (Fig. 7.8A–E):

(1) Major deposit in the right liver and small deposit in the left liver (Fig. 7.8A). This situation can be treated:
 • either by an extended right hepatectomy (Starzl's right trisegmentectomy) removing segments V, VI, VII, VIII and IV (8A1);
 • or by a right hepatectomy combined with a wedge resection in the left lobe (8A2);
 • or by one or more segmentectomies in the right liver combined with a wedge resection in the left lobe (8A3).

(2) Major deposit in the left liver and small deposit in the right liver (Fig. 7.8B). This situation can be treated by a left lobectomy (8B1) or a left hepatectomy (8B2 + 3) combined with a wedge resection in the right lobe. If the left liver is involved and also segments V and VIII, an extended left hepatectomy can be performed (8B4) removing segments II, III, IV, V and VIII.

(3) Major deposit located in the central part of the liver and involving both lobes (Fig. 7.8C). This presentation can be treated by a central hepatectomy removing segment IV (either totally (8C1) or only the anterior portion (8C2) if the posterior portion is not involved) and both segments V and VIII.

(4) Both lobes present, each with a major deposit (>5 cm) (Fig. 7.8D). This presentation can be treated by a left lobectomy combined with a bisegmentectomy in the right liver (segments VI and VII) (8D1), segments V and VI (8D2) or segments VII and VIII (8D3). In this last situation, venous drainage from segments V and VI

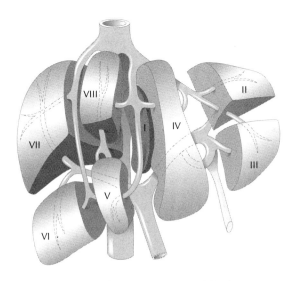

Figure 7.7 Couinaud's segmentation of the liver.

Table 7.4 **Bilobar liver colorectal metastases resections, 1985–1999 (segment I is not considered here)**

Type of bilobar hepatic resection[a]	Number of cases
A1	6
A2	8
A3	20
B1	10
B2	3
B3	2
B4	4
C1	1
C2	11
D1	5
D2	3
D3	1
E1	14
E2	4
	92

[a]As shown in Fig. 7.8

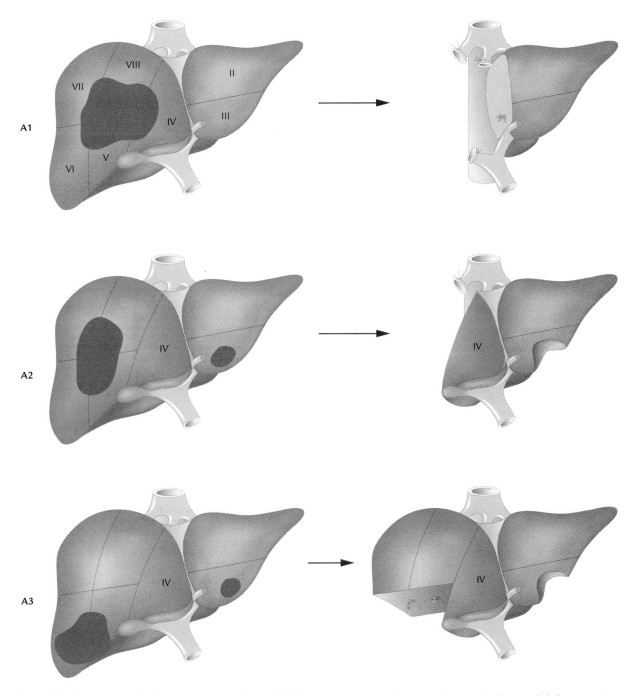

Figure 7.8 Five types of schematic presentation of bilobar metastases and various types of adequate bilobar resections. (A) Major deposit in the right liver and small deposit in the left liver.

continued

is maintained by one or more right inferior hepatic veins, if they are large enough.[80] (This can be assessed by ultrasound, Doppler and visual exploration along the inferior vena cava.) If not, reconstruction of the right hepatic vein can be performed.

(5) Both lobes present, each with several minor deposits (Fig. 7.8E). This presentation can be treated by several minor resections (segmentectomies or wedge resection) according to the location of the deposit (8E1, 8E2).

The various types of hepatectomies (Fig. 7.9A–D), following this classification, that we performed in 92 cases of resection of bilobar colorectal metastases are summarized in Table 7.4.

The possible involvement of the caudate lobe (segment I) must be systematically assessed. Located behind the hilum of the liver and in front of the inferior vena cava, this lobe is an independent functional and anatomical unit consisting of two parts. One is situated to the left of the vena cava

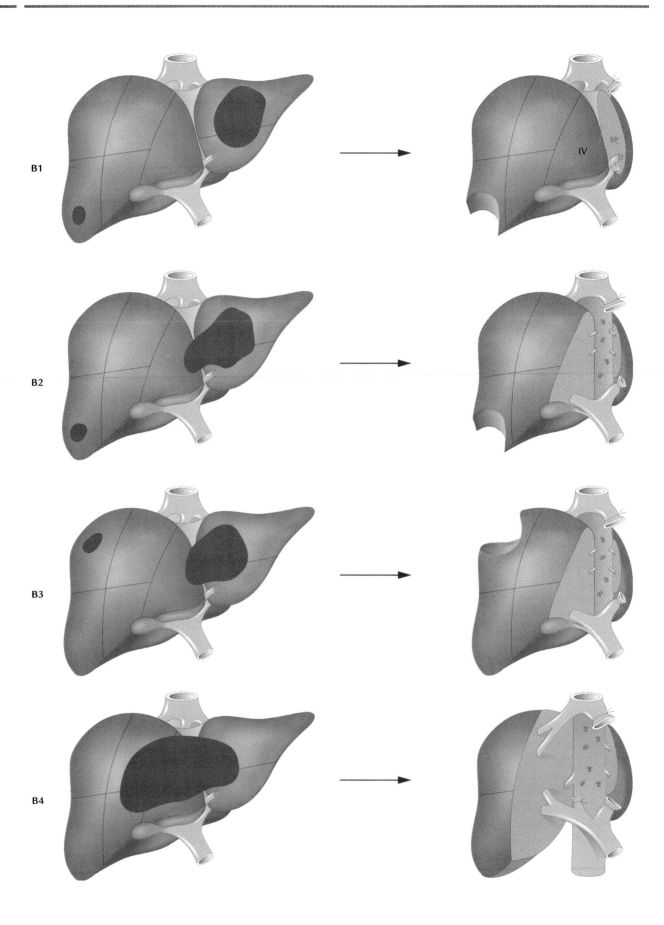

Figure 7.8 *continued* Five types of schematic presentation of bilobar metastases and various types of adequate bilobar resections. (B) Major deposit in the left liver and small deposit in the right liver.

continued

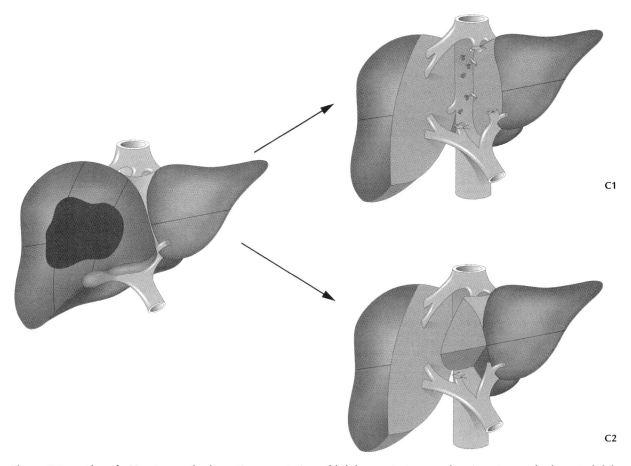

C1

C2

Figure 7.8 continued Five types of schematic presentation of bilobar metastases and various types of adequate bilobar resections. (C) Major deposit located in the central part of the liver, involving both lobes.

continued

which corresponds to the Spieghel lobe or Couinaud's segment I (Fig. 7.10). The second part, or right caudate lobe, is located in front and to the right of the vena cava, with an elevation situated between the right end of the hilum and the anterior aspect of the inferior vena cava called the caudate process or also Couinaud's segment IX.[77,78] In the case of large metastases located in the left liver and in the caudate lobe, left hepatectomy extended to the caudate lobe is necessary. At the opposite end of the scale in the case of small deposits in the caudate lobe, isolated resection of segment I is feasible after complete mobilization of the liver on both sides.[81–83] The inferior vena cava must be controlled for total vascular exclusion in the event of hemorrhage. In the case of infiltration of the caudate lobe by a large tumor which has developed in the posterior part of the right liver, a right hepatectomy extended to the caudate lobe is necessary.

A large variety of resections can be undertaken, following the distribution of the metastases. Usually true segmentectomies are suitable for the vast majority of situations and are technically easier. The liver parenchyma is separated along the lines of ischemic demarcations produced by selective clamping of the various glissonian pedicles. This procedure has been made much easier by the use of an ultrasonic dissector, which facilitates a quick separation of the parenchyma with elective control of vessels and bile ducts.

Clamping

The control and prevention of intraoperative hemorrhage is obtained by the use of pedicle clamping (Pringle maneuver). This procedure reduces the need for blood transfusion, which represents one of the main factors associated with postoperative morbidity[84,85] and also tumor recurrence rates. However, the relationship between pressure within the inferior vena cava and blood loss during liver resection has now been established, suggesting one should maintain low venous pressure (<5 mmHg) in the inferior vena cava.[86] There are several types of clamping:

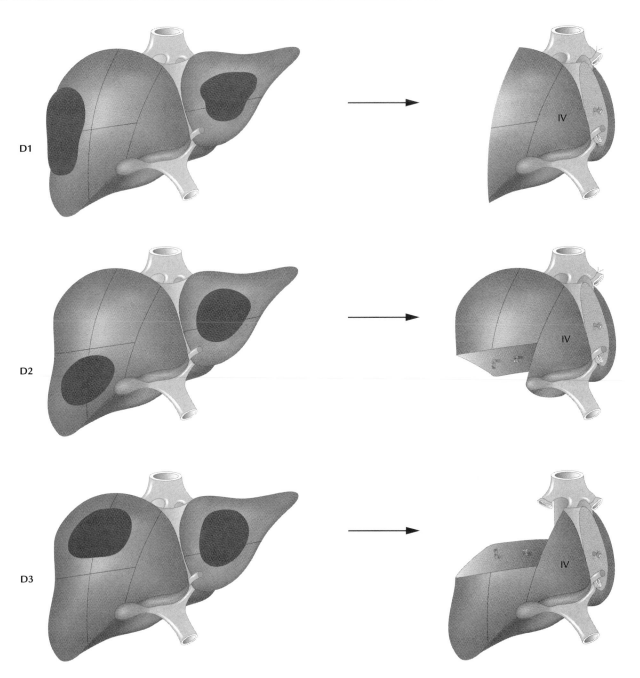

Figure 7.8 continued Five types of schematic presentation of bilobar metastases and various types of adequate bilobar resections. (D) Both lobes present, each with a major deposit (>5 cm).

continued

(1) Non-selective clamping, whereby the hepatic pedicle is clamped in order to limit bleeding as much as possible. A number of authors have shown that the liver has a good tolerance to normothermic ischemia, even for periods of more than 1 hour.[87–90] Intermittent clamping for periods of up to 15 minutes has been proposed in order to reduce the ischemic damage to the hepatocytes.[91,92]

(2) Hemihepatic vascular occlusion with selective clamping of the right or left glissonian pedicle, depending on the site of the parenchymal resection, has been advocated to increase the safety of the clamping maneuvers.[93] This policy can be followed in segmentectomies. However, before the type of clamping is chosen, several criteria have to be considered, such as the number and extent of resections, the quality of liver function

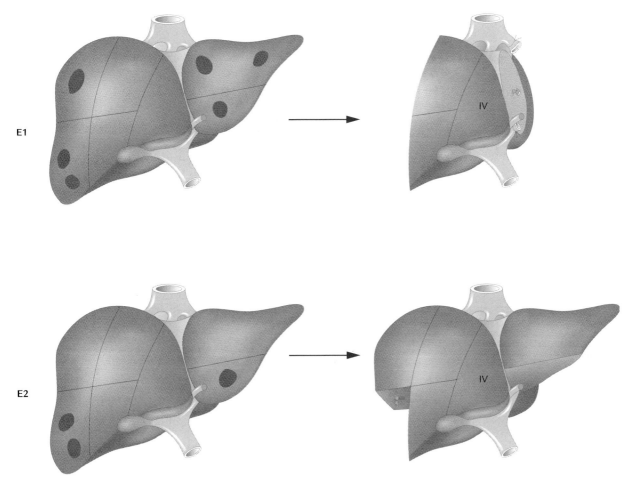

Figure 7.8 continued Five types of schematic presentation of bilobar metastases and various types of adequate bilobar resections. (E) Both lobes present, each with several minor deposits.

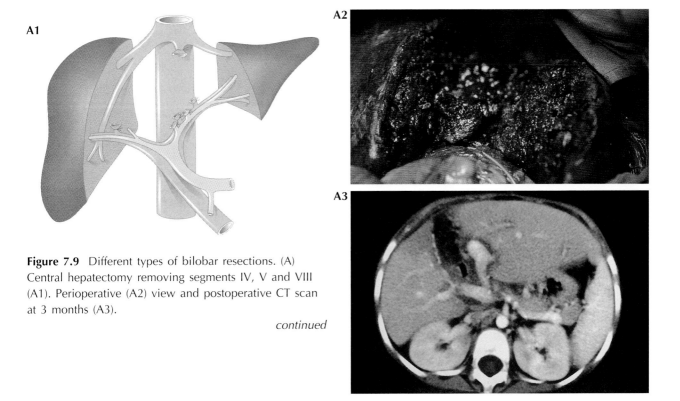

Figure 7.9 Different types of bilobar resections. (A) Central hepatectomy removing segments IV, V and VIII (A1). Perioperative (A2) view and postoperative CT scan at 3 months (A3).

continued

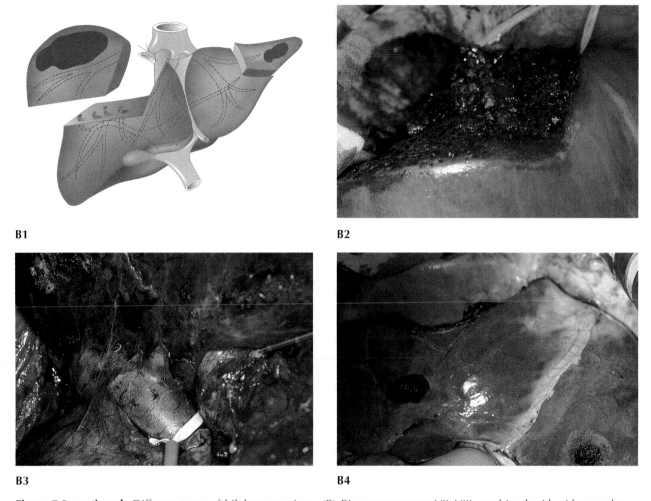

B1

B2

B3

B4

Figure 7.9 continued Different types of bilobar resections. (B) Bisegmentectomy VII–VIII combined with either wedge resections or left segmentectomy (B1,2,3). Right inferior hepatic vein(s) (B4) may achieve (if caliber large enough) the venous drainage of segments V and VI when right superior hepatic vein has to be resected.

continued

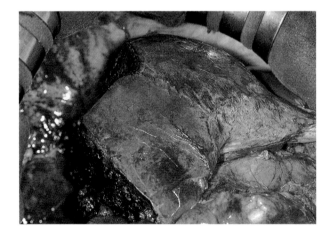

Figure 7.9 continued Different types of bilobar resections. (C) Right hepatectomy combined with partial resection of segment IV.

continued

(sometimes impaired by previous chemotherapy or associated chronic liver disease) and also the general condition of the patient (associated cardiovascular disease). Research is ongoing to evaluate a number of therapeutic substances

able to reduce the ischemic reperfusion injury to the liver.[94]

(3) Total vascular exclusion is particularly useful in cases of tumor infiltration of the vena cava or of the caval–hepatic vein confluence. If this

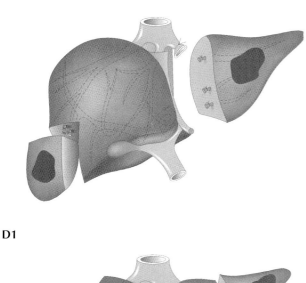

D1

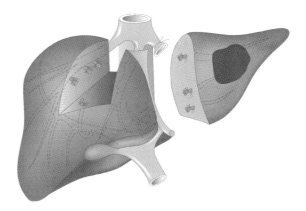

D2

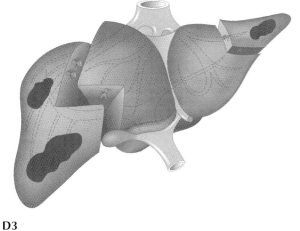

D3

Figure 7.9 continued Different types of bilobar resections. (D) Various types of bilobar segmentectomies preserving a maximum of healthy liver: D1: segmentectomy VI + left lobectomy; D2: segmentectomy VIII + left lobectomy; D3: segmentectomy V + VI + VII + segmentectomy II.

A

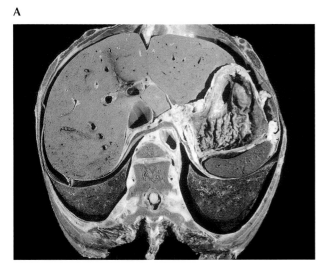

B

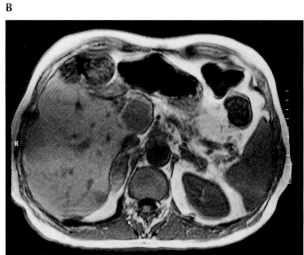

Figure 7.10 (A) Anatomical view of the Spieghel lobe. (B) Metastatic involvement of the Spieghel lobe (MRI imaging).

maneuver is not well tolerated then the use of a veno–venous bypass is indicated. However, in many other cases, total vascular exclusion of the liver with preservation of caval flow can be obtained by selectively controlling the hepatic veins by taping the right hepatic vein on one side and the middle and the left hepatic vein on the other side[95,96] (Fig. 7.11).

(4) Innovative techniques for major liver resections with hypothermic perfusion. These techniques

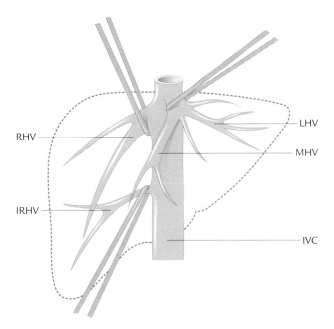

Figure 7.11 Selective control of the hepatic veins without clamping of the inferior vena cava.

were developed together with orthotopic liver transplantation and may be associated with vascular reconstruction, for instance in the case of invasion of the vena cava. Liver perfusion with a 4°C preservation solution has been used in three different approaches in major liver resections: ex vivo (bench procedure) (see Chapter 10),[97] in vivo in situ[98] or in vivo ex situ.[99–101]

• In the ex vivo technique, the liver is completely removed from the abdominal cavity by transection of afferent and efferent vessels, as well as the common bile duct; liver resections and vascular reconstruction are performed on the bench and the remnant liver is reimplanted as it would be done for a liver graft. Veno–venous bypass is used during the anhepatic phase (see Chapter 10).

• In the in situ procedure, after vascular exclusion, the liver is perfused in situ, and a draining cavotomy is performed on the infrahepatic IVC. When resection is complete, the preservative solution is flushed out of the remnant parenchyma by perfusing 4°C Ringer lactate or albumin solution. To avoid cardiac arrythmias the potassium level must be carefully controlled in the blood before reperfusion.

• The ex situ in vivo procedure has been proposed for very selected cases in which a long ischemia time is necessary (3–5 hours). Compared to the ex vivo technique, the significant advantage is to avoid the need to perform portal, arterial and biliary anastomoses. The application of these techniques may open a

different strategy in very selected cases for the treatment of multiple or huge tumors with extrahepatic vascular involvement. However, it is too early to evaluate the results of these procedures. It is very likely that, in most cases, low morbidity and low mortality can best be achieved with less sophisticated techniques avoiding too complex surgical conditions.

Liver parenchyma resection

The easiest way to carry out parenchymal division is to crush small portions of the liver tissue with a Kelly forceps. The smaller vessels are coagulated with unipolar or bipolar coagulation. The bigger ones as well as the biliary structures are either ligated with absorbable sutures or sutured or clipped. Use of the ultrasound dissector, in our experience, makes the exposure of the vascular and biliary intrahepatic pedicles easier and appears of particular help in segmentectomies. The waterjet dissection has been recently introduced and needs further evaluation.

Hemostasis and biliostasis must be achieved very cautiously to avoid any source of hemorrhage or bile leak. The Argon beam coagulator represents a significant advantage in performing coagulation without necrosis on small surface hemorrhage. In order to achieve biliostasis, the use of a dilute solution of methylene blue injected via the cystic duct facilitates detection of small bile leaks on the resected surface of the liver. In our experience, in accidental lesion of a main bile duct or in complex surgery with extended resected surface, external biliary drainage through a transcystic catheter in patients with dilated bile ducts can be quite useful.

Which other local treatments can be used?

Liver resection is the best treatment for liver colorectal metastases and the only therapy giving a chance of cure.[4] However, it may be achieved in only 10 to 20% of patients.[102,103] If curative liver resections cannot be performed, palliative resection shows no significant benefit.[1,5] Other local treatments have been evaluated in the treatment of these unresectable hepatic metastases which, in fact, represent the majority of secondary liver tumors.

Cryosurgery

Cryosurgery has been used with some interesting results.[104–106] This method is less limited than resection techniques by the anatomic distribution of liver metastases. Therefore, the addition of cryosurgery to surgical ablation could increase the number of patients rendered disease-free. The cryosurgical probes are placed into each lesion, which is frozen using liquid nitrogen to a temperature of −196°C for about 10–15 minutes. This is followed by a 10 minute thaw period and then a second 10–15 minute freeze. Usually, the size of the ice-ball achieved by the cryoprobe is visible as a hypoechogenic area with the intraoperative ultrasonography and exceeds by 1 cm the diameter of the lesion. In the case of bilobar metastases this procedure can be used to avoid extensive loss of parenchyma in combining resection of the lobe predominantly involved and freezing of lesion(s) in the remaining part. Unfortunately, the recurrence rate seems to be high, around 50%,[105,106] which suggests that cryosurgery does not achieve total destruction of the tumoral tissue in all cases. The effect on overall survival will require further evaluation. Rather than an alternative to resection, cryosurgery appears to offer a complementary strategy in achieving tumor eradication when total excision cannot be performed. Hewitt et al. have reported the use of cryotherapy to destroy residual metastases following liver resection in patients with multiple bilobar liver metastases, with promising results (2-year survival 60% and median survival 32 months).[107]

Other forms of local treatments

Other techniques which produce controlled hepatic destruction include thermotherapy, interstitial radiotherapy and ethanol injection.

Thermotherapy
The concept of heat destruction of tumors dates from antiquity. However, this approach requires extremely accurate localization to avoid injury of healthy tissue and of adjacent major vascular and biliary trunks, which are very heat sensitive. Thermotherapy may be achieved by saline-enhanced radiofrequency, by electromagnetic or microwave radiation or finally by laser.

During radiofrequency ablation (RFA) – or radiofrequency 'destruction' – a high frequency alternating current flows from the uninsulated tip of an electrode into the tissue. Several preliminary clinical and experimental reports suggest that this may be a safe and efficacious treatment for some liver tumors.[108–112] The debate whether RFA probes should be used percutaneously or at laparotomy or laparoscopy is only beginning. It has been suggested that RFA is more efficient when the blood flow through the liver is reduced by a Pringle maneuver.

The use of electromagnetic or microwave radiation has been advocated in the treatment of liver tumors.[113] The heat produced has to cross normal tissue before reaching the tumor and, again, the proximity of main vessels or biliary ducts may contraindicate the use of this method for a deeply located tumor.

Laser hyperthermia can be used intraoperatively or percutaneously under ultrasound control. The magnetic-resonance-guided laparoscopic approach has been studied experimentally for interstitial laser therapy of the liver.[114] At present, only a few reports are available concerning the results of laser-induced thermotherapy: they show partial and transitory benefit.[115,116] It is too early to draw conclusions from these series. Nonetheless, this method may be effective for the treatment of small superficial hepatic metastases; it does not seem applicable to large, deeply located tumors in the neighborhood of the main vascular and biliary trunks.

Interstitial radiotherapy
Radioactive implants have been used to treat gross residual disease or to sterilize positive margins following hepatic resection of colorectal metastases. The observed results were poor, with early as well as distant recurrence.[117] Intestinal radiotherapy has no advantage over other local treatments and its cost and inherent problems limit its usefulness.

Ethanol injection
Percutaneous alcohol injection has been used to treat unresectable colorectal liver metastases. Results are far from satisfactory as early recurrence and partial responses are commonly observed.[118] Morphologically the opposite of hepatocellular carcinoma, colorectal liver metastases present with dense stroma into which it is difficult to inject alcohol. Pain following the injection is common and the technique seems ineffective, as the alcohol spreads out into the normal parenchyma.

What results can be expected after surgery?

The mortality associated with elective liver resections for colorectal metastases is less than 5% in most recent series, even for bilobar liver involvement.[1,3,5,6,10,11,31,51] In the French Association of Surgery survey[1,11] there was a 2.4% postoperative death rate; these deaths were more frequent after a major resection (3%) than after a minor one (1–2%). An increased risk was also observed in older patients (median age of patients who survived was

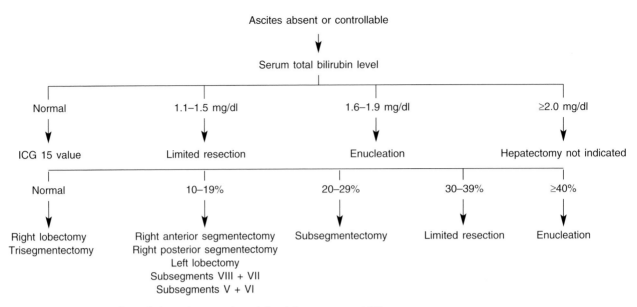

Figure 7.12 Criteria for safe hepatic resections (after Miyagawa et al.[121])

60 years compared to 68 years for the group of patients who died during the postoperative period ($P = 0.001$). The postoperative mortality rate was also higher in patients with the largest metastases (>5 cm) than in patients with smaller metastases (3.2% vs 1.3%; $P = 0.01$). The postoperative risk of major liver resections was greater when primary tumor resection and liver resection were performed at the same operation than when liver resection was postponed for more than one month (6.9% vs 2.3%; $P = 0.01$). Conversely, more recently, in our own experience in selected cases, we did not notice a higher mortality in the group of patients undergoing simultaneous resection;[119] we believe it is a safe strategy, especially for patients presenting with a primary tumor of the right colon with liver metastases resectable by means of a minor hepatectomy and through the same abdominal incision.

Reversible complications occured in 23% of the patients and were more frequent after major than after minor resections (26% vs 17%; $P = 0.001$). Among these complications observed with decreasing frequency: sepsis, biliary leaks, liver failure and bleeding. Most postoperative complications after liver resection can be managed without reoperation; percutaneous drainage of perihepatic collections and endoscopic stenting of biliary leaks are now used routinely.[5] If bleeding can be avoided during hepatic resection, this results in lower mortality. Excessive bleeding during hepatic resection is a major complication, associated with a perioperative mortality as high as 17%.[1] Hepatic failure occasionally occurs after liver resection for colorectal metastases and is often a lethal complication.[120] It is especially related to the extent of hepatic resection; its occurence is related to the quantity and quality of the remnant parenchyma. After prolonged chemotherapy the liver parenchyma is often more fragile and steatotic and the risk of bleeding is higher, which requires the use of the Pringle maneuver. The use of intermittent rather than continuous clamping, and also limiting the period of vascular occlusion, are safer procedures for these patients. Factors leading to higher morbidity after hepatic resection have been identified.[121] Among them are longer operation time, major hepatic resection, preoperative cardiovascular disease and the presence of chronic liver disease. When the liver is diseased, either due to chronic disease or to previous chemotherapy, serum total bilirubin level and plasma retention rate of indocyanine green at 15 minutes may be good predictors when deciding the volume of a safe hepatic resection[121] (Fig. 7.12).

The reported overall 5-year survival rates range from 25% to 50%.[1–6,10,31,51] Analysis of the various prognostic factors which were studied in the survey of the French Association of Surgery is shown in Table 7.5.[1,11] The survival for patients who were treated for bilobar metastases is summarized in Table 7.1. There is no difference from survival of patients with unilobar disease. The predictors of survival were also predictors of disease-free survival. Extension into serosa and lymphatic spread of the primary tumor were strong predictors. Other factors include a period of more or less than 2 years between treatment of the primary tumor and discovery of metastases, the size of the largest deposit (≥5 cm) and the number of metastases (≥4), which all correlated with survival as well as preoperative CEA level. On the other hand, distribution of resectable metastases on one or both liver lobes was not correlated with survival. Neither was extent of liver resection correlated with survival. However, clearance of normal parenchyma resected with the

Table 7.5 **Analysis of various prognostic factors studied in the survey of the French Association of Surgery:[11] relative risk of mortality and disease recurrence**

Variable	Relative risk of mortality			Relative risk of mortality or disease recurrence		
		Univariate			Univariate	
	RR	95% CI	P value	RR	95% CI	P value
Patient						
Sex (female)	1.1	0.9–1.3	0.25	1.0	0.9–1.2	0.66
Age (≥60 years)	1.2	1.0–1.3	0.06	1.0	0.8–1.1	0.46
Primary tumor						
Site of primary tumor (rectum)	1.1	0.9–1.3	0.25	1.2	1.0–1.3	0.03
Extension into serosa	1.4	1.2–1.6	<0.001	1.4	1.2–1.6	<0.001
Lymphatic spread	1.5	1.3–1.8	<0.001	1.4	1.2–1.6	<0.001
Hepatic metastases						
Delay from primary tumor (<3 months)	1.1	0.9–1.3	0.29	1.1	0.9–1.2	0.25
Delay from primary tumor (<2 years)	1.4	1.1–1.7	0.001	1.3	1.1–1.5	0.01
No of metastases resected (≥4)	1.6	1.3–2.0	<0.001	1.3	1.1–1.6	0.004
Size of the largest lesion (≥5 cm)	1.3	1.1–1.5	0.002	1.3	1.1–1.4	0.001
Location on liver (bilateral)	1.1	0.9–1.3	0.58	1.2	1.0–1.4	0.08
Type of resection (major)	1.1	0.9–1.3	0.36	1.0	0.9–1.1	0.95
Clearance of normal prenchyma (edge or <1 cm)	1.4	1.1–1.6	<0.001	1.3	1.1–1.6	<0.001
Adjuvant chemotherapy (No)	1.2	1.0–1.4	0.05	1.1	1.0–1.3	0.09

CI: confidence interval; RR: relative risk.

tumor was strongly correlated with prognosis. This means that surgical excision of two or three metastases, for example, should be undertaken, if technically feasible, whether they are located on one liver lobe and require one lobectomy or in two lobes and demand two separate resections. It also means that if complete resection of the tumors can be performed with wedge resections there is no need to perform larger hepatectomies, provided a 1 cm clearance of normal parenchyma is resected with the tumor.

What strategies are available in certain conditions, especially with a small left lobe?

One of the prerequisites for hepatectomy, particularly in case of bilobar metastatic disease, is the presence of enough remaining liver parenchyma to avoid life-threatening postoperative liver failure.[69] This concern may occur when there is a small left lobe and an extended right hepatectomy is mandatory or when major liver resection is necessary in patients with impaired liver function due, for instance, to previous prolonged chemotherapy. To render hepatectomy feasible and safe in such cases, preoperative portal vein embolization (PE) represents

a very helpful method which is able to redistribute portal blood flow rich in hepatotrophic substances toward the future remnant liver. At the same time it induces a slight shrinkage in the volume of the embolized liver for which resection is planned[48,52,53,122] (Fig. 7.13). In 1920, it was shown that portal branch ligation in the rabbit resulted in shrinkage of the affected lobe;[123] and the origin, nature and action of hepatotrophic substances in portal venous blood were largely investigated.[124] Hepatocyte growth factor has also been isolated and reported to increase after hepatectomy.[125] Portal embolization induces a decrease in hepatocyte growth factor clearance and reroutes hepatotrophic hormones to the unembolized liver. For these reasons, in patients with multiple bilobar colorectal liver involvement, metastases in the future remnant liver (non-embolized) should be resected before portal vein embolization, since growth rate of metastatic nodules in the remnant liver can be more rapid than that of non-tumoral liver parenchyma after portal vein embolization;[126] otherwise, progression of metastases in the remnant liver may result in non-resectable disease. A major hepatic resection (embolized liver) can then be performed after the period of liver regeneration. Our preliminary experience of this two-stage hepatectomy procedure combined with portal vein embolization has been recently reported[127], showing that surgical outcome

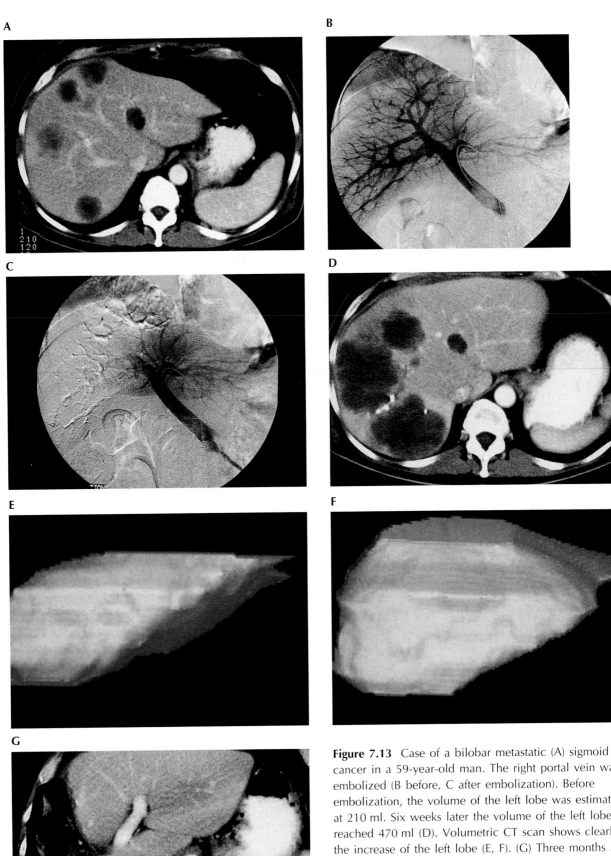

Figure 7.13 Case of a bilobar metastatic (A) sigmoid cancer in a 59-year-old man. The right portal vein was embolized (B before, C after embolization). Before embolization, the volume of the left lobe was estimated at 210 ml. Six weeks later the volume of the left lobe reached 470 ml (D). Volumetric CT scan shows clearly the increase of the left lobe (E, F). (G) Three months after right hepatectomy was extended to segment IV and combined wedge resection of deposit in the left lobe, CT scan shows the left lobe remnant.

and 3-year survival were similar to those of initially resectable patients (Figs. 7.14 and 7.15). However, occlusion of the portal branches has to be complete and durable. Therefore, at present, cyanoacrylate appears to be the most suitable agent for PE. Some necrotic reactions have been described after PE, but less severe than after hepatic arterial embolization, which could explain the good clinical tolerance of this procedure. Injection is performed under a percutaneous transhepatic approach with a Blue Histoacryl® and Lipiodol Ultrafluide® mixture. Liver volumetric measurements are obtained with three-dimensional, color-encoded CT, before portal embolization and before surgery. Expected hypertrophy of the future remnant liver is usually around 80 ± 50% after a 4–5 week interval between PE and surgery. Fewer than 20% of the patients develop insufficient hypertrophy of the future remnant liver and cannot undergo hepatic resection.[52,53] Clear criteria for the use of PE have not been established; however, it has been suggested that PE is indicated when the volume of the future remnant liver estimated by CT-scan volumetry is less than 40% in patients with normal liver tissue (ICG 15 between 10 and 20%).[51,52] Preoperative portal vein embolization widens the possibility of curative hepatectomies, particularly when extensive surgery is needed. It also appears effective for increasing the safety of hepatectomy for patients with multiple small metastases who require major right-sided resection combined with wedge resection of the left lobe[128] (Fig. 7.16).

Is there a place for adjuvant or neo-adjuvant chemotherapy?

After resection of hepatic metastases no study has shown that systemic chemotherapy prevents recurrence; however, controlled trials are currently ongoing to further answer this question.

Intra-arterial chemotherapy has a proven benefit on survival, but this is modest and the technique has important drawbacks (chemical hepatitis, sclerosing cholangitis, arterial thrombosis).[129–131]

Neo-adjuvant chemotherapy seems more promising. It has been shown that initially unresectable colorectal metastases could be debulked by chronomodulated chemotherapy,[132] using an association of 5-fluorouracil, folinic acid and oxaliplatin. Hepatic resection could then be performed using either major hepatectomy or minor resections. There was no operative mortality in this group of 53 patients and the cumulative 3- and 5-year survival rates were 54% and 40%, respectively. Two-staged hepatectomies were performed in some patients with large bilateral lesions

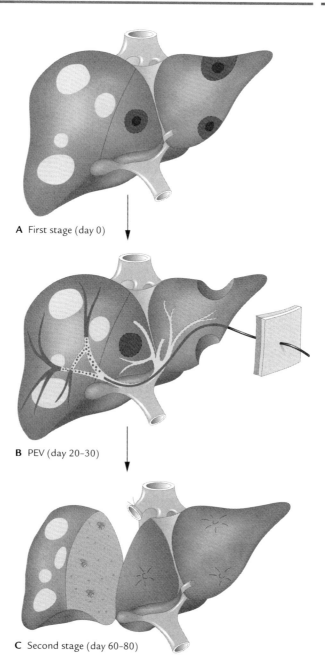

A First stage (day 0)

B PEV (day 20–30)

C Second stage (day 60–80)

Figure 7.14 Two-stage hepatectomy procedure combined with portal vein embolization. (A) first stage: resection of left liver nodules (day 0). (B) percutaneous right portal vein embolization (day 20–30). (C) second stage: right hepatectomy (day 60–80).

in which one-stage resection of all involved segments would have led to liver failure (e.g. segments V–VIII at the first operation and segments II–III thereafter). All the patients who underwent curative hepatic resection were treated by the same regimen of chronomodulated intravenous chemotherapy for at least 6 months. It must be emphasized that this now offers hope in treatment of patients who were initially considered unsuitable for radical surgery. The combined approach of neo-adjuvant systemic[132,133] or intra-arterial[134] chemotherapy followed by curative

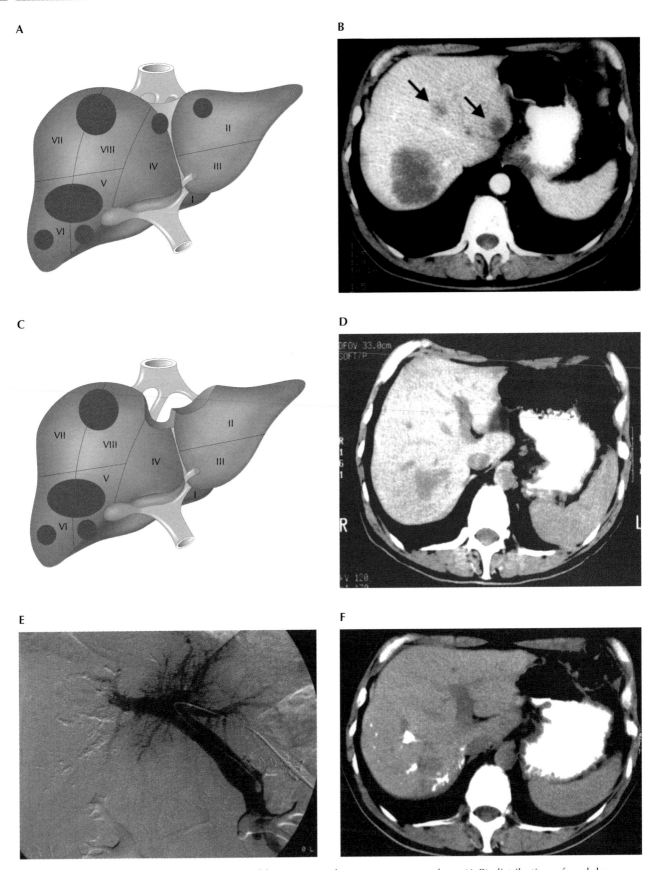

Figure 7.15 Case of bilobar metastases treated by two-stage hepatectomy procedure. (A,B) distribution of nodules before resection (arrows show nodules located in segment II and IV). (C,D) first stage hepatectomy: resection of the two left liver nodules. (E,F) right portal vein embolization. (E) portogram after embolization. (F) CT-scan five weeks after embolization shows lipiodol deposits in the right embolized atrophic liver and hypertrophy of the left liver.

continued

G

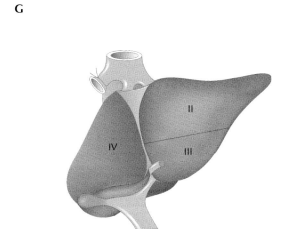

H

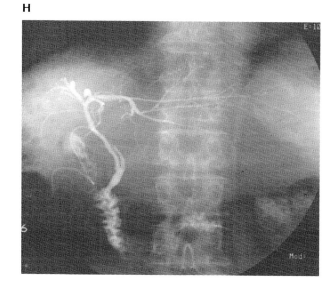

I

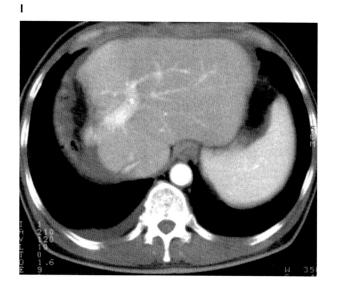

Figure 7.15 continued (G) second stage hepatectomy with right hepatectomy (day 72). (H) postoperative cholangiogram. (I) CT-scan 6 months after right hepatectomy showing hypertrophy of the left liver without nodule. (J,K) alternative to first stage hepatectomy: radiofrequency ablation is used as an alternative to left liver nodule resection or combined with left liver nodule resection.

J

K

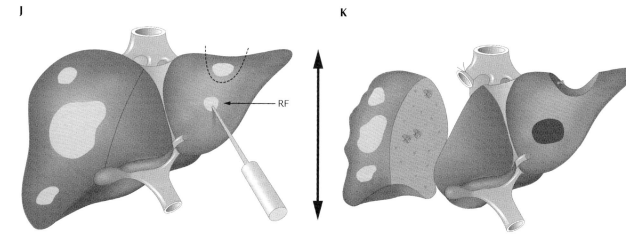

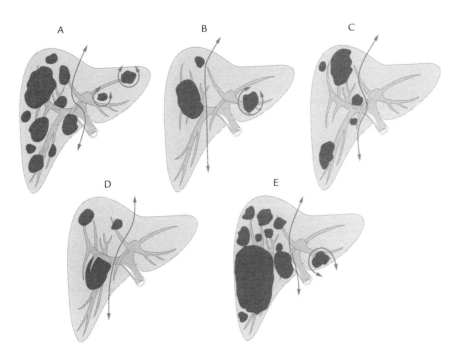

Figure 7.16 (A–E) Schematic representation of tumor location and type of liver resection in five patients with bilateral multiple liver metastases from colorectal cancer.

resection is a concept which may provide reasonable hope for long-term survival in some patients.

The follow-up: is repeat hepatectomy worthwhile?

After resection of colorectal liver metastases, it is estimated that unfortunately in about 60 to 70% of the patients, the disease will recur.[1,2,22–24,65,135–137] In approximately 30% of these cases, the disease will present as isolated liver metastases.[137,138] If metastases recur soon after surgery it is likely that, although not detected, they were already present during liver surgery.[139] In most cases they are diffuse and clearly unresectable. However, in a limited number of cases, recurrent metastases appear either solitary or localized and resectable. The results of the retrospective study of the French Association of Surgery are based on the data from 130 patients who received 143 repeat liver resections for recurrent liver metastases.[22] The operative mortality and morbidity rates were 0.9% and 24.7%, respectively. The 2- and 3-year survival rates were 57% and 33%, respectively, which were very similar to those obtained after first resections (57% and 38%, respectively). Twelve patients underwent more than two successive liver resections with some benefit. Other series have been reported with similar results,[23,24,140] encouraging an aggressive approach for selected patients. Combined extrahepatic surgery may sometimes be required to achieve tumor eradication.

The results of these studies suggest that very careful follow-up is recommended after resection of colorectal liver metastases with regular monitoring of CEA levels, liver ultrasound and CT imaging in order to detect recurrent disease.[141,142] In selected cases, repeat hepatectomy seems to be worthwhile.

Conclusions

The widest experience of hepatic surgery for metastatic disease has been gained with colorectal secondaries. Indeed, hepatic resection is currently the only form of treatment that offers both a chance of long-term survival, with rates ranging from 25 to 50% at 5 years and also a chance for cure: bilobar metastatic disease represents a clinical challenge that hepatic surgeons have to face up to more and more frequently. Without surgery the prognosis is so poor that patients have nearly no chance of long-term survival. The tremendous development of liver surgery techniques, assisted by the development of new strategies (portal vein embolization, two-stage hepatectomies, repeat hepatectomies, neo-adjuvant chemotherapy), has brought great enthusiasm in the treatment of patients with hepatic metastases from colorectal cancer. These new strategies have proven to be safe and postoperative mortality is now very low (around 1%). However, only a minority of patients (about 20%) can be considered for surgery and the first crucial point for the future is to increase the number of patients who will benefit from surgery. The second point is to develop efficient adjuvant treatments which will be able to reduce significantly the risk of recurrence after surgery. Progress will only be made through a multi-disciplinary approach.

Acknowledgements

The authors thank Professor Francis Veillon and Dr Bernard Woerly for their help in selecting X-ray illustrations. They express their gratitude to Mrs Véronique Rohfritsch for editing the manuscript and to Mrs Caroline Gstalter for processing the slides.

Key points

- Better prognostic factors:
  1–3 metastases
  <5 cm diameter
  No extrahepatic disease
  CEA <30 ng/l

  Detection >2 years after resection of primary tumor.
- French Association of Surgery Study of 1818 patients showed no difference in survival following resection of uni- versus bi-lobar disease.
- Preoperative assessment
  Spiral CT (dual phase) or MRI
  CT angio-portography
  Experimental: PET scanning.
- Evaluate residual hepatic reserve before considering resection.
- Consider:
  Two-stage procedure
  Combination of resection with residual tumor destruction.

REFERENCES

1. Nordlinger B, Jaeck D, Guiguet M et al. Surgical resection of hepatic metastases. Multicentric retrospective study by the French Association of Surgery. In: Nordlinger B, Jaeck D, eds. Treatment of hepatic metastases of colorectal cancer. Paris: Springer-Verlag, 1992: 129–61

2. Adson MA. Resection of liver metastases. When is it worthwhile? World J Surg 1987; 11: 511–20

3. Hughes KS, Simons R, Songhorabodi S et al. Resection of the liver for colorectal carcinoma metastases: a multi-institutional study of indications for resection. Registry of hepatic metastases. Surgery 1988; 103: 278–88

4. Jaeck D, Bachellier P, Guiguet M et al. Long-term survival following resection of colorectal metastases. Br J Surg 1997; 84: 977–80

5. Scheele J, Stangl R, Alterndorf-Hofmann A. Resection of colorectal liver metastases. World J Surg 1995; 19: 59–71

6. Nakamura S, Suzuki S, Baba S. Resection of liver metastases of colorectal carcinoma, World J Surg 1997; 21: 741–7

7. Scheele J. Hepatectomy for liver metastases. Br J Surg 1993; 80: 274–6

8. Steele G, Bleday R, Mayer RJ et al. A prospective evaluation of hepatic resection for colorectal carcinoma metastases to the liver (Gastrointestinal tumor study group protocol 6484). J Clin Oncol 1991; 9: 1105–12

9. Elias D, Ducreux M, Rougier P et al. Quelle sont les indications réelles des hépatectomies pour métastases d'origine colorectale? Gastroentérol Clin Biol 1998; 22: 1048–55

10. Minagawa M, Makuuchi M, Torzilli G et al. Extension of the frontiers of surgical indications in the treatment of liver metastases from colorectal cancer. Long-term results. Ann Surg 2000; 231: 487–99

11. Nordlinger B, Guiguet M, Vaillant JC et al. Surgical resection of colorectal carcinoma metastases to the liver. A prognostic scoring system to improve case selection, based on 1568 patients. Cancer 1996; 77: 1254–62

12. Bradpiece HA, Benjamin IS, Halevy A, Blumgart LH. Major hepatic resection for colorectal liver metastases. Br J Surg 1987; 74: 324–6

13. Ballantyne GH, Quin J. Surgical treatment of liver metastases in patients with colorectal cancer. Cancer 1993; 71 (Suppl): 4252–66

14. Gayowski TJ, Iwatsuki S, Madariaga JR et al. Experience in hepatic resection for metastatic colorectal cancer: analysis of clinical and pathological risk factors. Surgery 1994; 116: 703–11

15. Wanebo HJ, Chu QD, Vezeridis MP et al. Patient selection for hepatic resection of colorectal metastases. Arch Surg 1996; 131: 322–9

16. Bakalakos EA, Kim JA, Young DC et al. Determinants of survival following hepatic resection for metastatic colorectal cancer. World J Surg 1998; 22: 399–404; (discussion) 404–5

17. Rosen SA, Buell JF, Yoshida A et al. Initial presentation with stage IV colorectal cancer: how aggressive should we be? Arch Surg 2000; 135: 530–4; (discussion) 534–5

18. Cady B, Jenkins RL, Steele GD Jr et al. Surgical margin in hepatic resection for colorectal metastasis. A critical and improvable determinant of outcome. Ann Surg 1998; 227: 566–71

19. Elias D, Cavalcanti A, Sabourin JC et al. Resection of liver metastases from colorectal cancer: the real impact of the surgical margin. Eur J Surg Oncol 1998; 24: 174–9

20. Shirabe K, Takenaka K, Gion T et al. Analysis of prognostic risk factors in hepatic resection for metastatic colorectal carcinoma with special reference to the surgical margin. Br J Surg 1997; 84: 1077–80

21. Fong Y, Fortner J, Ruth L et al. Clinical score for predicting recurrence after hepatic resection for metastatic colorectal cancer. Analysis of 1001 consecutive cases. Ann Surg 1999; 230: 309–21

22. Nordlinger B, Vaillant JC, Guiguet M et al. Survival benefit of repeat liver resections for recurrent colorectal metastases: 143 cases. J Clin Oncol 1994; 12: 1491–6

23. Pinson CW, Wright JK, Chapman WC et al. Repeat hepatic surgery for colorectal cancer metastasis to the liver. Ann Surg 1996; 223: 765–76

24. Adam R, Bismuth H, Castaing D et al. Repeat hepatectomy for colorectal liver metastases. Ann Surg 1997; 225: 51–62

25. Yamamoto J, Kosuge T, Shimada K et al. Repeat liver resection for recurrent colorectal liver metastases. Am J Surg 1999; 178: 275–81

26. Bozzetti F, Gennari L, Regalia E et al. Morbidity and mortality after surgical resection of liver tumors. Analysis of 229 cases. Hepatogastroenterol 1992; 39: 237–41

27. Fong Y, Blumgart LH, Cohen AM et al. Repeat hepatic resections for metastatic colorectal cancer. Ann Surg 1994; 220: 657–62

28. Iwatsuki S, Dvorchik I, Madariaga JR et al. Hepatic resection for metastatic colorectal adenocarcinoma: A proposal of a prognostic scoring system. J Am Coll Surg 1999; 189: 291–9

29. Yamaguchi J, Yamamoto M, Komuta K et al. Hepatic resections for bilobar liver metastases from colorectal cancer. J Hepatobil Pancreatic Surg 2000; 7: 404–9

30. Imamura H, Kawasaki S, Miyagawa S et al. Aggressive surgical approach to recurrent tumors after hepatectomy for metastatic spread of colorectal cancer to the liver. Surgery 2000: 127: 528–35

31. Bolton JS, Fuhrman GM. Survival after resection of multiple bilobar hepatic metastases from colorectal carcinoma. Ann Surg 2000; 231: 743–51

32. Poupon MF. Biology of cancer invasion and liver metastases. In: Nordlinger B, Jaeck D, eds. Treatment of hepatic metastases of colorectal cancer. Paris: Springer-Verlag, 1992: 25–39

33. Shirai Y, Wakai T, Ohtani T et al. Colorectal carcinoma metastases to the liver. Does primary tumor location affect its lobar distribution? Cancer 1996; 77: 2213–6

34. Yasui K, Hirai T, Kato T et al. A new macroscopic classification predicts prognosis for patient with liver metastases from colorectal cancer. Ann Surg 1997; 226: 582–6

35. Rosen CB, Nagorney DM, Taswell HF et al. Perioperative blood transfusion and determinants of survival after liver resection for metastatic colorectal carcinoma. Ann Surg 1992; 216: 493–505

36. Sheu JC, Sung JL, Chen DS et al. Ultrasonography of small hepatic tumors using high-resolution linear-array real-time instruments. Radiology 1984; 150: 797–802

37. Chezmar JL, Rumancik WM, Megibow AJ et al. Liver and abdominal screening in patients with cancer: CT versus MR imaging. Radiology 1988; 168: 43–7

38. Strotzer M, Gmeinwieser J, Schmidt J et al. Diagnosis of liver metastasis from colorectal adenocarcinoma. Comparison of spiral-CTAP combined with intravenous contrast-enhanced spiral-CT and SPIO-enhanced MR combined with plan MR imaging. Acta Radiol 1997; 38: 986–92

39. Yamaguchi A, Ishida T, Nishimura G et al. Detection by CT during arterial portography of colorectal metastases to liver. Dis Colon Rectum 1991; 34: 37–40

40. Senéterre E, Taourel P, Bouvier Y et al. Detection of hepatic metastase: Ferumoxide-enhanced MR imaging versus unenhanced MR imaging and CT during arterial portography. Radiology 1996; 200: 785–92

41. Ward BA, Miller DL, Frank JA et al. Prospective evaluation of hepatic imaging studies in the detection of colorectal metastases. Correlation with surgical findings. Surgery 1989; 105: 180–7

42. John TG, Greig JD, Crosbie JL et al. Superior staging of liver tumors with laparoscopy and laparoscopic ultrasound. Ann Surg 1994; 220: 711–9

43. Rahusen FD, Cuesta MA, Borgstein PJ et al. Selection of patients for resection of colorectal metastases to the liver using diagnostic laparoscopy and laparoscopic ultrasonography. Ann Surg 1999; 230: 31–7

44. Vitola JV, Delbeke D, Sandler MP et al. Positron emission tomography to stage suspected metastatic colorectal carcinoma to the liver. Am J Surg 1996; 171: 21–6

45. Hustinx R, Paulus P, Daenen F et al. Intérêt clinique de la tomographie à émission de positrons dans la détection et le bilan d'extension des récidives des cancers colorectaux. Gastroentérol Clin Biol 1999; 23: 323–9

46. Stone HH, Long WB, Smith RB III et al. Physiological considerations in major hepatic resection. Am J Surg 1969; 117: 78–84

47. Okamoto E, Kyo A, Yamanaka N et al. Prediction of the safe limits of hepatectomy by combined volumetric and functional measurements in patients with impaired hepatic function. Surgery 1984; 95: 586–92

48. Kubota K, Makuuchi M, Kusaka K et al. Measurement of liver volume and hepatic functional reserve as a guide to decision-making in resectional surgery for hepatic tumors. Hepatology 1997; 26: 1176–81

49. Soyer P, Roche A, Elias D et al. Hepatic metastases from colorectal cancer: influence of hepatic volumetric analysis on surgical decision making. Radiology 1992; 184: 695–7

50. Kawasaki S, Makuuchi M, Matsunami H et al. Preoperative measurement of segmental liver volume of donors for living related liver transplantation. Hepatology 1993; 18: 1115–20

51. Azoulay D, Castaing D, Small A et al. Resection of nonresectable liver metastases from colorectal cancer after percutaneous portal vein embolization. Ann Surg 2000; 231: 480–6

52. Makuuchi M, Le Thai B, Takayasu K et al. Preoperative portal embolization to increase safety of major hepatectomy for hilar bile duct carcinoma: a preliminary report. Surgery 1990; 107: 521–7

53. De Baere T, Roche A, Elias D et al. Preoperative portal vein embolization for extension of hepatectomy indications. Hepatology 1996; 24: 1386–91

54. Abdalla EK, Hicks ME, Vauthey DN. Portal vein embolization: rationale, technique and future prospects. Br J Surg 2001; 88: 165–75

55. Hemming AW, Scudamore CH, Shackleton CR et al. Indocyanine green clearance as a predictor of successful hepatic resection in cirrhotic patients. Am J Surg 1992; 163: 515–8

56. Makuuchi M, Kosuge T, Takayama T et al. Surgery for small liver cancers. Semin Surg Oncol 1993; 9: 298–304

57. Ozawa K. Hepatic function and liver resection. J Gastroenterol Hepatol 1990; 5: 296–309

58. Ueda I, Mori K, Sakai Y et al. Noninvasive evaluation of cytochrome-C-oxidase activity of the liver. Its prognostic value for hepatic resection. Arch Surg 1994; 129: 303–8

59. Lau H, Man K, Fan ST et al. Evaluation of preoperative hepatic function in patients with hepatocellular carcinoma undergoing hepatectomy. Br J Surg 1997; 84: 1255–9

60. Jaeck D, Bachellier P. Quel traitement chirurgical proposer dans les cancers du colon avec métastases viscérales (synchrones et métachrones)? Conférence de consensus. Gastroentérol Clin Biol 1998; 22: S168–76.

61. Elias D, Saric J, Jaeck D et al. Prospective study of microscopic lymph node involvement of the hepatic pedicle during curative hepatectomy for colorectal metastases. Br J Surg 1996; 83: 942–5

62. August DA, Sugarbaker PH, Schneider PD. Lymphatic dissemination of hepatic metastases. Implications for the follow-up and treatment of patients with colorectal cancer. Cancer 1985; 55: 1490–4

63. Scheele J, Stangl R, Altendorf-Hofmann A et al. Indicators of prognosis after hepatic resection for colorectal secondaries. Surgery 1991; 110: 13–29

64. Beckurts KTE, Hölscher AH, Thorban St et al. Significance of lymph node involvement at the hepatic hilum in the resection of colorectal liver metastases. Br J Surg 1997; 84: 1081–4

65. Wagner S, Adson MA, Van Heerden JA et al. The natural history of hepatic metastases from colorectal cancer. Ann Surg 1984; 199: 502–7

66. Nakamura S, Yokoi Y, Suzuki S et al. Results of extensive surgery for liver metastases in colorectal carcinoma. Br J Surg 1992; 79: 35–8

67. Rafaelsen SR, Kronberg O, Larsen C et al. Intraoperative ultrasonography in detection of hepatic metastases from colorectal cancer. Dis Colon Rectum 1995; 38: 355–60

68. Bismuth H. Surgical anatomy and anatomical surgery of the liver. World J Surg 1982; 6: 3–9

69. Bismuth H, Houssin D, Castaing D. Major and minor segmentectomies 'réglées' in liver surgery. World J Surg 1982; 6: 10–24

70. Scheele J. Segment orientated resection of the liver: rationale and technique. In: Lygidakis NJ, Tytgat GNJ, eds. Hepatobiliary and pancreatic malignancies. Stuttgart: Thieme-Verlag, 1989: 219–47

71. Scheele J, Stangl R. Segment orientated anatomical liver resections. In: Blumgart LH, eds. Surgery of the liver and the biliary tract. Vol 2. London: Churchill Livingstone, 1994: 1557–78

72. Maziotti A, Cavallari A. II – Standard techniques of liver resection. III – Complex techniques of liver resection. In: Maziotti A, Cavallari A, eds. Techniques in liver surgery. London: Greenwich Medical Media, 1997: 15–116

73. Stone MD, Kane R, Bothe A et al. Intraoperative ultrasound imaging of the liver at the time of colorectal resection. Arch Surg 1994; 129: 431–45

74. Herman K. Intraoperative ultrasound in gastrointestinal cancer. An analysis of 272 operated patients. Hepatogastroenterology 1996; 43: 565–70

75. Couinaud C. Le foie: études anatomiques et chirurgiales. Paris: Masson, 1957

76. Couinaud C. Principes directeurs des hépatectomies réglées. Chirurgie 1980; 106: 103–8

77. Couinaud C. Secteur dorsal du foie. Chirurgie 1998; 123: 8–15

78. Couinaud C. The paracaval segments of the liver. J Hepatobil Pancr Surg 1994; 2: 145–51

79. Strasberg SM, Belghiti J, Clavien PA et al. The Brisbane 2000 terminology of liver anatomy and resections. HPB 2000; 2: 333–9

80. Makuuchi M, Hasegawa H, Yamazakis et al. Four new hepatectomy procedures for resection of the right hepatic vein and preservation of the inferior right hepatic vein. Surg Gynecol Obstet 1987; 164: 68–72

81. Bartlett D, Fong Y, Blumgart LH. Complete resection of the caudate lobe of the liver: technique and results. Br J Surg 1996; 83: 1076–81

82. Elias D, Lasser Ph, Desrennes E et al. Surgical approach to segment 1 for malignant tumors of the liver. Surg Gynecol Obstet 1992; 175: 17–24

83. Makuuchi M, Kawasaki S, Takayama T et al. Caudate lobectomy. In: Lygidakis NY, Makuuchi M, eds. Pitfalls and complications in the diagnosis and management of hepatobiliary and pancreatic disease. Stuttgart: Thieme-Verlag, 1993: 124–32

84. Gozzetti G, Maziotti A, Grazi A et al. Liver resections without blood transfusions. Br J Surg 1995; 82: 1105–10

85. Younes RN, Rogatko A, Brennan MF. The influence of intraoperative hypotension and perioperative blood transfusion on disease-free survial in patients with complete resection of colorectal liver metastases. Ann Surg 1991; 214: 107–13

86. Johnson M, Mannar R, Wu AVO. Correlation between blood loss and inferior vena caval pressure during liver resection. Br J Surg 1998; 85: 188–90

87. Huguet C, Nordlinger B, Galopin JJ et al. Tolerance of the human liver to prolonged normothermic ischemia. Arch Surg 1978; 113: 1448–51

88. Delva E, Camus Y, Nordlinger B et al. Vascular occlusions for liver resections: operative management and tolerance to hepatic ischemia. Ann Surg 1989; 209: 211–8

89. Hannoun L, Borie D, Delva E et al. Liver resection with normothermic ischemia exceeding 1 hour. Br J Surg 1993; 80: 1161–5

90. Huguet C, Gavelli A, Chicco A et al. Liver ischemia for hepatic resections: where is the limit? Surgery 1992; 11: 251–9

91. Makuuchi A, Mori T, Gunven P et al. Experimental study of protective effect of intermittent hepatic pedicle clamping in the rat. Br J Surg 1992; 79: 310–3

92. Belghiti J, Noun R, Malafosse R et al. Continuous versus intermittent portal triad clamping for liver resection. A controlled study. Ann Surg 1999; 229: 369–75

93. Makuuchi M, Mori T, Gunven P et al. Safety of hemihepatic vascular occlusion during resection of the liver. Surg Gynecol Obstet 1997; 164: 155–8

94. Nakano H, Nagasaki H, Barama A et al. The effects of N-acetylcysteine and anti-cellular adhesion molecule-1 monoclonal antibody against ischemia-reperfusion injury of the rat steatotic liver procuded by a choline-methionine-deficient diet. Hepatology 1997; 26: 670–8

95. Elias D, Lasser P, Debaene B et al. Intermittent vascular exclusion of the liver (without vena cava clamping) during major hepatectomy. Br J Surg 1995; 82: 1535–9

96. Cherqui D, Malassogne B, Cohen PI et al. Hepatic vascular exclusion with preservation of the caval flow for liver resections. Ann Surg 1999; 230: 24–30

97. Pichlmayr R, Grosse H, Hauss J et al. Technique and preliminary results of extracorporeal liver surgery (bench procedure) and of surgery on the in situ perfused liver. Br J Surg 1990; 77: 21–6

98. Fortner JG, Shin M H, Kinne DW et al. Major hepatic resection using vascular isolation and hypothermic perfusion. Ann Surg 1974; 180: 644–52

99. Hannoun L, Panis Y, Balladur P et al. 'Ex situ in vivo' liver surgery. Principle and first results. Lancet 1991; 337: 1616–7

100. Belghiti J, Dousset B, Sauvanet A et al. Résultats préliminaires de l'exérèse 'ex situ' des tumeurs hépatiques: place entre les traitements palliatifs et la transplantation. Gastroentérol Clin Biol 1991; 15: 449–53

101. Delrivière L, Hannoun L. 'In situ' and 'ex situ in vivo' procedures for complex major liver resections requiring prolonged hepatic vascular exclusion in normal and diseased livers. J Am Coll Surg 1995; 181: 272–6

102. Steele G, Ravikumar TS, Benotti PN. New surgical treatments for recurrent colorectal cancer. Cancer 1990; 65: 723–30

103. Stangl R, Altendorf-Hoffmann A, Chanley RM et al. Factors influencing the natural history of colorectal liver metastases. Lancet 1994; 343: 1405–10

104. Ravikumar TS, Kane R, Cady B et al. Hepatic cryosurgery with intraoperative ultrasound monitoring for metastatic colon carcinoma. Arch Surg 1987; 122: 403–9

105. Weaver ML, Altkinson D, Zemel R. Hepatic cryosurgery in treating colorectal metastases. Cancer 1995; 76: 210–4

106. Adam R, Akpinar E, Johann M et al. Place of cryosurgery in the treatment of malignant liver tumors. Ann Surg 1997; 225: 39–50

107. Hewitt PM, Dwerryhouse SJ, Zhao J et al. Multiple bilobar liver metastases: cryotherapy for residual lesions after liver resection. J Surg Oncol 1998; 67: 112–6

108. Nagata Y, Hiraoka M, Akuta K et al. Radiofrequency thermotherapy for malignant liver tumors. Cancer 1990; 65: 1730–6

109. Rossi S, Di Stasi M, Buscarini E et al. Percutaneous radiofrequency interstitial thermal ablation in the treatment of hepatic cancer. Am J Roentgenol 1996; 167: 759–68

110. Patterson EJ, Scudamore CH, Owen DA et al. Radiofrequency ablation of porcine liver in vivo. Ann Surg 1998; 227: 559–65

111. Curley SA, Izzo F, Delrio P et al. Radiofrequency ablation of unresectable primary and metastatic hepatic malignancy. Results in 123 patients. Ann Surg 1999; 230: 1–8

112. De Baere T, Elias D, Ducreux M et al. Ablathermie percutanée des métastases hépatiques. Expérience préliminaire. Gastroentérol Clin Biol 1999; 23: 1128–33

113. Hamazoe R, Hiraoka Y, Ohtani S et al. Intraoperative microwave tissue coagulation as treatment of patients with nonresectable hepatocellular carcinoma. Cancer 1995; 75: 794–800

114. Klotz HP, Flury R, Erhart P et al. Magnetic resonance-guided laparoscopic interstitial laser therapy of the liver. Am J Surg 1997; 174: 448–51

115. Masters A, Steger AC, Brown SG. Role of interstitial therapy in the treatment of liver cancer. Br J Surg 1991; 78: 518–23

116. Vogl TJ, Muller PK, Hammerstingl R et al. Malignant liver tumors treated with MR imaging-guided laser-induced thermotherapy. Technique and prospective results. Radiology 1995; 196: 257–65

117. Armstrong JG, Anderson LL, Harrison LB. Treatment of liver metastases from colorectal cancer with radioactive implants. Cancer 1994; 73: 1800–4

118. Amin Z, Brown SG, Lees WR. Local treatment of colorectal liver metastases. A comparison of interstitial laser photocoagulation (ILP) and percutaneous alcohol injection (PAI). Clin Radiol 1993; 48: 166–71

119. Jaeck D, Bachellier P, Weber JC et al. Le traitement chirurgical des métastases hépatiques synchrones des cancers colo-rectaux. Ann Chir 1996; 50: 507–16

120. Doci R, Gennari L, Begnami P et al. Morbidity and mortality after hepatic resection of metastases from colorectal cancer. Br J Surg 1995; 82: 377–81

121. Miyagawa S, Makuuchi M, Kawasaki S et al. Criteria for safe hepatic resection. Am J Surg 1995; 169: 589–94

122. Elias D, Cavalcanti A, De Baere T et al. Résultats carcinologique à long terme des hépatectomies réalisées après embolisation portale selective. Ann Chirurgie 1999; 53: 559–64

123. Rous P, Larimore L. Relation of the portal blood to liver maintenance. J Exp Med 1920; 31: 609–32

124. Starzl T, Trancavilla A, Halgrimson C et al. The origin, hormonal nature, and action of hepatotrophic substances in portal venous blood. Surg Gynecol Obstet 1973; 137: 179–99

125. Zarnegar R, Michalopoulos G. Purification and biological characterization of human hepatopoietin A, a polypeptide growth factor for hepatocytes. Cancer Res 1989; 49: 3314–20

126. Elias D, De Baere T, Roche A et al. During liver regeneration following right portal embolization the growth rate of liver metastases is more rapid than that of the liver parenchyma. Br J Surg 1999; 86: 784–8

127. Bachellier P, Nakano H, Weber JC et al. Two-stage hepatectomy procedure combined with portal vein embolization for initially unresectable multiple bilobar liver metastases from colorectal carcinoma. HPB Surg 2001; 3: 79A

128. Kawasaki S, Makuuchi M, Kakazu T et al. Resection for multiple metastatic liver tumors after portal embolization. Surgery 1994; 115: 674–7

129. Rougier P, Lasser Ph, Elias D. Systemic and local chemotherapy in palliative and adjuvant treatment of hepatic metastases of colorectal origin. In: Nordlinger B, Jaeck D, eds. Treatment of hepatic metastases of colorectal cancer. Paris: Springer-Verlag, 1992: 109–28

130. Hasuike Y, Yagyu T, Shih E et al. A new two-part therapy for multiple bilobar liver metastases for colorectal cancer – treatment of one lobe with partial hepatectomy and the other with arterial chemotherapy. Gan To Kagaku Ryoho 1997; 24: 1757–9

131. Lygidakis NJ, Vlachos L, Raptis S et al. New frontiers in liver surgery. Two-stage liver surgery for the management of advanced metastatic liver disease. Hepatogastroenterology 1999; 46: 2216–28

132. Bismuth H, Adam R, Lévi F et al. Resection of non-resectable liver metastases from colorectal cancer after neoadjuvant chemotherapy. Ann Surg 1996; 224: 509–22

133. Fowler WC, Eisenberg BL, Hoffmann JP. Hepatic resection folowing systemic chemotherapy for metastatic colorectal carcinoma. J Surg Oncol 1992; 51: 122–5

134. Elias D, Lasser Ph, Rougier Ph et al. Frequency, technical aspects, results and indications for major hepatectomy after prolonged intra-arterial chemotherapy for initially unresectable hepatic tumors. J Am Coll Surg 1995; 180: 213–9

135. Hughes KS, Simon R, Songhorabodi S. Resection of the liver for colorectal carcinoma metastases: a multi-institutional study of patterns of recurrence. Surgery 1986; 100: 278–84

136. Nordlinger B, Quilichini MA, Parc R et al. Hepatic resection for colorectal liver metastases. Influence on survival of preoperative factors and surgery for recurrence in 80 patients. Ann Surg 1987; 205: 256–63

137. Bozzetti F, Bignami P, Morabito A et al. Patterns of failure following surgical resection of colorectal cancer liver metastases. Rationale for a multimodal approach. Ann Surg 1987; 205: 264–70

138. Ekberg H, Tramberg KG, Anderson R et al. Patterns of recurrence in liver resection for colorectal secondaries. World J Surg 1987; 11: 541–7

139. Panis Y, Ribeiron J, Chrétien Y et al. Dormant liver metastases: demonstration by experimental study in rats. Br J Surg 1992; 79: 221–3

140. Suzuki S, Nakamura S, Ochiai H et al. Surgical management of recurrence after resection of colorectal liver metastases. J Hepato-Bil Pancr Surg 1997; 4: 103–12

141. Wanebo HJ, Chu QD, Avradopoulos KA et al. Current perspectives on repeat hepatic resection for colorectal carcinoma: a review. Surgery 1996; 119: 361–71

142. Elias D, Lasser Ph, Hoang JM et al. Repeat hepatectomy for cancer. Br J Surg 1993; 80: 1557–62

8 Non-resectional treatment of colorectal cancer metastases

David L Morris, Ian Finlay, Sivakumar Gananadha and Winston Liauw

Introduction

Between 25 and 35% of colorectal cancer patients will develop hepatic metastases.[1] However, only 25% of these patients will be suitable for potentially curative hepatic resection.[2]

Patients may be considered unsuitable for hepatic resection for a variety of reasons:

- The presence of extrahepatic disease.
- Bilobar distribution of disease (relative).
- Unilobar disease in an awkward location, e.g. hepatic vein/IVC confluence.
- A large number of metastases (most centres resect a maximum of four metastases).
- The remaining liver volume would be inadequate.
- The patient is unfit for major surgery.

Fifty per cent of patients who undergo hepatic resection will develop hepatic recurrence.[3] For these patients one should consider other treatment options, i.e. non-resectional treatment. Non-resectional treatments can be categorized into two groups: imaging controlled tumour destructive techniques and those employing chemotherapy.

Imaging controlled tumour destructive techniques

The purpose of these methods is to destroy metastatic disease leaving the surrounding normal hepatic parenchyma unaffected. Three techniques have been used widely: cryotherapy, which freezes tissue, and radiofrequency ablation and interstitial laser hyperthermia, which heat tissue. These methods are indicated only for relatively limited, well-defined disease and have no place in the treatment of patients with additional extrahepatic metastases.

Percutaneous ethanol injection is a further method of producing localized tissue destruction which has produced good results in the treatment of small (less than 2 cm diameter) hepatocellular tumours.[4–6] However, the technique has been shown to be relatively ineffective in treating colorectal hepatic metastases.[6]

Chemotherapy techniques

Two methods of delivering chemotherapy are currently employed in the treatment of colorectal hepatic metastases: regional delivery via the hepatic artery and systemic intravenous infusion. Both techniques are associated with particular complications and results differ between the techniques.

Regional chemotherapy treats only hepatic disease and has no role in the treatment of patients with extrahepatic disease. In such patients systemic intravenous chemotherapy is the only treatment option.

This chapter will review these various methods of non-resectional treatment for colorectal hepatic metastases, concentrating upon their relative results and complications. Figure 8.1 provides a brief overview of the indications for each of the treatment modalities later expanded upon in this chapter.

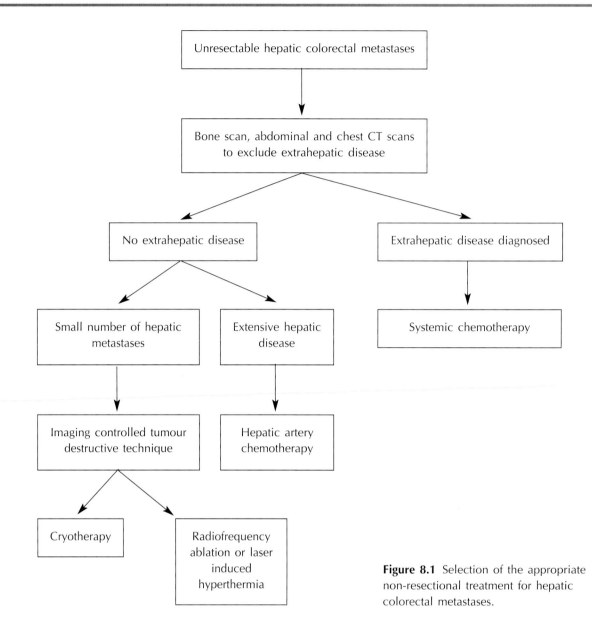

Figure 8.1 Selection of the appropriate non-resectional treatment for hepatic colorectal metastases.

Hepatic cryotherapy

Introduction

Cryotherapy is the most developed technique of imaging controlled tumour destruction. The currently used system of liquid nitrogen and trocar probes was first used in 1961,[7] and has since been employed in the treatment of lesions in various organs in addition to the liver. Figure 8.2 details the basic design of modern cryotherapy probes.

The mechanism of action of cryotherapy upon tumours is multifactorial. Rapid freezing results in the formation of intracellular ice crystals, which damage intracellular structures and cell membranes, resulting in cell death. Slower freezing to higher temperatures results in the formation of extracellular ice crystals, producing an osmolar gradient between the intra- and extracellular fluid compartments, and results in cellular dehydration. Extracellular ice crystals also expand and distort tissue architecture, particularly the microvasculature, which is also damaged by thrombus formation. Histologically cryolesions are very similar to areas of ischaemic necrosis.[8–12]

Indications

Current indications for hepatic cryotherapy include liver metastases of colorectal origin, neuroendocrine tumours and hepatoma. Patients should be free of extrahepatic disease, with liver disease judged to be unresectable due to multiple tumours of bilobar distribution. Cryotherapy may also be employed in patients with anatomically resectable disease in whom resection is not possible due to poor liver reserve (cirrhosis).

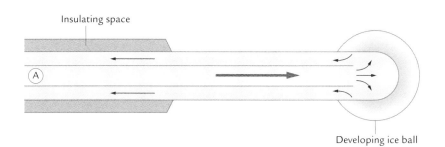

Insulating space

A

Developing ice ball

Figure 8.2 Cross-section of a cryoprobe. Liquid nitrogen is delivered through the inner tube (A) to the tip of the probe where it vaporizes, and travels back along the outer tube of the probe.

The number of lesions which can usefully be treated by cryotherapy depends on the tumour type, but in colorectal cancer is probably limited to six lesions.[13] There is no proven role for the debulking of colorectal liver metastases by cryotherapy, whereas in neuroendocrine cancers the destruction of most, but not all, disease can be of symptomatic and possibly survival benefit.[14]

There are currently few data to support the use of cryotherapy as an alternative to liver resection. Liver resection is associated with a perioperative mortality of below 2% and the long-term results are well established.[15,16] While the safety of cryotherapy is established, with a perioperative mortality less than 5%,[12] the long-term results are not established as being equivalent to liver resection.

Cryotherapy might be of use as an adjuvant to liver surgery. It can be used to treat an inadequate or involved resection margin[17] or synchronous lesions in the residual liver at the time of resection.[18] This approach is potentially capable of increasing the proportion of patients to whom resection can be offered.

The use of hepatic cryotherapy at the time of colonic resection of the primary tumour is dangerous, the combination of an area of necrosis (the cryolesion) and a contaminated peritoneum may cause liver abscess formation.

Technique

Cryotherapy is often a prolonged procedure, therefore careful attention should be paid to the positioning of the patient, and antithromboembolic measures (subcutaneous heparin, graded pressure stockings and calf compression) should be employed together with antibiotic prophylaxis. To prevent the development of hypothermia, warming devices such as the Bair Hugger should be used.

The liver is fully mobilized and a plan for probe placement is made. Probe positioning is sometimes easily achieved but may require the use of needle localization under ultrasound control, particularly if a lesion is impalpable. The use of a Seldinger technique with a dilator and sheath being passed over the localizing needle followed by insertion of the probe through the sheath is optimal. Ultrasound assessment is essential to confirm correct probe placement and it is important to examine placement in both longitudinal and transverse sections.

The diameter of the lesions to be treated is of principal importance, and the capability of the particular cryoprobe must be appreciated. In brief, a 5 mm liquid nitrogen cryoprobe might be expected to produce a 5 cm cryolesion. If a 1 cm cryomargin is required then one perfectly sited probe might adequately treat a 3 cm lesion.

The time of freezing is determined by the time taken to achieve an ice ball of adequate size. The proximity of the lesion to major vascular structures is of importance because of the heat sink effect. It may be necessary to position a probe eccentrically and closer to such a heat sink. When multiple probes are used to treat large lesions, this should be performed synchronously rather than serially. Portal inflow occlusion reduces the time required to achieve large ice ball diameters and probably increases efficacy. We limit inflow occlusion to a total of 60 minutes.

Careful intraoperative assessment using ultrasound is necessary to ensure that each boundary of a tumour is well enveloped by a margin of at least 1 cm.

We advise passive thawing of a 1 cm rim followed by refreezing. The destructive effects of a twin freeze thaw cycle appear to be greater than single cycle freeze. We are, however, concerned that double freeze thaw cycles are involved in the pathogenesis of the cryoshock phenomenon. The thaw and refreeze of the edge of the ice ball is intended to re-treat the least effectively treated part of the lesion – the peripheral rim. We do not know the critical temperature for the destruction of colorectal cancer metastases in the liver, but the edge of a large ice ball may only be exposed to a degree or two below zero because of the almost exponential fall of temperature around an ice ball.

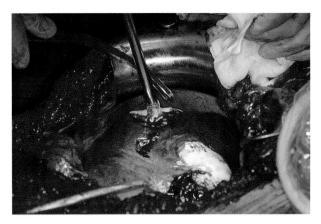

Figure 8.3 Hepatic cryotherapy in progress.

After thawing, a gelfoam plug is placed in the cryoprobe track to arrest any bleeding. Large parenchymal cracks can develop during freezing and, upon thawing, can cause significant bleeding which may require compressive sutures or packing until haemostasis is achieved. Such bleeding might not appear until the lesions have completely thawed, therefore the wound should not be closed until thawing is complete. We routinely place a catheter for hepatic artery chemotherapy following cryotherapy.

Care must be taken to avoid freezing the gut or any other extrahepatic structure. Injury to bile ducts within the liver seldom seems to be a problem, but one must avoid injury to the extrahepatic biliary tree.

Laparoscopic and percutaneous approaches to hepatic cryotherapy are currently under clinical evaluation, with encouraging results.

Figure 8.3 depicts cryotherapy in progress, with two probes being used to treat two individual lesions synchronously.

Complications

While serious complications are rare, good post-operative monitoring is important.

- *Postoperative haemorrhage* is a very rare event if the ice ball has fully thawed and any parenchymal cracks have been dealt with before closure of the abdomen.
- *Cryoshock* is perhaps the most important specific complication. This is very rare, but in a recent world questionnaire of surgeons employing cryotherapy 1% of hepatic cryotherapy patients had developed this syndrome and it

was responsible for six out of 33 perioperative deaths in 2173 patients.[19] Cryoshock is seen only in patients subjected to at least two freeze thaw cycles. The syndrome consists of renal impairment, ARDS-like pulmonary injury and coagulopathy and requires active supportive treatment with ventilation and replacement of coagulation factors.[20,21] We have not seen this complete syndrome in our experience of almost 200 patients.[13]

- *Thrombocytopenia* is common following large volume cryotherapy and may require platelet transfusion.[22]
- *Abscess:* subphrenic or hepatic abscesses are a rare complication of cryotherapy, except when it is performed at the time of colectomy.
- *Biloma* is a specific complication of the use of hepatic arterial 5-fluoro-2'-deoxyuridine (FUDR) chemotherapy following cryotherapy, perhaps as a result of chemical biliary sclerosis causing increased biliary pressure.
- *Pyrexia:* postoperative pyrexia is common and perhaps due to tissue necrosis. Septic screening in such cases is negative.
- *Deranged liver function tests:* there is often a striking but self limiting rise in serum hepatic transaminase levels, present by the first postoperative day and resolving within 7 days.

Imaging

CT portography

Hepatic cryotherapy is dependent upon accurate imaging. CT portography scanning is useful in the preoperative assessment of hepatic metastases necessary to plan treatment. CT scanning of the rest of the abdomen and the chest together with a bone scan is desirable to exclude extrahepatic disease.

Intraoperative ultrasound

Intraoperative ultrasound is indispensable at laparotomy. It can detect additional small tumours in 30% of patients compared to other imaging techniques. Cryotherapy trocars are inserted under two-dimensional ultrasound guidance, and once successfully placed the development and extent of the ice ball are monitored by ultrasound.

Colorectal malignancies are variable in their ultrasonic appearance between patients, being hyperechoic, hypoechoic or isoechoic compared to the surrounding normal liver. However, in any one patient all lesions should have a similar echogenic appearance. The position of the lesion in respect to hepatic veins can be distinguished from portal structures as the veins lack a hyperechoic sheath.

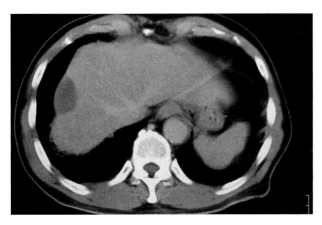

Figure 8.4 CT scan showing the 'golf ball in the sand' appearance of a cryolesion.

As freezing develops, the ice ball appears as a hypoechoic (black) area surrounded by a hyperechoic rim, and can be monitored in real time. When thawed the cytoplasm appears hypoechoic compared to the normal liver, and the extent of the treated area is readily assessed.

On postoperative CT the cryolesion initially appears as a large avascular lesion with gas in the probe track. This gradually involutes to leave a smaller fibrous retracted spherical lesion – the so-called 'golf ball in the sand' appearance, as illustrated in Fig. 8.4.[23]

Postoperative follow-up

Postoperatively we routinely use serial 3-monthly carcinoembryonic antigen (CEA) levels to monitor patients with CEA secreting tumours. CEA levels fall rather more slowly following cryotherapy than after hepatic resection, taking several weeks to decrease.[24] The percentage fall in CEA levels pre- and postoperatively may be prognostic for survival,[25,26] with some 60% of patients' CEA levels returning to the normal range.[13] CT scanning of the liver and abdomen is used only in the follow-up of non-secretors, or to assess patients with a CEA rise.

Results

A recent review of published clinical series found 14 postoperative deaths in 869 patients treated with cryotherapy, a 1.6% mortality rate. Reported rates of postoperative complications ranged from 0 to 45%, chest infection being the most common complication.[12]

Survival

The most striking survival results published are those of the Boston group.[27] They reported 5-year survival and disease-free survival rates of 78 and 39%, respectively. However, there were only 18 patients in this series, and only one to three lesions were treated in each patient. Our own 5-year survival data are more modest at 13%, but constitute a group of inoperable patients with a median of 3.9 lesions, 83% having bilobar disease. Other series tend to have short median follow-up times but report median survival times of 13.5–16 months, again with some patients surviving longer than 5 years.[12] These results certainly compare well with those of hepatic artery chemotherapy, but it is not yet clear whether cryotherapy is able to achieve results comparable to liver resection.

Interstitial laser hyperthermia (ILH)

Introduction and theoretical considerations

Lasers are particularly suitable to generate localized hyperthermia within the liver. They produce a highly collimated, coherent beam of light of a set wavelength and can be transmitted down thin, flexible optical fibres and directed towards a target area with great accuracy. Neodymium yttrium aluminium garnet (Nd YAG) laser is the most suitable for ILH,[28] as it produces light with a wavelength of around 1064 nm which is capable of penetrating tissue to a far greater depth than that produced by either CO_2 or argon lasers.

Nd YAG laser light can be delivered down thin (0.2–0.6 mm diameter), flexible, optical quartz fibres, and is emitted only at the tip of the fibre. This allows treatment to be performed percutaneously, the fibre being introduced via a 19 gauge needle under local anaesthetic with little chance of damage to major blood vessels or biliary structures, making it suitable for percutaneous application.

Mechanism of tissue destruction and techniques

When light from an Nd YAG laser at low (<2 W) power settings is emitted from the end of a single optical fibre embedded in tissue, it is scattered in multiple directions by the surrounding tissue. This results in an almost spherical distribution of the light around the fibre tip.[29] Light is absorbed and heating results; when the temperature exceeds 45°C coagulation of cellular proteins occurs and well-defined areas of necrosis ensue.

Early investigators employed modified tips on the fibres in an attempt to enhance diffusion of the light and maximize effects. However, these tips had no significant advantage over plain fibre tips,[30] they were too large in diameter to be safely used percutaneously[31] and required gas coolant, which was responsible for a fatal gas embolus.[32] When plain fibre tips are employed, light is transmitted throughout the tissue for around 20–30 seconds but then blood coagulation and charring occur around the tip. The charred area then strongly absorbs light and acts as a point heat source, diffusing heat into the surrounding tissue.[33]

Using plain fibres and low (<2 W) power laser energy for up to 2400 seconds a highly reproducible, near spherical area of necrosis is produced with a maximum diameter of 1.6 cm.[29] In order to increase the area of necrosis produced and treat larger diameter lesions, beam splitters have been employed to allow one laser to illuminate four optical fibres. These fibres can be placed no more than 1.5 cm apart around a lesion to allow the area of necrosis to overlap,[33] and treat tumours of up to 3 cm.[34,35] Larger lesions have been treated by repeated treatments with repositioning of the fibres within or around the tumours.[36]

More recently, investigators have returned to using diffuser tipped fibres; these diffusers are smaller than those used initially and can be placed percutaneously.[37,38] In contrast to bare fibre tips, diffusers do not produce charring, which absorbs light, and therefore allow deeper light penetration and more extensive and homogeneous heat distribution. Using this method tumours of diameter 2.4 cm can be ablated simply by placing the tip in the centre of the tumour, and larger lesions by using a beam splitter and/or fibre repositioning. This is a modest size compared with that achieved by modern RFA units.

Imaging

Accurate imaging is required at three stages: (a) placement of the fibres within the lesions, (b) real time monitoring of the treatment to ensure the whole lesion is treated and (c) follow-up assessment of the lesion to assess response to treatment.

Once lesions have been diagnosed on CT scanning, most studies of ILH have used ultrasound scanning to guide the placement of fibres within lesions.[34,35,37,39] Unfortunately, the resolution capability of percutaneous ultrasound scanning makes the detection and subsequent targeting of small (<2 cm) lesions difficult. Intraoperative ultrasound is capable of detecting additional liver tumours in 30% of patients compared to other imaging techniques,[40,41] and laparoscopic ultrasound scanning has been proposed as an alternative technique to guide the placement of fibres.[42]

During ILH of previously hypoechoic, mixed or isoechoic metastases a central bright hyperechoic region appears around the fibre tip. A hyperechoic ring then develops around this point, it radius expanding with the duration of treatment. This is thought to be due to the development of echogenic microbubbles.[37,43] These well-defined areas correlate well with the extent of necrosis produced.[44] The lesion changes in ultrasonic appearance within 24 hours, becoming a central hyperechoic point of charring surrounded by a hypoechoic ring. The margin of the treated area and normal liver becomes progressively less sharp in the months after treatment,[35,37] making detection of recurrence difficult by ultrasound scanning.

Dynamic CT scanning with intravenous contrast has been shown to be capable of distinguishing non-enhancing necrosis from enhancing viable tumour tissue, allowing assessment of the effectiveness in tumour destruction to be made post procedure.[43]

More recently, magnetic resonance imaging (MRI) scanning has been employed in an attempt to overcome the limitations of ultrasound scanning. Vogl et al.,[45] have used MRI scanning to guide fibre insertion, and by using a novel MRI protocol were able to perform real time thermometry to assess the extent of the treated area. Gadolinium enhanced MRI allowed early and late follow-up of treated lesions. The clinical application of MRI guidance for ILH appears to overcome most of the problems associated with percutaneous ultrasound guidance and results are promising.[46]

Results

Tumour response

The potential of ILH in the ablation of liver tumours was first investigated by Hashimoto et al.,[31] who demonstrated that ILH was capable of reducing the alpha feto protein levels of two hepatoma patients to the normal range, and produced similar dramatic falls in the carcinoembryonic antigen levels of patients with colorectal hepatic metastases. Masters et al.[34] subsequently demonstrated that, by using the four bare fibre tip technique, radiologically confirmed necrosis of tumours less than 3 cm diameter could be achieved, with 50% of these treated tumours remaining the same size or involuting over the ensuing 6 months. Others have evaluated the use of bare fibre tips by contrast enhanced CT scanning and found 100% necrosis could be produced in 38% of lesions, and greater than 50% necrosis in 82% of lesions, with metastases smaller than 4 cm being treated most effectively.[43]

When a diffuser tip was used 12 of 16 metastases were found on ultrasound scanning and guided fine needle aspiration biopsy to be completely destroyed. The successfully treated lesions ranged in diameter from 1 to 3.7 cm.[37] Vogl et al.[45] used MRI scanning both to position and monitor the progress of ILH with a diffuser fibre tip, and found that in 69% of lesions 2 cm or smaller 100% necrosis could be produced, and 44% of these did not progress within 12 months. However, in lesions over 2 cm complete necrosis was achieved in only 41%, with 27% of these remaining static at 12 months.

Survival

Amin et al.[43] reported basic survival data for a series of 21 patients treated by bare fibre tip ILH for metastases from colorectal and other cancers. Survival of the 15 colorectal cancer patients ranged from 4 to 40 months, with a median of 9 months. Subsequently, Vogl et al.[47] reported comprehensive survival data for a series of 99 patients with 282 hepatic colorectal metastases treated by diffuser tip ILH under MRI guidance and monitoring. Survival rates were 88% at 12 months, 70% at 24 months and 42% at 36 months, with a predicted median of 36.4 months. In both of these studies all patients were unsuitable for hepatic resection, and the survival data compare well with that of other treatments in similar patients.[48]

Complications and limitations

As ILH can be performed percutaneously under local anaesthetic the complications of laparotomy and general anaesthesia are avoided. Only one death has been reported and this was from a gas embolus from a gas-cooled system no longer employed.[32]

Mild abdominal discomfort is common both during and for 24–48 hours post-treatment. It is more common when treating peripheral lesions, presumably due to irritation of visceral or parietal peritoneum, but is easily controlled with simple analgesics. Bradycardia has been described during the procedure, presumably due to vagal stimulation. Asymptomatic sub- and extracapsular haemorrhage and small pleural effusions have also been seen to occur. No major biliary or vascular damage has been reported and most patients are able to leave hospital within 24 hours.[37,43,47]

The percutaneous approach does render a small number of lesions inaccessible to this method, in particular 9 deep right lobe lesions.[49] The limited resolution of percutaneous ultrasound makes localization and fibre insertion into small (<2 cm) lesions difficult, but the recent development of MRI guidance and monitoring may overcome this. However, interventional MRI is currently prohibitively expensive. For most centres the purchase cost of the laser is prohibitive, but can be justified to

some extent as it can also be used for other applications, particularly endoscopic procedures.

Radiofrequency ablation

Introduction

Radiofrequency waves are of lower energy and longer wavelength than conventional diathermy and result in the heat dissipating into the area that is close to the electrode–tissue interface. In the radiofrequency ablation of tissue, the frequency range used is between 400 and 500 kHz. At this frequency, stimulation of muscles and nerves does not occur.[50]

Mechanism of radiofrequency ablation

Radiofrequency ablation is produced by alternate current in the frequency range of 400–500 kHz delivered through an electrode tip. This current causes agitation of the particles of the surrounding tissues, which attempt to follow the alternate current, so generating frictional heat.[51] The heat generated is dependent on:

- *Current density:* this is the current divided by the area. As current density is highest at the tissue adjoining the electrode, the heat generated is the maximum at this plane.
- *Current intensity:* the heat generated is proportional to the square of the current. Therefore the more current delivered, the higher the heat generated. However, current that is too high or applied too rapidly results in overheating and charring of the tissue adjacent to the electrode, thus resulting in a rise of impedance and loss of efficacy.
- *Distance from the electrode:* as the distance increases the heat generated drops to the fourth power of the radius.

Indications

The current indications include patients with primary liver cancer and those with liver metastases from colorectal and neuroendocrine tumours.[52]

The size of these lesions has an important impact on the local recurrence rate, as larger lesions are more likely to develop local recurrence.[53] This is due to the fact that larger lesions require multiple overlapping electrode placements. The development of newer probe designs means that a 7 cm ablation is now possible in 20 minutes with a single probe placement.

In one reported series, patients with severe coagulation disorder and portal vein thrombosis were excluded from RFA.[52] Patients with tumours close to the hepatic hilum risk damage to the biliary structures and tumours adjacent to blood vessels may be inadequately heated due to the heat sink effect.[54]

Equipment

Probes

Early designs of probe had a single electrode but the size of the ablation was small (approximately 2 cm). Multiple arrays of conventional electrodes resulted in larger ablations. Expandable needle electrodes (4–10 electrodes) arranged as lateral hooks at 90° to each other are now used. Figure 8.5 shows a RITA 5 cm probe. The geometry of these electrodes is such that the separate elliptical lesions overlap to produce a spherical lesion.[55]

Internally cooled electrodes using chilled perfusate through the hollow electrode can be used to produce a larger ablation. The cooled electrode prevents overheating of the tissue adjacent to the electrode, thus preventing charring and a rise in impedance.[56]

Saline infusion through the hollow electrode has also resulted in larger ablation size. The proposed mechanism includes increased surface area and conductivity of the electrodes, reduced tissue vaporization and diffusion of the boiling saline into the tissue.[57]

Generator

The generator is used to deliver the radiofrequency energy in the range of 460–480 kHz. Figure 8.6 shows one of the commercially available generators and the computer used for data collection and display. There are currently three commercially available radiofrequency ablation devices. The RITA medical system (Mountain View, CA) uses a temperature thermocouple on the electrodes to monitor the temperature of the ablation. The electrodes are deployed partially until the target temperature is reached, then deployed fully until the target temperature is again reached, then maintained for a fixed duration of time.

The Radiotherapeutics (Mountain View, CA) device uses impedance to monitor the lesion size. After electrode deployment, the initial power is applied at 50 W and then the power increased at increments of 10 W at intervals of 1, 2, 3 and 4 minutes to 90 W. The treatment is continued until power roll-off occurs. After a 20 second pause the power is reapplied at 75% of maximum until power roll-off occurs again.[52]

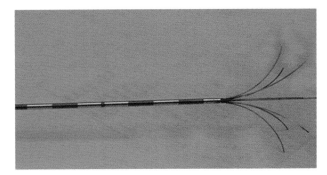

Figure 8.5 RITA radiofrequency probe when fully deployed.

The Radionics (Burlington, CA) system uses the cooled electrode tip to produce thermal ablation. A peristaltic pump is used to infuse saline at 0°C into the lumen of the electrode to maintain the electrode tip temperature at 20–25°C.[56]

Bipolar/monopolar mode

Radiofrequency energy can be delivered in either monopolar or bipolar mode. In the monopolar mode the current is delivered through the electrode and the return current is through a larger, dispersive, patient grounding pad. In the bipolar mode the current passes between two electrodes, separated by a distance of 1–4 cm, both of which are placed in the lesion. The bipolar mode results in larger ablation and the effect is greater than twice the size obtained by a single electrode as the entire energy is delivered to the tissue instead of a distant larger grounding pad.[58,59]

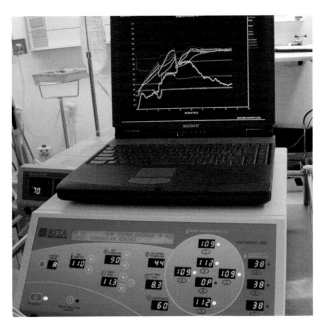

Figure 8.6 One of the commercially available generators for radiofrequency ablation. A laptop computer is used for data collection and display.

Technique

The main advantage of radiofrequency ablation is the ability to create thermal ablation by the percutaneous or laparoscopic approach. Patients having percutaneous RFA can be admitted as day surgery and the procedure can be performed under local anaesthetic, conscious sedation or a general anaesthetic. The patient is positioned either supine or in the left lateral position, depending on the site of the lesion. The patient grounding dispersive pads are applied if the monopolar mode is used. After preparation of the skin and draping, a small skin incision is made and the probe is inserted under ultrasound or CT guidance. Radiofrequency ablation is then performed.

Radiofrequency ablation can also be performed by the laparoscopic approach. The main advantage is easier probe placement in visible lesions, the ability to perform laparoscopy before the ablation to look for evidence of extrahepatic metastases and the ability to separate the liver from the diaphragm, stomach or bowel to prevent RF injury to these structures when the tumour is close to or involving the surface of the liver.[60] Laparoscopic intraoperative ultrasound facilitates intraparenchymal views of probe placement and monitoring of the ablation.

The advantage of using RFA during open surgery is that the Pringle manoeuvre (hepatic inflow occlusion) can be performed, which has been shown to increase the lesion size as well as the speed of the procedure.[55] Figure 8.7 shows radiofrequency ablation in progress via the open approach.

Imaging

Imaging is essential for the correct placement of the probe, monitoring of the ablation and follow-up of the patient. Imaging of the RF lesion can be by either ultrasound, CT scan or MRI. Ultrasound is the only method for laparoscopic as well as for open operation. Ultrasound shows a slowly enlarging speckled hyperechoic area.[61] It is considerably harder to judge the edge of the lesion during RFA than during cryotherapy, where the ice ball can be clearly seen.

The use of CT for monitoring the ablation gives better correlation as the RF lesion and liver–lesion interface is better demonstrated when compared to ultrasound.[62]

Both CT scan and MRI have been used in the follow-up and assessment of treatment efficacy. Contrast enhanced CT shows well-demarcated non-enhancing areas that correspond to the RF induced necrosis. A CT scan performed 1–3 days after treatment shows sharper margins between the RF treated and untreated regions of the lesion than scans performed immediately after the ablation.[63]

MRI images show a hypointense and unenhancing area representing the area of RF ablation. PET scan has also been used in the evaluation and follow-up of patients treated with RFA. It was found to be useful for distinguishing the inactive (RF treated) from the recurrent disease which CT was unable to do.[64]

Results

The use of radiofrequency ablation has now been reported in more than 500 patients with unresectable liver malignancies for both primary and metastatic tumours. RFA has been used in the treatment of hepatocellular carcinoma (HCC) in patients with cirrhosis and has been found to be safe with results that are comparable to those of cryotherapy.[65] In patients with colorectal metastases treated with RFA, the results are comparable to those of cryotherapy, with local recurrence rates of 1–30%. There are as yet no reports on 5-year survival and disease-free survival in these patients. RFA was found to be safer with fewer complications than cryoablation in a retrospective analysis of patients with HCC.[66] Comparison of alcohol injection to RFA showed a significantly lower local recurrence rate as well as higher 1- and 2-year disease-free survival rates in the RFA group after a median follow-up of 2 years.[67]

Local recurrence rates

Local recurrence is due either to inadequate heating of the tumour or to inadequate coverage of the tumour. As imaging of the radiofrequency ablation is not optimal, lesions requiring multiple electrode

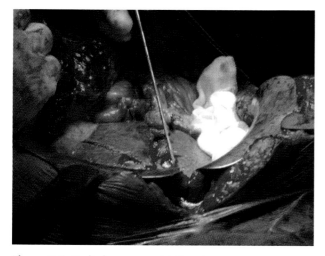

Figure 8.7 Radiofrequency ablation in progress.

placements are associated with higher local recurrence rates.[56] Probes that are capable of producing larger lesions are likely to decrease the local recurrence rates. Inadequate heating is another cause of local recurrence. Tumours that are situated near blood vessels are inadequately heated due to the heat sink effect as heat is conducted away by blood flow.[54]

Survival

There are few reports of the long-term follow-up of these patients. The median follow-up of patients in the reported series has been between 10 and 18 months. In 50 patients with HCC treated with RFA, the overall survival was 94% at 1 year, 86% at 2 years, 68% at 3 years and 40% at 4 and 5 years.[68] As yet, there are no randomised controlled trial data to show the benefit of RFA treatment.

Complications

Radiofrequency ablation has been found to be safe with few major complications. There have been only two reported deaths in over 500 patients who underwent RFA.[66,69] Major complications have been rare, with haemorrhage, haematoma and abscess formation accounting for the most of these complications.[52,65,66,69] Minor complications including fever, mild to moderate pain and pleural effusion were more common, but did not require any intervention in the majority of these patients.

Conclusions

Radiofrequency ablation is emerging as a new minimally invasive treatment modality for unresectable liver malignancies with low complication rates. The results appear to be better in patients with small lesions, but larger lesions are associated with higher local recurrence.

The main advantage is the facility to perform the procedure via the percutaneous or the laparoscopic route. The major disadvantages are the expense of the disposable probes and the need to treat multiple lesions concurrently.

Hepatic artery chemotherapy

Introduction

The regional delivery of cytotoxic drugs into the artery supplying malignant tumours was first described in 1950.[70,71] The infusion of chemotherapy to the liver via the hepatic artery was first reported by Sullivan et al. in 1964.[72] In the following 30 years hepatic artery chemotherapy evolved, with improved delivery technology and pharmacological understanding.[73]

The aim of any cancer chemotherapy regimen is to maximize its cytotoxic effect against tumour cells while minimizing the effects upon normal cells which result in side effects, in order to prolong survival and maintain quality of life. Two theoretical principles suggest that hepatic colorectal cancer metastases may be particularly suited to this method of cytotoxic administration.

(1) Drug targeting

Most cytotoxic agents have a steep dose response curve,[74] therefore the cytotoxic effect is enhanced by higher local drug concentrations. By targeting the administered drug to the diseased area, higher local levels can be achieved.

Widder et al.[74] described three distinct stages in the intravascular targeting of drugs:

- First order targeting – selective distribution of the drug into the capillary bed of the affected organ
- Second order targeting – the selective direction of the drug to tumour cells rather than normal cells
- Third order targeting – delivery of the drug into intracellular sites in tumour cells.

Hepatic colorectal metastases are particularly susceptible to such drug targeting. The arterial supply to the liver is well defined and easily accessed, allowing first order targeting. Both primary and metastatic hepatic neoplasms are supplied via the hepatic artery, unlike normal liver tissue which receives its blood supply predominantly from the portal vein, allowing second order targeting.[75–77] Hepatic arterial administration of chemotherapeutic agents can potentially expose the tumour to higher concentrations than could be achieved by systemic administration.

(2) Hepatic extraction

The fluoropyrimidines have been extensively used systemically in colorectal cancer and both 5-fluoro-2'-deoxyuridine (FUDR) and 5 fluorouracil (5 FU) are catabolized in vitro by hepatic enzymes. In 1978 Ensminger et al.[78] demonstrated that when administered as an infusion via the hepatic artery (even at very high doses), FUDR is efficiently extracted by the liver (92% of the administered dose being extracted on the first pass through the liver). 5 Fluorouracil was shown to be less efficiently extracted, but this is improved with longer duration infusions.[79] This high hepatic extraction of FUDR results in lower systemic drug levels – 60% of that seen with systemic administration. Lower systemic levels are associated with less systemic toxicity.

Results

Many studies have been published on the results of hepatic artery chemotherapy. Initial publications reported only patients given hepatic arterial chemotherapy and comparison of these results with those of patients in trials of systemic chemotherapy was difficult as hepatic artery patients tended to have liver only disease, compared to a more systemic distribution in the patients given intravenous therapy, and there was considerable variation between the treatment protocols used.[80]

Later, randomized controlled trials allowed direct comparisons to be made between the two delivery techniques, their merits being assessed in terms of tumour response rates, which are easy and quick to quantify, patient survival and the equally important effects upon patients' quality of life.

Tumour response rates

Early trials of hepatic artery chemotherapy reported response rates of 39 to 75%, which compare well with response rates seen in trials of systemic single agent chemotherapy of 9.5 to 44%,[80] although such comparisons are tenuous.

Later, randomized controlled trials[81–85] were able to compare response rates directly for patients with liver only disease. Hepatic artery chemotherapy produced partial or complete responses in 43–62%, compared to 17–21% response rates with systemic chemotherapy. In each trial the differences in response rates were statistically significant.

Survival

The clear differences in response rates between regional and systemic chemotherapy were not shown to translate into a significant survival advantage in early controlled trials.[81–84] These trials compared relatively small numbers of patients and were therefore of low power, and the largest[81] allowed patients to cross over from the systemic to hepatic artery arms if their disease progressed – potentially masking any survival advantage. Two later European trials did demonstrate clear survival advantages of hepatic artery chemotherapy over controls.[85,86] However, the control groups were

given systemic chemotherapy using regimens at the discretion of each patient's physician.

In a meta analysis of all controlled trials,[87] a significant survival advantage was seen when all trials were considered but not when restricted to trials in which the control arm received systemic chemotherapy. However, a later meta analysis using different statistical methods and incorporating the data of Hohn et al.[83] reported a small but statistically significant survival advantage for hepatic arterial over systemic chemotherapy. Further trials specifically designed to clarify the issue of survival are nearing completion.[88]

Quality of life

When treating hepatic metastases from colorectal cancer, in addition to improving crude survival time one must aim to improve the length of survival with a normal quality of life. Only one study has addressed this issue.[86] This trial found not only a significant improvement in crude survival over controls, but also improved survival with normal quality of life.

Adjuvant hepatic artery infusion chemotherapy

Adjuvant hepatic artery chemotherapy has been shown to decrease the incidence of liver recurrence after liver resection. Comparison of the outcome of patients undergoing liver resection with adjuvant hepatic artery chemotherapy and systemic chemotherapy has shown a significant improvement in the recurrence-free survival. Two-year recurrence-free survivals of 90% and 60% in the combined hepatic artery and intravenous group and the systemic group, respectively, have been reported.[89]

Surgical procedure and techniques

Preoperative work-up

The advantages of hepatic artery chemotherapy are proven only in patients with liver metastases from colorectal cancer. Patients must be screened to exclude extrahepatic disease. Locoregional recurrence or metachronous tumour should be excluded by colonoscopy or barium enema, and a computed tomographic (CT) scan of the abdomen performed to exclude intra-abdominal extrahepatic disease. In a patient with a histologically confirmed primary colorectal adenocarcinoma, an elevated carcinoembryonic antigen (CEA) level and characteristic lesions on a good quality CT scan, we do not biopsy the liver lesions.

As aberrant hepatic arterial anatomy is seen in about 33–40% of patients,[90,91] some authors advocate that a preoperative angiogram should always be performed in order to define the anatomy. However, this is unnecessary for surgeons experienced in this technique and familiar with the anatomical variations, which are easily defined at operation.

Catheter placement

The success of hepatic artery chemotherapy is dependent upon achieving uniform perfusion of the liver and avoiding perfusion of the gut.[90,92] In addition, cholecystectomy should be performed in all patients to avoid chemical cholecystitis.[93]

In patients with conventional anatomy (demonstrated in Fig. 8.8) the gastroduodenal artery is the ideal site for the insertion of a hepatic artery catheter. The common hepatic, gastroduodenal, hepatic and its division into right and left hepatic arteries are easily exposed and displayed by dividing the gastrohepatic ligament and mobilizing the duodenum. The right gastric artery and any other branches to the stomach or duodenum should be ligated and divided to avoid malperfusion of the gut.[94] The gastroduodenal artery should be ligated 3–4 cm distally with a non-absorbable tie and controlled proximally. A longitudinal arteriotomy allow a specially designed, beaded, silastic catheter to be advanced retrogradely into and along the artery up to its junction with the hepatic artery. The catheter is secured in place with non-absorbable ties – one each side of the catheter bead (Fig. 8.9). Care should be taken not to occlude the catheter by excessively tight securing ties.

By injecting 5–10 ml of methylene blue 1% down the catheter parenchymal hepatic perfusion can be assessed, and any malperfusion of the stomach or duodenum detected. Fluorescein and a UV lamp can be used instead of methylene blue; anaphylaxis has been reported with both compounds, but is rare. If the liver does not stain uniformly blue an aberrant accessory hepatic artery must be suspected, as demonstrated in Fig. 8.10. Failure of the right lobe of the liver to perfuse suggests the presence of an accessory right hepatic artery, which invariably arises from the superior mesenteric artery and lies behind the common bile duct on the right side of the portal vein anterior to the foramen of Winslow, as depicted in Figs 8.11 and 8.12. A failure of the left lobe to perfuse suggests an accessory left hepatic artery arising from the left gastric artery or a proximal origin of the left artery from the common hepatic artery before the gastroduodenal branch containing the catheter (Fig. 8.13). In most cases, ligation of the smaller aberrant vessel allows cross perfusion to occur from the contralateral lobe of the liver.[95,96] This can be confirmed prior to ligation of the vessel by occluding it with a vascular clamp and repeating the

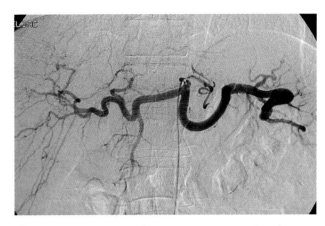

Figure 8.8 Arteriogram demonstrating conventional hepatic arterial anatomy.

methylene blue test. It is rarely necessary to insert a second catheter into a dominant aberrant vessel to achieve uniform perfusion.

Other anatomical variations are encountered in addition to aberrant right or left hepatic arteries. The most common of these is described as a trifurcation,

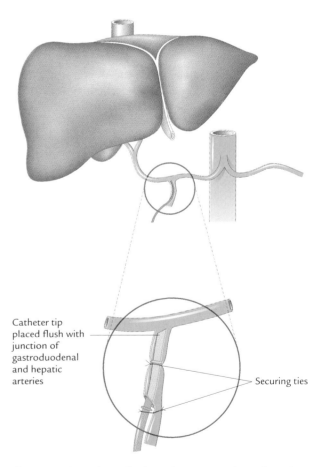

Catheter tip placed flush with junction of gastroduodenal and hepatic arteries

Securing ties

Figure 8.9 Insertion of a hepatic artery catheter into the gastroduodenal artery in a patient with conventional anatomy.

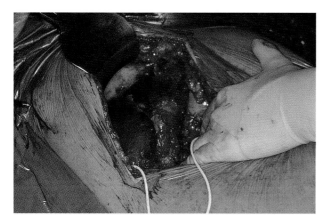

Figure 8.10 Methylene blue infused via a hepatic artery catheter demonstrating inadequate perfusion of the right liver, indicating an accessory right hepatic artery.

when the gastroduodenal artery arises from the common hepatic artery very close to its division into right and left hepatic arteries. Insertion of the catheter here would result in streaming of chemotherapy into one or other lobes of the liver. This can be overcome by inserting the catheter through a side arm of saphenous vein or prosthetic graft to the side of the proximal common hepatic artery.[97] Coeliac stenosis can be a difficult problem for hepatic artery catheter placement because the whole foregut may derive its blood supply via retrograde flow in the gastroduodenal artery. This should be suspected when one encounters an abnormally large calibre gastroduodenal artery, and can be confirmed by clamping the proximal (hepatic) end of the gastroduodenal artery and palpating distally for a pulse. Placing the catheter in the left hepatic

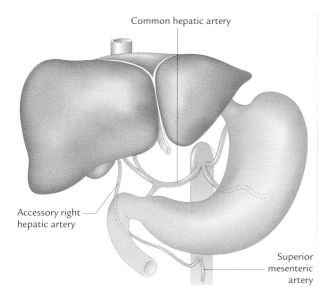

Figure 8.11 An accessory right hepatic artery arising from the superior mesenteric artery.

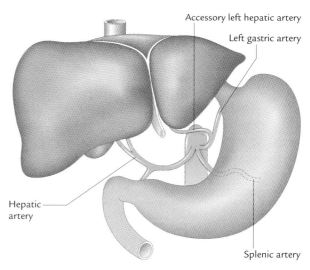

Figure 8.13 An accessory left hepatic artery arising from the left gastric artery.

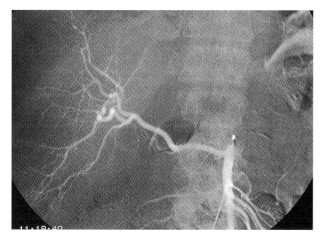

Figure 8.12 Arteriogram demonstrating an accessory right hepatic artery arising from the superior mesenteric artery.

artery and tying off the artery around the catheter, or putting a side arm on to the common or right hepatic artery distal to the gastroduodenal, may be required.

For aberrant anatomical variations, an appropriate catheter placement technique can result in the same response rate to chemotherapy as patients with normal anatomy.[98] Variant anatomy has been found to be associated with higher rates of complications, but this was much less of a factor than the experience of the operating surgeon.[90]

Delivery devices

Once inserted, hepatic artery catheters must be connected to a pump for chemotherapy delivery.

Several implantable systems are available: implantable refillable pumps such as the Infusaid 400 pump (Fig. 8.14) and implantable ports such as the Portacath port used with a connecting needle and external pump (Fig. 8.15). Both of these devices are inserted into subcutaneous pockets, the ports placed over the lower costal margin and pumps over the abdominal wall, and must be sutured in place to prevent them rotating in the pocket.

Ports must be accessed using special non-coring needles each time an infusion is given, the needle being connected to an external pump to deliver the infusion. In order to prevent thrombosis and occlusion of the catheter, it is essential to flush these systems with heparinized saline once every 2 weeks when they are not in use and to ensure that a positive pressure is always applied whenever the port is accessed.

Pumps are easier to manage and are associated with a lower occlusion rate than ports,[94] but are substantially more expensive. Pumps can be loaded with chemotherapy and run at a predetermined set rate, being refilled either with chemotherapy or heparinized normal saline to ensure that they never run dry.

Complications

Drug toxicity

Systemic and hepatic regional cytotoxic chemotherapy are both associated with toxicity. However, the patterns of toxic effects are different with the two methods. While systemic chemotherapy is associated with effects such as diarrhoea, mucositis and leucopenia, hepatic arterial chemotherapy results in more regional toxicity, namely hepatobiliary and upper GI toxicity.

When administered via the hepatic artery, FUDR can result in significant sclerosing cholangitis in 5–29% of patients,[93] which may require biliary stenting or external drainage. This serious complication should be suspected in any patient with a rise in serum hepatic transaminase, bilirubin or alkaline phosphatase levels, and may be averted by immediate cessation of treatment for a period. We would stop treatment if there were a doubling of any of these levels. Serious non-resolving cases are best investigated by endoscopic retrograde cholangiopancreatography (ERCP) as the ducts are sclerotic and undilated, making ultrasound diagnosis difficult.

Several techniques have been advocated to reduce the incidence of this complication. The first is dose reduction, either by using a lower dose from the onset of treatment, 0.2 mg/kg/day as opposed to the more usual 0.3 mg/kg,[86] or upon the development

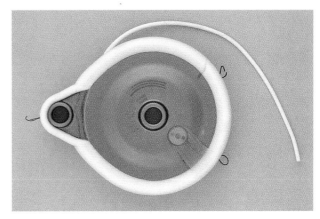

Figure 8.14 An Infusaid 400 implantable infusion pump.

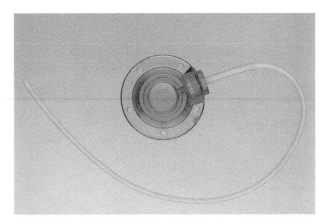

Figure 8.15 An implantable infusion port.

of biochemical changes. Using 5 FU instead of FUDR has been advocated, and may be more efficacious. Some centres use 5 FU alone in preference to FUDR,[99,100] and others advocate alternating infusions of FUDR with 5 FU infusions.[101] Recently, co-administration of dexamethasone with FUDR has been shown to reduce the incidence of sclerosing cholangitis.[102]

The preparations of 5 FU administered via the hepatic artery have a very alkaline pH and can result in arteritis of the hepatic artery in a minority of patients, as depicted in Fig. 8.16. This arteritis may be severe enough to occlude the vessel and is probably responsible for the pseudoaneurysms which can cause major gastrointestinal bleeding. 5 FU has been reported to result in impaired left ventricular function when given systemically,[103] and the possibility should be considered when treating patients with known cardiac disease.

Upper gastrointestinal complications encompass gastritis, ulceration and pain, but are best considered to be technical complications rather than toxic reactions.

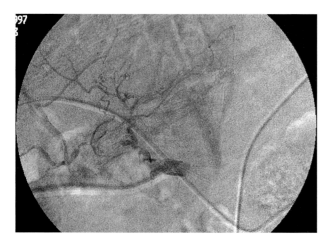

Figure 8.16 Arteriogram demonstrating arteritis of the hepatic artery following 5 FU infusion via a hepatic artery catheter.

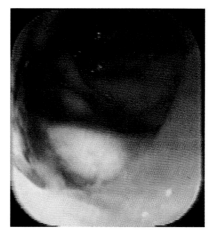

Figure 8.17 Endoscopic picture demonstration of malperfusion of the duodenum from a hepatic artery infusion; methylene blue has been injected via the hepatic artery catheter.

Technical complications

The rate of technical complications is higher with inexperienced surgeons. It is essential to be aware of the possible complications as they present in innocuous and non-specific ways, yet may be fatal.

1. Gastrointestinal mucosal damage

This encompasses the spectrum of peptic ulcer disease from gastritis to bleeding or perforation of duodenal ulcers. It is usually due to malperfusion of the lesser curve of the stomach or duodenum with chemotherapy via missed branches of the hepatic arterial tree. It typically presents as epigastric pain developing at or shortly after the start of a chemotherapy infusion, and can occur some months after the initiation of treatment. Pain may be absent altogether, upper gastrointestinal haemorrhage being the presenting feature, and can be life threatening. When malperfusion is demonstrated the responsible vessel can usually be embolized at angiography. Treatment can continue following repeated endoscopy with methylene blue perfusion to exclude malperfusion, as demonstrated in Fig. 8.17.

2. Hepatic artery aneurysm formation

This is an uncommon but potentially life threatening complication illustrated in Fig. 8.18, which usually presents with rupture into the duodenum and haematemesis. It is seen more commonly with 5 FU infusions and requires either urgent operation to remove the catheter and ligate the vessel, or radiological embolization using permanent metal coils.

3. Catheter leakage and extravasation

This is usually secondary to occlusion of the catheter or artery further upstream, and is easily diagnosed by a portocathogram (Fig. 8.19). It necessitates cessation

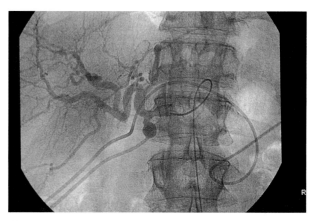

Figure 8.18 Arteriogram demonstrating a pseudoaneurysm at the site of insertion of a hepatic artery catheter into the gastroduodenal artery.

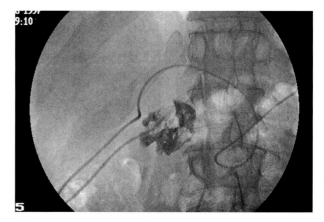

Figure 8.19 Arteriogram demonstrating extravasation from a dislodged hepatic artery catheter.

of the treatment and, if appropriate, replacement of the catheter, which may require an end to side anastomosis of vein or prosthetic vascular graft material onto the hepatic artery.

Abdominal pain in the hepatic arterial chemotherapy patient: methods of investigation

Endoscopy and methylene blue can demonstrate any areas of mucosal damage or loss together with any bleeding site which can then be treated by radiological embolization. By injecting 5–10 ml of 1% methylene blue down the hepatic artery catheter via the port while observing the gastroduodenal mucosa, areas of malperfusion are easily demonstrated, as seen in Figure 8.17.

Angiography of the coeliac and superior mesenteric vessels can demonstrate any aberrant vessels responsible for any gastroduodenal malperfusion or unequal hepatic perfusion, and any such vessels can be occluded with coils, gelfoam or similar material at the same time.

'Portocathogram' performed by injecting a contrast agent down the hepatic artery catheter under radiological screening to demonstrate catheter blockage, leakage and extravasation. Also useful to demonstrate hepatic artery aneurysms.

Figure 8.20 Investigation of the patient with abdominal pain.

4. Inadequate perfusion of one hepatic lobe

This occurs when an accessory vessel supplies an area of liver, and should be suspected when the response of metastases to treatment demonstrated by CT changes appears heterogeneous throughout the liver. Radionucleotide scanning via the port can confirm any perfusion defect, and responsible vessels may be identified and embolized at angiography.

5. Pump or port complications

Both are associated with similar complications, namely development of seromas, pocket infections and extrusion. Seromas are quite common and may require repeated aspiration. Infection is usually obvious and necessitates removal of the device, although we do have some experience of replacing infected ports. Pump malfunction is rare, but the septum is susceptible to damage if ordinary needles or high injection pressures are used when refilling.

Investigation of abdominal pain

As the more serious complications often present as vague epigastric pains, it is essential that all patients presenting with such pain are thoroughly investigated. Three investigations are indicated in all cases of pain in such patients as each investigation provides different information. The investigations are described in Fig. 8.20.

Chemotherapy: agents and regimens

Choice of agent

The theoretical advantages of FUDR over 5 FU in terms of hepatic extraction have been outlined previously. Consequently the majority of the early work and all of the randomized trials investigating hepatic artery chemotherapy used FUDR. More recently, the high rates of sclerosing cholangitis seen with FUDR use have prompted researchers to reconsider the use of regionally delivered 5 FU.

Studies using hepatic arterial 5 FU at various dosages and treatment schedules have produced response rates of 27.3 to 56%, and median survivals of 11–19 months.[99,100,104,105] These results are comparable to those seen with FUDR, with the advantage that sclerosing cholangitis is avoided. As a larger infusion volume is required to deliver an adequate dose of 5 FU, faster running implantable pumps or external pumps must be used.

The biomodulation of fluoropyrimidines by the addition of leucovorin-folinic acid increases the binding of their active metabolite to the target enzyme thymidylate synthase, resulting in enhanced cytotoxicity. When this was combined with systemic 5 FU chemotherapy it produced dramatically improved response rates[85] and enhanced survival in some studies.[106–108] These

Hepatic arterial 5 FU via a subcutaneous port and external pump

Drug	Dose	Route	Day
5 FU	4000 mg	IA	4 day continuous infusion
Heparin	20 000 units	IA	4 day continuous infusion
Dexamethasone	8 mg	IA	4 day continuous infusion
Folinic acid	3 × 15 mg	Oral	Daily on days 1–4, before food

Treatment administered every 2 weeks, may be reduced to every 4 weeks based on response

Hepatic arterial 5 FU via Infusaid implantable pump

Drug	Dose	Route	Day
5 FU	*2500 mg	IA	7 day continuous infusion
Folinic acid	3 × 15 mg	Oral	Daily on days 1–4, before food

Treatment administered every 2 weeks, may be reduced to every 4 weeks based on response

*Dose loaded must be adjusted according to flow rate of pump

Hepatic arterial FUDR via a subcutaneous port and external pump

Drug	Dose	Route	Day
5 FU	0.1–0.3 mg/kg/day	IA	7 day continuous infusion
Heparin	25 000 units	IA	7 day continuous infusion
Dexamethasone	8 mg	IA	7 day continuous infusion

Cycle repeats every 14 days

Hepatic arterial FUDR via a subcutaneous port and external pump

Drug	Dose	Route	Day
5 FU	*0.1–0.3 mg/kg/day	IA	14 day continuous infusion
Heparin	50 000 units	IA	14 day continuous infusion
Dexamethasone	20 mg	IA	14 day continuous infusion

Cycle repeats every 28 days

*Dose loaded must be adjusted according to response and flow rate of pump

Figure 8.21 Examples of hepatic artery chemotherapy protocols.

results prompted investigators to look at the addition of folinic acid to hepatic arterial chemotherapy regimens. The intra-arterial administration of low dose leucovorin with FUDR resulted in an improved response rate of 75%, but the risk of cholangitis was higher than with FUDR alone and others have demonstrated an increased risk of arterial thrombosis with intra-arterial leucovorin. The combination of intravenous leucovorin and intra-arterial 5 FU has been shown to produce good tumour response rates of 48%.[103]

The hepatic arterial chemotherapy protocols in use at our institution are reproduced in Fig. 8.21.

Systemic chemotherapy

Introduction

The majority of patients presenting with colorectal liver metastases will be unsuitable for resection, guided cytodestructive therapy or hepatic artery chemotherapy due to extensive liver involvement or the presence of extrahepatic disease. In addition, many of these patients may ultimately progress locally or systemically. For these patients palliative systemic therapy can be offered with the intent of prolonging survival and improving or maintaining quality of life.

The use of adjuvant systemic therapy following resection of primary colorectal tumours is well established for Dukes C patients, and is outside the scope of this chapter. Trials evaluating systemic chemotherapy for liver only disease have not been conducted. All trials have involved the entire spectrum of metastatic disease.

Progress in the development of systemic chemotherapy has been slow. 5 Fluorouracil has been the mainstay of chemotherapy for colorectal cancer since its synthesis in 1958.[109] More recently, the benchmarks for systemic therapy have changed with the introduction of several new agents including irinotecan, oxaliplatin, raltitrexed, trimetrexate and MTA. In addition, the need for intravenous treatment has been challenged by various strategies that enable the oral administration of fluorinated pyrimidines such as capecitabine, UFTx S-1 and eniluracil.

Indications

Evidence from randomized controlled trials and meta analysis of those trials support the use of systemic chemotherapy for the palliation of inoperable colorectal cancer. The meta analysis conducted by the Colorectal Cancer Collaborative Group reviewed 13 randomized trials involving 1365 patients.[110] These trials were reported prior to July 1998. Individual patient data for 866 patients were associated with a 35% reduction in risk of death (95% confidence interval 24 to 44%). This was equivalent to an absolute improvement in survival of 16% at 6 and 12 months and a median survival improvement of 3.7 months. There appeared to be no difference in benefit between age groups, but fewer than 2.5% of the patients were older than 75 years of age.

Despite small numbers, Scheithauer et al.[111] and Beretta et al.[112] were able to demonstrate in separate trials a survival advantage for chemotherapy over best supportive care. The Scheithauer study found 5 FU, folinic acid and methotrexate to produce a median survival of 11 months for the supportive care group (p = 0.006). Quality of life scores were no different between the groups overall, but patients with abnormal scores pretreatment fared better in the chemotherapy arm.

Cunningham et al. have demonstrated that after failure of 5 FU there is evidence to support second-line therapy with irinotecan.[113] This trial compared 3 weekly irinotecan to best supportive care and found a survival benefit (9.2 versus 6.5 months, p = 0.0001). Irinotecan appeared to delay time to deterioration in performance status, weight loss, pain control and global quality of life. These advantages were seen despite toxicity related to irinotecan.

The timing and duration of systemic chemotherapy are important considerations. The Nordic gastrointestinal tumour adjuvant therapy group[114] compared early versus delayed introduction of chemotherapy for asymptomatic patients. This study demonstrated a significant improvement in symptom-free survival (10 versus 2 months, p = 0.001) and a non-significant prolongation of survival (14 versus 9 months). An Australian and Canadian meta analysis has failed to confirm a survival benefit for early versus delayed chemotherapy.[115] The MRC Colorectal Cancer Group has investigated whether intermittent or continuous chemotherapy is preferable for responding or stable patients.[116] No survival difference was found between the groups but a quality of life disadvantage was seen in the continuous treatment arm.

One problem in interpreting the literature with respect to both intra-arterial and systemic chemotherapy is that although survival benefits have been demonstrated the principal determinants of enhanced survival are poorly understood. Buyse et al. have conducted a meta analysis to examine the relation between tumour response to first-line chemotherapy and survival in advanced colorectal cancer.[117] Survival was found to be associated with response, but the benefit in proportional terms was small. A treatment that lowered the odds of failure to respond by 50% would decrease the odds of death by 6%. The example offered by Buyse et al. is that a treatment that doubles the response rate of an agent from 20 to 40% would only increase median survival from 14 to 16 months. It is possible that delay in progression rather than objective response is a better surrogate marker for survival.

Agents, regimens and results

5 Fluorouracil

This has been the principal agent used to treat colorectal carcinoma for the past 40 years. 5 FU is a fluorinated pyrimidine antimetabolite prodrug that is converted intracellularly to 5-fluorouracil triphosphate (5 FUTP), 5-fluorodeoxyuridine triphosphate (5 FdUTP) and the principal cytotoxic agent 5-fluorodeoxyuridine monophosphate (5 FdUMP). 5 FdUMP inhibits thymidylate synthase (TS), so producing thymidine depletion, impaired DNA synthesis and apoptosis. 5 FUTP interferes with the nuclear processing of RNA and 5 FdUTP interferes with the nuclear processing of RNA and produces DNA strand breaks.

As a single agent 5 FU has antitumour activity of the order of 10–15%. This low activity is attributable to a number of factors including the pharmacokinetic profile, variable metabolism of 5 FU and intrinsic resistance to 5 FU. 5 FU has an extremely short half-life of 8–20 minutes. Assuming that its principal activity is as an inhibitor of thymidylate synthase, then 5 FU functions as an S phase specific agent. Therefore, at the time of any given bolus only a fraction of the tumour cells will be susceptible to 5 FU. 5 FU is metabolized by dihydropyrimidine dehydrogenase (DPD). This may be expressed variably between patients and between tumours. Approximately 2% of the population are DPD deficient and may experience severe toxicity with 5 FU administration. Tumours may overexpress both DPD and TS or have reduced intracellular folate pools leading to resistance to 5 FU.

A number of strategies have been used to overcome resistance to 5 FU and optimize response to treatment. Folinic acid (calcium folinate or leucovorin) increases intracellular levels of 5-10-methylene tetrahydrofolate. This is a co-factor necessary for the stabilization of FdUMP with thymidylate synthase. The results of nine clinical trials and a confirmatory meta analysis demonstrated that co-administration of folinic acid potentiates the cytotoxic activity of 5 FU, with tumour response rates of 23% compared to 11% for 5 FU alone.[118–127] This effect was seen in trials involving schedules of high dose folinic acid (Machover regimen: >200 mg/m^2/day) and low dose folinic acid (Mayo regimen: <25 mg/m^2/day), but each schedule had a different toxicity profile.[128]

Methotrexate is an antifolate agent that blocks dihydrofolate reductase. Inhibition of purine metabolism leads to accumulation of 5-pyrophosphate (PRPP) and enhanced conversion of 5 FU to 5 FUTP and 5 FdUMP. A meta analysis[129] has found that modulation of 5 FU by methotrexate almost doubled the response rate compared to 5 FU alone (19% versus 10%) and yielded a small but significant improvement in survival with median survival times of 10.7 versus 9.1 months.

An alternative strategy to biomodulation of 5 FU has been to alter the schedule of administration of 5 FU in order to overcome the short half-life and relative S phase selectivity of 5 FU. Delivery of 5 FU as a continuous infusion rather than a bolus injection has resulted in improved response (22%) and survival (12.1 months).[130] The Mayo regimen of bolus 5 FU 425 mg/m^2 daily for 5 days every 4 weeks has been regarded as the reference regimen for use as the control arm in randomized trials of new treatments for colorectal cancer. De Gramont et al. compared the Mayo regimen with a protocol of folinic acid 200 mg/m^2 as a 2 hour infusion followed by bolus 5 FU 400 mg/m^2 and 22 hour infusion of 5 FU 600 mg/m^2 for 2 consecutive days every 2 weeks.[131] The trial found in favour of the de Gramont regimen in terms of response rate (36.6% versus 14.4%, p = 0.0004) and progression-free survival (27.6 versus 22 weeks, p = 0.012); survival times were comparable (62 versus 56.8 weeks, p = 0.067). More grade 3–4 toxicity was experienced in the Mayo arm (23.9% versus 11.1%, p = 0.0004), in particular granulocytopenia, diarrhoea and mucositis. Infusion schedules tend to be associated with higher rates of cutaneous toxicity including plantar-palmar erythema (hand-foot syndrome).

Other groups have investigated chronomodulation of infusional chemotherapy in order to overcome circadian fluctuation in DPD activity. These studies have found increased response, decreased toxicity but no survival benefit for this strategy.[132] A further strategy has been pharmacokinetically guided dosage.[133] In a trial of the use of therapeutic drug monitoring in 117 patients, Gamelin et al. were able to produce 18 complete responses, 48 partial responses, 35 minor responses or stable disease and only 16 cases where progressive disease was the best response.[133] The median survival time was 19 months, comparable to the best multiagent therapy.

Irinotecan

Irinotecan (CPT-11) is a semi-synthetic derivative of the naturally occurring alkaloid camptothecin. Irinotecan is converted by carboxylesterases to SN-38, its principal active metabolite. Irinotecan and SN-38 inhibit the nuclear enzyme topoisomerase I. During the process of replication and transcription topoisomerase I relieves the torsional stress associated with the unwinding of DNA. It does this by creating a single strand break through which the intact strand can pass, and then by resealing the strand break. Topoisomerase I inhibitors block the reannealing of the strand break such that DNA fragmentation and cell death occur when the replication fork encounters the single-stranded break.

Irinotecan has been demonstrated to enhance survival compared with supportive care (9.2 versus 6.5 months, p = 0.0001)[113] or infusional 5 FU (10.8 versus 8.5 months, p = 0.35) in patients with 5 FU refractory colorectal cancer.[134]

In North America, Saltz et al. compared irinotecan 125 mg/m^2, 5 FU 500 mg/m^2 and folinic acid 20 mg/m^2 given weekly for 4 out of 6 weeks to single agent irinotecan and the Mayo regimen.[135] In Europe Douillard et al. compared irinotecan combined with infusional 5 FU to infusional 5 FU alone.[136] The physician could use either the weekly AIO regimen with 80 mg/m^2 irinotecan or the fortnightly de Gramont regimen with 180 mg/m^2 irinotecan. Both trials found statistically significant advantages for irinotecan in overall survival (p = 0.05), tumour response and progression-free survival. Whilst there was a tendency for increased toxicity with the irinotecan/5 FU combinations, at least with respect to diarrhoea, quality of life was not compromised in either of the trials. Douillard et al. demonstrated a delay to deterioration in performance status for the irinotecan recipients (11.2 versus 9.9 months, p = 0.046). The Mayo regimen exhibited increased mucositis and febrile neutropenia compared with the other treatments. Although not strictly comparable, these studies consistently demonstrate survival times that are two to three times greater than the 5-month survival observed in the supportive care arms of the Scheithauer and Beretta studies (Table 8.1).

Oxaliplatin

This is a novel platinum compound in which the platinum atom is associated with 1,2-diaminocyclo-hexane (DACH). Oxaliplatin forms inter- and intrastrand DNA adducts between adjacent guanines (GG or GNG) or between adjacent guanine adenine (GA) base pairs, so impairing DNA replication and inducing cell death. The chemistry of oxaliplatin may confer better DNA replication inhibition and cytotox-icity than cisplatin and may be responsible for the non-cross resistance seen when compared with cisplatin. Importantly, DNA mismatch repair complexes do not recognize DACH-Pt adducts, a major pathway of chemoresistance for colorectal cancer.

Oxaliplatin has low intrinsic activity against colorectal cancer, with response rates as a single agent of approximately 10%. Substantial synergy is seen when oxaliplatin is administered with 5 FU. De Gramont et al. studied the de Gramont regimen with and without oxaliplatin 85 mg/m^2 on day 1 in 420 patients.[137] An improved response rate (50.7% versus 22.3%, p = 0.0001) and progression-free survival (9.0 versus 6.2 months, p = 0.0003) were observed, but the median survival difference did not reach significance (16.2 versus 14.7 months). There were significantly increased rates of neutropenia, diarrhoea and the typical cold-exacerbated neuropa-thy of oxaliplatin, but there was no overall differ-ence in quality of life.

Recent studies from both France and the United States[138,139,140] have demonstrated that between 10 and possibly 33% of patients with colorectal liver metastases, previously deemed inoperable by experienced liver surgeons, can be resected after chemotherapy using oxaliplatin. Long-term survival for these patients following hepatectomy is virtually identical to those patients who were deemed resectable at the outset.[139] These observa-tions have formed the basis of an ongoing EORTC trial of neoadjuvant and adjuvant oxaliplatin combined with 5 FU around surgery versus surgery alone. In early 2002 the UK National Institute of Clinical Excellence advised that oxaliplatin-based treatment should be considered as first line chemotherapy for patients with non-resectable liver metastases who, in the opinion of an experi-enced liver surgeon, might be suitable for resection after successful treatment. If these data are correct, resectability rates for patients with colorectal liver metastases might rise from the current rate of 10% of all patients with disease confined to the liver to possibly over 30%.

Table 8.1 Results of irinotecan and 5 FU as first-line therapy for metastatic colorectal cancer

	Salt regimen, weekly irinotecan, 5 FU and folinic acid	Mayo regimen	Single agent weekly irinotecan	Irinotecan and infusional 5 FU	Infusional 5 FU AIO or de Gramont
Response rate	39%	21%	18%	35%	22%
Progression-free survival	7 months	4.3 months	4.2 months	6.7 months	4.4 months
Overall survival	14.8 months	12.6 months	12.0 months	17.4 months	14.1 months
Mucositis grade 3–4	2%	17%	2%	3%	3%
Emesis grade 3–4	10%	4%	12%	6%	3%
Diarrhoea grade 3	15%	6%	18%	17%	6%
Diarrhoea grade 4	8%	7%	13%	6%	5%
Neutropenia grade 4	24%	43%	12%	9%	1%
Febrile neutropenia	7%	15%	6%	5%	1%

Raltitrexed

This is a quinazoline folate analogue that specifically inhibits thymidylate synthase. A 3-weekly schedule is possible with this agent due to uptake and retention within cells by the reduced folate carrier system and subsequent polyglutamation by folyl polyglutamate synthetase. The development and acceptance of raltitrexed has been hampered by the determination in separate phase I studies of differing maximum tolerated doses. The North American phase III study compared raltitrexed at doses of 3 and 4 mg/m² every 21 days with the Mayo regimen.[141] The higher dose arm was closed due to excessive toxicity. The final results of this trial showed a survival benefit for the 5 FU arm. Two other phase III studies have been completed that have demonstrated comparable response and survival data to 5 FU.[142,143] Early toxicity appears greater with 5 FU due to the difficulty in dose selection mediated by variable DPD expression. Overall, raltitrexed is thought to be a useful substitute to 5 FU with comparable efficacy and toxicity and potential improvements in convenience and cost-effectiveness.[144]

Oral fluoropyrimidines

These have increasingly been investigated given the convenience of administration that would be achieved when compared with the cost and morbidity of infusional regimens that require placement of temporary or permanent venous access devices. While this has been demonstrated, the compounds developed to date have not demonstrated any survival advantage over conventionally administered 5 FU and, unexpectedly, severe gastrointestinal and haematologic toxicity has been observed with some agents.

The best established of these agents is capecitabine, a fluoropyrimidine carbamate prodrug. Capecitabine is converted by hepatic carboxylase to 5'-deoxy-5-fluorocytidine (5' DFCR). 5' DFCR is converted to 5'-deoxy-5-fluorouridine (5' DFUR) by cytidine deaminase and then 5' DFUR is converted to 5 FU by thymidine phosphorylase within the tumour cell. Hoff et al. have reported the phase III trial comparing the twice daily for 14 to 21 days schedule to the Mayo regimen.[145] The overall response rate was higher (24.8% versus 15.5%, p = 0.005), but no difference was observed for time to progression and overall survival, which was in the order of 12 to 13 months. The principal adverse effect of capecitabine is hand-foot syndrome.

UFT is a combination oral preparation of uracil and tegafur (ftorafur) in a molar ratio of 4:1. Tegafur is metabolized by CYP2A6 to 5 FU while uracil inhibits DPD, resulting in higher intratumoral exposure to 5 FU. Folinic acid is also administered to biomodulate the preparation further. In the phase II setting the response rate was 42.2%.[146] Diarrhoea is the main adverse effect.

Eniluracil is a DPD inhibitor that modifies the bioavailability of 5 FU to allow oral administration. The largest of the phase II trials demonstrated a 13% response rate and severe gastrointestinal and haematologic toxicity, including one treatment related death.[147] Further development will require an alternative schedule.

S-1 is an oral combination drug comprising tegafur, 5-chloro-2,4-dihydroxypyrimidine (CDHP) and potassium oxonate in a 1:0.4:1 molar ratio. Tegafur is metabolized to 5 FU, CDHP blocks DPD and potassium oxonate inhibits the phosphorylation of 5 FU by orotate phosphoribosyl transferase in the normal gastrointestinal mucosa. In the phase II setting S-1 has demonstrated a 35% partial response rate and median survival of 12 months.[148]

Antifolate agents

Such agents under development include trimetrexate and MTA (multitargeted antifolate). Trimetrexate enters cells by passive diffusion and inhibits dihydrofolate reductase. In the phase II setting the overall response rate to trimetrexate combined with 5 FU and folinic acid is 42% in untreated patients.[149] Phase III studies are in progress. MTA is transported by the reduced folate carrier and is retained within cells by polyglutamation via folypoly-γ-glutamate synthetase. It inhibits multiple enzymes including thymidylate synthase, dihydrofolate reductase, glycinamide ribonucleotide formyltransferase (GARFT) and aminoimidazole carboxamide ribonucleotide formyltransferase (AICARFT). The phase II response rate for MAT given as 500 mg/m² every 3 weeks is 17.2%.[150] Myelosuppression is common and a maculopapular rash can be treated or prevented with the co-administration of corticosteroids.

Which combination to use

Currently there is no consensus as to which of the available agents or combinations appears to confer a substantial advantage. The prescription for any given patient may depend on ease of administration, age and performance status. Tournigard et al. have conducted a trial that is likely to answer the number of questions related to the sequence of chemotherapy for patients with advanced colorectal cancer and good performance status.[151] This group has compared the sequence of irinotecan and infusional 5 FU (FOLFIRI) followed by oxaliplatin and infusional 5 FU (FOLFOX) at time of progression to the same schedules given in reverse sequence.

Weekly 5 FU/folinic acid adjuvant or palliative – weekly bolus

Drug	Dose	Route	Days
5 Fluorouracil	375–425 mg/m²	Slow IV push	1
Folinic acid	50 mg	Slow IV push	1
Capecitabine	1000–1250 mg/m² po bd	po	1–14 q21
Ralititrexed	3 mg/m²	IV	1 q2

Cycle repeats every week, folinic acid administered before 5 FU

Weekly 5 FU/folinic acid for palliative patients with disease progression on weekly bolus treatment

Drug	Dose	Route	Days
5 Fluorouracil	225 mg/m²/day	Continuous IV infusion	1–14
Folinic acid	15 mg tds	Oral, before food	Alternate days

Continuous infusion administered via external portable pump

FOLFOX4 regimen

Drug	Dose	Route	Days
Oxaliplatin	85 mg/m²	IV over 2 hours	1
Folinic acid	200 mg/m²	IV over 2 hours	1, 2
5 fluorouracil	400 mg/m²	IV bolus	1, 2
5 fluorouracil	600 mg/m²	22 hour infusion	1, 2

Irinotecan/De Gramont regimen

Drug	Dose	Route	Days
Irinotecan	160 mg/m²	IV over 90 mins	1
Folinic acid	200 mg/m²	IV over 2 hours	1, 2
5 fluorouracil	400 mg/m²	IV bolus	1, 2
5 fluorouracil	600 mg/m²	22 hour infusion	1, 2

Figure 8.22 Examples of systemic chemotherapy protocols.

Response rates were 57.5% for first-line FOLFIRI and 21% for second-line versus 56% for FOLFOX first-line and 7% for FOLFIRI second-line. Resection of inoperable hepatic metastases was possible in 15% after FOLFOX and 4% after FOLFIRI. Median survivals were 21.5 months for FOLFIRI first-line and 20.4 months for FOLFOX first-line. While no difference was seen in the survival the trial suggests that oxaliplatin may remain active after irinotecan failure, rather than vice versa.

A number of general conclusions can be drawn: irinotecan and oxaliplatin are best used in combination with 5 FU providing the toxicity observed is acceptable, infusional regimens of 5 FU confer an advantage over bolus 5 FU, folinic acid is an essential biomodulator of 5 FU and oral fluoropyrimidines are likely to be equivalent to, and substituted for, intravenous 5 FU. The systemic chemotherapy protocols used in our institution are detailed in Fig. 8.22.

Key points

- Cryotherapy and other imaging-controlled ablative techniques can be associated with long-term survival in patients with unresectable disease.
- Ablative techniques can be used as an adjunct to liver resection.
- Hepatic artery chemotherapy is associated with high response rates and significantly better survival, but has serious complications.
- Systemic chemotherapy for colorectal cancer has changed; several new active agents are reviewed here.
- Adjuvant hepatic artery chemotherapy after liver resection improves disease-free survival.

REFERENCES

1. Ballantyne GH, Quin J. Surgical treatment of liver metastases in patients with colorectal cancer. Cancer 1993; 71: 4252–66
2. Scheele J, Strangl R, Altendorf-Hofmann, Paul M. Resection of colorectal liver metastases. World J Surg 1995; 19: 59–71
3. Ohlsson B, Stenram U, Tranberg KG. Resection of colorectal liver metastases: 25 year experience. World J Surg 1998; 22: 268–77
4. Shiina S, Tagawa K, Unuma T et al. Percutaneous ethanol injection therapy of hepatocellular carcinoma: analysis of 77 patients. Am J Roentgenol 1990; 155: 1211–26

5. Livraghi T, Bolondi L, Lazzoroni S et al. Percutaneous ethanol injection in the treatment of hepatocellular carcinoma in cirrhosis. A study on 207 patients. Cancer 1992; 69: 925–9

6. Amin Z, Bown SG, Lees WR. Local treatment of colorectal liver metastases: a comparison of interstitial laser photocoagulation (ILP) and percutaneous alcohol injection (PAL). Clin Radiol 1993; 48: 166–71

7. Cooper IS, Lee ASJ. Cryostatic congelation: a system for producing a limited controlled region of cooling or freezing of biological tissues. J Nerv Ment Dis 1961; 133: 259–63

8. Gill W, Fraser J. A look at cryosurgery. Scot Med J 1968; 13: 268–73.

9. Mazur P. The role of intracellular freezing in the death of cells cooled at supraoptimal rates. Cryobiology 1977; 14: 251–72.

10. Whittaker DK. Mechanisms of tissue destruction following cryosurgery. Ann R Coll Surg 1984; 66: 313–17

11. Bischof J, Christou K, Rubinsky B. A morphological study of cooling rate response in normal and neoplastic human liver tumours: cryosurgical complications. Cryobiology 1993; 30: 482–92

12. Seifert JK, Junginger T, Morris DL. A collective review of the world literature on hepatic cryotherapy. J R Coll Surg Edin 1998; 43: 141–54

13. Seifert JK, Morris DL. Prognostic factors following cryotherapy for hepatic metastases from colorectal cancer. Ann Surg 1998; 228: 201–8

14. Cozzi PJ, Englund R, Morris DL. Cryotherapy treatment of patients with hepatic metastases from neuroendocrine tumours. Cancer 1995; 76: 501–9

15. Ballantyne GH, Qia T. Surgical treatment of liver metastases in patients with colorectal cancer. Cancer 1993; 71: 4252–66

16. Scheele J, Strong LR, Attendon F, Moffman A, Paul M. Resection of colorectal liver metastases. World J Surg 1995; 19: 59–71

17. Dwerryhouse SJ, McCall J, Iqbal J, Ross WB, Seifest J, Morris DL. Hepatic resection with cryotherapy to involved or inadequate resection margin (edge freeze) for metastases from colorectal cancer. Br J Surg 1998; 85: 185–7

18. Hewitt PM, Dwerryhouse SJ, Zhao J, Morris DL. Multiple bilobar liver metastases: cryotherapy for residual lesions after liver resection. J Surg Oncol 1998; 67: 112–16

19. Seifert JK, Morris DL. A world survey on the complications of hepatic and prostate cryotherapy. World J Surg 1999; 23: 109–14

20. Weaver ML, Atkinson D, Zemat R. Hepatic cryosurgery in treating colorectal metastases. Cancer 1995; 76: 210–14

21. Bagia JS, Perera DS, Morris DL. Renal impairment in hepatic cryotherapy. Cryobiology 1998; 36: 263–7

22. Cozzi PJ, Stewart GJ, Morris DL. Thrombocytopenia after hepatic cryotherapy for colorectal metastases correlates with hepatocellular injury. World J Surg 1994; 18: 774–7

23. King J, Glenn D, Morris DL. Computed tomography changes following cryotherapy for hepatic cancer. Aust Radiol 1997; 41: 22–7

24. Steele G, Ravikumar TS, Benotti PN. New surgical treatments for recurrent colorectal cancer. Cancer 1990; 65: 723–30

25. Preketis AP, King J, Caplehorn JRM et al. CEA reduction after cryotherapy for liver metastases from colon cancer predicts survival. Aust NZ J Surg 1994; 64: 612–14

26. Morris DL, Ross WB, Iqbal J, McCall JL, King J, Clinghan PR. Cryoablation of hepatic malignancy: an evaluation of tumour marker data and survival in 110 patients. GI Cancer 1996; 1: 247–51

27. Ravikumar TS, Kane R, Cady B, Jenkins R, Clouse M, Steel G, Jr. A 5 year study of cryosurgery in the treatment of liver tumours. Arch Surg 1991; 126: 1520–4

28. Bown SG. Phototherapy of liver tumours. World J Surg 1983; 7: 700–9

29. Matthewson K, Coleridge-Smith P, O'Sullivan JP, Northfield TC, Brown SG. Biological effects of intrahepatic neodymium:yttrium–aluminium–garnet laser photocoagulation in rats. Gastroenterology 1987; 93: 550–7

30. Van Eeden P, Steger AC, Bown SG. Fibre tip considerations for low power laser interstitial laser hyperthermia. Lasers Med Sci 1988; 3: abstract

31. Hashimoto D, Takami M, Idezuki Y. In depth radiation therapy by YAG laser for malignant tumours in the liver under ultrasonic imaging. Gastroenterology 1985; 88: 1663

32. Hahl J, Haapiainen R, Ovaksa J, Puolakkainen P, Schroder T. Laser induced hyperthermia in the treatment of liver tumours. Lasers Med Sci 1990; 10: 319–21

33. Steger AC. Interstitial laser hyperthermia for the treatment of hepatic and pancreatic tumours. Photochem Photobiol 1991; 53: 837–44

34. Masters A, Steger AC, Lees WR, Walmsley KM, Brown SG. Interstitial laser hyperthermia: a new approach for treating liver metastases. Br J Cancer 1992; 66: 518–22

35. Steger AC, Lees WR, Shorvon P, Walmsley KM, Brown SG. Multiple fibre low power interstitial laser hyperthermia: studies in the normal liver. Br J Surg 1992; 79: 139–45

36. Amin Z, Bown SG. Laser treatment of metastases. In: Morris DL, McArdle CS, Onik GM, eds. Hepatic metastases. Oxford: Butterworth-Heinemann, 1996: 148–59

37. Nolsoe CP, Torp-Pedersen S, Burcharth F et al. Interstitial hyperthermia of colorectal liver metastases with a US guided Nd–YAG laser with a diffuser tip: a pilot clinical study. Radiology 1993; 187: 333–7

38. Van Hillersberg R, Van Staveren HJ, Kort WJ, Zonderman PE, Terpstra OT. Interstitial Nd:YAG laser coagulation with a cylindrical diffusing fibre tip in experimental liver metastases. Lasers Surg Med 1994; 14: 14–38

39. Steger AC, Lees WR, Walmsley K, Bown SG. Interstitial laser hyperthermia: a new approach to local destruction of tumours. Br Med J 1989; 299: 363–5

40. Boldrini G, De Gaetano AM, Giovannini I et al. The systemic use of ultrasound for detection of liver metastases during colorectal surgery. World J Surg 1987; 11: 622–7

41. Hayashi N, Yamamoto K, Tamaki N et al. Metastatic nodules of hepatocellular carcinoma: detection with angiography, CT, and US. Radiology 1987; 165: 61–3

42. Germer CT, Albrecht D, Roggan A, Isbest C, Buhr HJ. Experimental study of laparoscopic laser induced thermotherapy for liver tumours. Br J Surg 1997; 84: 317–20

43. Amin Z, Donald JJ, Masters A et al. Hepatic metastases: interstitial laser photocoagulation with real time US monitoring and dynamic CT evaluation of treatment. Radiology 1993; 187: 339–47

44. Steger AC, Shorvon P, Walsmley K, Chisholm R, Brown SG, Lees WR. Ultrasound features of low power interstitial laser hyperthermia. Clin Radiol 1992; 46: 88–93

45. Vogl TJ, Muller PK, Hammerstingl R et al. Malignant liver tumours treated with MR imaging guided laser induced thermotherapy: technique and prospective results. Radiology 1995; 196: 257–65

46. Vogl TJ, Mack MC, Straub R, Roggan A, Felix R. Magnetic resonance imaging guided abdominal interventional radiology: laser induced thermotherapy of liver metastases. Endoscopy 1997; 29: 577–83

47. Vogl TJ, Mack MC, Straub R et al. Percutaneous MRI guided laser induced thermotherapy for colorectal cancer. Lancet 1997; 350: 29

48. Stagl R, Altendorf Hofman A, Charnley RM, Scheele J. Factors influencing the natural history of colorectal liver metastases. Lancet 1994; 343: 1405–10

49. Masters A, Steger AC, Bown SG. Role of interstitial therapy in the treatment of liver cancer. Br J Surg 1991; 78: 518–23

50. Siperstein AE, Gitomirski A. History and technological aspects of radiofrequency thermoablation. Cancer J 2000; 6(Suppl 4): 5293–303

51. Organ LW. Electrophysiologic principles of radiofrequency lesion making. Appl Neurophysiol 1976/77; 39: 69–76

52. Curley SA, Izzo F, Delrio P et al. Radiofrequency ablation of unresectable primary and metastatic hepatic malignancies. Results in 123 patients. Ann Surg 1999; 230: 1–8

53. Siperstein A, Garland A, Engle K et al. Local recurrence after laparoscopic radiofrequency thermal ablation of hepatic tumours. Ann Surg Oncol 2000; 7: 106

54. Scudamore CH, Lee SI, Patterson E et al. Radiofrequency ablation followed by resection of malignant liver tumors. Am J Surg 1999; 177: 411–17

55. Patterson EJ, Scudamore CH, Owen DA et al. Radiofrequency ablation of porcine liver in vivo: effects of blood flow and treatment time on lesion size. Ann Surg 1998; 227; 559–65

56. Solbiati L, Goldberg SN, Ierace T et al. Hepatic metastases: percutaneous radiofrequency ablation with cooled-tip electrodes. Radiology 1997; 205: 367–73

57. Livraghi T, Goldberg SN, Monti F et al. Saline enhanced radiofrequency tissue ablation in the treatment of liver metastases. Radiology 1997; 202: 205–10

58. Chang RJ, Stevenson WG, Saxon LA, Parker J. Increasing catheter ablation lesion size by simultaneous application of radiofrequency current to two adjacent sites. Am Heart J 1993; 125: 1276–84

59. Rossi S, Di Stasi M, Buscarini E et al. Percutaneous RF interstitial thermal ablation in the treatment of hepatic cancer. AJR 1996; 167: 759–68

60. Siperstein AE, Rogers SJ, Hansen PD, Gitomirsky A. Laparoscopic thermal ablation of hepatic neuroendocrine tumor metastases. Surgery 1997; 122: 1147–55

61. McGahan JP, Browning PD, Brock JM, Tesluk H. Hepatic ablation using radiofrequency electrocautery. Invest Radiol 1990; 25: 267–70

62. Cha CH, Lee FT, Gurney JM et al. CT versus sonography for monitoring radiofrequency ablation in aporcine liver. AJR 2000; 175: 705–11

63. Goldberg SN, Gazelle GS, Compton CC et al. Treatment of intrahepatic malignancy with radiofrequency ablation. Radiologic–pathologic correlation. Cancer 2000; 88: 2452–63

64. Ravikumar TS, Jones M, Serrano M et al. The role of PET scanning in radiofrequency ablation of liver metastasis from colorectal cancer. Cancer J 2000; 6: S330–43

65. Curley SA, Izzo F, Ellis L et al. Radiofrequency ablation of hepatocellular cancer in 100 patients with cirrhosis. Ann Surg 2000; 232: 381–91

66. Bilchik AJ, Wood TF, Allegra D et al. Cryosurgical ablation and radiofrequency ablation for unresectable hepatic malignant neoplasm. Arch Surg 2000; 135: 657–64

67. Lencioni RA, Cioni D, Paolicchi A et al. Percutaneous treatment of small hepatocellular carcinoma: radiofrequency thermal ablation versus percutaneous ethanol injection – a prospective randomized trial. Radiology 1998; 209: (P)174

68. Rossi S, Di Stasi M, Buscarini E et al. Percutaneous RF interstitial thermal ablation in the treatment of hepatic cancer. AJR 1996; 167: 759–68

69. Livraghi T, Goldberg SN, Lazzaroni S et al. Hepatocellular carcinoma: radiofrequency ablation of medium and large lesions. Radiology 2000; 214: 761–8

70. Klopp CT, Bateman J, Berry N et al. Fractionated regional cancer chemotherapy. Cancer Res 1950; 10: 229

71. Bierman HR, Byron RL, Miller ER, Shimkin MB. Effects of intra-arterial administration of nitrogen mustard. Am J Med 1950; 8: 535

72. Sullivan RD, Norcross JW, Watkins E. Chemotherapy of metastatic liver cancer by prolonged hepatic artery infusion. N Engl J Med 1964; 270: 321–7

73. Frei E. Effect of dose and schedule on response. In: Hollang JF, Frei E, eds. Cancer medicine. Philadelphia: Lea and Febiger, 1973: 717–30

74. Widder KJ, Senyei AE, Ranney DF. Magnetically responsive microspheres and other carriers for the biophysical targeting of antitumour agents. Adv Pharmacol Chemother 1979; 16: 213–71

75. Breedis C, Young G. The blood supply of neoplasms in the liver. Am J Path 1954; 30: 969–85

76. Lien WM, Ackerman NB. The blood supply of experimental liver metastases. II. A microcirculatory study of the normal and tumour vessels of the liver with the use of perfused silicone rubber. Surgery 1970; 68: 334–40

77. Ridge, JA, Bading JR, Gelbard AS et al. Perfusion of colorectal hepatic metastases. Relative distribution of flow from the hepatic artery and portal vein. Cancer 1987; 59: 1547–53

78. Ensminger WD, Rosowsky A, Raso V et al. A clinical pharmacological evaluation of hepatic arterial infusions of 5-fluoro-2-deoxyuridine and 5-fluorouracil. Cancer Res 1978; 38: 3784–92

79. Goldberg JA, Kerr DJ, Watson DG et al. The pharmacokinetics of 5-fluorouracil administered by arterial infusion in advanced colorectal hepatic metastases. Br J Cancer 1990; 61: 913–15

80. Huberman MS. Comparison of systemic chemotherapy with hepatic arterial infusion in metastatic colorectal carcinoma. Semin Oncol 1983; 10: 238–48

81. Kemeny N, Daly J, Reichman B et al. Intrahepatic or systemic infusion of fluorodeoxyuridine in patients with liver metastases from colorectal carcinoma. A randomised trial. Ann Int Med 1987; 107: 459–65

82. Chang AE, Schneider PD, Sugarbaker PH et al. A prospective randomised trial of regional versus systemic continuous 5-fluorodeoxyuridine chemotherapy in the treatment of colorectal liver metastases. Ann Surg 1987; 206: 685–93

83. Hohn DC, Stagg RJ, Freidman MA et al. A randomised trial of continuous intravenous versus hepatic intrarterial floxuridine in patients with colorectal cancer metastatic to the liver: the Northern California Oncology Trial Group. J Clin Oncol 1989; 7: 1646–54

84. Kirk Martin J, O'Connell MJ, Weiand HS et al. Intra-arterial floxuridine vs systemic fluorouracil for hepatic metastases from colorectal cancer. A randomised trial. Arch Surg 1990; 125: 1022–7

85. Rougier P, Laplanche A, Hugier M et al. Hepatic arterial infusion of floxuridine in patients with liver metastases from colorectal carcinoma: long term results of a prospective randomised trial. J Clin Oncol 1992; 10: 1112–18

86. Allen-Mersh TG, Earlam S, Fordy C et al. Quality of life and survival with continuous hepatic artery floxuridine infusion for colorectal liver metastases. Lancet 1994; 344: 1255–60

87. Meta Analysis Group in Cancer. Reappraisal of hepatic arterial infusion in the treatment of nonresectable liver metastases from colorectal cancer. J Natl Cancer Inst 1996; 88: 252–8

88. Kemeny MM. Hepatic artery infusion as a treatment of hepatic metastases from colorectal cancer. J Gastrointest Surg 1997; 1: 423–5

89. Kemeny N, Huang Y, Cohen AM et al. Hepatic arterial infusion of chemotherapy after resection of hepatic metastases from colorectal cancer. N Engl J Med 1999; 341: 2039–48

90. Campbell KA, Burns RC, Sitzmann JV et al. Regional chemotherapy devices: effect of experience and anatomy on complications. J Clin Oncol 1993; 11: 822–6

91. Michels NA. Newer anatomy of the liver and its variant blood supply and collateral circulation. Am J Surg Oncol 1966; 112: 337–47

92. Hohn DC, Stagg RJ, Price DC, Lewis BJ. Avoidance of gastrointestinal toxicity in patients receiving hepatic arterial 5-fluoro-2-deoxyuridine. J Clin Oncol 1985; 3: 1257–60

93. Kemeny MM, Battifora H, Blayney DW et al. Sclerosing cholangitis after continuous hepatic artery infusion of FUDR. Ann Surg 1985; 202: 176–81

94. Doci R, Bignami P, Quagliuolo V et al. Continuous hepatic arterial infusion with 5-fluorodeoxyuridine for the treatment of colorectal metastases. Reg Cancer Treat 1990; 3: 13–18

95. Chuang VP. Hepatic arterial redistribution for intraarterial infusion of hepatic neoplasms. Radiology 1980; 135: 295–9

96. Cohen AM, Higgins J, Waltman AC, Athanasoulis C. Effect of ligation of variant arterial structures on the completeness of regional chemotherapy infusion. Am J Surg 1987; 153: 378–80

97. Anderson JH, Goldberg JA, Leiberman DP et al. Saphenous vein grafts for anatomical variations encountered at surgical insertion of a hepatic artery catheter. Eur J Surg Oncol 1992; 18: 484–6

98. Doughty JC, Warren H, Anderson JH et al. Response to regional chemotherapy in patients with variant hepatic arterial anatomy. Br J Surg 1996; 83: 652–3

99. Sugihara K. Continuous hepatic arterial infusion of 5-fluorouracil for unresectable colorectal liver metastases: phase II study. Surgery 1995; 117: 624–8

100. Boyle FM, Smith RC, Levi JA. Continuous hepatic artery infusion of 5-fluorouracil for metastatic colorectal cancer localised to the liver. Aust NZ J Med 1993; 23: 32–4

101. Stagg RJ, Venook AP, Chase JL et al. Alternating hepatic intra-arterial floxuridine and fluorouracil: a less toxic regimen for treatment of liver metastases from colorectal cancer. J Natl Cancer Inst 1991; 83: 423–7

102. Kemeny N, Seiter K, Niedzwiecki D. A randomised trial of intrahepatic infusion of fluorodeoxyuridine with dexamethasone versus fluorodeoxyuridine alone in the treatment of metastatic colorectal cancer. Cancer 1992; 69: 327–34

103. Grandi AM, Pinotti G, Morandi PE et al. Non invasive evaluation of cardiotoxicity of 5-fluorouracil and low doses of folinic acid: a one year follow up study. Ann Oncol 1997; 8: 705–8

104. Warren HW, Anderson JH, O'Gorman PO et al. A phase II study of regional 5-fluorouracil infusion with intravenous folinic acid for colorectal liver metastases. Br J Cancer 1994; 70: 677–80

105. Schlag P, Hohenberger P, Holting T et al. Hepatic arterial infusion chemotherapy for liver metastases of colorectal cancer using 5-FU. Eur J Surg Oncol 1990; 16: 99–104

106. Erlichman C, Fine S, Wong A et al. A randomised trial of fluorouracil and folinic acid in patients with metastatic colorectal carcinoma. J Clin Oncol 1988; 3: 469–75

107. Valone FH, Friedman MA, Wittlinger PS et al. Treatment of patients with advanced colorectal carcinoma with flourouracil alone, high dose leucovorin plus flourouracil, or sequential methotrexate, flourouracil and leucovorin. J Clin Oncol 1989; 7: 1427–36

108. Advanced Colorectal Cancer Meta Analysis Project. Modulation of fluorouracil by leucovorin in patients with advanced colorectal cancer: evidence in terms of response rate. J Clin Oncol 1992; 10: 896–903

109. Heidelberger C, Chanakari NK, Danenberg PV. Fluorinated pyrimidines: a new class of tumour inhibitory compounds. Nature 1957; 179: 663–6

110. Colorectal Cancer Collaborative Group. Palliative chemotherapy for advanced colorectal cancer: systematic review and meta-analysis. Br Med J 2000; 321: 531–5

111. Scheithauer W, Rosen H, Kornek GV et al. Randomised comparison of combination chemotherapy plus supportive care with supportive care alone in patients with metastatic colorectal cancer. Br Med J 1993; 306: 752–55

112. Beretta G, Bollina R, Martignoni G et al. Flourouracil + folates (FUFO) as standard treatment for advanced/metastatic gastrointestinal carcinomas (AGC). Ann Oncol 1994; 5 (Suppl 8): 48

113. Cunningham D, Pyrohonen S, James RD et al. Randomised trial of irinotecan plus supportive care versus supportive care alone after fluorouracil failure for patients with metastatic colorectal cancer. Lancet 1998; 352: 1413–18

114. Nordic Gastrointestinal Tumour Adjuvant Therapy Group. Expectancy or primary chemotherapy in patients with advanced asymptomatic colorectal cancer: a randomised trial. J Clin Oncol 1992; 10: 904–11

115. Ackland SP, Moore M, Jones M et al. A meta-analysis of two randomized trials of early chemotherapy in asymptomatic metastatic colorectal cancer. Proc Am Soc Clin Oncol 2001; 20: 526 (abstract)

116. Maughan TS, James RD, Kerr DJ et al. Continuous versus intermittent chemotherapy for advanced colorectal cancer: preliminary results for the MRC Cr06B randomised trial. Proc Am Soc Clin Oncol 2001; 20: 498 (abstract)

117. Buyse M, Thirion P, Carlson RW et al. Relation between tumour response to first-line chemotherapy and survival in advanced colorectal cancer: a meta-analysis. Lancet 2000; 356: 373–8

118. Doroshow JH, Multhauf P, Leong L et al. Prospective randomised comparison of fluorouracil versus fluorouracil and high-dose continuous infusion leucovorin calcium for the treatment of advanced measurable colorectal cancer in patients previously unexposed to chemotherapy. J Clin Oncol 1990; 8: 491–501

119. Erlichman C, Fine S, Wong A et al. A randomised trial of fluorouracil and folinic acid in patients with metastatic colorectal carcinoma. J Clin Oncol 1988; 6: 469–75

120. Petrelli N, Doudlass HO, Herrera L et al. The modulation of fluorouracil with leucovorin in metastatic colorectal carcinoma: a prospective randomised phase III trial. J Clin Oncol 1989; 7: 1419–26

121. Petrelli N, Herrera L, Rustum Y et al. A prospective randomised trial of 5 fluorouracil versus 5 fluorouracil and high dose leucovorin versus 5 fluorouracil and methotrexate in previously untreated patient with advanced colorectal carcinoma. J Clin Oncol 1987; 5: 1559–69

122. Valone FH, Friedman MA, Wittlinger PS et al. Treatment of patients with advanced colorectal carcinomas with fluorouracil alone, high dose leucovorin plus fluorouracil, or sequential methotrexate, fluorouracil, and leukovorin. A randomised trial of the Northern California Oncology Group. J Clin Oncol 1989; 7: 1427–36

123. Cricca A, Martoni A, Guaraldi M et al. Randomised clinical trial of 5 FU plus folinic acid vs 5 FU in advanced gastrointestinal cancers. Proc ESMO 1988; 13: 427

124. Nobile MT, Vidili MG, Sobrero A et al. 5 Fluorouracil alone or combined with high dose folinic acid in advanced colorectal cancer patients. Proc Am Soc Clin Oncol 1988; 7: 371 (abstract)

125. Di Costanzo F, Bartolucci R, Sofra M et al. 5 Fluorouracil alone versus high dose folinic acid and 5 FU in advanced colorectal cancer: a randomised trial of the Italian oncology group for clinical research (GOIRC). Proc Am Soc Clin Oncol 1989; 8: 410 (abstract)

126. Labianca R, Pancera G, Aitini E et al. Folinic acid plus 5 fluorouracil (5 FU) versus equidose 5 FU in advanced colorectal cancer. Phase II study of 'GISTAD' (Italian group for the study of digestive tract cancer). Ann Oncol 1991; 2: 673–9

127. Advanced Colorectal Cancer Meta Analysis Project. Modulation of fluorouracil by leucovorin in patients with advanced colorectal cancer: evidence in terms of response rate. J Clin Oncol 1992; 10: 896–903

128. Machover D. A comprehensive review of 5 fluorouracil and leucovorin in patients with metastatic colorectal carcinoma. Cancer 1997; 80: 1179–87

129. Advanced Colorectal Cancer Meta Analysis Project. Meta-analysis of randomised trials testing the biochemical modulation of fluorouracil by methotrexate in metastatic colorectal cancer. J Clin Oncol 1994; 12: 960–9

130. Meta Analysis Group in Cancer. Efficacy of continuous intravenous infusion of fluorouracil compared with bolus administration in advanced colorectal cancer. J Clin Oncol 1998; 16: 301–8

131. de Gramont A, Bosset J-F, Milan C et al. Randomised trial comparing monthly low-dose leucovorin and fluorouracil bolus plus continuous infusion for advanced colorectal cancer: a French intergroup study. J Clin Oncol 1997; 15: 808–15

132. Levi F, Zidani R, Misset J-L. Randomised multicentre trial of chemotherapy with oxaliplatin, fluorouracil, and folinic acid in metastatic colorectal cancer. Lancet 1997; 350: 681–8

133. Gamelin E, Boisdron-Celle M, Delva R et al. Long-term weekly treatment of colorectal metastatic cancer with fluorouracil and leucovorin: results of a multicentric prospective trial of fluorouracil dosage optimization by pharmacokinetics monitoring in 152 patients. J Clin Oncol 1998; 16: 1470–8

134. Rougier P, Van Cutsem E, Bajetta E et al. Randomised trial of irinotecan versus fluorouracil by continuous infusion fluorouracil failure in patients with metastatic colorectal cancer. Lancet 1998; 352: 1407–12

135. Saltz LB, Cox JV, Blanke C et al. Irinotecan plus fluorouracil and leucovorin for metastatic colorectal cancer. N Engl J Med 2000; 343: 905–14

136. Douillard JY, Cunningham D, Roth AD et al. Irinotecan combined with fluorouracil compared with fluorouracil alone as first-line treatment for metastatic colorectal cancer: a multicentre randomised trial. Lancet 2000; 355: 1041–7

137. de Gramont A, Figer A, Seymour M et al. Leucovorin and fluorouracil with or without oxaliplatin as first-line treatment in advanced colorectal cancer. J Clin Oncol 2000; 18: 2938–47

138. Bismuth H, Adam R, Levi F et al. Resection of nonresectable liver metastases from colorectal cancer after neoadjuvant chemotherapy. Ann Surg 1996; 224: 509–20

139. Giacchetti S, Itzhaki M, Gruia G et al. Long-term survival of patients with unresectable colorectal cancer liver metastases following infusional chemotherapy with 5-fluorouracil, leucovorin, oxaliplatin and surgery. Ann Oncol 1999; 10: 663–9

140. Alberts SR, Horvath WL, Donohue JH et al. Oxaliplatin (OXAL), 5-Fluorouracil (5FU) and leucovorin (CF) for patients (pts) with liver only metastases (mets) from colorectal cancer (CRC): A North Central Cancer Treatment Group (NCCTG) phase II study. Proc Am Soc Clin Oncol 2001; 551

141. Pazdur R, Vincent M. Raltitrexed (Tomudex) vs 5-fluorouracil + leucovorin (5-FU + LV) in patients with advanced colorectal cancer (ACC); results of a randomised multicentre North American trial. Proc Am Soc Clin Oncol 1997; 16: 801 (abstract)

142. Harper P, on behalf of the Tomudex Study Group. Advanced colorectal cancer: results from the latest raltitrexed comparative study. Proc Am Soc Clin Oncol 1997; 16: 228 (abstract)

143. Cunningham D, Zalcberg JR, Rath U et al. Final results of a randomised trial comparing 'Tomudex®' (raltitrexed) with 5-fluorouracil plus leucovorin in advanced colorectal cancer. Ann Oncol 1996; 7: 961–5

144. Cunningham D. Mature results from the three large controlled studies with raltitrexed ('Tomudex'). Br J Cancer 1998; 77 (Suppl 2): 15–21

145. Hoff PM, Amsaro R, batost G et al. Comparison of oral capecitabine versus intravenous fluorouracil plus leucovorin as first-line treatment in 605 patients with metastatic colorectal cancer: results of a randomised phase III study. J Clin Oncol 2001; 19: 2282–92

146. Pazdur R, Lassere Y, Rhodes V et al. Phase II trial of uracil and tegafur plus oral leucovorin: an effective oral regimen in the treatment of metastatic colorectal carcinoma. J Clin Oncol 1994; 12: 2296–300

147. Meropol NJ, Niedzweicki D, Hollis D et al. Phase II study of oral eniluracil, 5-fluorouracil, and leucovorin in patients with advanced colorectal carcinoma. Cancer 2001; 91: 1256–63

148. Ohtsu A, Baba H, Sakara Y et al. Phase II study of S-1, a novel oral glucopyrimidine derivative, in patients with metastatic colorectal carcinoma. Br J Cancer 2000; 83: 141–5

149. Blanke CD, Kasimis B, Schein P et al. Phase II study of trimetrexate, fluorouracil, and leucovorin for advanced colorectal cancer. J Clin Oncol 1997; 15: 915–20

150. Cripps C, Burnell M, Jolivet J et al. Phase II study of first-line LY231514 (multi-targeted antifolate) in patients with locally advanced or metastatic colorectal cancer: a NCIC Clinical Trials Group study. Ann Oncol 1999; 10: 1175–9

151. Tournigard C, Ouvet C, Quinaux E et al. FOLFIRI followed by FOLFOX versus FOLFOX followed by FOLFIRI in metastatic colorectal cancer (MCRC): final results of a phase III study. Proc Am Soc Clin Oncol 2000; 20: 494 (abstract)

9 Management of neuroendocrine tumours

Ian Pope and Graeme J Poston

Neuroendocrine gastrointestinal tumours are derived from the neuroendocrine cell system. These tumours have widely differing clinical presentations that reflect both their organ of origin and syndromes related to excess hormone production. The neuroendocrine gastrointestinal tumours are divided into two main groups, carcinoid tumours and endocrine pancreatic tumours. Carcinoid tumours are now described according to their organ of origin, whereas pancreatic endocrine tumours are described according to their main hormone production and related clinical syndrome (insulinomas, gastrinomas, VIP-omas, glucagonomas, somatostatinomas and non-functioning endocrine pancreatic tumours). The first part of this chapter considers the clinical presentation and metastatic potential of primary neuroendocrine tumours. Given the rarity of these tumours, the experience of treatment of liver metastases from individual tumours is limited. Most studies combine carcinoid tumours derived from various organs of origin together with pancreatic endocrine tumours. The second part of this chapter is therefore devoted in general to the diagnosis and management of neuroendocrine hepatic metastases, albeit from a wide variety of primary tumours.

Neuroendocrine tumours: historical perspective

The diffuse neuroendocrine system was first described by Feyrter in 1938 (diffuse endokrine epithelail organe). The term 'carcinoid' was first introduced by Oberndorfer in 1907 to describe a morphologically distinct class of intestinal tumours that behave less aggressively than the more common intestinal adenocarcinomas. Lubarsh originally described this tumour in 1888. Multiple small tumours were observed at autopsy in the distal ileum of two patients. Microscopic examination revealed the absence of glandular structures, suggesting development of these tumours from epithelial cells within the glands of Leiberkuhn. The first case of metastatic disease, and indeed the carcinoid syndrome, was described by Ranson in 1890 who reported a patient with ileal carcinoma and multiple liver metastases who experienced diarrhoea and dyspnoea after eating.[1] In 1914, Gosset and Masson, using silver impregnation techniques, demonstrated that carcinoid tumours arose from the enterochromaffin cells of the glands of Leiberkuhn, thereby establishing their endocrine origin. In 1953, Lembeck demonstrated the presence of serotonin in carcinoid tumours and in 1954 Waldenstrom described the carcinoid syndrome, reporting a series of patients with small intestinal carcinoids and liver metastases with symptoms of diarrhoea, flushing, asthma, cyanosis and right-sided valvular heart disease.[2] In 1955, Page et al. demonstrated increased urinary 5-hydroxyindoleacetic acid (5-HIAA) in patients with carcinoid syndrome, thereby defining a relationship between carcinoid syndrome and tumour serotonin secretion. Finally, in 1969, Pearse showed that similar cells could be found in organs outside the gastrointestinal tract with the common capacity for amine precursor uptake and decarboxylation (APUD system). As described today, the diffuse neuroendocrine system includes all neuronal and endocrine cells that share a common phenotype characterized by simultaneous expression of general neuroendocrine markers and cell type specific regulatory peptides. It is now recognized that neuroendocrine cells are involved in a wide variety of tumours. The majority occur as primary tumours of the gastrointestinal tract; however, they can also be found in locations such as the lung, ovary, thymus and kidney. Tumours are found to have different hormonal profiles depending on their site of origin (Fig. 9.1). In addition, neuroendocrine tumours show great heterogeneity with respect to both histological and endocrinological

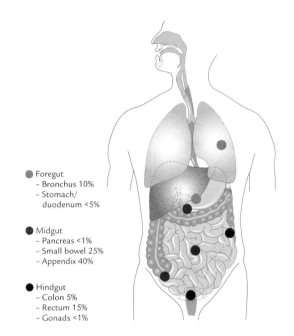

Figure 9.1 Location of carcinoid tumours which may be derived from the foregut (blue), midgut (red), or hindgut (green).

Foregut
– Bronchus 10%
– Stomach/ duodenum <5%

Midgut
– Pancreas <1%
– Small bowel 25%
– Appendix 40%

Hindgut
– Colon 5%
– Rectum 15%
– Gonads <1%

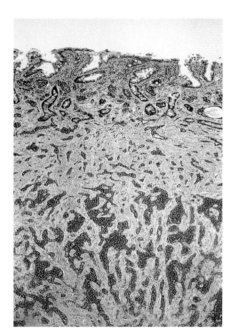

Figure 9.2 Haematoxylin and eosin (H&E) stained micrograph of a gastric carcinoid tumour showing cluster of neuroendocrine cells within the gastric stroma.

features and also clinical presentation and metastatic potential.

Gastrointestinal neuroendocrine (carcinoid) tumours

Stomach

In early studies, gastric neuroendocrine tumours accounted for only 3% of neuroendocrine tumours of the gut. However, according to later series their incidence ranges from 11% to 41%.[3] In part, this is due to an increased use of endoscopy, though many tumours are now seen in association with hypergastrinaemia. Three types of gastric neuroendocrine tumours are now recognized.[3] Type I tumours (80%) are associated with chronic atrophic gastritis. These tumours are usually multiple and arise against a background of gastrin-induced enterochromaffin-like (ECL) cell hyperplasia. They are generally small (<1 cm) and rarely metastasize. Type II tumours (6%) are associated with hypertrophic gastropathy due to multiple endocrine neoplasia (MEN) type 1 and Zollinger–Ellison syndrome (ZES). These tumours again are usually small, but are more aggressive than type I tumours and are somewhat more likely to metastasize. In general though, type I and type II tumours are considered to be benign. Endoscopic removal is recommended for tumours less than 1 cm, whereas surgical excision is recommended for lesions greater than 1 cm. Type III tumours (14%) are

sporadic lesions that are not associated with hypergastrinaemia. These tumours are considered malignant (Fig. 9.2). Regional lymph node metastases have been described in 20 to 50% of patients and liver metastases have ultimately developed in as many as two-thirds of patients.[4] Rindi et al. described 32 sporadic gastric neuroendocrine tumours, with liver metastases present in 52%.[5] Patients with type III disease will usually require formal gastrectomy and lymph node clearance.

Duodenum

Neuroendocrine tumours of the duodenum represent 1–2% of neuroendocrine gastrointestinal tumours. Five main types of tumour are recognized in the duodenum: gastrin producing tumours, somatostatin producing tumours, gangliocytic paragangliomas, serotonin/calcitonin/PP producing tumours and poorly differentiated carcinomas.[6,7] Gastrin producing tumours are the most frequent (60%) and these are found as small, sessile submucosal nodules in the first or second parts of the duodenum (Fig. 9.3). They may be associated with a sporadic ZES or as part of MEN-1 syndrome. Somatostatin producing tumours (20%) generally present as bulky lesions in the ampulla of Vater. These tumours are considered of low grade malignancy and although metastasis to regional lymph nodes may occur, liver metastases are rare. Gangliocytic paraganglionomas occur in the ampullary region and are considered to be benign. The serotonin, calcitonin or PP producing tumours

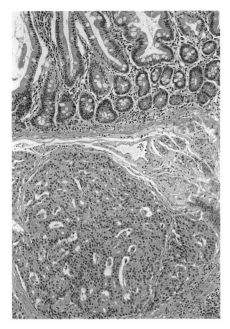

Figure 9.3 H&E stained micrograph of a duodenal gastrinoma lying beneath the duodenal mucosa.

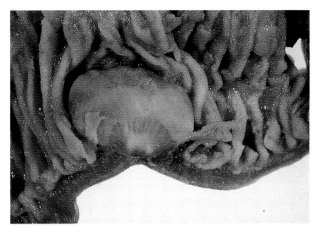

Figure 9.4 Macroscopic view of a surgically resected small bowel (terminal ileum) carcinoid tumour. The patient presented with the carcinoid syndrome due to liver metastases.

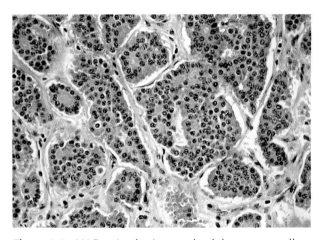

Figure 9.5 H&E stained micrograph of the same small bowel carcinoid demonstrated in Figure 9.4.

that occur outside the ampullary region are benign. However, about half of these tumours found in the ampulla are considered to be of low grade malignancy.

Small bowel

Neuroendocrine tumours of the jejunum and ileum account for 20 to 30% of neuroendocrine tumours of the gut. The majority of tumours are found in the terminal ileum and these are generally of the classic argentaffin carcinoid type. Most tumours are associated with the production of serotonin and substance P. Small bowel carcinoids are rarely diagnosed prior to surgery,[8] and patients are frequently treated conservatively for an extended period of time.[9] Patients usually present with bowel obstruction or ischaemia due either to the mechanical effects of tumour or due to a marked desmoplastic reaction involving the mesentery (Figs 9.4 and 9.5). Optimal treatment involves small bowel resection, together with resection of draining lymph nodes. However, this might not be easily achieved in the presence of extensive mesenteric desmoplastic reaction and in this situation a surgical bypass of the obstructing tumour may be the only possible palliative procedure. A careful laparotomy should be performed. Small bowel carcinoids are frequently multiple and are often also associated with a second primary gastrointestinal malignancy.[10] As with other gastrointestinal neuroendocrine tumours, there is a positive correlation between tumour size and the

risk of metastases. Tumours less than 1 cm have a 20 to 30% incidence of nodal and hepatic metastases. Tumours between 1 and 2 cm have a 60–80% incidence of nodal metastases and a 20% incidence of hepatic metastases. Tumours greater than 2 cm have an 80% incidence of nodal metastases and a 40–50% incidence of hepatic metastases.[8,11,12] Overall 5-year survival rates are 75% for node negative patients, 59% in patients with positive lymph nodes and 20 to 30% if liver metastases are present.[12,13] However, Thompson et al. have reported a 53% 5-year survival rate when hepatic metastases are present.[8]

Appendix

Approximately 40 to 50% of gut neuroendocrine tumours (Figs 9.6 and 9.7) are found in the appendix. These tumours have a good prognosis and the

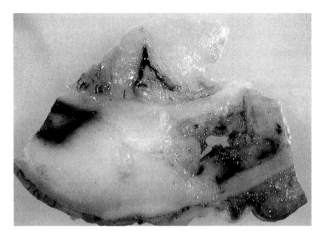

Figure 9.6 Macroscopic view of an appendix carcinoid removed because of acute appendicitis.

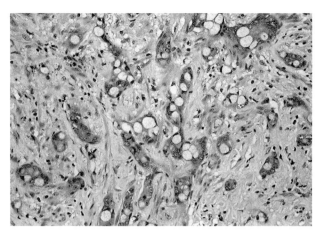

Figure 9.7 H&E stained micrograph of the same appendix carcinoid demonstrated in Figure 9.6.

risk of metastases is between 1.4 and 8.8%.[10,14–18] Tumours that metastasize are usually greater than 2 cm. Tumours between 1 and 2 cm rarely metastasize, but lymph node metastases have been shown in some cases.[8,16] Tumours less than 1 cm were said never to metastasize. Size of tumour is clearly related to risk of malignancy. However, mesoappendix invasion has also been shown to be predictive of an increased risk of metastases for tumours less than 2 cm.[19] Thus tumours greater than 2 cm should be treated by right hemicolectomy, whereas appendicectomy is usually adequate for tumours less than 1 cm. For tumours between 1 cm and 2 cm, treatment should be determined by tumour site, the patient's age and health and the presence of mesoappendix invasion or vascular and lymphatic invasion.

Colon

Colonic neuroendocrine tumours represent 2.8% of all of all gastrointestinal neuroendocrine tumours.[13] Tumours are found predominantly in the right colon and usually present with abdominal pain and weight loss.[20,21] Tumours often present at an advanced stage with distant metastases.[22,23] Colonic neuroendocrine tumours should be treated by standard colonic resection, as would be performed for adenocarcinomas of the colon. Overall 5-year survival rates for colonic neuroendocrine tumours are approximately 37%.[20,23]

Rectum

Rectal neuroendocrine tumours share similarities with neuroendocrine carcinomas of the appendix in that they are often found incidentally and usually have a good prognosis. Tumours may present with rectal bleeding, constipation, tenesmus or pruritis. Mayo Clinic experience suggests that one tumour will be found for every 2500 sigmoidoscopies performed.[24] Again, there is a correlation between tumour size and the risk of metastases. For tumours less than 1 cm, metastases only occur in 3% of cases. For tumours between 1 and 2 cm, metastases

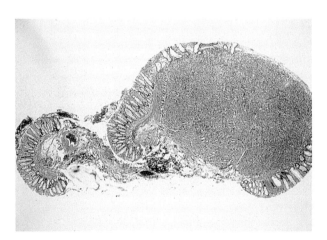

Figure 9.8 H&E stained low power micrograph of a rectal carcinoid tumour.

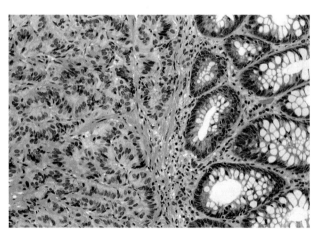

Figure 9.9 High power view of the same rectal carcinoid tumour shown in Figure 9.8.

occur in 11% of cases.[25] However, for tumours greater than 2 cm, metastases are found to occur in 11% of cases. However, for tumours greater than 2 cm, metastases are found to occur in 74% of cases.[25] Invasion of the muscularis propria has also been identified as an additional risk factor.[25] Small tumours, less than 1 cm, are usually treated by local excision. Tumours between 1 and 2 cm may be treated by local excision, but muscular invasion should be considered a further indication for radical surgery (Figs 9.8 and 9.9). Tumours greater than 2 cm should generally be treated by anterior or abdominoperineal resection. Five-year survival rates are 92% in the absence of metastases, 44% when lymph node metastases are present and 7% when distant metastases are present.[13,25]

Pancreatic endocrine tumours

Gastrinoma

Gastrinoma is the most common malignant endocrine tumour of the pancreas, with an incidence of 0.1–3 per million.[26] Although the majority of gastrinomas arise within the pancreas (Fig. 9.10), it is now recognized that up to 40% of gastrinomas may arise in the duodenum (Table 9.1). Gastrin overproduction results in ZES.[27] Approximately 20% of patients with ZES will also have MEN-1.[28] Patients present with peptic ulceration, gastritis, diarrhoea and malabsorbtion (Table 9.2). Severe peptic ulceration is now seen less commonly due to the widespread use of H2 receptor blockers and proton pump inhibitors. With improved medical treatment, the development of liver metastases has become an important determinant of long-term survival (Table 9.3). The overall 5-year survival rate for patients with liver metastases is 20–38%.[29] In a series published in 1994, hepatic metastases developed in 3 of 98

Table 9.1 Gastrinoma syndrome (Zollinger–Ellison 1955)

Fulminating ulcer diathesis
Recurrent ulceration despite therapy
Non-beta cell pancreatic islet tumour
Incidence 1:1 000 000
60% Malignant
30% MEN-1
20–40% Duodenal microgastrinomas

Table 9.2 Gastrinoma syndrome: clinical features

- Peptic ulceration
    Multiple
    Atypical sites: oesophagus, jejunum
    Complications: perforation, haemorrhage, obstruction
- Diarrhoea/steatorrhoea
    Enzyme inactivation
    Mucosal damage

Table 9.3 Gastrinoma syndrome: diagnosis

- Gastrin >40 pmol/l
    Fasted sample
    Off antisecory medication
    Other causes of elevated gastrin:
        Achlorhydria
        Hypercalcaemia
        Chronic renal failure
        ?G-cell hyperplasia
- Basal acid output >10 mmol/hour
- Secretin test
    Equivocal cases
    Not able to stop antisecory medication

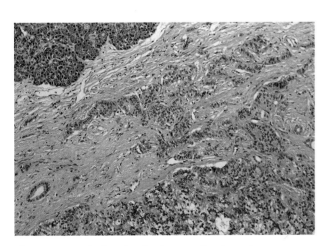

Figure 9.10 H&E stained micrograph of a primary pancreatic gastrinoma.

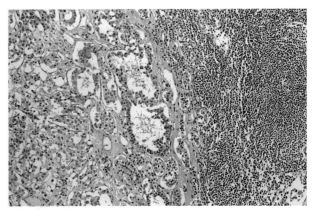

Figure 9.11 H&E stained micrograph showing metastatic gastrinoma in a lymph node adjacent to the pancreas of the same patient demonstrated in Figure 9.10.

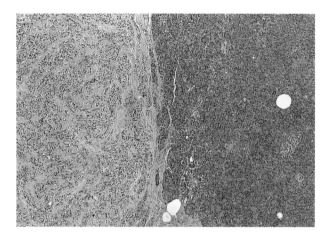

Figure 9.12 H&E stained micrograph of a primary pancreatic insulinoma.

patients (3%) treated by gastrinoma excision compared to 6 of 26 patients (23%) managed medically.[30] The goals of surgery have therefore now shifted from the control of gastric acid hypersecretion to resection of the primary tumour and any involved lymph nodes. Surgery is also the most effective treatment for patients with liver metastases. Aggressive resection of metastases results in a 5-year survival of 79%, compared to 28% in patients with inoperable metastases (Fig. 9.11).[29,31]

Insulinoma

The incidence of insulinoma is approximately one per million.[28] In contrast to gastrinomas, only approximately 5–10% of insulinomas are malignant (Figs 9.12 and 9.13) (Table 9.4).[32] Patients present with symptoms of acute hypoglycaemia with anxiety, dizziness, confusion, loss of consciousness and seizures (Tables 9.5 and 9.6). Treatment is surgical and the majority of tumours exist as small solitary benign tumours distributed uniformly within the pancreas. Dranoth et al. have reviewed 62 cases of malignant insulinoma.[33] Tumours are usually larger and approximately 6 cm in size. The median disease-free survival after resection of malignant tumours was approximately 5 years. Recurrence was observed in 63% of cases at a median interval of 2.8 years, followed by a median survival of only 19 months. Re-resection resulted in a median survival of 4 years, compared to 11 months for biopsy alone. Hepatic resection has rarely been reported for malignant insulinomas, however, surgery remains the optimal treatment for recurrent disease.

Other endocrine tumours of the pancreas

Other endocrine tumours of the pancreas (Table 9.7) include vasoactive intestinal peptide (VIP)-oma,

---

Table 9.4 Insulinoma syndrome

- Incidence 1:1 000 000
- 90% Benign
    10% Multiple – microadenomas
    10% MEN-1
    Pancreatic
- Nesidioblastosis
    Neonatal hypoglycaemia

Table 9.5 Insulinoma syndrome: clinical features

- Neuroglycopenic symptoms
    'Funny turns'/faints, especially after fasting
    Altered mood, behaviour, personality
    Neurological disturbance
- Autonomic symptoms
    Palpitations, tremors, sweating

Table 9.6 Insulinoma syndrome: biochemical diagnosis

- 3 × 15-hour fast or single 72-hour fast
    Hypoglycaemia: glucose <2.5 mmol/l
    Suppressed ketones (hydroxybutyrate)
    Elevated insulin and C-peptide ± proinsulin
- Negative sulphonylurea screen

Table 9.7 Other functioning tumour syndromes

- Glucagonoma
    Incidence 1:20 000 000
    Invariably pancreatic
    75% Malignant
- VIP-oma (Verner–Morrison syndrome)
    Incidence 1:10 000 000
    10% Extrapancreatic – neural crest tissue
    (usually children)
    50% Malignant
- Somatostatinoma
    Incidence 1: 40 000 000
    50% Pancreatic – 90% malignant
    50% Duodenal – 50% malignant (NF 1)

Table 9.8 **VIP-oma syndrome**

- Secretory diarrhoea
  Usually >3 l/day
  Severe dehydration and weakness
- Hypokalaemic acidosis
  Stool loss – may also cause hypomagnesaemia
- Hypochlorhydria 50%
  Inhibition of gastric acid
- Hypercalcaemia 50%
  ? PTHrP
- Glucose intolerance 50%
  Glucagon-like action
- Flushing 20%

Table 9.9 **VIP-oma syndrome: diagnosis**

- Elevated VIP
  Usually 60 pmol/l
- Associated increase in circulating PHM
NB Other causes of elevated VIP
      Bowel ischaemia
      Hepatic cirrhosis
      Renal impairment

Table 9.10 **Glucagonoma syndrome**

- Necrolytic migratory erythema
  Mucous membrane involvement
- Impaired glucose tolerance 90%
- Weight loss 90%
- Normochromatic normocytic anaemia
- Depression (5%) and mental slowness
- Severe venous thrombosis 15%
- Bowel disturbance

Table 9.11 **Glucangonoma syndrome: diagnosis**

- Elevated glucagon (usually 10–20-fold)
- Decreased amino acid levels
- Impaired glucose tolerance
- Coagulation abnormalities
NB Other causes of elevated glucagon
      Hepatic or renal failure
      Oral contraceptive pill, danazol
      Stress
      Prolonged fast
      Familial

Table 9.12 **Somatostatinoma syndrome**

- Impaired carbohydrate metabolism
  Hyperglycaemia – 90% pancreatic tumours
  Hypoglycaemia – rare
- Steatorrhoea (90%)
- Gallbladder disease (90% pancreatic, 40% duodenal)
- Duodenal tumours
  Local symptoms: obstruction, haemorrhage

glucagonoma, somatostatinoma and non-functioning islet cell tumour or pancreatic polypeptide (PP)-oma. Other hormones produced by functional pancreatic endocrine tumours include growth hormone releasing factor (GRF), adrenocorticotropic hormone (ACTH), parathyroid hormone (PTH) and neurotensin. These tumours have a combined incidence of less than 0.2 per million. They behave in a similar fashion to gastrinoma and they are usually malignant.[26] VIP-omas are associated with watery diarrhoea, hypokalaemia, hypochlorhydria and acidosis (WDHHA syndrome or Vernal–Morrison syndrome (Table 9.8). Tumours are usually confined to the pancreas, but may be found in the lung or sympathetic ganglia (Table 9.9).[34] Glucagonomas may present with a characteristic rash (necrolytic migratory erythema), diabetes, weight loss and venous thrombosis (Tables 9.10 and 9.11). Somatostatinomas may present with diarrhoea, malabsorbtion, gallstones and diabetes (Table 9.12). Somatostatinomas may also occur in the duodenum and present with symptoms related to location such as jaundice, pancreatitis or bleeding. Pancreatic polypeptide has no known biological function and so symptoms are usually due to mass effect and include abdominal pain, biliary obstruction and gastrointestinal bleeding. Tumours should be managed by surgical resection.

Hepatic metastases

Diagnosis

Clinical features
Neuroendocrine hepatic metastases may be diagnosed preoperatively following investigation and diagnosis of a specific neuroendocrine hormonal syndrome. Patients may also be diagnosed following the incidental finding of hepatomegaly or an abdominal mass. Liver metastases may be discovered at laparotomy following the acute presentation of carcinoid disease. Up to 45% of patients with

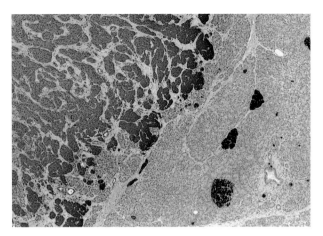

Figure 9.13 Photomicrograph of a pancreatic insulinoma stained using antibodies for insulin.

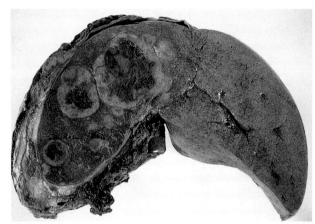

Figure 9.14 Macroscopic view of a post-mortem specimen of liver from a patient who died from the carcinoid syndrome.

Table 9.13 **Carcinoid tumours**

• Incidence 1:150 000
• Derived from embryonic gut
    Foregut: 5-hydroxytryptamine-producing,
        argyrophilic
    Midgut: serotonin-producing, argentaffin-positive
    Hindgut: non-secreting, non-staining
• Carcinoid syndrome
    10% of cases
    Almost invariably metastasized
    Usually small bowel
    Aetiology: serotonin, histamine, bradykinin,
        substance P

Table 9.14 **Carcinoid syndrome**

• Flushing 95%
    Site-specific flush – ? different mediators
    Carcinoid crises
• GI manifestations
    Secretory diarrhoea
    Cachexia
• Endocardial fibrosis 50%
    Tricuspid incompetence 50%
    Pulmonary valve lesions 50%
• Respiratory complications
    Bronchospasm
    Pleural fibrosis
• Pellagra 10%
• Arthropathy, myopathy

abdominal carcinoid will present with bowel obstruction and between 50 and 65% of patients are found to have liver metastases at the time of diagnosis (Fig. 9.13; Table 9.13).[35]

Carcinoid syndrome occurs when 5-hydroxytryptamine and other hormonal products are secreted directly into the systemic circulation. The carcinoid syndrome is therefore usually only seen in patients with liver metastases. Common symptoms and signs typically include cutaneous flushing (80%) (Fig. 9.14), diarrhoea (76%), hepatomegaly (71%), carcinoid heart disease (41–70%) and asthma (25%);[36–39] the cause of the different features of the carcinoid syndrome is not fully understood (Table 9.14). Serotonin may be responsible for the diarrhoea whereas tachykinins such as neuropeptide K may be involved in the symptoms of flushing. Carcinoid heart disease with pulmonary stenosis and tricuspid regurgitation may also be due to excess hormone

production. Levels of both 5-hydroxyindoleactic acid (5-HIAA) and neuropeptide K are higher in patients with carcinoid heart disease and the increased fibrosis seen in the heart is thought to be due to increased expression of transforming growth factor (TGF)-B.[39]

The features of this syndrome are well known; however, a diagnosis of carcinoid disease is rarely made preoperatively. Typically, the development of flushing and diarrhoea is preceded by a long history of vague abdominal pain.[40] Many patients have been diagnosed as having irritable bowel syndrome, peptic ulcer disease or Crohn's disease. Flushing attacks are usually confined to the face and chest. They may occur spontaneously or may follow a specific stimulus such as drinking alcohol or eating a particular food. Eventually patients may develop a permanent flush across the face which may vary from mild telangectasia to a deep cyanotic discoloration. Cardiac manifestations of carcinoid syndrome may be detected by echocardiography in 60 to 70% of patients.[39] The three most common abnormalities are pulmonary stenosis, tricuspid regurgitation and tricuspid stenosis.

The carcinoid syndrome may occur in up to one-third of patients with gastric carcinoid, although this is generally of an atypical type with a bright red severe flush, cutaneous oedema, lacrimation and bronchoconstriction. Diarrhoea is episodic and may be associated with abdominal pain and urgency; nocturnal diarrhoea is unusual. This syndrome is related to histamine secretion and urinary estimates of the histamine metabolite MeImAA may serve as a useful tumour marker. 5-HIAA is also often excreted, although this is less so than for midgut carcinoids.

Carcinoid crisis may be precipitated by anaesthesia or by surgical procedures in patients with carcinoid tumours. This occurs when large amounts of hormonal products are suddenly released into the systemic circulation. Clinical features include hypotension, tachyarrhythmias, bronchospasm and CNS abnormalities. Carcinoid crisis is treated by the intravenous administration of somatostatin (50–100 μg). Further boluses may be given or a somatostatin infusion set up as required.

Laboratory investigations

Blood
Following a suspected diagnosis of neuroendocrine liver metastases, radioimmunoassays may be performed in order to search for the products of specific pancreatic endocrine tumours. Otherwise, there are no blood tests diagnostic of hepatic metastases, although plasma alkaline phosphatase and gamma glutamyl transferase may be elevated in the presence of advanced disease. The plasma concentration of chromogranin A is a non-specific marker for neuroendocrine tumours, but this test is not in widespread clinical use.[41,42]

Urine
The 24-hour urinary excretion of the serotonin metabolite 5-HIAA is the most valuable biochemical screening test for the presence of metastatic carcinoid tumours. The level is usually calculated as the mean value of two 24-hour urine collections. Elevated levels are typical of metastases of small bowel origin. Gastric carcinoid tumours may have relatively small amounts of 5-HIAA in the urine but a marked excess of 5-HTP. This is thought to be due to a lack of aromatic amino acid decarboxylase. In addition, urinary estimates of the histamine metabolite MeImAA may serve as a useful marker for metastases secondary to gastric carcinoid tumours.

Pathology
Neuroendocrine tumours are characterized by uniform round cell nuclei and regular growth patterns (Fig. 9.15). A number of distinct histological growth patterns have been described (insular, trabecular, glandular, mixed and undifferentiated) and it has been suggested that morphology may influence survival.[43–45] Tumours are further classified on the basis of silver staining. Neoplasms that can directly deposit soluble silver salts are termed argentaffin positive. Tumours requiring an exogenous reducing agent for silver salt deposition are classified as argyrophil positive. Argyrophil staining by the Grimelius method is a general marker for neuroendocrine differentiation. Carcinoids of midgut origin also show an argentaffin reaction, reflecting the presence of serotonin.

Immunohistochemistry is now commonly used for the diagnosis of neuroendocrine tumours. Tumours are classified according to their expression of neuroendocrine markers. These markers are divided into cytosolic markers (neurone specific enolase), small vesicle associated markers (synaptophysin) and secretory granule associated markers (chromogranins). Cell specific or secretory neuroendocrine products are peptides or amines that normally act as hormones or neurotransmitters. However, elevated levels are usually responsible for the systemic symptoms or syndromes associated with neuroendocrine tumours.

Historically, gastrointestinal carcinoid tumours were classified according to their embryonic origin into foregut, midgut and hindgut tumours, the embryological foregut including respiratory tract and thymus. Foregut carcinoids were described as producing low levels of serotonin and sometimes secreting 5-hydroxytryptophan (5-HTP) or adrenocorticotrophic hormone (ACTH). Midgut carcinoids

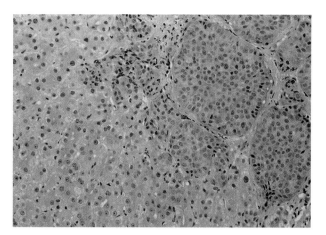

Figure 9.15 H&E stained micrograph of a surgically resected hepatic carcinoid metastasis.

were described as having high serotonin production, whereas hindgut carcinoids were hardly ever found to secrete serotonin, 5-HT or ACTH. Later, a new classification of neuroendocrine tumours was proposed whereby tumours are distinguished according to their site of origin.[6] Thus tumours of the stomach, duodenum, jejunum–ileum, appendix, colon and rectum are considered separately. The second principle is to subdivide neoplasms into (I) tumours with benign behaviour, (II) tumours with uncertain behaviour, (III) tumours with low-grade malignant behaviour and (IV) high-grade malignant tumours exhibiting angioinvasion, invasion of neighbouring structures or the presence of metastases. Tumour size has also been established as a reliable prognostic indicator for a number of tumours. The third principle is to incorporate hormonal function. Tumours causing an endocrine syndrome are designated as 'functioning', whereas those without a hormonal syndrome are called 'nonfunctioning'. The classic endocrine tumours of the pancreas are not included in this classification of neuroendocrine tumours. Insulinomas and glucagonomas arise from the islets of Langerhans. From an embryological point of view, the pancreatic islets are not part of the diffuse neuroendocrine system. They first occur as a separate islet organ and are later included in the pancreas as disseminated, minute endocrine glands. In contrast, gastrinomas and somatostatinomas, which may occur in the duodenal wall, are included.

Diagnostic imaging

Radiology

Ultrasound, CT and MRI are all used in the diagnosis of neuroendocrine hepatic metastases. Relatively few studies have compared the sensitivity of these techniques. In one study from Sweden, 84 patients with neuroendocrine tumours were identified. Seven patients had single liver metastases, 44 patients had multiple metastases. Ultrasound and CT showed similar sensitivities of 57% and 53%, respectively.[46] A study by the National Institutes of Health (NIH) prospectively evaluated 80 consecutive patients with ZES. In 24 patients with histologically proven liver metastases, the sensitivities for the detection of metastatic liver lesions were 46% for US, 42% for CT and 71% for MRI (Fig. 9.16).[47]

There has been some controversy regarding the optimal CT technique for the evaluation of neuroendocrine hepatic metastases. In contrast to colonic carcinoma metastases, neuroendocrine metastases are often hypervascular relative to the background hepatic parenchyma (see Fig. 9.5). It has been suggested that the administration of intravenous contrast may render metastases isoattenuating or

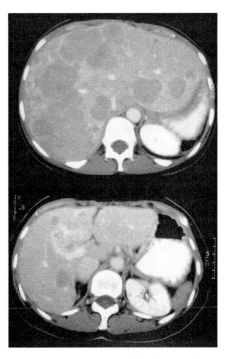

Figure 9.16 CT scan of the liver of a patient with carcinoid syndrome showing widespread multiple bilobar tumours clearly not suitable for any surgical intervention.

hyperattenuating when compared to the background liver. This may obscure metastases and complicate the assessment of tumour size. Some authors have therefore recommended the use of non-contrast enhanced CT for the evaluation of patients with suspected neuroendocrine metastases.[48] With the development of spiral CT, it is now possible to image the liver twice following the administration of intravenous contrast, once during the early hepatic arterial dominant phase (HAP) and again during the portal venous dominant phase (PVP) of enhancement. Paulson et al.[49] have evaluated triple phase spiral CT in 31 patients with proven neuroendocrine

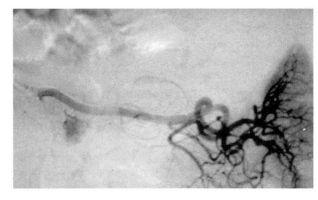

Figure 9.17 Visceral angiogram (splenic artery injection) showing a tumour 'blush' in the pancreas at the site of a primary insulinoma.

liver metastases. In this study, each phase identified metastatic lesions that were not seen in the other images. The HAP images showed more lesions than either the non-contrast or PVP images and in two patients lesions were only seen on the HAP images. The authors therefore recommend triple phase spiral CT for the evaluation of patients with suspected neuroendocrine hepatic metastases. Visceral angiography may also be useful in the localization of pancreatic tumours (Fig. 9.17).

Radionuclear investigations

Somatostatin receptor scintography
Neuroendocrine tumours have a high density of somatostatin receptors.[50] Somatostatin is a 14 amino acid peptide that acts as both a hormone and a neurotransmitter. Its main physiological role is to inhibit the release of growth hormone. Somatostatin was first isolated from hypothalamic extracts and shown to inhibit the release of growth hormone.[51] However, somatostatin has also been shown to inhibit the release of other anterior pituitary hormones, including adrenocorticotropic hormone (ACTH), prolactin and thyroid stimulating hormone (TSH). Somatostatin also inhibits the release of a number of gastrointestinal peptides including insulin, glucagon, gastrin motilin, gastric inhibitory peptide (GIP), vasoactive intestinal peptide (VIP), secretin, cholecystokinin and gastrin releasing peptide (GRP). GRP stimulates proliferation of normal and malignant intestinal epithelium. Somatostatin may also inhibit epidermal growth factor (EGF) induced cell proliferation. Somatostatin analogues have been used in the treatment of neuroendocrine tumours. Antiproliferative effects may be mediated by a number of different mechanisms including the inhibition of regulatory peptide release and the direct antagonism of growth factor effects on tumour cells.[52] Somatostatin has an extremely short half-life and this has limited its therapeutic applications. Octreotide is a somatostatin analogue with a much longer half-life, now used for the treatment of patients with metastatic neuroendocrine tumours. Radiolabelling of octreotide has allowed the development of somatostatin receptor scintography (SRS). Initially octreotide was labelled with ^{123}I and the first localization of a neuroendocrine tumour by this technique was reported by Krenning et al. in 1989.[53] Although initial results were encouraging, there were a number of problems with ^{123}I-labelled octreotide including cost and inefficient labelling. However, the main problem was the fact that this compound is rapidly cleared by the liver and excreted into the biliary system and intestines, thereby interfering with images of the abdomen and pelvis. These problems have been overcome by the introduction of

^{111}In-DTPA labelled octreotide, which has a longer half-life and is excreted by the kidneys. This Dutch group have subsequently published their experience of SRS in over 1000 patients.[54]

A number of groups have now reported their experience of SRS for the imaging of primary and metastatic neuroendocrine tumours (Fig. 9.18). Kwekkeboom et al.[55] have studied a group of 52 patients diagnosed as, or suspected of having carcinoid tumours. Accumulation of labelled octreotide was found in 86% of patients with histologically proven carcinoid tumours. However, in 27 patients (52%) accumulation of radioactivity was found at previously unsuspected sites not identified by conventional imaging techniques (Fig. 9.19). Joseph et al.[56] have reported positive findings in 81% of patients with carcinoid tumours, with additional tumour deposits identified in one-third of patients. Westlin et al.[57] detected tumour sites in 78% of

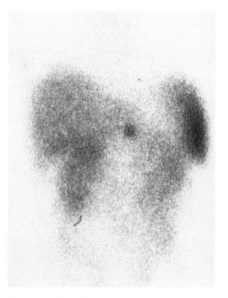

Figure 9.18 Octreotide scintogram showing uptake of radionucleotide by the same pancreatic insulinoma shown in Figure 9.17.

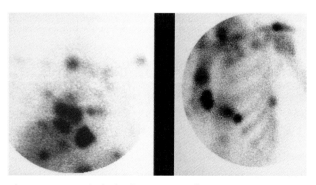

Figure 9.19 Whole-body scintography using radiolabelled octreotide to demonstrate multiple hepatic and bone carcinoid metastases.

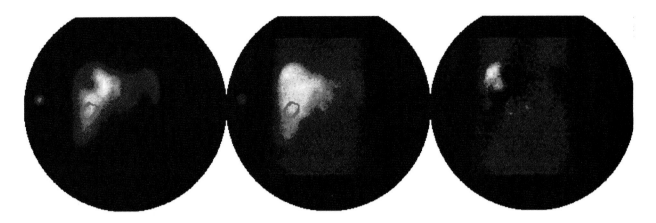

Figure 9.20 (A–C) Diagnostic hepatic scintography using ^{131}I-metaiodobenzylguanidine (MIBG) and demonstrating uptake in multiple hepatic carcinoid metastases. This patient suffered from the carcinoid syndrome and went on to be successfully relieved of her symptoms by a therapeutic course of MIBG treatment.

patients with carcinoid tumours, with additional tumour localizations in 32% of patients. In a study from the National Institute of Health, SRS was used to evaluate 80 consecutive patients presenting with ZES.[47] Primary tumours were detected in 9% of patients by ultrasound, in 31% of patients by CT, in 30% of patients by MRI and in 28% of patients by angiography. However, the sensitivity of SRS for the detection of primary tumours was 58%. Metastases were identified by ultrasound in 19% of patients, by CT in 38% of patients, by MRI in 45% of patients, by angiography in 40% of patients and by SRS in 70% of patients. In 24 patients with histologically proven liver metastases, the sensitivity of SRS for the detection of liver metastases was 92%.[47]

It seems likely that the widespread introduction of SRS will dramatically influence patient management. Ahlman et al.[58] have reported a sensitivity of 84% for octreotide scintography in 27 patients with carcinoid tumours. Tumour deposits not identified by US or CT were found in 19 patients and 8 patients underwent further surgery. Lebtahi et al. have assessed the clinical impact of SRS in 160 consecutive patients with gastrointestinal neuroendocrine tumours.[59] On the basis of conventional imaging, patients were divided into three groups according to the presence or absence of liver and/or extrahepatic metastases. Group 1 included 90 patients with no detected metastases. Group 2 included 59 patients with liver metastases but no extrahepatic metastases. Group 3 included 11 patients found to have extrahepatic metastases. Patients were then restaged following SRS. In group 1, 17 patients were found to have extrahepatic metastases, one patient was found to have extrahepatic and liver metastases and seven patients were found to have metastases confined to the liver. Six

of these seven patients were found to have only one liver metastasis and these patients were considered for liver resection. In group 2, SRS confirmed the presence of liver metastases in 56 patients, but new liver metastases were found in 5 patients and 13 patients (22%) were found to have previously undetected extrahepatic metastases. As a result, two proposed hepatic resections were cancelled and in three patients liver transplantation was cancelled. In group 3, SRS missed tumour deposits in three patients, but discovered new metastatic deposits in a further three patients. Clearly conventional imaging dramatically underestimates tumour burden and SRS is now frequently recommended as the first line imaging technique for patients with neuroendocrine tumours. However, SRS is dependent on the density and subtype of somatostatin receptors and large tumours are sometimes missed by SRS. Therefore, when patients are considered for curative surgery, SRS and conventional imaging techniques will probably remain complementary.

Metaiodobenzylguanidine (MIBG) scintography
Radiolabelled metaiodobenzylguanidine (MIBG) was initially introduced for the localization of phaeochromocytomas.[60] Since then, MIBG has been used to image a variety of endocrine tumours such as neuroblastoma, medullary thyroid cancer and paraganglioma. These tumours all arise from the neural crest and, in common with gastrointestinal neuroendocrine tumours, they share the specific amine precursor uptake and decarboxylase (APUD) pathway. MIBG is taken up by the same pathway and so may be used for imaging. Fisher et al. reported the first case of neuroendocrine hepatic metastases detected using MIBG.[61] A number of other groups have subsequently reported the use of ^{123}I-labelled MIBG for imaging.[62–64]

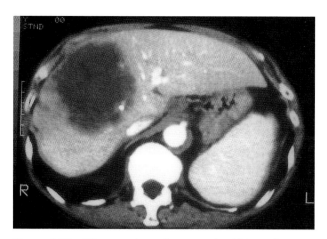

Figure 9.21 CT scan of a solitary carcinoid hepatic metastasis in a patient with carcinoid syndrome. This is suitable for surgical resection with potentially curative intent.

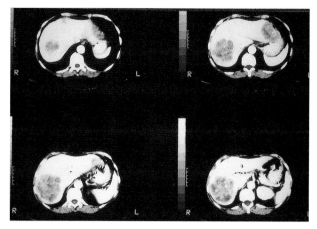

Figure 9.22 CT scan of the liver of a patient suffering from the carcinoid syndrome and showing several tumour deposits. These tumours would be suitable for surgical resection with the intention of debulking for relieving symptoms.

Few studies have compared the relative sensitivities of MIBG and somatostatin receptor scintography for the detection of neuroendocrine hepatic metastases.[65] In a review of all published series up to 1994, Hoefnagel identified a sensitivity of 86% for Octreoscan and 70% for labelled MIBG (Fig. 9.20).[66] One study from King's College Hospital, London, showed a sensitivity of 94% for Octreoscan and only 30% for MIBG. In this study, no previously occult primary sites were identified by either modality; however, two patients who had previously undergone orthoptic liver transplantation were found to have hepatic recurrence and bony metastases using Octreoscan.[67] It is likely that SRS will supersede imaging with labelled MIBG. However, in some circumstances the techniques may be complementary and imaging with MIBG may be useful in the identification of patients likely to respond to therapy with ^{131}I MIBG.[68,69]

Treatment

Liver resection

Liver resection is now considered potentially curative for selected patients with colorectal liver metastases.[70] In the majority of series, hepatic resection is performed with an operative mortality of less than 5%. Neuroendocrine hepatic metastases are generally slow growing and surgery is therefore an attractive therapeutic option. In addition, palliative resection of hepatic metastases may result in the relief of debilitating symptoms related to hormone overproduction (Fig. 9.21).

A number of early reports described the potential benefits of hepatic resection. Norton et al. reported three patients who underwent curative resection for metastatic gastrinoma.[71] Two of the three patients were alive at 22 and 32 months. Martin et al.[72] reported five patients who had undergone hepatic resection for metastatic carcinoid tumours. Three were alive with no evidence of disease at 12, 39 and 45 months. One patient developed recurrence at 19 months and one died at 31 months. In a collective series of 54 patients with hepatic resection for metastatic neuroendocrine tumours, Hughes and Sugarbaker found an operative mortality of 7% with palliation of symptoms in 33 of 36 of patients available for follow-up.[73] Survival ranged from 2 months to 10 years, with palliation lasting up to 78 months. These findings suggested that hepatic resection should be the first-line treatment for patients with operable hepatic neuroendocrine metastases.

McEntee et al. have published the Mayo Clinic experience of hepatic resection for metastatic neuroendocrine tumours.[74] Between 1970 and 1989, 37 patients underwent hepatic resection. Seventeen resections were considered curative, with no evidence of gross residual disease. In this group, 11 patients were disease-free with a median follow-up of 19 months. Two patients were alive with recurrence at 59 and 92 months. The remaining 20 resections were considered palliative (Fig. 9.22). In this group, 16 patients had symptomatic endocrinopathies and eight patients had complete relief of symptoms. However, the mean duration of response was only 6 months. The authors recommended that palliative resection should only be performed when at least 90% of the tumour bulk can be safely excised. This group subsequently published a retrospective series of 74 patients with neuroendocrine hepatic metastases undergoing resection between

1984 and 1992.[75] Twenty-eight patients underwent curative resection, whereas 46 patients had palliative or incomplete resections. The overall survival at 4 years was 74%. Median survival had not been reached with a mean follow-up of 2.2 years. The overall postoperative symptomatic response rate was 90%, with a mean duration of 19.3 months. This study did not compare survival with unresected patients. However, historical series suggest that the 5-year survival of patients with untreated carcinoid or islet cell hepatic metastases is 30 to 40%.[76,77]

Carty et al. have prospectively evaluated 42 patients presenting to the National Institute of Health with metastatic pancreatic neuroendocrine tumours.[29] Twenty-five patients were found to have inoperable disease with diffuse hepatic and distant metastases. This group had a 60% 2-year survival and a 28% 5-year survival. The remaining 17 patients were thought to have resectable disease on the basis of preoperative imaging studies. Of these, 13 patients underwent potentially curative resection; four patients were found to have unresectable disease at operation. In the 17 patients who underwent surgery, the 2-year survival was 87%, with a 5-year survival of 79%. The majority of patients subsequently developed recurrent disease. However, four patients remained disease free at 51, 39, 22 and 14 months. Thus hepatic resection appeared to offer a potential cure in selected patients and, in addition, long-term survival occurred despite the presence of recurrent disease.

Dousset et al. have published their experience of 34 patients with bilateral neuroendocrine hepatic metastases treated by either surgical resection, liver transplantation or medical management.[78] Seventeen patients underwent hepatic resection and in 12 patients resection was considered curative. Overall, the 2-year and 5-year actuarial survival rates were 87% and 46%, with disease-free survival rates of 43% and 36%. However, for patients considered to have undergone curative surgery, the 5-year survival rate was 62%, with a disease-free survival of 52%.

Chen et al. have published a further series suggesting that hepatic resection may prolong survival.[79] In this study, between 1984 and 1995, 38 patients with neuroendocrine metastases confined to the liver were assessed for hepatic resection. The survival of a group of patients with localized disease, treated by complete resection, was compared to that of a group of unresectable patients with a similar tumour burden. Twenty-three patients were found to have unresectable disease. Fifteen patients underwent curative resection. In the unresected group, the median survival was 27 months, with a 5-year actuarial survival of 29%. In the resected group, the median survival had not been reached and the 5-year actuarial survival was 73%. However, in this group, only five patients remained disease free, with a median time to recurrence of 21 months.

To date, no prospective randomized trial has compared hepatic resection to either no treatment or to best medical therapy. Given the rarity of these tumours and the long natural history of neuroendocrine hepatic metastases, definite evidence for the role of hepatic resection in these patients is only likely to come from multicentre national and international trials. However, at present, the available evidence suggests that all patients with resectable liver metastases should undergo hepatic resection.

Unfortunately, relatively few patients are likely to be suitable for hepatic resection. Carty et al.[29] and Dousset et al.[78] found, respectively, that only 40% and 35% of patients with metastatic disease were candidates for hepatic resection. Preoperative imaging dramatically underestimated tumour burden and, overall, only 30% and 35% of patients underwent curative resection. In the initial series from the Mayo Clinic,[74] only 9% of patients referred with metastatic disease were considered candidates for hepatic resection. Galland and Blumgart also found that only 2 of 30 patients with neuroendocrine hepatic metastases were suitable for resection.[80] Thus the majority of patients presenting with hepatic neuroendocrine metastases will not be suitable for hepatic resection. Alternative therapies will be required for these patients.

Hepatic artery embolization

It has long been known that primary and secondary hepatic tumours receive most of their blood supply from the hepatic artery, whereas the hepatic parenchyma is predominately supplied by the portal venous system. Hepatic metastases may therefore be treated by interruption of hepatic arterial blood supply. This was initially performed by formal hepatic artery ligation; however, hepatic artery embolization is now the method of choice. A number of embolic agents have been used including gelatin sponge, polyvinyl alcohol foam and absolute alcohol. Embolization is frequently associated with right upper quadrant pain and nausea. Most patients experience a pyrexia and transient elevation of liver enzymes. More serious complications include gallbladder ischaemia, liver abscess, acute pancreatitis, acute renal failure and carcinoid crisis. Patients are usually managed with intravenous fluids, somatostatin analogues and opiate analgesia. Some authors also recommend the use of prophylactic antibiotics. Contraindications to hepatic artery embolization include excessive tumour burden, persistently abnormal liver function and portal vein thrombosis. (Figs 9.23 and 9.24).

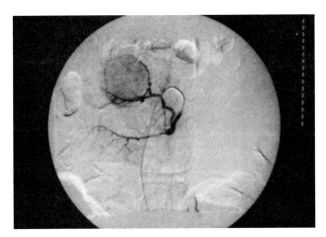

Figure 9.23 Hepatic angiogram showing a tumour 'blush' in a carcinoid metastasis prior to therapeutic embolization.

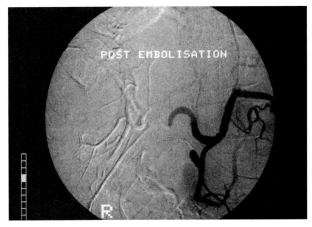

Figure 9.24 Angiogram of the same patient shown in Figure 9.23 after completion of a successful embolization.

Hepatic artery embolization was first used for the treatment of neuroendocrine metastases in 1977. Allison et al.[81] reported a series of two patients with carcinoid tumours embolized a total of four times. These patients had complete palliation of their symptoms during a follow-up of 6 months. Maton et al.[82] treated nine patients by hepatic artery embolization. They reported one death and one liver abscess. All surviving patients experienced symptomatic relief. Mean survival following embolization was 19 months. Carrasco et al.[83] treated 25 patients with hepatic carcinoid metastases by embolization. This study demonstrated an 87% symptomatic response rate and a median response duration of 11 months; however, this was associated with a 9% mortality secondary to complications of embolization. As yet there is little evidence that hepatic artery embolization improves survival. Mitty et al.[84] reported a 9-year follow-up of 18 patients treated with embolization. In this study mean survival was prolonged by 2 years compared with that of historical controls. However, Coupe et al.[85] reported a series of 63 consecutive patients from the Hammersmith Hospital, 30 of whom underwent embolization. No difference in survival was seen between these two groups of patients.

A mixture of cyanoacrylate and ethiodized oil has been used for embolization. Cyanoacrylate is a low viscosity liquid that polymerizes on contact with blood or endothelium. The use of this mixture allows peripheral, complete and permanent arterial occlusion. Winkelbauer et al. have used this technique to treat six patients with hepatic carcinoid metastases.[86] All patients achieved a complete symptomatic response and all were alive at a mean duration of 17 months following the procedure.

Chemoembolization involves the use of ethiodized oil as a carrier for various cytotoxic drugs. Hepatic arterial infusion is followed by arterial embolization. The encapsulation of drugs in microcapsules capable of slow deterioration is also of interest. In addition to vascular occlusion, encapsulation allows the slow release of cytotoxic agents in direct proximity to tumour deposits. A number of authors have reported their experience of these techniques, although it is uncertain whether there is any advantage over embolization alone.[87–89]

Hepatic cryotherapy

Cryotherapy was initially developed for the treatment of skin tumours. However, the development of modern cryotherapy delivery systems, together with the introduction of intraoperative ultrasound, has allowed the application of cryotherapy techniques for the treatment of hepatic tumours. Hepatic cryotherapy involves the delivery of liquid nitrogen to the tip of relatively thin insulated probes. Intraoperative ultrasound guides probe placement and the monitoring of ice formation during the freezing process. Cryotherapy has been widely used for the treatment of primary[90] and secondary hepatic tumours, predominately colorectal metastases.[91,92]

The first series describing the use of cryotherapy for the treatment of neuroendocrine hepatic metastases was published by Cozzi et al. in 1995.[93] A total of six patients were treated. Four patients were symptomatic and three of these patients had elevated tumour markers. All patients were alive and asymptomatic with a median follow-up of 24 months. Patients with elevated preoperative markers showed a dramatic reduction in tumour markers following treatment. In addition, all patients had a complete radiological response. This group published their experience of a total of 13 patients with neuroendocrine hepatic metastases treated by hepatic cryotherapy.[94] Twelve patients were alive with a median follow-up of 13.5 months. One patient died of bronchopneumonia 45 months following cryotherapy, but without evidence of tumour recurrence. Three patients had developed recurrent disease. One patient developed a recurrence in one of seven liver metastases and this was subsequently treated by hepatic resection 13 months following hepatic cryotherapy. This patient went on to develop a sacral recurrence of his rectal carcinoid which was also resected. Two other patients had developed recurrent liver metastases. However, the remaining nine patients were alive with no evidence of recurrent disease. Seven of these 13 patients had had symptoms related to ectopic hormone production. In all patients symptoms were significantly alleviated and postoperatively five patients were completely asymptomatic. In this series, two patients with carcinoid metastases developed a coagulopathy postoperatively and required further laparotomy together with the replacement of clotting factors.

Bilchik et al. have reported a series of 19 patients with neuroendocrine hepatic metastases treated by hepatic cryotherapy.[95] All patients were referred because of persistent endocrine related symptoms refractory to other treatments. All patients had advanced disease and cryosurgery was considered palliative as evidenced by residual liver disease, lymph node involvement, residual primary disease or unknown primary site. The median duration of symptom-free survival was 10 months. The median duration of overall survival was greater than 49 months. Recurrent symptoms following cryotherapy were effectively palliated in three patients using somatostatin and in five patients by chemotherapy. All these patients had previously been refractory to treatment.

Cryotherapy has the advantage of being able to treat bilobar disease and lesions close to major blood vessels. This treatment appears to be safe and to provide good palliation of symptoms related to ectopic hormone production. In some patients it appears that long-term disease-free survival may be obtained. However, given the long natural history of neuroendocrine tumours and the relatively short follow-up of patients treated by hepatic cryotherapy, evidence for prolonged survival is as yet unavailable.

Liver transplantation

Malignant tumours initially represented one of the main indications for orthoptic liver transplant (OLT). However, it rapidly became clear that this was associated with high rates of disease recurrence. The results of hepatic transplantation for metastatic tumours are particularly poor. The two largest series describe 2-year survival rates between 14% and 19%, with 5-year survival rates not exceeding 5%.[96,97] In contrast, patients with hepatic neuroendocrine metastases have been considered more likely to benefit from hepatic transplantation. In 1989, the Pittsburgh group reported a series of five patients with neuroendocrine hepatic metastases, three of whom were alive at 7, 16 and 34 months following surgery.[98] That same year, the group at King's College, London, reported a series of four patients with two patients alive and well 38 and 22 months following surgery.[99] Routley et al. subsequently described a series of 11 patients who had undergone OLT for neuroendocrine hepatic metastases.[100] In six patients the indication for transplantation was pain due to hepatomegaly and in five patients symptoms due to excess hormone production. All patients initially obtained complete relief of symptoms. However, six patients developed tumour recurrence at a median of 11 months. Five patients had died, four from recurrent disease and one from chronic rejection. Four patients were alive with no evidence of disease recurrence. Overall actuarial survival was 82% at 1 year and 57% at 5 years. In this study, tumour recurrence for patients with carcinoid tumours was more frequent. The reasons for this were unclear. However, it was thought that this may have reflected the fact that transplantation was carried out later in the course of the disease process in carcinoid patients or due to differential effects of immunosuppression on tumour growth.

Dousset et al.[79] reported their experience from Hôpital Cochin in Paris. They describe the results of OLT in nine cases. One patient underwent upper abdominal exenteration with liver replacement for a large pancreatic tumour. With this exception, all patients had previously undergone resection of the primary tumour. In this series, despite extensive preoperative imaging, extrahepatic tumour was found in four patients and this was resected. There were a total of five deaths related to transplant surgery. One patient died from primary nonfunction. Two patients died as a result of portal vein thrombosis and one patient died at day 7 from overwhelming septicaemia. A further patient died at 8 months from chronic rejection. Of the remaining patients, one patient died at 17 months as a result of bone and liver recurrence. Three patients were alive at 15, 24 and 62 months, but the longest survivor had developed bone and liver metastases. In some patients long-term palliation was achieved. However, clearly there was a high operative morbidity and mortality. Many patients considered for OLT will have undergone previous upper abdominal surgery or arterial embolization, adding to the technical difficulties of the procedure. The authors have recommended that transplantation should only be offered to patients with symptomatic disease that has failed to respond to all other therapies. In addition, they conclude that the finding of extra-hepatic disease at laparotomy should probably result in the abandoning of the transplant procedure.

More encouraging results have been reported from the Hanover group.[101] In this series, 12 patients underwent OLT. There was one operative death. Two patients died from tumour recurrence, one at 6 months, the other at 5 years post-transplantation. Nine patients were alive with a median survival of 55 months. Four of these patients were disease-free 2, 57, 58 and 103 months post-transplantation. All patients experienced good symptomatic relief and postoperative hormone levels were within normal ranges.

The largest series of patients undergoing liver trans-plantation for the treatment of neuroendocrine hepatic metastases comes from France. Le Treut et al. have published the results of a multicentre review including all cases of OLT for metastatic neuroendocrine tumours performed in France between 1989 and 1994.[102] The cases of Dousset et al. described above were included in this series. A total of 31 patients were treated by OLT. Six patients (19%) died following surgery. Twelve patients subsequently died; four of these deaths were due to delayed technical or other non-tumour complica-tions. All seven patients that had undergone upper abdominal exenteration died from immediate or delayed surgical complications. At the time of their publication, 13 patients were alive and in eight of these there was no evidence of recurrent disease. The overall actuarial 1- and 5-year survival was 58% and 36%, respectively. Disease-free survival was 45% and 17% at 1 and 5 years, respectively. However, the survival rate for carcinoid tumours was significantly higher with a 5-year survival rate of 69%. This reflected a lower postoperative mortal-ity for patients with carcinoid tumours and the fact that disease recurrence was more compatible with long-term survival. Overall survival figures are not dissimilar from the 25 to 35% 5-year survival reported for non-transplant treatments.[76,103,104] However, direct comparisons may be misleading, given that liver transplant is generally performed only when other therapies have become ineffective.

There is now a broad consensus regarding the indications and timing of liver transplantation for patients with neuroendocrine hepatic metastases. In general, the primary tumour should be removed before liver transplantation. This allows a full laparotomy to be performed and extrahepatic disease may be identified at this time. Patients with stable or controlled disease should be excluded.

Inevitably some patients may present later with extrahepatic disease and then no longer be candi-dates for transplantation. However, transplantation continues to be associated with high surgical mortal-ity and many patients can be maintained on medical therapy for a prolonged period of time. Finally, if extrahepatic disease is identified at the time of transplant, the procedure should probably be abandoned. Thus patients with symptomatic disease that have failed to respond to all other treatments may be considered candidates for hepatic trans-plantation. In selected patients transplantation offers good palliation and for a small proportion of patients there may be the possibility of cure.

Medical treatment

Chemotherapy

Chemotherapy has only a very limited role to play in the treatment of patients with neuroendocrine hepatic metastases. For patients with endocrine pancreatic tumours, single agent chemotherapy generally has poor response rates of between 7 and 25%. The combination of streptozotocin and doxiru-bicin has been more effective, with tumour regres-sion observed in up to 69% of patients.[105] This was often associated with sustained regression with a median duration of regression of 18 months. When the same combination of chemotherapeutic drugs was applied to patients with carcinoid tumours, response rates were generally only 10–20% with only a very brief response. All patients suffered serious and severe side effects including nausea, vomiting, neutropaenia and cardiomyopathy. Given that many patients are relatively asymptomatic and the range of alternative therapies available, chemotherapy should not generally be recom-mended for patients with metastatic carcinoid tumours.

There may be a role for chemotherapy for the treat-ment of anaplastic neuroendocrine tumours. Moertel et al. have treated 18 patients with anaplastic neuroendocrine tumours using a combination of etoposide and cisplatin. An objective tumour response was observed in 12 of 18 patients (67%). The median duration of response was 8 months. Thus, the overall regression rate was similar to that observed for small cell lung cancer, although again severe side effects were observed.[106]

Hepatic artery embolization has been combined with the administration of systemic chemotherapy. Moertel et al. found a response rate of 60% in 23 patients treated by embolization alone compared to 80% in 42 patients treated by hepatic artery embolization and sequential chemotherapy. The median duration of response with occlusion alone was 4 months, compared to 18 months with combined treatment. The median survival was 27 months with embolization compared to 49 months for patients treated with sequential chemotherapy. Although this was a non-randomized study, the results do suggest that there may be a role for chemotherapy when combined with other treatment modalities.[107]

Somatostatin analogues

The somatostatin analogue octreotide is now widely used for the treatment of patients with carcinoid syndrome. Somatostatin inhibits the release of hormones from the tumour and also directly inhibits gastric, pancreatic and intestinal secretion. Somatostatin has a half-life of approximately 2 minutes and so is not suitable for clinical use. Octreotide has a half-life of approximately 2–3 hours when given by subcutaneous injection. Octreotide has been shown to be effective in the treatment of both carcinoid diarrhoea and flushing.[108] Objective and symptomatic improvement occurs in over 70% of patients for a median duration of 12 months. Loss of therapeutic response eventually occurs and this is thought to be due to either downregulation of somatostatin receptors or the development of receptor-negative tumour clones. Doses of 50–200 µg usually allow symptomatic control, although higher doses may be required as treatment progresses. Octreotide is usually well tolerated. However, side effects do occur and these include diarrhoea, steatorrhea, flatulence, nausea, vomiting, impaired glucose tolerance and the development of gallstones. Octreotide therapy may also influence tumour growth. Evidence comes from the results of two prospective studies.[109,110] In the first ot these, 34 patients with carcinoid and pancreatic neuroendocrine metastases were shown to have progressive disease on the basis of CT scan. All patients were treated with octreotide. No objective tumour regression was observed. However, following repeat CT scans, 50% of patients were found to have stable disease. The median duration of response was only 5 months.[110] In a further study, 52 patients with progressive diseases were similarly treated with octreotide.[111] Again no objective tumour regression was observed. However, 36% of patients showed stabilization of disease with a median duration of response of 18 months.

One of the main disadvantages of octreotide is the need for frequent subcutaneous injections. New long acting preparations are now available and are clinically effective.[112] Lanreotide is a recently developed somatostatin analogue which also has a slow release formulation. It is administered as an intramuscular injection every 2 weeks. Lanreotide has been shown to be as effective as octreotide in controlling symptoms and it may also have some antitumour activity.[113–115]

Interferon

Interferon was first used for the treatment of patients with neuroendocrine metastases in 1982. The mechanism of action of interferon is thought to involve cell cycle blocking in G0 and G1 phase, induction of 2′-5′-A-synthetase and a reduction of mRNA for the synthesis of hormones and growth factors. In addition, alpha-interferon induces increased MHC class I expression of tumour cells together with a generalized upregulation of the immune system. The majority of experience comes from the endocrine oncology unit in Uppsala, Sweden.[115] This group have treated over 350 patients with alpha-interferon. Of 111 patients with carcinoid tumours, a biochemical response was noted in 42% of patients, tumour size was reduced in 15% of patients and stabilization of tumour growth was seen in 39% of patients. The median duration of response was 34 months. Of 47 patients with metastatic endocrine pancreatic tumours, 51% of patients showed a biochemical response, 12% showed tumour reduction and disease stabilization was observed in 24.5% of patients. The median duration of response was 20 months. The main side effects of interferon are flu-like symptoms such as myalgia, fever and fatigue.

Receptor targeted therapy

The uptake of ^{111}In-labelled octreotide and ^{123}I-labelled MIBG for scintographic scanning has led to the development of receptor targeted therapy. Carcinoid tumours have shown a biochemical response and reduction in size following treatment with repeated high dose ^{111}In-octreotide.[116] Similar results have been achieved with ^{123}I MIBG.[68,69,117] The choice of agent may be guided by uptake at diagnostic imaging. These therapies appear highly specific, are tolerated with minimal side effects and patients are able to undergo repeated treatments, followed by further scanning. The development of these therapies is likely to hold significant promise for the treatment of patients with disseminated neuroendocrine metastases.[118]

Summary

There are an increasing number of diagnostic procedures and therapeutic options available for the management of patients with neuroendocrine metastases. At present, all patients should be considered for liver resection. However, only a relatively small proportion of patients will be suitable for resectional surgery. Hepatic arterial embolization or hepatic cryotherapy should then be considered. Liver transplant should be considered for patients with progressive symptomatic disease confined to the liver when all other treatment options have failed.

Accurate staging is of critical importance when considering patients for any form of surgical intervention. Octreotide receptor scintography is therefore likely to have a major impact on the management of these patients. For patients with disseminated disease, chemotherapy has relatively little role to play. Symptomatic patients may benefit from octreotide therapy; however, receptor targeted therapies are likely to hold promise for the future.

Patients with neuroendocrine tumours are rare and the experience of individual centres is therefore limited. Randomized trials will be required to define more clearly the role of each of the above treatment modalities and the role of multimodality therapies. Given the long natural history of the disease, such trials are likely to require large numbers of patients. Optimum therapy will require a multidisciplinary team approach involving a physician, an oncologist, an interventional radiologist, a nuclear medicine physician and a surgeon. All patients with neuroendocrine metastases should therefore be cared for in centres of expertise and every effort should be made to enter patients into nationally or internationally co-ordinated clinical trials.

Key points

- Diagnostic imaging includes:
  Ultrasound
  CT (± arterio portography)
  MRI
  Radiolabelled octreotide scintography
  MIBG scintography.
- Surgical strategies include:
  Resection
  In situ ablation
  Liver transplantation.
- Non-surgical strategies include:
  Hepatic arterial embolization
  Symptom control with octreotide
  Therapeutic radionucleotide-MIBG ablation
  Therapeutic radionucleotide-octreotide ablation.
- Non-proven or therapies of little benefit:
  Hepatic artery surgical ligation
  Cytotoxic chemotherapy
  Interferon.

REFERENCES

1. Ranson WB. A case of primary carcinoma of the ileum. Lancet 1890; 2: 1020

2. Thorson A, Bjork G, Bjorkman G, Waldenstrom J. Malignant carcinoid of the small intestine with metastases to the liver, valvular heart disease of the right heart (pulmonary stenosis and tricuspid regurgitation without septal defect), peripheral vasomotor symptoms, bronchoconstriction and an unusual type of cyanosis. Am Heart J 1954; 47: 795

3. Rindi G, Bordi C, Rappel S et al. Gastric carcinoids and neuroendocrine carcinomas: pathogenesis, pathology and behaviour. World J Surg 1996; 20: 168–72

4. Gough DB, Thompson GB, Crotty TB et al. Diverse clinical and pathological features of gastric carcinoid and the relevance of hypergastrinaemia. World J Surg 1994; 18: 473

5. Rindi G, Luinetti O, Cornaggia M et al. Three subtypes of gastric argyrophil carcinoid and the gastric neuroendocrine carcinoma: a clinicopathological study. Gastroenterology 1993; 104: 994

6. Kloppel G, Heitz PU, Capella C, Solcia E. Pathology and nomenclature of human gastrointestinal neuroendocrine (carcinoid) tumours and related lesions. World J Surg 1996; 20: 132–41

7. Akerstrom G. Management of carcinoid tumours of the stomach, duodenum and pancreas. World J Surg 1996; 20: 173–82

8. Thompson GB, Van Heerden JA, Martin JK et al. Carcinoid tumours of the gastrointestinal tract: presentation, management and prognosis. Surgery 1985; 98: 1054–63

9. Mir Madjlesi SH, Winkleman EI, Davis GA et al. Carcinoid tumours of the terminal ileum simulating Crohn's disease. Cleve Clin J Med 1988; 55: 527–62

10. Memon MA, Nelson H. Gastrointestinal carcinoid tumours. Current management strategies. Dis Colon Rectum 1997; 40: 1101–18

11. Eller R, Frazee R, Roberts J. Gastrointestinal carcinoid tumours. Am Surg 1991; 57: 434–7

12. Srodel WE, Talpos G, Eckhauser F, Thompson N. Surgical therapy for small bowel carcinoid tumours. Arch Surg 1993; 118: 143–54

13. Godwin JD. Carcinoid tumours: an analysis of 2837 cases. Cancer 1975; 36: 560

14. Moertel CG, Weiland LH, Nagourney DM, Dockerty MB. Carcinoid tumour of the appendix: treatment and prognosis. N Engl J Med 1987; 317: 1699–701

15. Bowman GA, Rosenthal D. Carcinoid tumours of the appendix. Am J Surg 1983; 146: 145–53

16. Anderson JR, Wilson BG. Carcinoid tumours of the appendix. Br J Surg 1985; 72: 545–6

17. Syracruce DC, Perzin KH, Price JB et al. Carcinoid tumours of the appendix: mesoappendiceal extension and nodal metastases. Ann Surg 1979; 190: 28–63

18. Thirlby RC, Kasper CS, Jones RC. Metastatic carcinoid tumour of the appendix: report of a case and review of the literature. Dis Colon Rectum 1984; 27: 42–6

19. MacGillivray D, Heaton KB, Rushin JM, Cruess DF. Distant metastases from a carcinoid tumour of the appendix less than 1cm in size. Surgery 1992; 111: 466

20. Ballantyne GH, Savoca PE, Flannery JT et al. Incidence and mortality of carcinoids of the colon: data from the Connecticut tumor registry. Cancer 1992; 69: 2400

21. Disario JA, Burt RW, Kendrick ML et al. Colorectal cancers of rare histological types compared with adenocarcinomas. Dis Colon Rectum 1994; 37: 1277

22. Spread C, Berkel H, Jewell L et al. Colon carcinoid tumours: a population based study. Dis Colon Rectum 1994; 37: 482–91

23. Rosenberg JM, Welch JP. Carcinoid tumours of the colon: a study of 72 patients. Am J Surg 1985; 149: 775–9

24. Caldarola VT, Jackman RJ, Moertel CG, Dockerty MB. Carcinoid tumours of the rectum. Am J Surg 1964; 107: 844–9

25. Naunheim KS, Zeitals J, Kaplan EL et al. Rectal carcinoid tumours – treatment and prognosis. Surgery 1983; 94: 670–6

26. Peplinski GR, Norton JA. Gastrointestinal endocrine cancers and nodal metastases: biological significance and therapeutic implications. Surg Oncol Clin North Am 1996; 5: 159–71

27. Zollinger RM, Ellison EC, Fabri PJ et al. Primary peptic ulceration of the jejunum, associated with islet cell tumours. Twenty five year appraisal. Ann Surg 1980; 192: 520–30

28. Norton JA. Neuroendocrine tumours of the pancreas and duodenum. Curr Probl Surg 1994; 31: 77–164

29. Carty S, Jensen RT, Norton JA. Prospective study of aggressive resection of metastatic pancreatic endocrine tumours. Surgery 1992; 112: 1024–31

30. Fraker DL, Norton JA, Alexander HR et al. Surgery in Zollinger–Ellison syndrome alters the natural history of gastrinoma. Ann Surg 1994; 220: 320

31. Norton JA, Sugarbaker PH, Doppman JL et al. Aggressive resection of metastatic disease in selected patients with malignant gastrinoma. Ann Surg 1986; 203: 352

32. Service FJ, McMahon MM, O'Brien PC, Ballard DJ. Functioning insulinoma–incidence, recurrence and long term survival of patients: a 60-year study. Mayo Clin Proc 1991; 66: 711–9

33. Dranoth DN, Gorden P, Brennan MF. Metastatic insulin secreting carcinoma of the pancreas. Clinical course and the role of surgery. Surgery 1984; 96: 1027

34. Long RG, Bryant MG, Mitchell SJ et al. Clinicopathological study of pancreatic and ganglio-neuroblastoma tumours secreting vasoactive intestinal polypeptide (VIPomas). Br Med J 1981; 282: 1767

35. Buchanan KD, Johnston CF, O'Hare MMT et al. Neuroendocrine tumours: a European view. Am J Med 1986; 81 (Suppl 6B): 14–22

36. Grahame Smith DG. The carcinoid syndrome. Am J Cardiol 1968; 21: 376–87

37. Feldman JM. Carcinoid tumours and the carcinoid syndrome. Curr Probl Surg 1989; 26: 335–85

38. Tilson MD. Carcinoid syndrome. Surg Clin North Am 1974; 54: 409–23

39. Lundin L. Carcinoid heart disease: a cardiologist's viewpoint. Acta Oncol 1991; 30: 499–502

40. Vinik AI, Thompson N, Eckhauser E, Moattari AR. Clinical features of carcinoid disease and the use of somatostatin analogue in its management. Acta Oncol 1989; 28: 389

41. O'Connor DT, Deftos LJ. Secretion of chromogranin A by peptide producing endocrine neoplasms. N Engl J Med 1986; 314: 1145–51

42. Stridsberg M, Oberg K, Li Q et al. Measurements of chromogranin A, chromogranin B (secretogranin 1), chromogranin C (secretogranin II) and pancreastatin in plasma and urine from patients with carcinoid tumours and endocrine pancreatic tumours. J Endocrinol 1995; 144: 49–59

43. Soga J, Tazawa K. Pathologic analysis of carcinoids: histologic re-evaluation of 62 cases. Cancer 1971; 28: 990–8

44. Martin ED, Potet F. Pathology of endocrine tumours of the GI tract. Clin Gastroenterol 1974; 3: 511–32

45. Johnson LA, Lavin P, Moertal CG, Weiland L, Dayal Y. Carcinoids: the association of histologic growth pattern and survival. Cancer 1983; 51: 882

46. Eriksson B, Arnberg H, Lindgren PG et al. Neuroendocrine pancreatic tumours: clinical presentation, biochemical and histopathological findings in 84 patients. J Intern Med 1990; 228: 103–13

47. Gibril F, Reynolds JC, Doppman JL et al. Somatostatin receptor scintography: its sensitivity compared with that of other imaging methods in detecting primary and metastatic gastrinomas. A prospective study. Ann Intern Med 1996; 125: 26–34

48. Breeler EL, Alpern MB, Glazer GM et al. Hypervascular hepatic metastases: CT evaluation. Radiology 1987; 162: 49–51

49. Paulson EK, Mcdermott VG, Keogan MT et al. Carcinoid metastases to the liver: role of triple phase helical CT. Radiology 1998; 206: 143–50

50. Reubi JC, Hacki WH, Lamberts SWJ. Hormone producing gastrointestinal tumours contain a high density of somatostatin receptors. J Clin Endocrinol Metab 1987; 65: 1127

51. Brazeau P, Vale W, Burges R et al. Hypothalamic polypeptide that inhibits the secretion of immunoreactive pituitary growth hormone. Science 1973; 179: 77–9

52. Lamberts WJ, Krenning EP, Reubi JC et al. The role of somatostatin and its analogues in the diagnosis and treatment of tumours. Endocr Rev 1991; 12: 450–82

53. Krenning EP, Bakker WH, Breemon WAP et al. Localisation of endocrine related tumours with radio iodinated analogue of somatostatin. Lancet 1989; 1: 242–4

54. Krenning EP, Kwekkeboom DJ, Bakker WH et al. Somatostatin receptor scintography with (^{111}IN-DTPA-D-Phe) and (^{123}I-Try3)-octreotide: the Rotterdam experience

with more than 1000 patients. Eur J Nucl Med 1993; 20: 716–31

55. Kwekkeboom DJ, Krenning EP. Somatostatin receptor scintography in patients with carcinoid tumours. World J Surg 1996; 20: 157–61

56. Joseph K, Stapp J, Reinecke J et al. Receptor scintography with ^{111}In-pentreotide for endocrine gastroenteropancreatic tumours. Horm Metab Res 1993; 27 (Suppl): 28

57. Westlin JE, Janson ET, Arnberg H et al. Somatostatin receptor scintography of carcinoid tumours using the (^{111}In-DTPA-D-Phe)10-octreotide. Acta Oncol 1993; 32: 783

58. Ahlman H, Tisell LE, Wanberg B et al. Somatostatin receptor imaging in patients with neuroendocrine tumours: preoperative and postoperative scintography and intraoperative use of a scintillation detector. Semin Oncol 1994; 21 (Suppl 13): 21

59. Lebtahi R, Cadiot G, Sarda L et al. Clinical impact of somatostatin receptor scintography in the management of patients with neuroendocrine gastroenteropancreatic tumours. J Nucl Med 1997; 38: 853–8

60. Sisson JC, Frager MS, Valk TW et al. Scintographic localization of phaeochromocytoma. N Engl J Med 1981; 305: 12–7

61. Fischer M, Kamanabroo D, Sonderkamp H et al. Scintigraphic imaging of carcinoid tumours with ^{131}I-metaiodobenzylguanidine. Lancet 1984; 2: 165

62. Bomanji J, Levision DA, Zuzarte J et al. Imaging of carcinoid tumours with I-123-metaiodobenzylguanidine. J Nucl Med 1987; 28: 1907

63. Hanson MW, Feldman JM, Blinder EL et al. Carcinoid tumours: iodine-131-MIBG scintography. Radiology 1989; 172: 699

64. Wantabe N, Seto H, Ishiki M et al. I-123 MIBG imaging of metastatic carcinoid tumour from the rectum. Clin Nucl Med 1995; 20: 357–60

65. Bomanji J, Mather S, Moyes J et al. A scintographic comparison of iodine-123-metaiodobenzylguanidine and an iodine labeled somatostatin analog (Tyr-3-octreotide) in metastatic carcinoid tumours. J Nucl Med 1992; 33: 1121–4

66. Hoefnagel CA. Metaiodobenzylguanidine and somatostatin in oncology: role in the management of neural crest tumours. Eur J Nucl Med 1994; 21: 561–81

67. Ramage JK, Williams R, Buxton-Thomas M. Imaging secondary neuroendocrine tumours of the liver: comparison of I[123] metaiodobenzyle guanidine (MIBG) and In[111]-labelled octreotide (Octreoscan). Q J Med 1996; 89: 538–42

68. Hoefnagel CA, Den Hartog Jager FCA, Van Gennip AH et al. Diagnosis and treatment of a carcinoid tumour using 131-I-meta-iodobenzylguanidine. Clin Nucl Med 1986; 11: 150

69. Prvulovich EM, Stein RC, Bomanji JB et al. Iodine-131-MIBG therapy of a patient with carcinoid liver metastases. J Nucl Med 1998; 39: 1743–5

70. Hughes KS, Simon R, Songhorabodi S et al. Resection of the liver for colorectal carcinoma metastases: a multi-institutional study of patterns of recurrence. Surgery 1986; 100: 278–84

71. Norton JA, Doppman JL, Gardner JD et al. Aggressive resection of metastatic disease in selected patients with malignant gastrinoma. Ann Surg 1986; 203: 352–9

72. Martin JK, Moertel CG, Adson MA, Schutt AJ. Surgical treatment of functioning metastatic carcinoid tumours. Arch Surg 1983; 118: 537–43

73. Hughes KS, Sugarbaker PH. Resection of the liver for metastatic solid tumours. In: Rosenberg SA, ed. Surgical treatment of metastatic cancer. Philadelphia: JB Lippincott, 1987: 125–64

74. McEntee GP, Nagorney DM, Kvols LK et al. Cytoreductive hepatic surgery for neuroendocrine tumours. Surgery 1990; 108: 1091–6

75. Que FG, Nagorney DM, Batts KP et al. Hepatic resection for metastatic neuroendocrine carcinomas. Am J Surg 1995; 169: 36–43

76. Moertel CG. An odyssey in the land of small tumours. J Clin Oncol 1987; 5: 1053–522

77. Thompson GB, Van Heerden JA, Grant CS et al. Islet cell carcinomas of the pancreas: a twenty year experience. Surgery 1988; 104: 1011–7

78. Dousset B, Saint-Marc O, Pitre J et al. Metastatic endocrine tumours: medical treatment, surgical resection or liver transplantation. World J Surg 1996; 20: 908–15

79. Chen H, Hardacre JM, Uzar A et al. Isolated liver metastases from neuroendocrine tumours: does resection prolong survival? J Am Coll Surg 1998; 187: 88–93

80. Galland RB, Blumgart LH. Carcinoid syndrome: surgical management. Br J Hosp Med 1986; 35: 166–70

81. Allison DJ, Modlin IM, Jenkins WJ. Treatment of carcinoid liver metastases by hepatic artery embolization. Lancet 1977; 2: 1323–5

82. Maton PN, Camilleri M, Griffen et al. Role of hepatic arterial embolisation in the carcinoid syndrome. Br Med J 1983; 287: 932–5

83. Carrasco CH, Charnsangavei C, Ajani J et al. The carcinoid syndrome: palliation by hepatic artery embolization. AJR 1986; 147: 149–54

84. Mitty HA, Warner RRP, Newman LH et al. Control of carcinoid syndrome with hepatic artery embolisation. Radiology 1985; 155: 623

85. Coupe MO, Hodgson HJF, Hemingway A et al. The effect of hepatic artery embolisation on survival in the carcinoid syndrome. J Int Radiol 1989; 4: 179

86. Winkelbauer FW, Niederle B, Pietschmann F et al. Hepatic artery embolotherapy of hepatic metastases from carcinoid tumours: value of using a mixture of cyano-acrylate and ethiodized oil. AJR 1995; 165: 323–7

87. Ruszniewski P, Rougier P, Roche A et al. Hepatic arterial chemoembolization in patients with liver metastases of endocrine tumours. A prospective phase II study in 24 patients. Cancer 1993; 71: 2624–30

88. Therasse E, Breittmayer F, Roche A et al. Transcatheter chemoembolisation of progressive carcinoid liver metastases. Radiology 1993; 189: 541–7

89. Diamandidou E, Ajani JA, Yang DJ et al. Two phase study of hepatic artery vascular occlusion with micro-encapsulated cisplatin in patients with liver metastases from neuroendocrine tumours. AJR 1998; 170: 339–44

90. Zhou XD, Yu YQ, Tang ZY, Ma ZC. Clinical evaluation of cryosurgery in the treatment of primary liver cancer. Report of 60 cases. Cancer 1988; 61: 1889–92

91. Charnley RM, Doran J, Morris DL. Cryotherapy for liver metastases: a new approach. Br J Surg 1989; 76: 1040–1

92. Ravikumar TS, Steele GD. Hepatic cryosurgery. Surg Clin North Am 1989; 69: 433–9

93. Cozzi PJ, Englund R, Morris DL. Cryotherapy treatment of patients with hepatic metastases from neuroendocrine tumours. Cancer 1995; 76: 501–9

94. Seifert JK, Cozzi PJ, Morris DL. Cryotherapy for neuroendocrine liver metastases. Semin Surg Oncol 1998; 14: 175–83

95. Bilchik AJ, Saratou T, Foshag LJ et al. Cryosurgical palliation of metastatic neuroendocrine tumours resistant to conventional therapy. Surgery 1997; 1229: 1040–8

96. Penn I. Hepatic transplantation for primary and metastatic cancers of the liver. Surgery 1991; 110: 726–35

97. Pichlmayr K. Is there a place for liver grafting for malignancy? Transplant Proc 1988; 20: 478–82

98. Makowka L, Tzakis AG, Mazzaferro V et al. Transplantation of the liver for metastatic endocrine tumours of the intestine and pancreas. Surg Gynecol Obstet 1989; 168: 107

99. Arnold JC, O'Grady JG, Bird GL, Calne RY, Williams R. Liver transplantation for primary and secondary hepatic apudomas. Br J Surg 1989; 76: 248–9

100. Routley D, Ramage JK, McPeake, Tan KC, Williams K. Orthoptic liver transplant in the treatment of metastatic neuroendocrine tumours of the liver. Liver Transplant Surg 1995; 1: 118–21

101. Lang H, Oldhafer KJ, Weinman A et al. Liver transplantation for metastatic neuroendocrine tumours. Ann Surg 1997; 225: 347–54

102. Le Treut YP, Delpero JR, Dousset B et al. Results of liver transplantation in the treatment of metastatic neuroendocrine tumours: a 31 case French multicentric report. Ann Surg 1997; 225: 355–64

103. Ihse I, Persson B, Tibblin S. Neuroendocrine metastases of the liver. World J Surg 1995; 19: 76–82

104. McDermott EWM, Guduric B, Brennan MF. Prognostic variables in patients with gastrointestinal carcinoid tumours. Br J Surg 1994; 81: 1007–9

105. Moertel CG, Lefkopoulo M, Lipsitz S et al. Streptozotocin–doxorubicin, streptozotocin–fluorouracil or chlorozotocin in the treatment of advanced islet cell carcinoma. N Engl J Med 1992; 326: 519

106. Moertel CG, Kvols LK, O'Connell MJ, Rubin J. Treatment of neuroendocrine carcinomas with combined etoposide and cisplatin: evidence of major therapeutic activity in the anaplastic variants of these neoplasms. Cancer 1991; 68: 227

107. Moertel CG, Johnson CM, McKusick MA et al. The management of patients with advanced carcinoid tumours and islet cell carcinomas. Ann Intern Med 1994; 120: 302–9

108. Kvols LK, Moertel CG, O'Connel MJ et al. Treatment of the malignant carcinoid syndrome: evaluation of a long acting somatostatin analogue. N Engl J Med 1986; 315: 663

109. Saltz L, Trochanowsky G, Buckley M et al. Octreotide as an anti-neoplastic agent in the treatment of functional and non-functional neuroendocrine tumours. Cancer 1993; 72: 244–8

110. Arnold R, Neuhaus C, Benning R et al. Somatostatin analogue octreotide and inhibition of tumour growth in metastatic endocrine gastroenteropancreatic tumours. Gut 1996; 38: 430–8

111. Rubin J, Ajani J, Schirmer W et al. Octreotide acetate long acting formulation versus open-label subcutaneous octreotide acetate in malignant carcinoid syndrome. J Clin Oncol 1999; 17: 600–6

112. Ruszniewski P, Ducreux M, Chayvialle JA et al. Treatment of the carcinoid syndrome with the long acting somatostatin analogue lanreotide: a prospective study in 39 patients. Gut 1996; 39: 279–83

113. Tomassetti P, Migliori M, Gullo L et al. Slow release lanreotide treatment in endocrine gastrointestinal tumors. Am J Gastroenterol 1998; 93: 1468–71

114. Wymerga ANM Eriksson B, Salmela P et al. Efficacy and safety of prolonged-release lanreotide in patients with gastrointestinal neuroendocrine tumors and hormone related symptoms. J Clin Oncol 1999; 17: 1111–7

115. Oberg K. Neuroendocrine gastrointestinal tumours. Ann Oncol 1996; 7: 453–6

116. Krenning EP, Valkema P, Kooil PPM et al. Peptide receptor radionuclide therapy with (Indium-111-DTPA-Phe)-octreotide. J Nucl Med 1997; 38: 47

117. Taal BG, Hoefnagel CA, Olmos RA et al. Palliative effect of metaiodobenzylguanidine in metastatic carcinoid tumours. J Clin Oncol 1996; 14: 1829–38

118. Frank M, Klose KJ, Wied M et al. Combination therapy with ocreotide an α-interferon. Am J Gastroenterol 1999; 94: 1381–7

10 Diagnosis and management of haemangiomas of the liver

Enrique Moreno Gonzalez, JC Meneu Diaz and A Moreno

Introduction

The first description of the morphology of a hepatic haemangioma was made by Amboise Paré in 1570,[1] and nearly 300 years later it was fully characterized by Frerich.[2]

Haemangiomas are the most frequently found benign tumours in the liver,[3–16] and these are usually congenital.[17]

Over the last decade there has been growing interest in an understanding of the aetiological and epidemiological factors involved in the development of haemangiomas, as well as those factors which have an influence on their growth.[18] Due to progressively better knowledge of surgical techniques for resecting solid hepatic tumours, indications for surgical excision have increased, thus reducing options for conservative therapy. However, until 1963 there were only 80 reports of resection of hepatic haemangiomas in the medical literature.[6] More recently, minimally invasive surgical procedures have spurred interest in more patient acceptable types of treatment. Similarly, non-surgical techniques have gained protagonists due to their simplicity, although their effect is often short-lived combined with a high number of tumour relapses that then ensue.

Presentation

Haemangiomas are one of the most frequently observed lesions found in autopsy studies, appearing on average in 0.7% to 7.3% of cases,[19,20] with an overall average of 3.3% out of 50 000 autopsies.[21,22] In 1910, Adami[23] observed 20 cases in a total of 1400 autopsies (1.4%).

Unsuspected haemangiomas which have been identified during surgery undertaken for other conditions constitute from 0.30% to 3% of cases. However, this incidence depends on the age and sex of those groups studied. For example, Moreaux,[22] reporting on 3800 cholecystectomies found the proportion to be 0.23%. However, by the fifth decade the female/male ratio, initially 4:1, rises to 9:1.[4,11,24] If we disregard age, and consider women only, the percentage is 4%. Between 2%[22] and 10% of haemangiomas are multiple.[20]

Haemangiomas present most often between the third and sixth decade of life, with a predominance in the fourth decade. Without doubt, this condition is more frequent in women than in men (ratio 4:1–6:1),[24] and the main reason for this finding is female hormone activity, which explains the increase in size of haemangiomas seen during pregnancy.[25] Furthermore, there is a greater incidence of intratumoural haemorrhage or tumour rupture with haemorrhage in the free abdominal cavity during pregnancy, and when there is increased hormonal activity during the menstrual cycle, an increase in tumour diameter has been observed at this time.[26]

The relationship between hormonal activity and changes in the development of haemangiomas has been shown after the administration of oestrogens and progestogens.[21,27–29] This influence was observed not only on tumour growth, but also with the link to tumour relapse after surgical excision.[18,26,28] In spite of all the above, there is still a great deal of scepticism about the role of hormonal effects on morphological changes in these tumours.

Another explanation for volumetric changes in these tumours is related to changes in arterial flow and greater vascular stasis in the capillary bed of haemangiomas,[30–32] which could also be related to physiological, cyclical hormonal activity in women, or new states of greater hormonal activity such as pregnancy.[33,34] In any case, it is not scientifically proven that organs which may change vascular flow—or in which this may be altered—change diameter during these two stages in female physiology.[27,29]

Pathological anatomy: macroscopic and morphological features

Generally, haemangiomas are tumours with a red wine colouring which are elevated on the hepatic capsule. They have a shiny, smooth but irregular surface which, when large in diameter, has a lobulated appearance. Clearly delineated on the adjacent hepatic surface, from which they are separated, they are contained within their own capsule. They become depressed and reduce their size on manual compression, recovering their appearance and diameter when this pressure is removed.[30]

Haemangiomas may measure in size from a few millimetres up to several centimetres, and are generally single, less frequently multiple, and are distributed in random manner. Where multiple tumours are seen they are most often bilobar. Large haemangiomas are located most often on the right hepatic lobe, often concomitantly with others of smaller diameter in the contralateral lobe. Nevertheless, the presentation of large haemangiomas in both lobes is not exceptional.[14,35]

The definition of giant haemangioma is accepted when the tumour diameter reaches 10 cm.[36,37] Nevertheless, haemangiomas of more than 30 cm have been observed which occupy up to half the abdomen, displacing other intra-abdominal viscera towards the opposite side. The weight of these haemangiomas varies widely, with one haemangioma of 18.16 kg having been described, and frequently weighing 5 to 6 kg.[11] Even in cases of large tumours, diagnosis is, or may be, quite fortuitous.[13,38–42]

On cross-section, the tumour has a fibrous capsule and septae which produce a lobulated appearance on the cut surface. In small tumours the appearance is homogeneous and the consistency firm, with greater elasticity than the normal surrounding hepatic parenchyma. Large haemangiomas have a recognizable conjunctive central vascular pedicle.[30]

On the cut surface, giant haemangiomas frequently have areas of intense fibrosis which are hard in consistency and which may represent evolution towards cicatrization or the substitution of extensive areas of intratumoural infarct.

Similarly, giant haemangiomas may be found to contain a cavity, which is generally single, clearly delineated by a fibrous surface, and filled by a transparent fluid of low density which is odourless and sterile. The presence of this cavity is generally explained by the transformation of areas of extensive intratumoural haemorrhage which later involute towards liquefaction and breakdown of accumulated blood.

Microscopic examination of these tumours generally reveals vascular spaces in the form of large capillary lakes which form a confluence at their centre point and are lined with flat endothelial cells. In the septa, formed by the joining of the fibrous surfaces, vascular structures in the form of blood vessels can be identified. Biliary canals which do not show any morphological or microscopic anomaly can also be observed. Most often these walls are thick, less frequently revealing myxoid structures.[43]

From the microscopic and ultrastructural point of view, large haemangiomas possess cavernous loculi which have given rise to the name of 'cavernous' lobules. Other haemangiomas, generally smaller in size, have the typical characteristics of simple haemangiomas.[43]

The association between hepatic and cutaneous haemangiomas[44] and those found in other visceral locations, either hollow organ (oesophagus, stomach, jejunum–ileum, colon and rectum) or solid organ (spleen, kidney, brain) is not unusual, forming part of specific syndromes such as the Kasabah–Merrit syndrome.[45,46] These are generally identified early in life and are exceptional in adults. Another specific hereditary syndrome is the Osler–Weber–Rendu syndrome, in which the association of hepatic haemangiomas with angiomatous multiple telangiectases define this syndrome. In addition, an association has been identified between hepatic or pancreatic cysts[47,48] and other benign tumours, mainly adenomas[17] particularly after use of the oral contraceptive.[29,49] An association with endometriosis has also been identified.

Evolution

Haemangiomas generally tend to grow slowly and progressively, in an irregular way, perhaps subject to the influence of hormonal steroids or to changes in blood flow.[50] It is not possible, however, to explain the exceptional cases of spontaneous regression which have been documented.

Due to the high risk factor, there is much interest in the possibility of surface rupture of the haemangioma, reported in 19.7% cases,[51] which may cause severe intra-abdominal haemorrhage. This complication is less frequently spontaneous (2–6%),[52,53] mainly post-traumatic[10] or iatrogenic, and in this case may be caused by attempted diagnosis using FNA (fine needle aspiration).[54,55]

Isolated descriptions of spontaneous tumour rupture have related this to administration of oestrogens or progestogen.[17] However, although this association is accepted in hepatic adenoma, at the present time there is an on-going debate with some authors rejecting the concept of evolution of haemangiomas being related to hormonal and steroid action drugs.[56] In any event, spontaneous rupture is relatively frequent (5%), 28 cases having been published by Yamamoto et al.[53]

Traumatic rupture—generally in traffic accidents—is also rare, although it is more common than the spontaneous variety. Nevertheless, it should be remembered that the accentuated elasticity of the tumour parenchyma makes it more resistant to contusions than the liver tissue which surrounds it.

Puncture biopsy does, indeed, present a major risk of intratumoural and intra-abdominal haemorrhage, especially when the capsule is ruptured for some distance during puncture. For this reason, given the radiological suspicion of haemangioma, histological examination is contraindicated as it often produces a significant number of false negatives or positives due to the extraction of just fibrous tissue and cellular blood, without offering any other more characteristic histology.[55]

In general, the importance of rupture of a haemangioma is not in the frequency of its occurrence (historically 1.8%).[17,21] At present, the frequency of rupture is accepted as being between 3% and 4%. More importantly, rupture is associated with an average mortality rate of 50%, which is higher in spontaneous cases and those which are secondary to abdominal trauma (86%) than after puncture biopsy (47%),[6] or biopsy due to excision.[17]

Tumour recurrence is not frequent, but has been documented.[29,57] The most frequent cause is incomplete excision of the haemangioma, which occurs after inadequate enucleation or tumour excision when the plane corresponding to the tumour surface is used to facilitate excision. This explains why it is exceptional after anatomical hepatic resection, in which a resection margin of over 15 to 20 mm is always obtained. In these cases it is accepted that further haemangiomas appear as a result of the increase in size of others of smaller diameter which

had gone unnoticed during surgery. In any case, in order to avoid tumour recurrence after excision of a haemangioma, the surgeon should ensure that resection is complete, examining both the tumour surface and the surface corresponding to the adjacent hepatic bed, extending resection of hepatic tissue to its anatomical limits and removing small remaining haemangiomas, or others of larger size, in spite of their location on the contralateral hepatic lobe.[14,56]

The relationship of recurrence to administration of oestrogens or progestogens has been documented, especially in the case of tumour relapse or growth of small unapparent haemangiomas.[18]

In giant cavernous haemangiomas, their histological characteristics, and tendency to extensive growth have led to thoughts about possible malignant transformation.[17] Nevertheless, of the three patients with possible malignant transformation identified,[58] in none of these was there prior histological diagnosis of haemangioma, the subsequent diagnoses being haemangioendothelioma, haemangioendothelio-sarcoma and haemangiosarcoma, respectively. Logically, malignant transformation of haemangiomas cannot be accepted, as there is no evidence of this development elsewhere.[59]

Clinical practice

Most haemangiomas evolve silently with no clinical symptoms, even when they eventually acquire such a large volume that they occupy 60 to 70% of the abdominal cavity. Indeterminate symptoms are related to the finding of a haemangioma, but frequently they have nothing to do with the existence of the tumour, so that these symptoms remain even after excision.[35] Less frequently, patients from whom large haemangiomas have been removed may sometimes admit to improved symptoms and which are more closely related to the reduction of gastric capacity, gastro-duodenal emptying, intestinal transition, bowel habit, capsular adherence to the diaphragm or parietal peritoneum.[14,60]

More often than not, haemangiomas are diagnosed by chance. This may occur during abdominal palpation during an examination for no specific reason, as can happen in the case of giant haemangiomas which occupy a large part of the right hemi-abdomen. Currently transabdominal ultrasound[42,61–65] frequently detects small and middle-sized haemangiomas which had not previously produced any conditions,[66] such as gynaecological disease, or in the search for secondary hepatic lesions. They may also be detected during investigation of other intestinal diseases (gastric tumours, diverticulosis, alterations in bowel habit,[67] and have even been seen during the work-up of prostatism when pelvic ultrasound extends to the abdominal cavity.[41] A hepatic haemangioma has even been diagnosed in a foetus before birth.[68,69]

Pain is usually the main symptom, and this is probably due to these factors: changes produced during growth, adherence of the tumour surface to the diaphragmatic or parietoabdominal peritoneum and intratumoural haemorrhage due to rupture of vascular elements, which then gives rise to capsular distension.[70] Another factor which may cause tumour increase is the action of hormones, in particular steroids. Increase in tumour size is generally rapid in these cases, sometimes intermittent, with regression noted during menstruation. Less frequently, pain is related to compression of adjacent viscera.[71]

It is generally accepted that pain is the presenting symptom in 28% of patients, beginning in the epigastrium and right hypochondrium, extending to the ipsilateral iliac fossa or radiating to all abdominal quadrants in a diffuse manner.

Whether or not there are referred symptoms, during physical examination an enlargement of the hepatic lobules, or an overall increase in liver size, may be noted. Generally there is a smooth regular hepatomegaly, of soft consistency, with loss of the liver edge which is replaced by the tumour surface.[17]

Not exceptionally in these large size haemangiomas audible murmurs may be heard on the abdominal wall overlying the tumour surface, and, on occasions a thrill may be palpated. More unusual is the appearance of collateral circulation (portacaval) over ipsilateral hemiabdomen. This may appear at any stage, which further complicates the clinical differential diagnosis.[21,34]

There are a number of differential characteristics of complications which may arise during the development of haemangiomas. Tumour rupture in the abdominal cavity generally occurs spontaneously with no background history, presenting with extremely severe pain at right hypochondrium and with shoulder tip pain due to phrenic irritation and haemodynamic instability. Intratumoural rupture may produce fever and respiratory disorders due to ipsilateral pleural effusion.

Haemobilia has been described as a complication of tumour haemorrhage. Although very infrequent, its possible existence should be borne in mind due to the seriousness of its presentation which gives rise to right upper quadrant pain with jaundice and is accompanied by melaena but no associated splenomegaly or portal hypertension.

Jaundice may also appear without tumour rupture, due to compression of the extrahepatic bile duct or tumour confluence as a result of the growth of tumours located within the central liver. Nevertheless, due to the adaptation of adjacent structures which the haemangioma compresses during its slow growth, this presentation is exceptional.

Severe fever may appear in cases of extensive tumour thrombosis, or as a consequence of large-scale infarcts, followed by liquefication of extravasated blood, and the cavity may become infected in exceptional cases.[72]

Cavernous haemangiomas represent massive arteriovenous fistulae. This is demonstrated by the observation of the large diameter of the hepatic artery itself, and its branches which supply the tumour, or the segmental or named hepatic vein draining the tumour, as well as the significant increase in blood flow through the tumour. Nevertheless, only isolated, exceptional cases of heart failure, or aneurysmal dilatation of the draining veins, or retrohepatic vena cava have been described, in spite of frequent evidence of intense intratumoural arteriovenous shunting.

Of lesser importance is the association of joint pain due to rheumatoid arthritis in patients with hepatic haemangiomas treated with azathioprine.[73]

Laboratory investigations

Generally, laboratory investigations do not contribute much which could be of diagnostic assistance, or, more particularly, contribute to a differential diagnosis. It has been observed that anaemia is frequent, but only occurs in intratumoural bleeding.[70] Similarly, in spite of the extraordinary size of hepatic haemangiomas, the biochemical liver function tests are always normal, as well as serum tumour markers.[10,31,35,74,75]

More frequently, especially in large hemangiomata, alterations in blood coagulation have been reported. Generally this is a consumption-based coagulopathy, the most evident example of which is the Kasabach–Meritt syndrome, in which thrombocytopaenia prevails. This appears more frequently in giant haemangiomas as a result of platelet sequestration. It should be said, however, that no haematological alterations of any type are normally shown.[45,46,60,76]

Radiological diagnosis

Simple radiography

Plain abdominal radiography may show elevation of the right hemidiaphragm related to the overall increase in liver size. This is due to the displacement caused when the tumour is located in the upper level of the right hepatic lobe, or of upper middle segments. In addition, displacement of adjacent hollow viscera, the stomach, the hepatic angle of the transverse or ascending colon may also be observed. Similarly, but more difficult to detect due to their small size, phleboliths may be evident in the form of rounded calcifications which are sometimes arranged in line, following a vascular pathway, but with no anatomical reference. These are characterized by their very small size.

More frequently calcifications can be seen which adopt the form of a central mass, large in size, and surrounded by satellite microcalcifications, which may take on the form of a crown or a radial arrangement. Calcification is present in 6 to 10% of cases and is interpreted as calcium deposit at the level of the septae, corresponding to the walls used by the arterial branches for their intratumoural arterio-capillary distribution.[4,10,22,60,66,77]

Perhaps the diagnostic sign of greatest importance in giant haemangioma is the existence of a large soft tissue shadow, which displaces the air pattern of adjacent hollow viscera towards a non-anatomical position.

Ultrasound

The first examination which should be undertaken is abdominal ultrasound. This will show an overall increase in liver size, and the existence of one or several tumours within. In the case of small haemangiomas the distinct margin is of great importance with regard to adjacent hepatic parenchyma, as well as their homogeneous character. In giant haemangiomas tumour heterogeneity may be noted due to the existence of septae, fibrosis, intratumoural cavitation and possible evidence of fluid content in the interior of the cavities.[61,78]

Haemangiomas are often homogeneous, observed as a well-defined hyperechoic mass in 77–92% of cases.[79] In almost 80% posterior acoustic highlighting can be seen,[39] present in lesions of 25 mm upwards. Due to their increase in size, more than 80% of haemangiomas maintain their ultrasound characteristics, the most specific characteristic being progressive increase in size.[7,60,79]

Nevertheless, occasionally a central hypoechoic nucleus may be observed, though with no hypoechoic halo on the tumour periphery. Atypically, hypoechogenicity may extend to the whole of the tumour mass, if this is homogeneous, then it is surrounded by intense fatty deposits in the surrounding hepatic parenchyma.

In any case, ultrasound is an important method of diagnosis, and will help to differentiate haemangiomas from primary and secondary tumours, especially when the tumour mass may be compressed by the ultrasound probe. The haemangioma becomes increasingly isoechoic with this procedure, as echogenicity decreases due to compression of the cavernous sinuses. Such changes cannot be observed in solid malignant tumours.[41,62,78]

Abdominal CT scan

This is not the most appropriate study for diagnosis of haemangiomas; however, this is a method which can go hand in hand with ultrasound, so its indication is not controversial[62] (Figs 10.1 and 10.2).

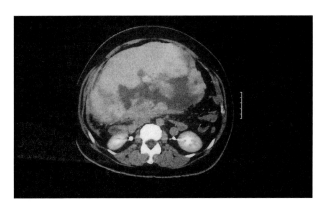

Figure 10.1(A) CT scan. Large haemangioma localized in the right lobe of the liver. Central areas of connective tissue can be seen.

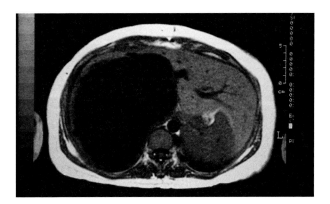

Figure 10.1(B) Large hypervascular mass in the right lobe of the liver. Homogeneous contrast distribution in all the haemangioma tissue is shown.

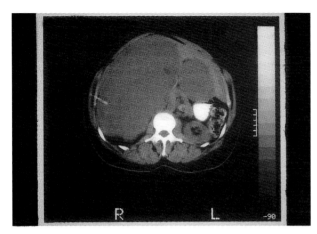

Figure 10.2 Bilateral haemangioma. CT scan. Large mass in the right lobe of the liver also occupying segment IV of the left. Small mass in the left lobe of the liver, posterior part of segment II and III. In the right lobe needle biopsy is being performed.

Four rigorous diagnostic criteria have been described in between 50 and 55% of haemangiomas studied:[38] (1) relative hypoattenuation in comparison with the hepatic parenchyma which surrounds the lesion before administering contrast; (2) perilesional increase in contrast in the early phase; (3) progressive opacification from the periphery to the centre of the lesion, and (4) isoattenuation, which occurs between 3 and 60 minutes after administration of intravenous contrast.[80] Nevertheless, hypoattenuation is frequently seen. These findings depend, as in the case of ultrasound, on the degree of fatty infiltration within the peritumour hepatic parenchyma, as the existence of diffuse steatosis may give rise to images of isoattenuation or hypoattenuation before administration of intravenous contrast,[8,81] which is of special importance in dynamic CT.[82]

From the morphological point of view, haemangiomas are clearly delineated tumours which show their richness of intratumoural capillaries after administration of contrast. After several minutes, the contrast is seen generally to be located peripherally, with either larger or smaller stellar images in the centre of the tumour, which represents the central axis of the lesion where actual walls or septa may be seen. This central portion markedly alters the level of attenuation where cavitated areas usually exist. In general, large haemangiomas can be diagnosed using an abdominal CT scan, which gives 70% sensitivity and a specificity of 65% to 75%.

MR imaging

This very safe test provides higher resolution than abdominal CT scans.[83] From the morphological point of view, haemangiomas are spherical in 90% of cases, much less frequently ovoid, and clearly delineated from the proximal hepatic parenchyma by well-defined edges which represent the fibrous capsular sheath. MR imaging gives 90% sensitivity, 95% specificity and 93% accuracy.[84,85]

Haemangiomas show marked hyperintensity during T_2 imaging (light-bulb sign). The imaging of greatest use for diagnosis is obtained using multiecho techniques (ET: 120 milliseconds). Nevertheless, light-bulb sign specificity is not 100%, as it may be present in any hypervascular lesion, such as adenoma, hepatocellular carcinoma and endocrine tumour metastasis. The greatest use of this technique is in a differential diagnosis between haemangioma and primary hepatic tumours, especially hepatoma, as these tumours are heterogeneous in 70% of cases.[86] A low intensity signal is observed at the level of the tumour capsule in more than half of examinations, which, in contrast, is not seen in haemangiomas. In addition, in hepatoma the signal during T_2 is less prolonged.

Giant haemangiomas are most often heterogeneous in images obtained during both T_1 and T_2 imaging. In almost all cases, images appear to be similar to septae, in the form of low intensity areas during T_1, with a high intensity signal during T_2. Septal areas were identified in more than 50% of cases as a low intensity signal during both T_1 and T_2.[87]

Due to the largely vascular composition, administration of contrast provides greater possibilities for diagnosis of haemangiomas. Intravenous bolus administration of gadolinium (gadopentate dimeglumine; diethylene triaminepentacetic acid) is used with a dynamic gradient of echosequences which show peritumour reinforcement after 2 minutes, which persists in late images in a similar way to that which occurs after administration of contrast in abdominal CT scan.[38,87]

Gamma camera imaging after administration of Tc99m-labelled red blood cells (SPECT: single photon emission CT)

At present, conventional gamma camera imaging with Tc99m-labelled red blood cells is being indicated less, due to the fact that there is no great difference in its results when compared with hepatic magnetic resonance imaging. Moreover, MRI has shown greater sensitivity, detecting lesions of less than 2 cm in diameter. It is true, however, that SPECT, in contrast, has greater specificity and predictive value than MRI, as this is practically 100%.[84] In the case of haemangiomas this is more valuable than the detection of small diameter

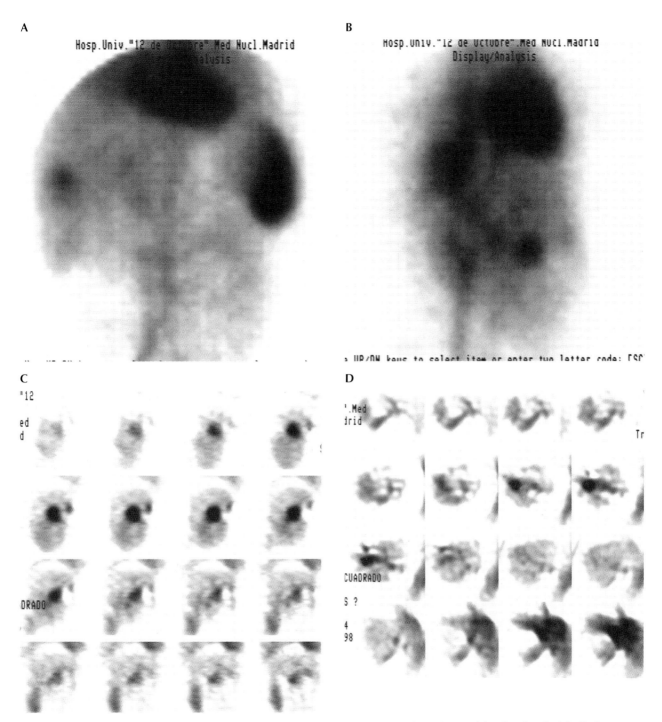

Figure 10.3 Hepatic gammagraphy performed 60 minutes after injection of autologous blood red cells labelled 'in vitro' with PYP^{99m}Tc. Radiological (A,B) and tomographic/SPECT (C,D) imaging. In a different projection (A,B) a focus of enlargement of the vascular pool in the right hepatic lobe is observed, anterolateral, typical of angioma and a smaller one, previously located (more anterior), suspicious of another similar lesion. Tomographic imaging (C,D) showing two angiomas.

lesions, as the latter are benign lesions which would remain under observation only,[62] once a correct diagnosis has been confirmed. Less specificity is shown in cirrhotics with portal hypertension[88] (Fig. 10.3).

Gamma camera examination (SPECT) has 90% sensitivity, 100% specificity and precision close to

100%, which provides a higher safety level in the diagnosis of haemangiomas. In these tumours a decrease in activity and an accumulation of labelled red cells is shown immediately after perfusion, with this activity increasing to its maximum in later images. Other very highly vascularized tumours such as adenomas and focal nodular hyperplasia also show progressive accumulation of labelled red cells. Nevertheless, the difference between these and haemangiomas is that in the latter case, the increase in activity is shown at the earliest stages.[63,84,86,89]

In most giant haemangiomas (65–70%), a significant increase in perfusion can be seen in dynamic imaging. Nevertheless, in a not insignificant percentage (20–25%) this hyperperfusion is seen only in the most peripheral part of haemangiomas, the central part appearing hypoperfused, perhaps as a consequence of less capillary richness in the central portion of the lesion or the existence of extensive areas of fibrosis or cavitation. False positives also occur.[90]

A great difference between conventional gamma camera imaging and single photon emission CT has been demonstrated, particularly as regards sensitivity, as lesions of around 3 cm in diameter may be detected with the latter technique.[74,91,92]

Vascular examination

Arteriography shows the intense and extensive uptake of contrast within the tumour parenchyma, persisting in the interior of the lesion much longer than in the surrounding parenchyma. The distribution of contrast is uniform in giant cavernous haemangiomas, provided that there has been no fibrosis or cavitation in its interior. There is no evidence of particular vascular activity within the tumour capsule. Consequently, the periphery of the lesion is less easily appreciated[6,10,14,35] (Figs 10.4–10.6).

Specific characteristics of haemangiomas are displacement of the intratumoural vascular trunks towards the peripheral areas of the tumour, as well as the thick diameter of the feeding branches of the hepatic artery and changes in the anatomical position of arterial and venous trunks which are displaced by tumour growth.

In multiple haemangiomas even lesions of a few centimetres may be demonstrated. In this situation all lesions within the liver will have similar characteristics, regardless of which lobule they are located in.[21,81]

One of the advantages of visceral angiography is access for embolization of the arterial branches feeding the tumour, especially in the case of haemangioma.[93] However, this procedure may be ineffective, even in cases when it has been undertaken prior to surgical excision. However, embolization has a role in the management of haemangioma.[93–95] Exceptional cases have been published on the use of embolization in the treatment of spontaneous rupture of the tumour[53] or intratumoural haemorrhage.[70]

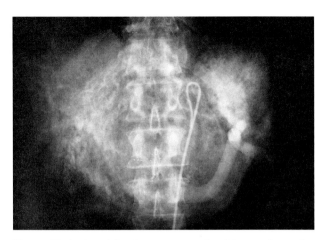

Figure 10.4 Arterial splenoportography. Venous face of splenic arteriography. Very wide splenic vein. Hypervascular large mass is localized in the left lobe of the liver, producing reduction of right lobe.

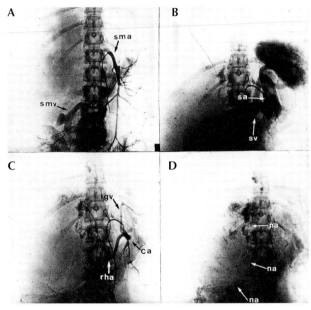

Figure 10.5 Angiographic examination of large right lobe haemangioma. (A) sma: superior mesenteric artery, displaced to the left side. smv: superior mesenteric vein, displaced by the tumour mass to the midline (B) Venous phase of splenic arteriography, sa: splenic artery. sv: splenic vein. Both vessels are displaced to the left side by the tumour mass. (C) lgv: left gastric vein, rha: right hepatic artery, ca: celiac trunk. Celiac trunk and its branches are displaced to the left side about 7 cm. (D) Capillary phase hepatic arteriography, na: limits of the internal surface of the large haemangioma localized in the right lobe of the liver.

At present there are few indications for angiographic examination in this disease, which, in our opinion also goes for laparoscopy,[77] first due to the fact that there is little gained from this procedure and, second, because angiography is being substituted by MRI,

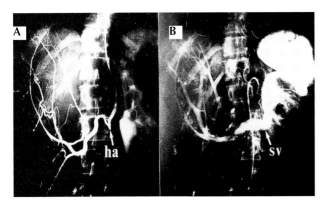

Figure 10.6 (A) Large haemangioma localized in the right lobe of the liver following resection. Branches of hepatic artery (ha) and portal vein surround the surface of the haemangioma. The gallbladder can be seen on the lower part of the tumoural surface. (B) SV, splenic vein. Aspect of the right lobe of the liver after resection of a large haemangioma.

which is much more innocuous.[38,84,87] Less important, but also less aggressive, are Doppler,[42] colour Doppler,[68,96], scintigraphy[91] and renoscintigraphy.[92]

Percutaneous biopsy

In general, in hepatic tumours, percutaneous biopsy can only be indicated when there are difficulties in establishing a differential diagnosis between primary or secondary malignant tumours; i.e. this will never be established as a routine or necessary diagnostic test to confirm clinical and/or radiological diagnosis,[61] although several groups consider percutaneous cytology very helpful.[66]

First, if undertaken, histological diagnosis of the tumour will alter or establish the correct course of treatment, as, if it is not going to influence the final decision, it should never be indicated.[66] Moreover, one should carefully consider all possible complications which this test may cause, such as tumour rupture, intratumoural haemorrhage either in the abdominal cavity or in the case of a malignant lesion, tumour spread along the path followed by the needle during extraction across the abdominal cavity (exceptional) or in the abdominal wall.[6,66]

In general, interpretation of material extracted by fine needle aspiration is not easy. In the case of haemangiomas, diagnosis is generally reached by exclusion, as the sample extracted shows only red cells and fibrosis, often making several more attempts at puncture essential to ensure the correct histological diagnosis,[55] with the corresponding risk of haemorrhage.[14,55,97]

Finally, we should be aware of the possibility, already described, of rupture—especially in the case of giant haemangioma with a very fine capsule, most often as a consequence of repeated puncturing, but also due to tumour fragility or subcapsular haemorrhage. We are not in favour of biopsy puncture, except in a few very specific exceptional cases. Diagnosis, in most cases, can be undertaken by morphological tests which are less invasive,[14] both in the case of haemangiomas and in the other types of benign or primary or secondary malignant tumours.

Surgical treatment

Indications

Although it was initially considered necessary to excise these tumours regardless of their diameter or location[3,5,98] at the present time there are selective criteria which are sufficiently robust to avoid unnecessary operations. These operations do not incur any benefit for most patients,[14] and may, indeed, involve unnecessary risk—however small this may appear—or unjustified morbidity. There is also the possibility of greater complications to which the patient should not be exposed. No matter how expert the team of surgeons may be in liver surgery, there can be no argument for the treatment of patients without absolute indications for surgery.[14,57,99–101]

It is accepted that small size haemangiomas (2 to 4 cm) diagnosed by chance should not be removed, but should merely undergo periodic review in order to gain a more adequate knowledge of their behaviour and thus act accordingly.[5,32,56] Nevertheless, it is essential to be absolutely certain of their nature, with no doubt whatsoever as to whether they are benign or not, and to their histological diagnosis.[49,102] Haemangiomas detected during the follow-up of a patient who has undergone removal of a malignant tumour of another abdominal organ, especially colon or rectum, may be candidates for surgical treatment when the liver lesion is not clearly characterized and elevation of a specific tumour marker (CEA) is detected.

Previous history, lack of morphological identification or negative cytology following puncture aspiration (although infrequent, if indicated at all), must be factors when considering any eventual surgical treatment.[10,12,61]

There may be doubt in the case of small size haemangiomas detected in the course of a surgical operation undertaken for another reason.[20,103] If a possible haemangioma is detected, located on the liver edge or on its surface in an easily accessible area due to the type of incision made, excision is justified. However, if the appearance of the lesion leaves no doubt about the diagnosis of haemangioma, it could be left alone, with a description in the operative note, along with the reasons for not removing the lesion. We believe that such haemangiomas should be excised, as a removal in our hands does not increase the risk of the operation. It is clear that incision biopsy of the tumour should not be undertaken, as the risk of haemorrhage,[104] even in small lesions, is very high.[105]

Currently, accepted indications for surgical treatment of haemangiomas are as follows: (1) tumours of diameter over 6 cm, (2) haemangiomas causing episodes of pain of great intensity in the area of the tumour which occur spontaneously and which can be correlated with intratumoural bleeding, (3) giant tumours which cause symptoms by reducing the capacity of the abdominal cavity, (4) hypotension and inexplicable anaemia, which sometimes may coincide with an increase in the size of a hepatic lobule, signs which may be secondary to intratumoural rupture with capsular distension and (5) tumours which are difficult to diagnose, with a well-documented suspicion of malignancy, and which, even after inconclusive aspiration cytology, due to their diameter (5 to 7 cm) cannot be left without any treatment.[32,102,106]

At present it seems difficult to be able to justify surgical treatment for large asymptomatic haemangiomas,[24,107] first because it is not known how long it has taken to reach this size and, second, because most asymptomatic giant haemangiomas do not give rise to any special symptoms. Moreover, they do not produce complications and spontaneous rupture is exceptional, as is traumatic rupture.[14,36,108] Special care should be taken in childhood when indications for surgical treatment are exceptional.[109]

Preoperative tumour embolization

As previously stated, embolization will reduce tumour mass, as well as its arterial input, making any surgical operation easier by reducing blood loss and demarcating the border between the tumour capsule and the underlying liver parenchyma.

Nevertheless, embolization of these tumours has a short-lived effect.[18] Arterial flow is quickly re-established by other routes, and the tumour rapidly recovers its original morphology and size.[12,53,70,93,109] In spite of this, preoperative embolization has nevertheless been indicated in giant haemangiomas[95] to facilitate surgical manoeuvres.

It should be remembered that large haemangiomas which consequently have a very intense arterio-portal flow are difficult to embolize. This is the main contraindication for embolization. Our experience of this technique is minimal, and reports from other authors do not back up this practice. In addition, there is the additional risk of vascular occlusion progressing back along the arterial branches corresponding to the adjacent segments or contralateral hepatic lobule.

Surgical excision

At the present time the accepted procedure is tumour resection or enucleation,[99] as it is not necessary to include any resection margin of healthy liver tissue to avoid tumour recurrence. The margin between hepatic haemangiomas and healthy hepatic tissue is minimal, with no infiltration or satellite nodules which would justify the inclusion of a healthy margin of tissue covering the resected tumour to ensure greater safety.[110] This criterion is accepted equally for small surface haemangiomas or those on the anterior edge of the liver if, despite their small diameter, excision is indicated.

Anatomical resections (segmentectomies, lobectomies and extended lobectomies)[3,111,112] are only indicated in exceptional cases of unilobular multiple hepatic haemangiomas, or those confined to several segments in which multiple tumourectomy would leave areas of the hepatic parenchyma poorly vascularized with the danger of biliary leaks, increasing postoperative morbidity and hindering the process of liver regeneration.[35,40,76]

Total hepatectomy and liver replacement by orthotopic homotransplant is not indicated in hepatic haemangiomas in spite of their frequent occurrence.[113] Nevertheless, in exceptional cases which may markedly affect liver function, or give rise to serious haemodynamic alterations as a consequence of the presence of innumerable arteriovenous fistulae, liver transplant may be absolutely necessary as well as urgent. Perhaps the best example is the Kasabach–Merritt syndrome,[45,46] provided that there are no multiple cerebral haemangiomas which are generally incompatible with survival. In our experience in 625 hepatic transplants undertaken between April 1986 and September 1998, we have seen two cases, although in the case of an adult patient the histopathological diagnosis was a haemangioendothelioma, whereas in the case of a baby girl with Kasabach–Merritt syndrome, the patient was a 39-day-old neonate weighing 2.2 kg, born after a 24 week pregnancy. While still in the incubator, she underwent surgery on the twenty-first day after birth because of a patent ductus. At the preagonal phase,

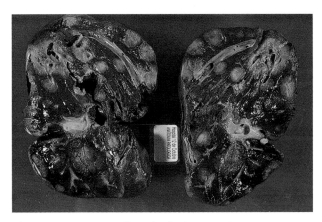

Figure 10.7 Liver with multiple haemangiomas (Kasabach–Merrit syndrome). The liver was removed and replaced by total graft in a premature baby, after a 24-week pregnancy, at 2.2 kg birth weight.

she became haemodynamically unstable, and required liver transplantation. As can be seen in Fig. 10.7, the hepatic parenchyma is replaced by multiple haemangiomas of differing diameters.

Nevertheless, the indication for hepatic transplantation in the Kasabach–Merritt syndrome is dubious, as haemangiomas tend to disappear or lead to thrombosis and resolution, as happens in cutaneous haemangiomas. For this reason, it is only indicated in particularly acute situations in order to save the patient's life. The existence of a giant haemangioma, in this syndrome could in exceptional circumstances indicate a liver transplantation.[46]

In cases of diagnostic doubt, excision could be extended to obtain a sufficient resection margin. Biopsy by excision in these cases is advisable but not compulsory, especially given the complications this produces.[14,17]

Surgical excision technique

Incision
Surgical incision should always be abdominal, with right subcostal laparotomy being favoured, extended laterally under the tenth rib, in order to extirpate the

A

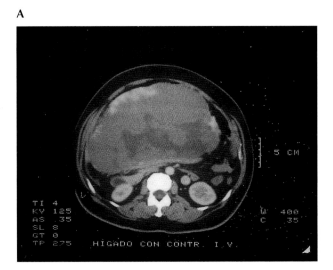

B

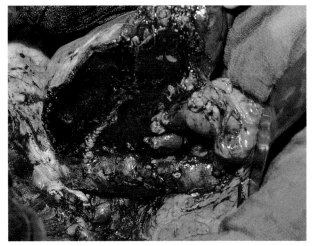

C

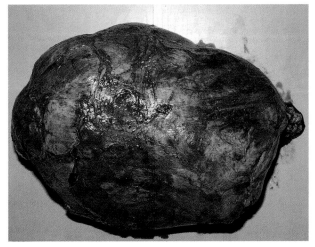

Figure 10.8 (A) CT scan showing large haemangioma localized in the right lobe of the liver. (B) Same patient after resection of the right lobe haemangioma; the surface of the normal liver and retrohepatic vena cava can be seen. (C) Haemangioma of 32 cm diameter (same patient as in Fig. 10.9).

A

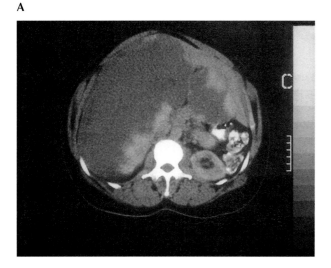

B

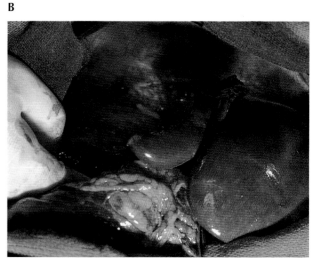

C

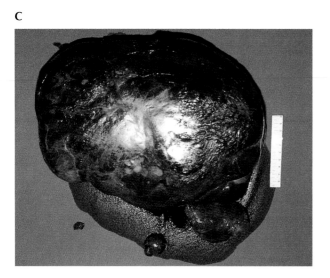

Figure 10.9 (A) CT scan showing very large haemangioma localized in the right lobe of the liver. (B) Aspect of the anterior surface of the liver after removal of a haemangioma (same patient as in (A)). (C) Large haemangioma resected on same patient as in (A) and (B). The gallbladder can be seen in the inferior limit of the tumour.

cartilage and medial end of the rib (respecting the perichondral sheath and periosteum which will allow osteocartilaginous regeneration) in bulky haemangiomas which occupy the hepatic dome, sometimes with firm adhesions to the diaphragm surface, and which may be intensely vascularized (Figs 10.8 and 10.9).

In cavernous haemangiomas located on the left hepatic lobule, the most commonly accepted incision is an upper midline extended inferiorly to improve access. These tumours are large in diameter and impossible to resect through a smaller incision (Figs 10.10–10.12).

Bilateral subcostal incision is necessary in giant haemangiomas which affect central segments of the liver (IV, V, VIII). Thoracoabdominal incisions (thoracophrenolaparotomy) are not indicated. Between 10 and 20 years ago, Japanese surgeons were keen on the use of thoracolaparotomy during

transplantation of hepatomas, however this incision has now fallen into disuse, and is only used in exceptional cases (Fig. 10.11A,B).

In spite of the advance of laparoscopy over the last few years, this technique is not indicated in the surgical treatment of giant haemangiomas due to risk of rupture, and consequent haemorrhage. Similarly, laparoscopic examination and biopsy by excision, along with direct laparoscopic ultrasound, do not offer any therapeutic benefit to these patients. In the future the possibility of undertaking laparoscopic arterial ligation, sclerotherapy and/or cryotherapy may arise. However, these procedures at present remain theoretical.

Vascular control
The reduction in size which occurs following arterial ligation can be dramatic, and is maximized by extending this ligature to involve the trunk of the portal vein entering the tumour.

A

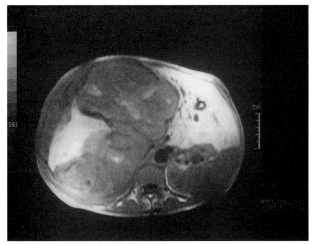

Figure 10.10(A) CT scan. Large haemangioma localized in the centre of the liver.

B

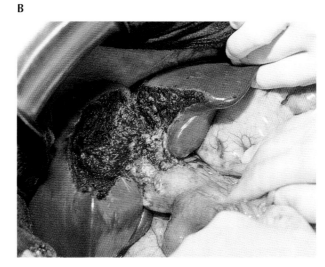

Figure 10.10(B) Aspect of the central area of the liver after resection of the haemangioma diagnosed in the patient in (A). Mesohepatectomy.

A

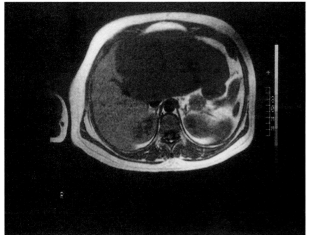

Figure 10.11(A) CT scan showing large haemangioma localized in the left lobe of the liver.

B

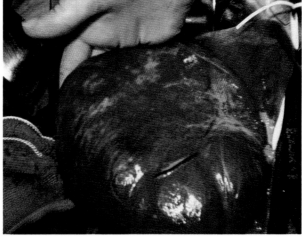

Figure 10.11(B) Haemangioma in the left lobe (same patient as in (A)).

A

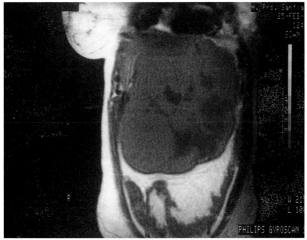

Figure 10.12(A) CT scan showing very large haemangioma in the left of the liver, occupying almost 60% of the abdominal cavity.

B

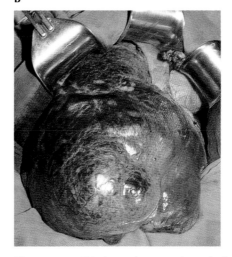

Figure 10.12(B) Large haemangioma before resection.

A

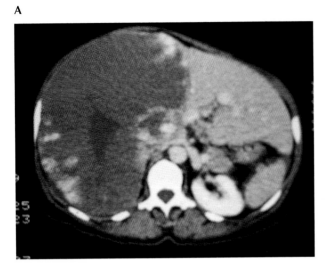

B

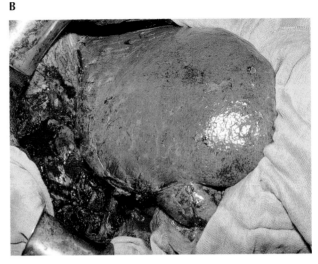

C

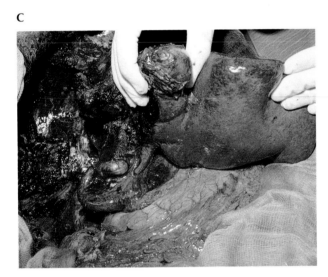

Figure 10.13 (A) CT scan. Large mass localized in the right lobe of the liver, occupying all the right segments and segment IV. (B) After removal of a right side haemangioma, segments II and III of the left lobe can be seen. Enlargements of these two segments can be seen, giving the appearance of a complete liver. (C) Same patient as in (A) and (B), showing the enlargement of segments II and III and the normal aspect of the inferior surface. The subphrenic space can be seen after removal of the large haemangioma localized in the right lobe of the liver.

Ligation of a main branch of the hepatic artery (right or left), and of the portal vein is essential in most cases of giant haemangioma that require anatomical resection. For this reason, control must be prehepatic using a vascular clamp or vessel loop which permits arterial and venous blood flow to re-establish itself after tumour enucleation[14] (Fig. 10.13).

The fastest and easiest method of preventing afferent blood flow is complete vascular occlusion of the liver at the hepatoduodenal ligament.[114] Nevertheless, the success of this manoeuvre depends on the response of the rest of the hepatic parenchyma to ischaemia.[115] In our experience the Pringle[114] manoeuvre can be maintained for up to 90 minutes without any serious functional effects, with only a discrete rise in hepatic enzyme levels, and a very limited drop in prothrombin factors.[116] Nevertheless, in giant cavernous haemangiomas, this is only indicated when it is necessary to shorten operating time, or in cases of bleeding through the hepatic surface in contact with the tumour, when the tumour capsule is ruptured and penetrates into the remaining liver.[117]

Total vascular isolation is less frequently indicated. Vascular occlusion is achieved at the level of the hepatoduodenal ligament and supra and infrahepatic vena cava.[99,118] The haemodynamic changes which occur in the splenic and lower abdomen, along with the greater seriousness of the reperfusion syndrome, make this procedure too dangerous for routine use in this disease.[115] In addition, this technique, while questionable in malignant hepatic tumours, is absolutely unnecessary in cavernous haemangiomas. Similarly, ex vivo procedures of bench resection,[119] which occasionally play a role in the resection of malignant hepatic tumours, offer no advantage while they do give rise to a number of possible complications.[14,56,106]

Dissection and tumour removal

Enucleation is characterized by dissection and separation of the tumour capsule from the adjacent hepatic parenchyma. Similarly, the whole of the tumour must be removed, with no residual tumour capsule.

During dissection vascular elements can be seen which enter the tumour structure. These should be ligated and divided. The segmental branches of the intrahepatic biliary tree should be preserved and small vessels displaced by tumour growth may be ligated and divided by suture-ligature stitches. Accidental ligature of larger intrahepatic vascular structures must be avoided as these could give rise to biliary fistulae. Unrecognized small biliary leaks are the most frequent cause of perihepatic infection, giving rise to subphrenic abscesses.

Dissection of the tumour surface may be undertaken by ultrasonic dissection (CUSA, Ultrajet, etc), harmonic scalpel or electrocautery. Nevertheless, in attempting to simplify the procedure we prefer to use clips to dissect through liver tissue.

Maintaining the integrity of the biliary tree

For several years cholangiography after tumour excision had been the rule for many surgeons to ensure the absence of biliary fistulae. Nevertheless, this procedure usually involves a cholecystectomy which is unnecessary, particularly when the bile duct is far from the tumour. Less frequently this is undertaken by transhepatic puncture, afterwards compressing the parenchyma in order to force the passage of contrast into the bile duct, or by direct puncture of the common hepatic or bile duct. Both procedures avoid cholecystectomy.

Nevertheless, identification of a biliary fistula on the raw liver surface—even if this is small in diameter—may be done by wiping with a surgical gauze. By moving this slowly away from the liver surface a small stain of bile can be seen which indicates its exact location.

Assisting biliary drainage with a T-tube is not indicated for any type of liver resection, considering the fact that this increases the morbidity of the procedure. None of the theoretical advantages of T-tube placement in fact justify it.

The raw surface is fulgurated by argon beam coagulation, thus removing any microscopic capsular remains which could have been left behind. Nevertheless, caution is necessary, as this may disrupt small suture-ligatures. This is because reabsorbable polyglycolic acid is sensitive to the high temperatures of fulguration.

Drainage in the residual cavity

The use of postoperative intra-abdominal drainage has been questioned over the last few years. The basis for avoiding drainage is that perfect haemostasis, absence of biliary fistula, and the avoidance of poorly vascularized tissues will reduce the risk of postoperative collections. For this reason, once confirmed by waiting a few minutes and rinsing with warm saline, it is not necessary to drain the operative field.

In addition, the surgical field is located in the free abdominal cavity, so that the transudate produced may be reabsorbed through the peritoneal mesothelium. On the other hand, drainage keeps the external space in contact with the inside of the abdominal cavity, with the attendant risk of subsequent infection.

Operative mortality

Enucleation or resection of cavernous haemangiomas can only be undertaken in the absence of serious complications and mortality. However, there are reports of between 2 and 5% operative mortality at 30 days after operation. These figures seem excessive, as there is no justifiable reason for mortality, i.e. the mortality rate should be as close to 0% as possible.

These patients have normal hepatic parenchyma, and are generally between the third and sixth decade of life, without any deranged hepatic function and with normal coagulation studies. If patients are selected correctly, there should be no operative deaths.

Factors which may be related to postoperative mortality are: co-existence of cirrhosis of the liver, respiratory failure, kidney failure and/or cardiopathy. For this reason it is questionable whether patients in poor physical condition at an advanced age, or those with cardiopulmonary disease or kidney or liver failure, even if moderate, should be treated or not.

In our experience, out of a total of 78 giant cavernous haemangiomas, no patients died in the postoperative period.

Tumour recurrence

Provided the considerations described above are observed, recurrence of the excised lesion within the liver is exceptional and must not be confused with the appearance of a haemangioma in the remaining hepatic tissue, far from the surgical field.

We have never observed a case of tumour recurrence, and we advise surgical treatment whenever possible.[15]

Other therapeutic options

Prevention of further growth

This is advisable in the case of giant cavernous haemangiomas in which, for the reasons mentioned above, excision is not indicated (small diameter tumours, asymptomatic patients or considerable risk factors).

This approach applies to the majority of patients. Complications relating to growth of haemangiomas occur in approximately 20% of patients, resulting in subsequent excision when symptoms occur. The occurrence of rupture and haemorrhage is exceptional, and malignant transformation does not occur.

One of the dangers of not monitoring these tumours is, without doubt, erroneous diagnosis, since the image of a cavernous haemangioma may be confused with other very vascularized tumours, such as hepatoma when located on a non-cirrhotic liver, when there is no background of viral infection and plasma levels of alpha1-phetoprotein are normal. These conditions are not frequent in hepatomas, nor are they, however, exceptional.

However, conservative management is acceptable when the diagnosis is absolutely clear and there are no indications to operate. Nevertheless, in spite of most surgeons agreeing with this approach, the reality is that even among experienced liver surgeons, 20–40% of haemangiomas remain undiagnosed with excisional biopsy.

Radiotherapy

This has been advocated in diffuse haemangiomas or in unresectable voluminous haemangiomas.[120] Until 1970, before the advent of modern liver surgery, this form of therapy was still indicated, based on the possibility of provoking sclerosis of the tumour parenchyma with consequent reduction in its volume. For this reason it was used in patients who complained of pain in upper right quadrants due to capsular distension as a result of progressive tumour growth, or following episodes of intratumoural haemorrhage.[121]

Initially conventional external beam radiotherapy was used, with the risk of radiation hepatitis or centrilobular thrombosis when dosage exceeded 2500 to 2800 rds. For this reason it was superceded first by cobalt therapy and then subsequently by the linear accelerator. Use of the linear accelerator enables better limitation of the field, both on the surface and deeper within the liver, thus reducing undesirable effects on the surrounding healthy liver parenchyma.

Following radiotherapy, reductions in volume of haemangiomas ranged between 20% and 40%, with approximately 30% improvement in symptomatology. For this reason, some authors continue to advocate its use.

However, radiotherapy is associated with a high rate of complications such as radiation hepatitis, and tumour rupture only a few months after completion of treatment, probably due to the increase in capsular fragility. Isolated cases of malignant transformation induced by radiotherapy have been described, as well as the development of malignant tumours at other sites after administration.[122]

Selective hepatic dearterialization

Although the role of hepatic dearterialization was described 20 years ago, at present it is not widely indicated for the treatment of liver tumours.[70,123]

The demonstration of intense vascularity in liver tumours logically leads to selective, permanent occlusion, which both decreases the arterio-venous shunt and reduces the size of the tumour.

However, the effect of dearterialization is temporary, and blood flow is re-established through an intricate network of collateral branches.[17]

Embolization

Apart from its transitory nature, morbidity of embolization is high because of tumour necrosis, sometimes even leading to the formation of intrahepatic abscesses.

Short-term results are difficult to evaluate, but in the long term tumour size may be reduced, with a reduction in symptomatology as well, although only in exceptional cases. For this reason, at present embolization is not a procedure that can be widely recommended.[17,53,109]

Sclerosing by means of direct injection of hypertonic solutions is of only historical value.[124]

Key points

*   Presentation of hepatic haemangiomas:
    Incidental finding (US or CT)
    Pain (28%)

Spontaneous or post-traumatic rupture
Fever, jaundice, cholangitis uncommon
Cardiac failure due to A-V fistula (rare).
- Investigation of hepatic haemangioma:
    US
    CT
    MRI
    Technetium-labelled red cell scan
    Angiography.

- Do not biopsy.
- Indications for surgical resection:
    >6 cm diameter
    Pain not responding to analgesic drugs
    Risk of spontaneous rupture
    Giant tumours compressing other viscera
    Anaemia
    To exclude malignancy.

REFERENCES

1. Paré A. Formaciones vasculares visibles en la superficie hepática. Paris. 1509–90

2. Frerich FI. A clinical treatise on disease of the liver. Vol 2. London: New Sydenham Society, 1861

3. Adam YG, Huvos AG, Fortner JG. Giant hemangioma of the liver. Ann Surg 1970; 172: 239–45

4. Baer HV, Schweizer W, Gertsch Ph, Blumgart LH. Klinik, diagnostic und therapie von 'frossen' leber hämangiomen. Helv Chir Acta 1987; 54: 387–9

5. Berloco P, Borzomati D, Altomare V et al. Surgical treatment of hepatic angiomas: the experience at the Campus Bio Medico. Hepato-Gastroenterology 1998; 45 (Suppl II): 120–1

6. Berman JK, Kirkoff P, Levine N. Liver hemangiomas. Diagnosis and treatment. Surgery 1955; 71 (2): 249–53

7. Boldrini G, Giovannini I, De Gaetano AM et al. Clinical patterns of liver hemangioma. Hepato-Gastroenterology 1998; 45 (Suppl II): 120

8. Cuevas-Ibañez A, Santos-Cores J, Molina-Lopez-Nava P, Fernandez-Iglesias P, Bones-Purkis J. El hemangioma, tumor hepático mas frecuente. Diagnóstico con TAC dinámico. An Med Interna 1994; 11: 385–8

9. Fagarasanu I, Ionescu-Bujor C, Aloman D, Albu E. Surgery of the liver and intrahepatic bile ducts. St Louis: Warren H Green, 1972: 366–79

10. Foster JH, Berman M. Solid liver tumors. Vascular tumors. Philadelphia: WB Saunders, 1977: 185–92

11. Henson SW, Gray HK, Dockerty MB. Benign tumours of the liver. Surg Gynecol Obstet 1956; 103: 327–31

12. Jenkins RL, Johnson LB, Lewis WD. Surgical approach to benign liver tumors. Semin Liver Dis 1994; 14: 178–89

13. Malt RA. Current concepts surgery for hepatic neoplasms. N Engl J Med 1985; 313: 1591–6

14. Moreno González E, Calleja Kempin J, Santoyo Santoyo J et al. Indicationen un resultate der chirurgischen behandlung von Kavernöses Hämangiomen. Der Chirurg 1988; 59: 338–40

15. Nichols FC, Van Heerden JA, Weiland LH. Benign liver tumors. Surg Clin North Am 1989; 69: 297

16. Wills JA, Lally JF. Incidental hepatic hemangioma. Del Med J 1992; 64: 589–94

17. Foster JH. Benign liver tumours. In: Blumgart LH, ed. Surgery of the liver and biliary tract, Vol 2. London: Churchill Livingstone, 1988: 1115–27

18. Conter RL, Longmire WP Jr. Recurrent hepatic hemangiomas: possible association with estrogen therapy. Ann Surg 1988; 207: 115–9

19. Belghiti J, Vilgrain V. Management of hemangiomas. In: Lygidakis NJ, Makuuchi M, eds. Pitfalls and complications in the diagnosis and management of hepatobiliary and pancreatic diseases. Stuttgart: G. Thieme Verlag, 1993: 78–85

20. Ishak KG, Rabin L. Benign tumours of the liver. Med Clin N Am 1975; 59: 995–1013

21. Mouiel J, Mazarguil P, Teboul J, Bruneton JN, Huguet C. L'Hemangiome. In: Huguet CL, Mouiel J, eds. Les tumours primitives du foie chez l'adulte. Monographies de L'Association Française de Chirurgie. Paris: Masson, 1983: 47–71

22. Oschner JL, Halpert B. Cavernous hemangioma of the liver. Surgery 1958; 43: 577–82

23. Adami GL. Principles of pathology. Philadelphia: Lea & Febiger, 1910

24. Kawarada Y, Mizumoto R. Surgical treatment of giant hemangioma of the liver. Am J Surg 1984; 148: 287–91

25. Reyes M, Monsalve V, Hepp J, Vaccaro H. Hemangioma hepático gigante y embarazo. Rev Chil Obstet Ginecol 1992; 57: 359–61

26. Losa Garcia JE, Sanchez Sanchez R, García Iglesias MC, González Villaron L. Asociacion de endometriosis con afección urinaria y hemangioma hepático. Med Clin Barc 1993; 27, 100: 318

27. Fost NC, Esterly NB. Successful treatment of juvenile hemangiomas with prednisone. J Pediat 1968; 72: 55–7

28. Klatskin G. Hepatic tumours: possible relationship to oral contraceptives. Gastroenterology 1977; 73: 386–94

29. Mays ET, Christopherson WM, Mahr MM. Hepatic changes in young women ingesting contraceptive steroids: hepatic hemorrhage and primary hepatic tumors. JAMA 1976; 235: 730–2

30. Letulle M. Anatomie pathologique. Vol I. Masson Ed, 1931: 130

31. Rios L, Gajardo P, Olea E, Orellana P, Marinovic I. Pool sanguineo en el estudio del hemangioma hepático. Rev Med Chil 1993; 121: 1149–53

32. Trastek VF, Van Heerden JA, Sheedy T, Adson MA. Cavernous hemangiomas of the liver: resect or observe? Am J Surg 1983; 145: 49–53

33. Shimada M, Matsumata T, Ikeda Y et al. Multiple hepatic hemangiomas with significant arterioportal venous shunting. Cancer 1994; 73: 304–7

34. Winograd J, Palubinskas A. Arterial–portal venous shunting in cavernous hemangioma of the liver. Radiology 1977; 122: 331–2

35. Bornman PC, Terblanche J, Blumgart RL, Harris-James EP, Kalvaria I. Giant hepatic hemangiomas: diagnostic and therapeutic dilemmas. Surgery 1987; 101: 445–9

36. Grieco MB, Miscall BC. Giant hemangiomas of the liver. Surg Gynecol Obstet 1978; 147: 783–7

37. Paksoy N. Giant hemangioma of the liver. An observation from Samoa Islands. Trop Geogr Med 1992; 44: 69–71

38. Nelson RC, Chezmar JL. Diagnostic approach to hepatic hemangiomas. Radiology 1990; 176: 11–21

39. Tsai MK, Lee PH, Tung BS, Yu SCh, Lee ChS, Wei TCh. Experiences in surgical management of cavernous hemangioma of the liver. Hepato-Gastroenterology, 1995; 42: 988–92

40. Belli L, De Carlis L, Beatin C, Rondicara G, Sansalone V, Brambilla G. Surgical treatment of symptomatic giant hemangiomas of the liver. Surg Gynecol Obstet 1992; 174: 474–8

41. Bruncton JN, Dravillard J, Fenart D, Roux P, Nicolay A. Ultrasonography of hepatic cavernous hemangiomas. Br J Radiol 1985; 56: 791–5

42. Weimann A, Repp H, Klempnauer J et al. Diagnostic value of colour Doppler sonography in primary liver tumors – a trend study. Bildgebung 1993; 60: 140–3

43. Kojimahara M. Ultrastructural study of hemangiomas. Acta Pathol Jn 1986; 36: 1477–85

44. Larcher VF, Howard ER, Mowat AP. Hepatic haemangioma: diagnosis and management. Arch Dis Child 1981; 65: 7–14

45. About I, Capdeville J, Bernard P, Lazorthes F, Beneu B. Hemangiome hepatique geant inextirpable et syndrome de Kasabach-Merritt. Rev Med Interne 1994; 15: 846–50

46. Longeville JH, De la Hall P, Dolan P et al. Treatment of a giant haemangioma of the liver with Kasaback-Meritt syndrome by orthotopic liver transplant, a case report. HPB Surg 1997; 10 (3): 159–62

47. Feldman M. Hemangioma of the liver. Special reference to its association with cysts of the liver and pancreas. Am J Clin Pathol 1958; 29: 160–2

48. Foster JH. History of liver surgery. Arch Surg 1991; 126: 381–7

49. Michter LS, Tompkins RK. Three histologically different benign liver tumours in a single patient. Surg Gastroenterol 1982; 2: 277–88

50. Mungovan JA, Cronan JJ, Vacarro J. Hepatic cavernous hemangiomas: lack of enlargement over time. Radiology 1994; 191: 111–3

51. Shumaker HB. Hemangioma of the liver. Discussion of symptomatology and report of patient treated by operation. Surgery 1942; 11: 209–22

52. Wewell JH, Weiss K. Spontaneous rupture of hemangioma of the liver: a review of the literature and presentation of illustrative case. Arch Surg 1981; 83: 729–33

53. Yamamoto T, Kawarada Y, Yano R, Noguchi T, Mizumoto R. Spontaneous rupture of hemangioma of the liver: treatment with transcatheter hepatc arterial embolization. Am J Gastroenterol 1990; 14: 468–71

54. Faure JL. Tumeurs du foie. In: Traité de chirurgie clinique et opératoire. Vol VIII. Paris: Baillière, 1899; 239

55. Taavitsainen M, Airaksinen T, Krevla J, Paivansali M. Fine-needle aspiration biopsy of liver hemangioma. Acta Radiol 1990; 31: 69–74

56. Schwartz SI, Cowles Husser W. Cavernous hemangioma of the liver: a single institution report of 16 resections. Ann Surg 1987; 205: 456–65

57. Hobbs KEF. Hepatic hemangiomas. World J Surg 1990; 14: 468–71

58. Dubois M. La radiotherapie dans le traitement de l'hemangiome caverneux du foie. These Lyon, 1982

59. Farlow DC, Little JM, Gruenewald SM, Antico VG, O'Neill P. A case of metastatic malignancy masquerading as a hepatic hemangioma of labeled red blood cell scintigraphy. J Nucl Med 1993; 34: 1172–4

60. Zafrani ES. Update on vascular tumours of the liver. J Hepatology 1989; 8: 125–30

61. Bree RL, Schwab RE, Neiman HC. Solitary echogenic spot in the liver: is it diagnostic of a hemangioma? AJR 1983; 140: 41–5

62. Itai Y, Ohtomo K, Araki R, Furvi S, Ilo M, Atomi Y. Computed tomography and sonography of cavernous hemangioma of the liver. Am J Radiol 1983; 141: 315–20

63. Jacobson AF, Teefey SA. Cavernous hemangiomas of the liver. Association of sonographic appearance and results of Tc-99m labeled red blood cell SPECT. Clin Nucl Med 1994; 19: 96–9

64. Moody AR, Wilson SR. Atypical hepatic hemangioma: a suggestive sonographic morphology. Radiology 1993; 188: 413–7

65. Patiel HJ, Patriquin HB, Keller MS, Babcock DS, Leithiser RE. Infantile hepatic hemangioma: Doppler US. Radiology 1992; 182: 735–42

66. Ferrucci TJ. Liver tumor imaging. Cancer 1991; Suppl 67: 1189–95

67. Okai T, Mouri I, Yamaguchi Y, Ohta H, Motoo Y, Sawabu N. Hepatic hemangioma showing a mass effect on the stomach well: endosonographic differentiation from submucosal tumor of the stomach. J Clin Gastroenterol 1993; 16: 168–70

68. Abuhamad AZ, Lewis D, Inati MN, Johnson DR, Copel JA. The use of colour flow Doppler in the diagnosis of fetal hepatic hemangioma. J Ultrasound Med 1993; 12: 223–6

69. Sepulveda WH, Donetch G, Giuliano A. Prenatal sonographic diagnosis of fetal hepatic hemangioma. Eur J Obstet Gynecol Reprod Biol 1993; 48: 73–6

70. Graham E, Cohen AW, Soulen M, Faye R. Symptomatic liver hemangioma with intra-tumor hemorrhage treated by angiography and embolization during pregnancy. Obstet Gynecol 1993; 81 (5, part 2): 813–16

71. Paolillo V, Sicuro M, Nejrotti A, Rizzetto M, Casaccia M. Pulmonary embolism due to compression of the inferior vena cava by a hepatic hemangioma. Tex Heart Inst J 1993; 20: 66–8

72. Lee CW, Chung UH, Lee GC, Kim JY, Lee JS. A case of giant hemangioma of the liver presenting with fever of unknown origin. J Korean Med Sci 1994; 9: 200–4

73. Linana Santafe JJ, Calvo Catala FJ, Hortelano Martínez E, González Cruz I, Martínez San Juan V. Hemangiomas hepáticos y artritis reumatoide en pacientes tratados con azatioprina. An Med Interna 1992; 9: 498–500

74. Kudo M, Ikekubo K, Yamamoto K et al. Distinction between hemangioma of the liver and hepatocellular carcinoma: value of labeled RBC-SPELT scanning. 1989; AJR Am J Roentgenol 152(5): 977–1002

75. Tang DJ, Lang YM, Feng YZ. Evaluation of combined assays of serum ferritin, alpha-1-antitrypsin and alpha-fetoprotein in liver cancer. Chin Med J Engl 1992; 105: 900–4

76. Iwatsuki S, Todo S, Starzl TE. Excisional therapy for benign hepatic lesions. Surg Gynecol Obstet 1990; 171: 240–6

77. Kato M, Sugawara I, Okada A et al. Hemangioma of the liver. Diagnosis with combined use of laparoscopy and hepatic arteriography. Am J Surg 1975; 129: 698–704

78. Dong BW, Wang M, Zie K, Chen MH. In vivo measurements of frequency-dependent attenuation in tumors of the liver. J Clin Ultrasound 1994; 22: 167–74

79. Vecherko UN, Gredzhev FA, Konoplia PP. Diagnostika, Khirurgicheskoe lechenie kavernoznykh hemangiom pecheni. (Diagnosis and surgical treatment of cavernous hemangioma of the liver.) Khirurgiia Mosk 1996; 2: 22–3

80. Duan CW, Lu TZ, Tao WZ, Wang JJ, Han XY. Hepatic cavernous hemangioma. CT findings and pathological basis. Chin Med J Engl 1992; 105: 771–4

81. Johnson CM, Sheedy PF, Stanson AV, Stephens DH, Hattery RR, Adson MA. Computed tomography and angiography of cavernous hemangiomas of the liver. Radiology 1981; 138 (1): 115–21

82. Ito K, Honjo K, Matsumoto T, Tanaka R, Nakada T, Nakanishi T. Distinction of hemangiomas from hepatic tumors with delayed enhancement by incremental dynamic CT. J Comput Assist Tomogr 1992; 16: 572–7

83. Rodriguez Balderrama I, Rodriguez Juarez DA, Rodriguez Bonito R, Quiroga Garza A. Hemangioma hepático en un recien nacido prematuro. Imágenes por resonancia magnética. Bol Med Hosp Infant Mex 1993; 50: 121–4

84. Birnbaum BA, Weinreb JC, Mengibow AJ et al. Definitive diagnosis of hepatic hemangiomas: MR imaging versus Tc-99m labeled red blood cell SPECT. Radiology 1990; 176: 95–102

85. Choi BI, Shin YM, Chung JW, Kim SH, Park JH, Han MC. MR findings of hepatic cavernous hemangioma after intraarterial infusion of iodized oil. Abdom Imaging 1994; 16: 507–11

86. Ito K, Choji T, Nakada T, Nakanishi T, Kurokawa F, Okita K. Multislice dynamic MRI of hepatic tumors. J Comput Assist Tomogr 1993; 17: 390–6

87. Mahfouz AE, Hamm B, Taupitz M, Wolf KJ. Hypervascular liver lesions: differentiation of focal nodular hyperplasia from malignant tumors with dynamic gadolinium-enhanced MR imaging. Radiology 1993; 186: 133–42

88. Auchog DM, Oates E. Hepatic hemangioma in cirrhotics with portal hypertension: evaluation with Tc-99m red blood cell SPECT. Radiology 1994; 191: 115–7

89. Hanafusa K, Ohashi I, Himeno Y, Suzuki S, Shibuya H. Hepatic hemangioma: findings with two-phase CT. Radiology 1995; 196: 465–9

90. Ali A, Berg R, Fordhm EW. False-positive hepatic blood pool SPECT study for hepatic hemangioma. Clin Nucl Med 1994; 19: 687–8

91. Rubin RA, Lichtenstein GR. Scintigraphic evaluation of liver masses: cavernous hepatic hemangioma (clinical conference). J Nucl Med 1993; 34: 2278

92. Yamazaki T, Maruoka S, Takahashi S, Sakamoto K. Incidentally visualized hepatic hemangioma during dynamic renoscintigraphy. Clin Nucl Med 1995; 20: 373–4

93. Vomberg PP, Buller HA, Marsman JWP, Lam J, Van Zaane DJ, Heymans HSA. Hepatic artery embolization: successful treatment of multinodular hemangiomatosis of the liver. Eur J Pediatr 1986; 144: 472–4

94. Hivet M, Elbaz C. Angiome mostreaux du foie traite sans succes par la ligature de l'artere hepatique. Sem Hop Paris 1973; 49, 41: 2681–3

95. Suzuki H, Nimura Y, Kamiya J et al. Preoperative transcatheter arterial embolization for giant cavenous hemangioma of the liver with consumption coagulopathy. Am J Gastroenterol 1997; 92: 688–91

96. Maresca G, Barbaro B, Summaria V et al. Color Doppler ultrasonography in the differential diagnosis of focal hepatic lesions. The 5H U 508A (Levovist) experience. Radiol Med (Torino) 1994; 87 (5 Suppl 1): 41–9

97. Foster JH, Adson MA, Schwartz SI, Starzl ET, Tompkins RK. Symposium: benign liver tumours. Contemp Surg 1982; 21: 67–102

98. Delbet P, Hemangiomes. In: Traité de chirurgie clinique et operatoire. Vol I. Paris: Baillière, 1896: 439–42

99. Baer HU, Dennison AR, Mouton W, Stain SC, Zimmerman A, Blumgart LH. Enucleation of giant hemangiomas of the liver. Ann Surg 1992; 216: 673–6

100. Blumgart LH. Liver resection: liver and biliary tumours. In: Blumgart LH, ed. Surgery of the liver and biliary tract, Vol II. New York: Churchill Livingstone, 1988: 1251–80

101. Farges O, Daradketh S, Bismuth H. Cavernous hemangiomas of the liver: are there any indications for resection? World J Surg 1995; 19: 19

102. Yamagata M, Kanematsu T, Marsumata T, Utsonomiya T, Ikeda Y, Sugimachi K. Management of hemangioma of the liver: comparison of results between surgery and observation. Br J Surg 1991; 98: 1223–5

103. Iwatsuki S, Starzl TE. Personal experience with 411 hepatic resections. Ann Surg 1988; 208: 412–34

104. Alter AJ, Prucell RH, Sh JW. Detection of antibody to hepatitis C virus in prospectively followed transfusion recipients with acute and chronic non-A non-B hepatitis. N Engl J Med 1989; 231: 1494–1500

105. Weimann A, Ringe B, Klempnaver J et al. Benign liver tumours: differential diagnosis and indications for surgery. World J Surg 1997; 21: 983–91

106. Starzl TE, Koep LJ, Neil R III. Excisional treatment of cavernous hemangioma of the liver. Ann Surg 1980; 192: 25–7

107. Pietrabissa A, Giulianotti P, Campatelli A et al. Management and follow-up of 78 giant haemangiomas of the liver. Br J Surg 1996; 83: 915–7

108. Lambilliotte JP. Hepatic resections for benign and malignant tumors. Acta Gastro-Enterol Belg 1980; 43 (7–8): 329–40

109. Nguyen L, Shandling B, Ein S, Stephens C. Hepatic hemangioma in childhood. Medical management or surgical management? J Pediat Surg 1982; 17: 576–9

110. Miyagawa S, Makuuchi M, Kawasaki S, Kakazu T. Criteria for safe hepatic resection. Am J Surg 1995; 169: 586–94

111. Borgonomo G, Razzetta F, Arezzo A, Torre G, Matioli F. Giant hemangiomas of the liver: surgical treatment by liver resection. Hepato-Gastroenterology 1997; 44: 231–4

112. Mercadier M, Pernod R. Hepatectomies et lobectomies reglees pour hemangiomes massifs. Mem Acad Chir 1962; 88: 723–31

113. Jimenez Romero C, Moreno González E, García García I et al. Successful transplantation of a liver graft with a calcified hydatid cyst after back-table resection. Transplantation 1995; 60 (8): 883–4

114. Pringle JH. Notes of the arrest of hepatic hemorrhage due to trauma. Ann Surg 1908, 48: 542–50

115. Huget C, Gavelli A, Chieco A. Liver ischemia for hepatic resection. Where is the limit? Surgery 1992; 111: 251–9

116. Shimada M, Matsumata T, Akazawa K et al. Estimation of risk of major complications after hepatic resection. Am J Surg 1994; 167: 399–403

117. Rees M, Plant G, Wells J, Bygrave S. One hundred and fifty hepatic resections: evolution of technique towards bloodless surgery. Br J Surg 1996; 83: 1526–9

118. Huget C, Gallot D. Les ligatures de l'artere hepatique. Med Chir Dig 1972; 117: 313–5

119. Delriviere L, Hannoun L. In situ and ex situ in vivo procedures for complex major liver resections requiring prolonged hepatic vascular exclusion in normal and diseased livers. J Am Coll Surg 1995; 181: 272–6

120. Issa P. Cavernous hemangiomas of the liver. The role of radiotherapy. Br J Radiol 1968; 41: 26–32

121. Park WC, Phillips R. The role of radiation therapy in the management of hemangiomas of the liver. J Am Med Assoc 1970; 212: 1496–8

122. Okazaki N, Yoskino M, Yoshido T, Ohno T, Kilagania T, Hatto N. Radiotherapy of hemangioma cavernosum of the liver. Gastroenterology 1977; 13: 353–6

123. Nishida O, Satoh N, Alam AS, Uchino J. The effect of hepatic artery ligation for unresectable cavernous hemangioma of the liver. Am Surg 1988; 54: 483–8

124. Magnenat P, Delaloye B, Couinaud C. Angiomes diffus inextirpables du foie: une 3e. observation d'hemangiome diffus du foie traite par injections sclerosantes. Rev Med Chir Mal Foie 1962; 37: 102–6

11 Management strategies for benign cysts and polycystic disease of the liver

Francis Sutherland and Bernard Launois

Biliary cysts and polycystic liver disease were for a long time relatively unknown; they were only discovered when symptoms or complications occurred. With the development of improved imaging techniques the asymptomatic forms of this disease were first appreciated.

Simple biliary cysts and polycysts have in common three characteristics: they are cysts that normally do not communicate with the biliary tract; the surface of the cysts is composed of cuboidal or columnar epithelium, identical to normal biliary epithelium, resting on thin connective tissue and without precise separation from displaced hepatic parenchyma; the intracystic liquid is relatively acellular and the composition is similar to independent secretions of biliary cells.[1,2] These criteria facilitate separation from the other intrahepatic cystic formations, in particular hydatid cysts and biliary cystadenomas.

The congenital origin of biliary cysts is the same for the simple cysts and the polycysts of polycystic liver disease. They develop from embryonic canalicular vestiges formed by an excess of progenitor cells from the cranial hepatic pouch at the time of their differentiation towards biliary cells and hepatocytes. These vestiges are known under the name biliary microhamartomas or von Meyenburg complexes.[3]

Natural history of simple biliary cysts

Simple biliary cysts are found in 1.6 to 3.6% of subjects during ultrasound examination for other indications.[4,5] Their frequency increases with age; simple biliary cysts are unusual before the age of 10 years, and attain the maximum frequency between 50 and 60 years. They are more frequent in women by a 5:1 ratio. This female predominance is even more accentuated for very large cysts and cysts that are symptomatic or complicated.[6,7] The majority of cysts detected by ultrasound are small; 60% have a diameter less than 2 cm and fewer than 20% are more than 1 cm in diameter. In 30% of cases the cysts are multiple, from two to five, without systematic topography.[7] Giant cysts are rare.

Simple biliary cysts are lesions that may or may not increase in size. During successive ultrasound examination fewer than 20% of cysts are noted to have an increase in their volume and only one time in four does growth attain double the initial volume estimate. Only in rare cases does size increase occur rapidly, in less than a year.[8]

The majority of biliary cysts are asymptomatic and their discovery is incidental. The relationship between symptoms of abdominal pain and the presence of a biliary cyst must be accepted with caution and one must consider this only for large cysts where the diameter exceeds 8 cm.[6,7] The temporary disappearance of the symptoms after needle aspiration can serve as an argument in favor of responsibility of the cyst for symptoms. Otherwise it is a diagnosis of exclusion after ruling out biliary, stomach and colon pathology. Complications are unusual: compression of the biliary tree, vascular compression (vena cava or hepatic veins), intracystic hemorrhage, biliary fistula, rupture and cyst infection. Malignant degeneration is extremely rare because, unlike cystadenomas, the epithelial borders of the biliary cysts do not undergo active proliferation.

In summary, one can emphasize that simple biliary cysts are common, with little or very slow growth, and they rarely produce symptoms or complications.

The factors that cause the development of subsidiary small cysts, giant cysts, symptomatic cysts and the complicated cysts have not been established.

Natural history of the polycystic liver in the adult

This term is designated for the presence of more than three cysts and is often reserved for the genetic forms of the illness in the setting of polycystic liver and kidney disease. In fact, polycystic liver disease can be observed in the absence of renal cysts or can be associated with benign kidney cysts, of which the prevalence is equally increased. In the course of genetic polycystic disease the kidney disease always proceeds the hepatic disease.

The appearance of the liver cysts generally occurs after the renal cysts and the liver cysts are never detected before the age of 15 years. The number of cysts and their size increases progressively with age. The percentage of patients suffering from symptoms is less than 20% before the age of 30 and exceeds 75% after the age of 60 years.[9]

Three factors are associated with an increased number of cysts and progressive disease: female sex, number of pregnancies and presence of polycystic kidney disease. The severity of the polycystic renal disease correlates with the expansion of liver cysts explaining the frequency of symptomatic polycystic liver disease in dialysis patients.[10]

In the absence of biliary or vascular compression or other associated hepatic disease the development of cysts in not accompanied by a reduction in the volume of liver parenchyma quantified by CT scan, even when the cystic volume surpasses the liver parenchyma volume.[11] This preservation of the liver parenchymal mass explains the absence of liver function abnormalities. Complications like biliary compression with cholestasis, vascular compression and intraperitoneal rupture are unusual. Like the simple biliary cyst, the alteration in the tissue covering the epithelium with atrophy and then erosion of the epithelium are probably responsible for intracystic hemorrhage, biliary connections and bacterial infection with suppuration. The last problem is serious; it is the major cause of death from liver disease in adult patients suffering from polycystic kidney disease on dialysis.[10]

Diagnosis of biliary cysts

The diagnosis of biliary cysts is usually simple and relies on ultrasound (or the CT scan) examination that shows a round clear image, without septae, strictly anechoic, and with accentuation of echoes beyond the cyst. The differential diagnosis includes a young hydatid cyst, non-calcified and not containing daughter cysts. The hydatid serology is negative in 10 to 15% of hydatid cysts, and this occurs more frequently in the young forms. The diagnosis rests on the search for scoleces in the cystic liquid removed by a fine needle under ultrasound control after 3 weeks of treatment with albendazole. An intracystic hemorrhage modifies the ultrasound appearance of biliary cysts. False septae can appear after hemorrhage that correspond to fibrinous deposits; the contents of the cyst are then not strictly anechoic. Magnetic resonance imaging gives an excellent evaluation of liver cysts, permitting differentiation of complicated biliary cysts from hydatid cysts and cystadenomas. Biliary cystadenomas without septa can occasionally appear identical to a simple cyst. Cyst fluid analysis for tumor markers CEA and CA 19–9 can distinguish the difference.[12]

Certain hepatic metastases appear cystic, particularly neuroendocrine tumors, sarcomas and epidermoid carcinomas. These cystic lesions are always associated with tissue lesions, and this allows differentiation from simple biliary cysts.

Management of simple biliary cysts

No treatment

The best treatment is no intervention in cases of asymptomatic, moderately symptomatic or non-complicated disease. The discovery by imaging of an asymptomatic cyst can result in the demand for intervention from a hypochondriac patient. It is important to resist the temptation to offer these patients surgery.

Sclerotherapy

The non-surgical treatment is needle puncture; however, aspiration alone results in recurrence of all cysts within 2 years.[13] More recently, the use of aspiration followed by sclerotherapy has gained popularity. A number of sclerosants have been tried including pantopaque,[14] tetracycline, minocycline and alcohol.[15–17] The use of formalin has been abandoned because of reports of sclerosing cholangitis in cases of bile duct communication. Good success has been reported with alcohol.[16,18–23]

This technique produces a chemical cystitis which destroys the epithelial layer of the cyst wall and results in a secondary reactive sclerosis. Epithelial lining cells are fixed and non-viable after 1–3 minutes of contact with 95% alcohol.[16] Inflammatory cells have been noted as deep as 0.5 mm from the surface.[16]

The technique most often reported involves ultrasound or CT guided placement of a pigtail catheter in the cyst, followed by a cystogram to rule out biliary communications. The cyst fluid is usually completely clear, 'sweetwater cyst', and in such a circumstance the chance of biliary communication is low. However, because any communication risks catastrophic sclerosis of the biliary tree, a radiograph is prudent.[18] A cystogram may also demonstrate if there is a significant leak that could result in spillage of the sclerosant into the peritoneal cavity. If the cyst fluid is not clear the diagnosis should be questioned, as this suggests infection or malignancy. Fluid should routinely be sent for cytology to rule out cancer, culture to rule out infection, and microscopy to rule out hydatid scolicies. As much of the fluid as possible should be removed from the cavity to prevent dilution of the ethanol. Ninety-five per cent ethanol is utilized and the amount recommended varies in the different studies; usually about 10–30% of the aspirated volume up to 100 ml is instilled. The alcohol is left for 20–30 minutes and then drained, during which the patient's position is changed to allow complete contact of the sclerosant with the cyst endothelium.

Most authors recommend immediate removal of the catheter and report successful treatment of the cyst with one treatment.[16,18,20] These procedures can be performed on an outpatient basis or with overnight stay. Immediate follow-up usually reveals a residual cyst cavity that may increase in size for several weeks but thereafter either remains stable or decreases in size for up to 2 years.[18] The walls of the cyst are thickened and infolded. Repeat sessions for large cysts may be necessary and some authors report leaving the catheter in place and using the amount of drainage to guide the number of trials of sclerotherapy to use (up to 11 repeat sessions).[19,24]

Pain is reported as the most frequent complication, present in up to 100% of patients.[18] This has resulted in modification of technique in some series by either premedicating the patient with pethidine[18] or the use of a local anesthetic agent either injected before or mixed with the sclerosant. The presence of pain may be the indicator of a significant leak into the peritoneal cavity. In this circumstance postponing the procedure

for 24 hours will allow the leak to seal and the sclerotherapy to proceed uneventfully. The catheter may be either left in situ or removed and reinserted the following day. Because of the leakage problem, pigtail catheters placed by the Seldinger technique are preferable to simple needle puncture. Some authors report placing the catheter through liver tissue to reduce the possibility of leakage from the cyst.[18]

Postsclerotherapy infection has been reported in the literature[16,19,22] and we have seen infection in two patients that eventually required operative intervention. Because treatment involves a large dead space the risk of infection is real and strict aseptic technique must be followed. Antibiotic prophylaxis should be considered. The longer the catheter is left in place, the increased likelihood of contamination of the cyst cavity. For this reason we feel immediate removal after sclerotherapy is best. Treatment of a postsclerotherpy infection in the residual cyst cavity can be effected by replacement of the drain and intravenous antibiotics. Infection and recurrence may be related to the size of the cysts, with the very large cysts more susceptible to both. After these problems surgical treatment is made more difficult.

Other problems with percutaneous therapy include bleeding and bile duct fistulization. Indeed, any connection with the biliary tree from this procedure likely occurs by transgression of the bile duct during needle placement. At the first sign of bile or significant bleeding the procedure should be terminated and open surgical management considered if problems progress. Histologic examination of previously resected cysts that have been treated with alcoholization demonstrates pronounced fibrosis of the cyst wall.[18] This raises the theoretical question of possible damage to the compressed vasculobiliary structures in the cyst wall; however, to date this kind of problem has not been reported.

Elevation in the blood alcohol level after sclerotherapy has been investigated by a number of authors.[18–20] Most report very low or negligible ethanol levels.[18] Repeated application of alcohol, prolonged procedures or the use of a large amount of alcohol in a large cyst may result in more elevated levels.[20] At the termination of the procedure maximal amounts of alcohol should be removed from the cyst cavity and the patients should be advised not to drive a vehicle.[19]

Perhaps the major problem with cyst alcoholization is the inadvertent treatment of malignancy as a result of the inability to histologically confirm the diagnosis, as reported by vanSonnenberg et al.[19] Almost all reports of hepatic cyst treatment contain cases of simple cysts being mistaken for malignant cysts, either cystadenomas or cystic metastasis. The Lahey clinic series found two out of 18 non-parasitic cysts were neoplastic.[25] Furthermore, 3% of all liver metastases are cystic.[26,27] After successful sclerotherapy the cyst may appear as a convoluted, echodense network,[18] that may make differentiation from a malignancy difficult. Careful preoperative screening will diminish but not eliminate this problem.

The results of percutaneous sclerotherapy are promising, with most authors reporting an initial success rate from 80 to 100%.[16,18–23] The analysis of the different studies is complicated by a number of factors. Many series include patients with polycystic liver disease and hydatid disease where the outcomes are likely to be different. Most series are small, ranging from 10 to 30 patients. How success is defined varies from symptomatic relief, to ablation of the cyst, to a reduction in volume.[18] Serious complications are rare but a number of patients do go on to surgical therapy.[18] Follow-up ranges from 6 months to 2 years and small residual cystic cavities occur in up to 28% of patients.[18] Larger studies with long follow-up and standardized outcome measures including quality of life scales will help establish the usefulness of this technique.

How to decide which patients are candidates for percutaneous sclerotherapy is at present unclear. Patients with contraindications to surgery, including poor cardiopulmonary tolerance, are among the best candidates. It should also be considered in patients who have had extensive previous upper abdominal surgery, where adhesions may make laparoscopy or open surgery difficult. Futhermore, in this situation surgical fenestration may be predisposed to recurrence because of early isolation of the cyst cavity and a limited resorptive surface area. Another situation where alcohol sclerotherapy offers an advantage is in the patient with failed surgical management of a large cyst, a cyst that is situated deep in the hepatic parenchyma or a cyst that is located in segments VII and VIII.

Open surgical treatment

Until recently problematic large hepatic cysts have been exclusively treated by open surgery. It has been recognized that external drainage or aspiration is associated with complications and recurrence.[13,28] Unroofing/fenestration of the cyst has emerged as the most popular treatment.[28] Initially the cyst should be aspirated and the contents examined for hydatid scolicies; cytology and culture should also be performed. Cloudy fluid should be sent for gram stain to rule out infection. The unroofing technique involves removal of the protruding dome of the cyst back to hepatic parenchyma, exposing the secretory epithelium to the peritoneal cavity. As much cyst wall as possible should be removed and results are best when at least one third of the cyst wall is excised.[29] The edges should be sutured to prevent bleeding and bile leakage. The fluid is usually absolutely clear unless there has been previous bleeding, infection or biliary communication. Careful inspection of the inside of the cyst wall and biopsy of any irregular, papillary or solid elements is essential to rule out malignancy.[28] Several series have included cases of previously unrecognized malignancies that were diagnosed at surgery and treated with resection rather than unroofing.[25,26,28] The resected specimen of cyst wall should be examined histologically to rule out unusual malignancies such as cystadenomas or cystic liver metastasis. Electrocoagulation of the remaining cyst wall may decrease secretory epithelium and prevent recurrence. However, it carries with it a risk of damaging underlying blood vessels or bile ducts. Argon beam electrocautery is safer as thermal damage is more superficial; care should still be taken as there is still a theoretical risk of injuries.[30] Because success depends on creating a permanent communication between the cyst and the peritoneal cavity, the placement of omentum in the cyst cavity may facilitate drainage and prevent recurrence. This is particularly applicable in posteriorly placed cysts where peritoneal drainage may be interrupted by the formation of adhesions to the diaphragm.

The abdomen should be closed tightly and in most cases drains are not necessary. Significant ascites is rarely a problem and results of this procedure are generally reported as excellent, with only rare recurrences in most series.[28,29,31] The unusual discovery of bile within the cyst cavity should prompt a search for the leaking ductule and closure with oversewing. Cyst jejunostomy is not indicated as it is associated with significant septic complications.[28]

Other therapy recommended for symptomatic solitary cysts has included local excision (cystectomy) and anatomic or non-anatomic hepatic resection.[25,26,32–34] This form of therapy is still recommended by some authors who cite high radiologic recurrence rates with unroofing.[26] However, radiologic recurrence must not be confused with symptomatic recurrence. The presence of a small residual cyst cavity is common and the significance in terms of symptomatic recurrence is unproven. Morbidity and mortality rates for major hepatic resections are well established: approximately 30% and 5%, respectively.[35] Hepatic cystectomy performed on large cysts is risky as the surrounding parenchyma is compressed and vasculobiliary structures are often in the walls, as shown in Fig. 11.1. With a cyst deep in the liver it may not be obvious on initial inspection that part of its wall contains one or two hepatic veins or the inferior vena cava. The possible place for resection may be when there

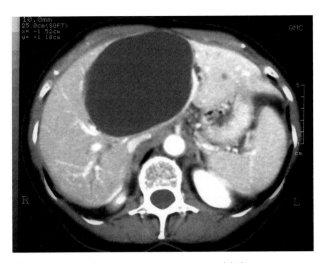

Figure 11.1 A large symptomatic central biliary cyst with glissonian sheath in the left wall. It was treated successfully with unroofing.

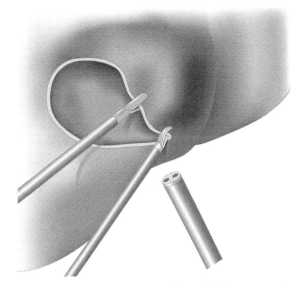

Figure 11.2 Laparoscopic unroofing of a large central simple biliary cyst.

is suspicion that the cyst is neoplastic in origin, or if it is in a superficial location where it can be wedged out. When treating a benign disease that does not affect the patient's longevity one must be careful not to utilize therapy that is riskier than the disease.

The best opportunity to discover malignancy within a simple cyst is by careful inspection of the cyst wall at open surgery. The risk of malignancy in a simple biliary cyst is small, but eight cases of adenocarcinoma and five cases of squamous cell carcinoma have been reported.[36] Most patients present late with jaundice from invasion of the biliary tree.[37] Prognosis in these circumstances is very poor, with no survivor beyond 14 months.[34]

The recurrence of a 'simple biliary cyst' after adequate treatment must raise the possibility that the initial diagnosis was incorrect and a cystadenoma or other tumor was actually present. While this may be more frequent in situations where the cyst was managed without histologic evaluation, it may also occur where the initial histology showed a flat cuboidal epithelium without papillary projections. For this reason all patients should be followed long term.

Laparoscopic surgical treatment

Laparoscopic management of the hepatic cysts is emerging as a new, less invasive therapeutic option. This procedure, as in open surgery, involves wide unroofing of all non-parenchymal cyst wall to allow fluid produced from the epithelial cells of the cyst wall to drain into the free peritoneal cavity where it

can be absorbed, as shown in Fig. 11.2. The cyst edges are more difficult to secure than in open surgery. They can be cauterized and sutured[38] or, alternatively, the endoscopic vascular stapler can be used to resect the cyst wall. This technique is perhaps technically easier and faster than intracorporeal suturing and secures blood vessels and bile ducts effectively. The creation of a flap of omentum off the transverse colon to pack in the cyst cavity may decrease the risk of recurrence.[30] Drainage of the cavity has been suggested to help diagnose and treat bile leakage, with many authors removing drains early after only 24 hours.[30,39] However, bile leakage is rare and drainage is probably not necessary, as with the open procedure.[40]

The gallbladder should be removed if it contains stones or is adjacent to the cyst wall being resected. The rationale for cholecystectomy is to prevent the need for reoperation in a scarred area and eliminate the risk of torsion of a free-floating gallbladder. Furthermore, a symptomatic gallstone can produce pain that is indistinguishable from hepatic cystic disease. An intraoperative cholangiogram is useful in identifying any connection with the biliary tree, which can then be oversewn.

The selection of patients with symptomatic hepatic cysts for laparoscopic treatment is important. Extensive previous upper abdominal surgery is a relative contraindication. The position of the cyst is paramount. Cysts accessible for laparoscopic therapy are located in segments II, III, IVb, and V. Cysts in segments VI and IVa are more difficult to access and conversion may be required.[39] Cysts in the upper segments of the right liver (VII and VIII) are difficult to approach and are associated with a higher rate of recurrence.[39] Cysts in these locations may best be approached by the open technique. Watson and Jamieson have reported successful treatment of a patient with a posterolateral cyst by placing the patient in the lateral position to gain access to the cyst wall.[41]

One of the limitations of laparoscopic unroofing is a restricted examination of the interior of the cyst wall. Visual inspection without palpation may not be adequate to rule out malignancy. This problem may be partly resolved by the use of laparoscopic ultrasound to image the cyst wall.[42] However, in any case where there is a possible diagnosis of a cystadenoma or other malignancy, an open technique with direct examination and biopsy or the cyst wall may be preferable.

The results of laparoscopic unroofing of liver cysts are encouraging. Nevertheless, symptomatic recurrence can occur and complication rates of around 10% are reported.[40,43] However, as with sclerotherapy, most studies have only a few patients and follow-up is short (usually less than 12 months). Strict outcome measures are lacking.

Management of polycystic liver disease

Most frequently multiple cysts in the liver present with a variable number of very large cysts (in general from one to five) associated with much smaller cysts. In the patients with isolated symptomatic large cysts symptoms are comparable to the patients with simple biliary cysts. The treatment consists of treating each one of these voluminous cysts the same as for the isolated simple biliary cysts. The treatment of deep small cysts is often ineffective: alcoholization of each of these cysts is possible but surgical fenestration is simpler and more adaptable.

The fenestration operation was first proposed by Lin in 1968.[44] The procedure involves progressive unroofing of liver cysts, starting on the surface and working to the cysts placed deep in the parenchyma. It is generally reported as successful in relieving symptoms, but is associated with a significant postoperative morbidity of around 50%.[44,45] Recurrence of symptoms is not unusual as cysts in the remaining liver reform and grow.

The situation is different when all the liver is occupied by multiple small cysts, because it is not possible on the preoperative examination to identify which of the cysts are responsible for the symptoms. The symptomatology of these patients is very different and is associated with painful abdominal distention, early

satiety associated with vomiting, loss of muscle bulk and sometimes profound malnutrition. Dyspnea, ascites and edema of the lower extremities may also occur.[45] The treatment consists of fenestration of as many cysts as possible to obtain a total collapse of the liver. This intervention is long because it is necessary to fenestrate the deep cysts pocket by pocket by traversing the more superficial cysts. It must be done very delicately because the vasculobiliary structures are distorted between the cystic layers. It is almost always followed by ascites that can be prolonged and must be accompanied by a rigorous fluid and electrolyte replacement that can attain several liters. The laparoscopic approach is not adaptable to this approach. Surgical fenestration of polycystic liver disease is efficacious in about 75% of patients over the short term; it is accompanied by parenchymal hypertrophy in the remaining liver. Failures are observed in patients where there is no zone of non-cystic hepatic parenchyma and/or a very active cyst secretory epithelium.

In the past, several authors have reported success with the fenestration/resection surgical approach.[46–48] This technique usually involves a non-anatomic resection of either the right or left lobe of the liver, with the addition of unroofing the remaining cyst on the opposite side. The operation is tailored to the patient's anatomy in an attempt to preserve hepatic parenchyma. This is particularly useful when the cyst distribution is asymmetrical, as shown in Fig. 11.3.

Proponents of resection/fenestration report very adequate reduction of liver volume and prolonged relief of symptoms.[46–48] However, there is significant risk of intraoperative hemorrhage. The most dangerous structures are the hepatic veins. Anatomy is always very distorted with intrahepatic and extrahepatic bile ducts and blood vessels

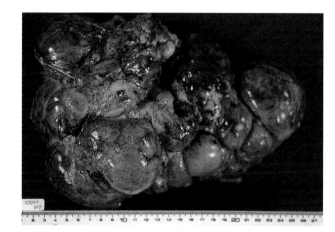

Figure 11.3 Pathological specimen from a left hepatectomy/fenestration for asymmetrical type II polycystic liver disease.

Table 11.1 **Gigot classification of adult polycystic liver disease**
Type I: limited number (<10) of large cysts (>10 cm)
Type II: diffuse involvement of liver parenchyma by multiple, medium-sized cysts with remaining large areas of non-cystic liver parenchyma
Type III: diffuse involvement of liver parenchyma by small- and medium-sized liver cysts and only a few areas of normal liver parenchyma between cysts

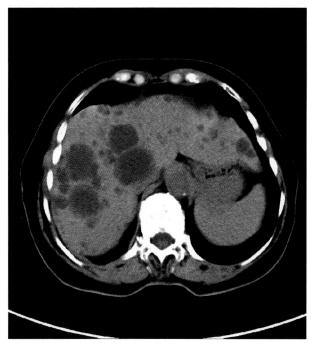

Figure 11.4 Mild type II polycystic liver disease.

compressed between contiguous cyst walls. While control of the hepatic pedicle with a Pringle maneuver is usually possible, control of the hepatic veins from above may be impossible because of intervening liver and cyst tissue. Because of difficulty with exposure once hemorrhage begins it may be very hard to control. With the absence of landmarks there is also the ever present danger of occluding the remaining hepatic vein, creating the acute Budd–Chiari Syndrome.[49] These resections should be performed with care by experienced liver surgeons; intraoperative ultrasound can be a useful tool for choosing safe sites for fenestration or identifying hepatic veins. Collapse of as many superficial liver cysts as possible before the resection is started may aid in exposure. The advantage is more prolonged relief of symptoms with the reduction of cyst surface area and less difficulty with postoperative ascites.

Gigot et al. have produced a useful classification scheme of adult polycystic liver disease according to the number and size of liver cysts and the distribution of liver parenchyma,[50] as shown in Table 11.1. The classification is based on the preintervention CT scan. Therapy should be tailored to the classification. Type I patients have a minimal number of large cysts; Bismuth classified these patients as 'multicystic liver disease', as opposed to polycystic liver disease (types II and III). These patients may benefit from a laparoscopic unroofing with omental interpositions, as in patients with solitary cysts. This minimally invasive approach offers immediate relief of symptoms and is probably associated with the least postinterventional problems. Patients that have a single dominant cyst that can be accessed by percutaneous needle insertion may also benefit from alcohol sclerotherapy. This approach is particularly attractive in elderly patients with co-morbidities, where surgical intervention may be hazardous.

Patients with type II cysts (diffuse involvement of the liver by medium-sized cysts) can benefit from either fenestration or fenestration/resection (Fig. 11.4). Both approaches have their proponents. Fenestration has the advantage of being perhaps a less aggressive and easier approach. The risk of massive intraoperative hemorrhage may be less than with resection, and if the cyst walls are thin there is a satisfactory reduction in size that can result in prolonged relief of symptoms. Problems do exist in that some patients have a relatively rigid liver skeleton, probably based on fibrotic reaction, that does not allow collapse after decompression (type III). Furthermore, extensive fenestration without resection exposes large amounts of a secretory biliary type of endothelium to the free peritoneal surface.[45,48] The resulting fluid load may overwhelm the peritoneal cavity's absorptive capacity and result in ascites. The long-term results are probably not as favorable as resection/fenestration.[48]

Patients with the most severe form of adult polycystic liver disease are the patients with Gigot type III anatomy. Here no part of the liver is spared from involvement and the cysts are small, making fenestration difficult. There are often no large areas of uninvolved hepatic parenchyma. Furthermore, the liver is often quite rigid, with significant fibrosis of cyst walls, limiting the amount of collapse that occurs with fenestration.[50] Gigot et al. have demonstrated a significant post-therapy increase in size of residual cysts over the long term in type III disease.[50] Farges and Bismuth reported recurrence of symptoms in three out of five patients they treated with numerous small cysts and no large areas of parenchyma (Gigot type III).[45] Resection has been shown to effectively decrease liver volume in these patients, however, the risks are high. Turnage reported significant morbidity and postoperative death in three out of five patients with this type of polycystic liver disease treated with resection and/or fenestration.[51]

There are several reports of successful transplantation of patients with polycystic liver disease.[52,53] This therapy has been generally reserved for end stage patients with a syndrome described as lethal exhaustion.[52] These patients have reached the end of their functional lives and can no longer carry the weight of their enlarged livers. Fatigue, cachexia and narcotic addiction are often present. Many of these patients present late or after a series of partially successful fenestration operations. Renal failure and a need for kidney transplantation may also prompt the decision to transplant the liver, using the same donor for both organs. Postoperative morbidity with these type of procedures is high and mortality is 25–30%.[52,53] Patients are often in poor condition for this type of major surgical intervention and this is a persuasive argument for more aggressive therapy earlier in the course of their treatment. Recent reports suggest improvement in survival following transplantation.[54] Successful living donor liver transplantation has now been reported in a patient with polycystic liver disease.[55] These are among the most difficult and rare cases and should be handled in experienced centers that can offer both forms of therapy, resection and transplantation.[56]

The decision on the best type of therapy for each patient depends very much on the stage at which the patient presents and the type of cysts present, including size and position. Clearly, patients that are presenting late after previous surgical interventions, with massively enlarged livers and/or chronic renal insufficiency, should be treated differently from the patient presenting for the first time with pressure symptoms from a large dominant cyst.

Prevention and management of biliary complications

Biliary complications are among the most frequent postoperative problems. They most commonly present in the early postoperative period with a bile leak and/or biliary ascites. These leaks no doubt result from an inability to secure small bile ducts in the resected cyst walls. They also appear to occur with equal incidence with fenestration and fenestration/resection procedures.[47,50] Their prevention starts with meticulous surgical technique which includes oversewing any thick cyst wall. Leakage

can be assessed intraoperatively by applying dry sponges on the raw areas and looking for bile staining, or by performing an intraoperative cholangiogram after cholecystectomy (a recommended procedure in all cases). Very small leaks may not be discovered on cholangiogram so injecting air or a dilute solution of methylene blue into the bile duct with direct vision of the resected area may be efficacious. Fibrin glue (Tissucol) may also be applied to large areas to prevent small leaks.[47]

In rare circumstances a cyst may be found to contain bile stained fluid, indicating a biliary connection. Some authors in this circumstance have recommended cyst jejunostomy.[31,33] We feel this is inappropriate and can be associated with significant infectious complications. Sewing a piece of bowel to a cyst creates a large, contaminated, poorly drained cavity that connects with the biliary tree. It predisposes the patient to developing abscesses and/or cholangitis.[28,57] In the same manner that cyst jejunostomies for choledocal cysts have been abandoned so should this practice with biliary cysts. Direct suture closure of the connection with the biliary tree and decompression of the common bile duct with a T-tube, transcystic duct drain or internal biliary stent are preferred. If the cyst is superficial consideration should be given to a non-anatomical resection of the entire cyst area.

Once a biliary leak has been detected postoperatively management begins with fluid and electrolyte resuscitation and intravenous antibiotic therapy. CT or ultrasound guided placement of a percutaneous drain may be the only therapy required. Endoscopic retrograde cholangiography has proven very useful in these circumstances, first in diagnosing the site of leakage and then treating the leak by placing an endoscopic stent to reduce bile duct pressure.

Prevention and management of postoperative ascites

Postoperative ascites has emerged as a significant problem in the therapy of polycystic liver disease. It is present in up to 70% of cases and may be more common in patients with renal insufficiency and in patients with the type III disease.[45] This may be the result of a higher secretion rate and a larger exposed surface area and/or blockage of diaphragmatic lymphatics from the extensive fibrosis associated with this disease type.

Minor postoperative ascites is best ignored as the absorptive capacity of the peritoneum will increase and the fluid will likely resorb within one or two weeks. Massive ascites, however, presents a significant problem. It can compromise respiration and postoperative mobilization. There is an ever present risk of infection. Furthermore, it may have deleterious effects on already compromised renal function. For this reason several groups do not offer surgical therapy to patients with renal insufficiency until after correction with kidney transplantation.[46]

Awareness of the problem is probably most important. One should attempt to minimize the amount of residual epithelium by extensively removing as much of the cyst walls as possible or by resecting a segmental area. Postoperative ascites is probably reduced in the resection/fenestration operation compared to fenestration alone, as less of the secretory epithelium is left in contact with the peritoneal cavity. Cyst cavities exposed to the peritoneum can be fulgurated by electrocautery or argon beam coagulation (Bard Electromedical Systems, Englewood, CO). Que et al.[48] reported only mild postoperative ascites in 7 of 31 of their patients treated with resection/fenestration and fulguration. There is an undefined risk of causing damage to the bilio-vascular elements in the cyst wall, so care should be taken.

Secretion from biliary epithelium may be pharmacologically reduced with either H2 antagonists (ranitidine) or somatostatin and its analogs. Several groups have reported a beneficial effect of these drugs in decreasing postoperative ascites,[47] however, this therapy remains unproven. Other groups have reported treating this problem with repeated peritoneal tapping.[58] There is also a report of placement of a LeVeen shunt for intractable ascites.[19] Tapping and draining should be used as a last resort as this risks infection. Letting time pass will often solve this problem.

Summary

Benign cysts of the liver are common, but rarely cause problems requiring surgery. However, where cysts or polycysts produce disabling symptoms, or if a cystic malignancy is suspected, intervention is required. Because of the rareness of these lesions most clinical series are small and there are no randomized or case-control trials of the different treatment options. Thus, clinical decisions must be based on the lowest level of evidence, the case report or small clinical series. In this situation one must rely on reports from referral institutions with the largest numbers of patients treated. One must also rely on one's own clinical judgment and experience. When subjecting these patients to surgery, extensive liver resection and biliary reconstruction may be required. Referring a patient with one of these rare conditions to a center with specialized expertise may be in the patient's best interest.

Key points

- The vast majority of simple hepatic cysts are small and asymptomatic and should be left alone.
- Abdominal pain should only be attributed to large (>8 cm) cysts.
- Indications for drainage/resection of simple cysts include:
    Resolution of pain after aspiration
    Compression of biliary tree, cava or portal system
    Intracystic hemorrhage
    Biliary fistula
    Spontaneous/traumatic rupture
    Infection.
- Indications for fenestration in polycystic liver disease:
    Painful abdominal distension
    Early satiety associated with vomiting
    Malnutrition, loss of muscle bulk
    Dyspnea, ascites and ankle edema.

REFERENCES

1. Comfort MW, Gray HK, Tahlin D et al. Polycystic disease of the liver: a study of 24 cases. Gastroenterology 1952; 20: 60–78

2. Patterson M, Gonzales-Vitale JC, Fagam CJ. Polycystic liver disease. A study of cyst fluid constituents. Hepatology 1982; 2: 475–8

3. Melnick PJ. Polycystic liver. Analysis of seventy cases. Arch Pathol 1955; 59: 162–72

4. Bruneton JN, Eresue J, Caramella E et al. Les kystes congenitaux du foie en echographie. J Radiol 1983; 64: 471–6

5. Kunstlinger E. Decouverte echographique fortuite des lesions focalises du foie. Gastroenterol Clin Biol 1983; 7: 951–4

6. Huguier M, Chergui D, Houry S et al. Kysts biliares du foie. Presse Med 1986; 15: 827–9

7. Moreaux J, Block P. Les kystes biliares solitaires du foie. Arch Franc Mal App Digest, 1971; 60: 203–24

8. Griffe J, Crespy C, Lesaut J. Kyst solitaire du foie; evolution rapide (1 an). Presse Med 1975; 4: 32

9. Paliard P, Valette PJ, Bretagnolle M. Kysts biliare et polykystose hepatique. Actualities digestives medicale chirurgicales. Paris: Hansen, 1992: 104–8

10. Grunfeld JP, Albouze G, Jungers P et al. Liver changes and complication in adult polycystic kidney disease. Adv Nephrol 1985; 14: 1–20

11. Everson GT, Emmett M, Brown WR et al. Functional similarities of hepatic cysts and biliary epithelium: studies of fluid constituents and in vivo secretion in response to secretin. Hepatology 1990; 11: 557–65

12. Dixon E, Sutherland FR, Mitchell P et al. Cystadenomas of the liver: a spectrum of disease. Can J Surg 2001; 44: 371–6

13. Saini S, Mueller PR, Ferrucci JT et al. Percutaneous aspiration of hepatic cysts does not provide definitive therapy. AJR 1983; 141: 559–60

14. Goldstein HM, Carlyle DR, Nelson RS. Treatment of symptomatic hepatic cyst by percutaneous instillation of Pantopaque. AJR 1976; 127: 850–3

15. Rosenberg GV. Solitary non-parasitic cysts of liver. Am J Surg 1956; 91: 441–4

16. Bean WJ, Rodan BA. Hepatic cysts: treatment with alcohol. AJR 1985; 144: 237–41

17. Hagiwara H, Kasahara A, Hayashi N et al. Successful treatment of a hepatic cyst by one-shot instillation of minocycline chloride. Gastroenterology 1992; 103: 675–7

18. Larssen TB, Viste A, Jenssen DK et al. Single-session alcohol sclerotherapy in benign symptomatic hepatic cysts. Acta Radiol 1997; 38: 993–7

19. vanSonnenberg E, Wroblicka JT, D'Agostino HB et al. Symptomatic hepatic cysts: percutaneous drainage and sclerosis. Radiology 1994; 190: 387–92

20. Kairaluoama MI, Leinonen A, Stahlberg M et al. Percutaneous aspiration and alcohol sclerotherapy for symptomatic hepatic cysts: an alternative to surgical intervention. Ann Surg 1989; 210: 208–15

21. Montorsi M, Torzilli G, Fumagalli U et al. Percutaneous alcohol sclerotherapy of a simple hepatic cyst. Results from a multicentre survey in Italy. HPB Surg 1994; 8: 89–94

22. Simonetti G, Profili S, Sergiacomi GL et al. Percutaneous treatment of hepatic cysts by aspiration and sclerotherapy. Cardiovasc Intervent Radiol 1993; 16: 81–4

23. Furuta T, Yoshida Y, Saku M et al. Treatment of symptomatic non-parasitic liver cysts—surgical treatment versus alcohol injection therapy. HPB Surg 1990; 2: 269–79

24. Andersson R, Jeppsson B, Lunderquist A et al. Alcohol sclerotherapy of non-parasitic cysts of the liver. Br J Surg 1989; 76: 254–5

25. Jones WL, Moutain JC, Warren KW. Symptomatic non-parasitic cysts of the liver. Br J Surg 1974; 61: 118–23

26. Sanchez H, Gagner M, Rossi R et al. Surgical management of nonparasitic cystic liver disease. Am J Surg 1991; 161: 113–9

27. Federle MP, Filly RA, Moss AA. Cystic hepatic neoplasms: complementary roles of CT and sonography. AJR 1981; 136: 345–8

28. Litwin DEM, Taylor BR, Langer B, Greig P. Nonparasitic cyst of the liver. The case for conservative surgical management. Ann Surg 1987; 205: 45–8

29. Wellwood JM, Madara JL, Cady B, Haggitt RC. Large intrahepatic cysts and pseudocysts. Pitfalls in diagnosis and treatment. Am J Surg 1978; 135: 57–64

30. Emmermann A, Zornig C, Lloyd DM et al. Laparoscopic treatment of nonparasitic cysts of the liver with omental transposition flap. Surg Endosc 1997; 11: 734–6

31. Koperna T, Vogl S, Satzinger U et al. Nonparasitic cyst of the liver: results and options of surgical treatment. World J Surg 1997; 21: 850–5

32. Sanfelippo PM, Beahrs OH, Weiland LH. Cystic disease of the liver. Ann Surg 1974; 179: 922–5

33. Longmire WP, Mandiola SA, Gordon HE. Congenital cystic disease of the liver and biliary system. Ann Surg 1971; 174: 711–5

34. Madariaga JR, Iwatsuki S, Starzl TE et al. Hepatic resection for cystic lesions of the liver. Ann Surg 1993; 218: 610–4

35. Steele G, Ravikumar TS. Resection of hepatic metastases from colorectal cancer. Ann Surg 1989; 210: 127–38

36. Le Borgne J, Lehor PA, Guiberteau-Canfrere V et al. Complications des kystes biliares. A propos de 10 observations. Chirurgie 1994–1995; 120: 181–6

37. Lynch MS, Mcleod MK, Weatherbee L et al. Squamous cell cancer of the liver arising from a solitary benign non-parasitic hepatic cyst. Am J Gastroenterol 1988; 83: 426–31

38. Krahenbuhl L, Baer HU, Renzulli P et al. Laparoscopic management of nonparasitic symptom-producing solitary hepatic cysts. J Am Coll Surg 1996; 183: 493–8

39. Gigot JF, Legrand M, Hubens G et al. Laparoscopic treatment of nonparasitic liver cysts: adequate selection of patients and surgical technique. World J Surg 1996; 20: 556–61

40. Fabiani P, Mazza D, Toouli J et al. Laparoscopic fenestration of symptomatic non-parasitic cysts of the liver. Br J Surg 1997; 84: 321–2

41. Watson DI, Jamieson GG. Laparoscopic fenestration of giant posterolateral liver cyst. J Laparoendosc Surg 1995; 5: 255–7

42. Marvik R, Myrvold HE, Johnson G et al. Laparoscopic ultrasonography and treatment of hepatic cysts. Surg Laparosc Endosc 1993; 3: 172–4

43. Hansman MF, Ryan JA, Holmes JH et al. Management and long-term follow-up of hepatic cysts. Am J Surg 2001; 181: 404–10

44. Lin TY, Chen CC, Wang SM. Treatment of non-parasitic cystic disease of the liver: a new approach to therapy with polycystic liver. Ann Surg 1968; 168: 921–7

45. Farges O, Bismuth H. Fenestration in the management of polycystic liver disease. World J Surg 1995; 19: 25–30

46. Newman KD, Torres VE, Rakela J et al. Treatment of highly symptomatic polycystic liver disease. Ann Surg 1990; 212: 30–7

47. Vauthey JN, Maddern GJ, Blumgart LH. Adult polycystic disease of the liver. Br J Surg 1991; 78: 524–7

48. Que F, Nagorney DM, Gross JB et al. Liver resection and cyst fenestration in the treatment of severe polycystic liver disease. Gastroenterology 1995; 108; 487–94

49. Ambrosetti P, Widmann JJ, Robert J et al. Syndrome aigu de Budd-Chiari apres traitement chirurgical d'une polykystose hepatique. Gastroenterol Clin Biol 1992; 16: 894–6

50. Gigot JF, Jadoul P, Que F et al. Adult polycystic liver disease. Is fenestration the most adequate operation for long-term management? Ann Surg 1997; 225: 286–94

51. Turnage RH, Eckhauser FE, Knol JA et al. Therapeutic dilemmas in patients with symptomatic polycystic liver disease. Am Surg 1988; 54: 365–72

52. Starzl TE, Reyes J, Tzakis A et al. Liver transplantation for polycystic liver disease. Arch Surg 1990; 125: 575–7

53. Lang H, Woellwarth Jv, Oldhafer KJ et al. Liver transplantation in patients with polycystic liver disease. Transplant Proc 1997; 29: 2832–3

54. Pirenne J, Aents R, Yoong K et al. Liver transplantation for polycystic liver disease. Liver Transpl 2001; 7: 238–48

55. Takegoshi K, Tanaka K, Nomura H et al. Successful living donor liver transplantation for polycystic liver in a patient with autosomal-dominant kidney disease. J Clin Gastroenterol 2001; 33: 229–31

56. Henne-Bruns D, Klomp HJ, Kremer B. Non-parasitic liver cysts and polycystic liver disease: Results of surgical treatment. Hepato-Gastroenterol 1993; 40: 1–5

57. Lewis WD, Jenkins RL, Rossi RL et al. Surgical treatment of biliary cystadenoma. Arch Surg 1988; 123: 563–8

58. Huguet C, Hecht Y, Ricordeau P et al. Les enormes polykystoses hepatiques. Med Chir Dig 1973; 2: 227–30

12 Management of choledochal cysts

Matthew Jones and David Lloyd

Incidence

Cystic dilatation of the extrahepatic bile ducts is a rare abnormality in Western countries, with an incidence which has been estimated at around 1 in 15 000 live births.[1] The incidence is much higher in the Far East, and in Japan choledochal cysts may account for up to 1 per 1000 hospital admissions. The male to female ratio has been variably reported as being between 1:2 and 1:4.[2,3] More than 60% of cases present before the age of 10,[4,5] and an increasing number are presenting antenatally as a result of routine ultrasound scanning.[6-8]

History

Abnormalities in the anatomy of the common bile duct were originally described by Vater,[9] but Douglas[10] gave the first detailed account of a patient with massive dilation of the bile duct. He described a 17-year-old girl with the now classic triad of pain, jaundice and a right-sided abdominal mass. This was managed by percutaneous aspiration of 900 ml of bile, but unfortunately the girl died 1 month later. The subsequent postmortem examination confirmed the presence of a choledochal cyst.

Aetiology

The liver and biliary tree arise as a ventral outgrowth (the hepatic diverticulum) of the endodermal epithelium from the caudal part of the foregut early in the fourth week of gestation. The hepatic diverticulum initially consists of solid endodermal cell strands, which later canalize to form the biliary tree. It is widely accepted that the majority of choledochal cysts are congenital lesions,[4] and this is supported by the increasing number which are being detected by antenatal ultrasound scanning, sometimes as early as 17 weeks of gestation.[4,6,11]

There are several theories as to the aetiology of these lesions, but the most popular concerns the presence of an abnormality at the pancreaticobiliary junction. This was first proposed by Babbitt[12] who found that there was a common channel between the lower end of the common bile duct and pancreatic duct, in 19 cases of choledochal cyst. He suggested that this predisposal to reflux of pancreatic secretions up the biliary tree might lead to chronic mucosal damage and thus ductal dilatation. This finding has been corroborated by several other authors,[2,4,13,14] who have shown that a common channel may be present in as much as 75% of choledochal cysts.[2] In such cases the biliary amylase is usually elevated.[15] Babbitt's theory is further supported by an experiment in dogs,[16] in which the pancreatic duct was anastomosed to the gall bladder, resulting in dilatation of the biliary tree and mucosal destruction. A study of human foetuses by Wong[17] showed that the pancreaticobiliary junction does not become incorporated in the duodenal wall until the eighth week of gestation. It is clear that any arrest in this process would tend to result in the creation of a common channel and thus pancreaticobiliary reflux. However, it is unlikely that a common channel is the sole explanation for choledochal cysts as there are many of these lesions in which it is not present.

Other aetiologies which have been suggested include 'weakness of the bile duct wall', 'a primary abnormality of ductal proliferation' and 'congenital duct obstruction'. Such theories are largely speculative, but they are supported by a study in newborn lambs, which showed that lesions similar to choledochal cysts could be produced by simple ligation of the bile duct.[18] Moreover, it has been shown that biliary amylase is not elevated in choledochal cysts which present as a result of antenatal diagnosis,[15] implying the absence of pancreaticobiliary reflux in these patients. This would tend to suggest that such cysts are truly congenital, as opposed to those cysts which present later, and are therefore 'acquired' as a consequence of a common channel anomaly.

Petersen et al[19] created a murine model for extrahepatic biliary atresia by infecting newborn mice with rotavirus group A. Amongst the various pathological

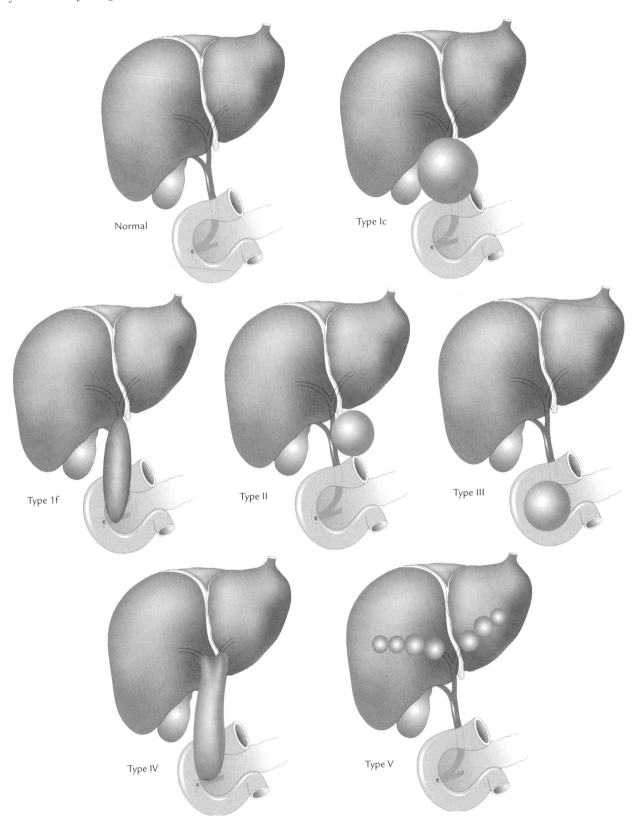

Figure 12.1 Classification of choledochal cysts.

features produced by this model was a single mouse, which developed a ballooning dilatation of the biliary tree. This model is particularly interesting in that it suggests a possible infectious aetiology for some of these lesions. On balance, however, it seems likely that there are a number of possible mechanisms, any or all of which might result in the formation of choledochal cysts.

Pathology

Macroscopic

The macroscopic appearance of choledochal cysts differs widely. They may affect any part of the biliary tree, and the bile duct dilatation may vary from no more than 2 cm, to a giant cyst containing more than a litre of bile. A number of schemes have been devised to classify these lesions, the most widely used of which is that proposed by Alonso-Lej et al. in 1959.[1] They divided the cysts as follows (Fig. 12.1):

- Type Ic: cystic
- Type If fusiform
- Type II: diverticulum
- Type III: choledochocoele (dilatation of intraduodenal bile duct)
- Type IV: extra and intrahepatic dilatation
- Type V: intrahepatic dilatation.

The relative frequency of different cyst types varies from series to series, but there is a general consensus that type Ic accounts for about 50%, type If for 25%, type IV for 10% and type V for 5% of cysts.[2,4,8,14] Types II and III are very rare. Since then, other authors have devised classifications based on the cholangiographic findings of intrahepatic duct or pancreaticobiliary malunion, i.e. the so-called common channel.[3,20,21] These later classifications have the merit of relating the anatomical findings to a possible underlying aetiology, however in practice the choice of classification has little impact on subsequent patient management.

A number of unclassified anatomical variants have been described, most of which relate to the presence of aberrant hepatic ducts,[22,23] cysts without apparent connections to the biliary tree,[24] and associated hepatic duct strictures.[25] The existence of these variants emphasizes the importance of adequate peroperative investigations, in order that they be identified and treated appropriately.

Microscopic

The wall of a choledochal cyst is thickened and may vary from 2.0 to 7.5 mm in thickness. It is composed of fibrous tissue with scanty fibres of smooth muscle and elastic tissue. The cuboidal biliary epithelium may be present, but typically there is extensive ulceration, and only small patches of cells remain. The degree of histological damage appears to correlate with age.[4] In infants with asymptomatic cysts there is fibrosis and epithelial loss, but relatively little inflammation. However, in longstanding cysts there is a marked acute and chronic inflammatory infiltrate. In some of the oldest patients the cysts may show evidence of metaplasia, dysplasia and early adenocarcinoma.[26]

Immunohistochemical studies[27] in 'cystic' choledochal cysts have shown a reduced number of ganglion cells, irrespective of the diameter of the cyst. By contrast, in 'fusiform' cysts, the number of ganglion cells varies according to the severity of the clinical presentation and the age of the patient. This would tend to support the hypothesis that 'cystic' cysts are truly congenital, whilst 'fusiform' cysts are generally acquired.[15,27]

Presentation

Choledochal cysts may present at any age, but the majority (up to 60%) are diagnosed before the age of 10.[2–4,28] The clinical manifestation of choledochal cysts differs according to the age of presentation.

Choledochal cysts used to be uncommon in neonates, but more recently the incidence has been increasing owing to the widespread use of antenatal ultrasound scanning.[6–8,11,15,29] These infants are initially asymptomatic, although a mass may be palpable in the right upper quadrant. For a while there was some question as to whether such cysts might be managed non-operatively.[29] However, it has become increasingly apparent that early intervention is the best course of action, as the majority of these infants go on to develop cyst enlargement and/or obstructive jaundice.[3,8,29] In some cases this may be due to ductal obstruction by an inspissated bile plug.[30]

In older children, the commonest presenting symptoms are jaundice (75%), abdominal pain (50%) and an abdominal mass (30%),[2,4,15] although the classic triad of all three occurs in less than half of cases.[2,4,31–33] In general children tend to present in one of two ways: children with 'cystic' choledochal cysts usually present with a palpable right upper quadrant mass and intermittent obstructive jaundice, whilst those with 'fusiform' choledochal cysts usually present with recurrent abdominal pain due to pancreatitis.[3] It has been reported that the bile ducts are significantly more dilated during the symptomatic phase than the asymptomatic phase, and that this may be the result of acute ductal obstruction by protein plugs.[34] In 1–2% of cases, choledochal cysts may present acutely as a result of cyst rupture with subsequent bile peritonitis.[35] The cause of rupture is usually unknown, and is thought to be spontaneous.[35–37]

Choledochal cysts in adults appear to behave somewhat differently. Although adults may still present with typical features, they are more likely to have developed such complications as calculi, cirrhosis, portal hypertension, hepatic abscesses, bleeding cyst erosions,[38] cholangitis and adenocarcinoma,[39] any of which may be the presenting feature.[4,40,41]

The differential diagnosis of choledochal cysts depends upon the mode and timing of presentation, and includes duplication cysts, biliary atresia, spontaneous perforation of the common bile duct, rhabdomyosarcoma,[42] simple hepatic cysts, mucocoele of the gallbladder, hepatic tumours and lesions of the pancreas, kidney and adrenal gland.

Diagnosis

The diagnosis of choledochal cyst is generally straightforward once the possible diagnosis is considered.

Ultrasonography is usually the first-line investigation of choice. As has been previously mentioned, an increasing number of cysts are being detected antenatally as a result of routine antenatal scanning, and some cysts are being detected as early as 17–19 weeks of gestation.[4,11] Ultrasonography can determine the size, position and shape of the cyst, as well as the anatomy of related structures (Fig. 12.2). However, it is less useful in the case of fusiform cysts, as there

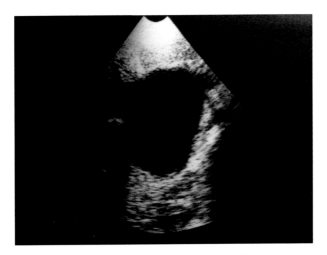

Figure 12.2 Ultrasonography of choledochal cyst.

are limitations in its ability to demonstrate the ductal anatomy at the pancreaticobiliary junction.

A plain abdominal radiograph may show a right upper quadrant mass which displaces bowel, and may reveal some radio-opaque calculi if these are present. Cholangiography provides the most accurate information about the cyst and its associated ductal anatomy. A cholangiogram may be obtained either by the 'percutaneous transhepatic' route (PTC) or by the endoscopic retrograde route (ERCP). However, these are invasive investigations with a significant complication rate, and although they provide excellent anatomical delineation, they rarely produce information which alters the subsequent management of the cyst. The risk of developing necrotizing pancreatitis after ERCP is such that this investigation is contraindicated in patients with active pancreatitis.[3] Most surgeons agree that it is essential to have highly accurate information about the ductal anatomy, and that such information can only be obtained through some form of cholangiography.[43,44] However, this information is best obtained by operative cholangiography, which is simple, safe and accurate. These studies are usually best performed by injecting contrast material directly into the common hepatic and distal common bile ducts, since contrast which is injected directly into the cyst itself tends to be excessively diluted and may not adequately display the ductal anatomy.[4]

Computerized tomography (CT) scanning provides clear images of the cyst and adjacent structures. Its particular value is that it may reveal associated pathology within the parenchyma of related organs. Recent advances in spiral CT cholangiography may enable 3D reconstruction of the biliary tree and provide further anatomical information.[45]

Hepatobiliary scintigraphy with technetium-99m labelled iminodiacetic acid (IDA) derivatives will often show the cyst, and is particularly helpful at establishing that the cystic structure is an intrinsic part of the biliary tree. A typical scan shows an initial filling defect in the liver, followed by a gradual increase in concentration within the cyst, which may take up to 24 hours to become apparent in patients with obstructive jaundice. IDA scanning is also helpful at assessing hepatobiliary function and anastomotic patency postoperatively.

Magnetic resonance imaging (MRI) has been used with increasing success (Fig. 12.3). MR cholangiopancreatography (MRCP) is non-invasive and will produce clear images of the biliary tree (Fig. 12.4), which may even demonstrate the 'common channel'.[5,46,47] At present most images lack the clarity and definition of those obtained by conventional cholangiopancreatography, although this is likely to become less of a problem as technology improves.

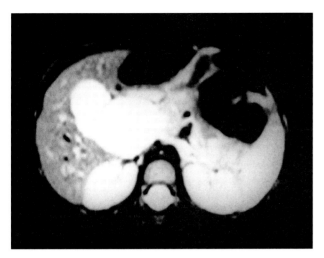

Figure 12.3 MR scan of choledochal cyst.

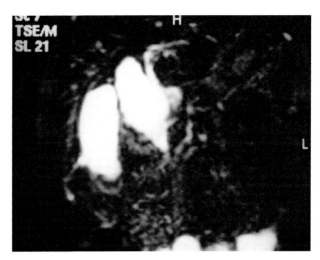

Figure 12.4 MR cholangiogram of choledochal cyst.

A variety of other diagnostic modalities have been suggested, including endoscopic ultrasonography,[48] angiography, laparoscopy and intraoperative cyst endoscopy.[40] All of these may provide useful information in selected cases, but in general they add little to the sum total of information available by more conventional means. Our preferred investigations are ultrasonography and MRCP, with an on-table cholangiogram where necessary.

Treatment

All choledochal cysts will require operative treatment. There is no role for long-term observation because of the risk of gallstones, pancreatitis, cholangitis, cirrhosis and malignancy. The theoretical requirements of an ideal operation are:

(1) To allow free hepato–enteric bile flow.
(2) To remove all cyst mucosa (with its associated malignant potential).
(3) To exclude any 'common channel' and prevent pancreaticobiliary reflux.
(4) To minimize the subsequent risk of cholangitis.

These criteria are met by the operation of 'cyst excision and hepaticojejunostomy', which has become the mainstay of choledochal cyst surgery. This operation is not suitable for all cases of choledochal cyst and may not always be possible in the acute situation, however there are many large series which testify to its continuing success.[2,4,5,8,49–51]

Cyst excision and hepaticojejunostomy

Preparation
The patient will require a full preoperative work-up, which should include a full blood count,

coagulation profile, liver function tests and cross-matching. Any abnormalities in the above will need to be corrected in so far as this is possible. A full bowel preparation should be carried out, and systemic antibiotics should be commenced prior to starting surgery.

Access
Optimal access can be had with the patient placed in a supine position and with his/her back slightly extended. This can be achieved by placing a small radiolucent roll under the small of the back. A high transverse or subcostal incision provides excellent exposure. If possible, this incision should not cross the midline in order to reduce postoperative discomfort.

Procedure
A laparotomy is carried out, in which the appearance of the liver, spleen, pancreas and biliary tree are noted (Fig. 12.5). Fluid may be aspirated from

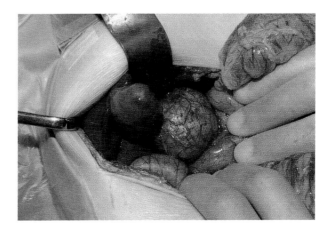

Figure 12.5 Operative field prior to dissection of choledochal cyst.

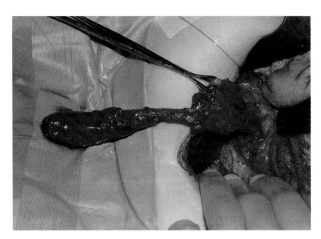

Figure 12.6 Operative field following dissection of choledochal cyst.

the choledochal cyst for evaluation of microbial content and estimation of biliary amylase, elevation of which implies the presence of a common channel.[4,15] Operative cholangiography[4,22,52] and/or cyst endoscopy[5,33,40] will help to define the anatomy of the cyst, and is particularly useful at revealing the presence of proximal ductal stenoses,[25] calculi and aberrant ducts.[27]

The choledochal cyst and gall bladder are mobilized, keeping to a plane of dissection which lies between the peritoneum and cyst wall. This plane is entered anteriorly, and is then extended around the sides of the cyst, taking great care to avoid damaging the hepatic artery, which may be very adherent to the cyst wall. The cyst is lifted forwards from the portal vein and is encircled proximally and (where possible) distally. The common hepatic duct is then divided at the level of the bifurcation and the cyst and gallbladder are reflected forwards (Fig. 12.6). This allows the dissection to proceed distally, as far towards the pancreaticobiliary junction as possible, whilst avoiding damage to the pancreas and related structures. At this point the bile duct is divided and the cyst and gallbladder are removed en bloc. The distal end of the common bile duct is either ligated or oversewn, depending on size.

The common hepatic duct is carefully examined to exclude any proximal stenoses. If these are present, they can usually be resected from the divided end of the duct.[25] The common hepatic duct is then anastomosed to a 40 cm retrocolic roux loop of jejunum with interrupted absorbable sutures. It is important to achieve a wide anastomosis, which is proximal to any ductal strictures.[25,52] The abdomen is then closed, leaving a small suction drain in place.

Alternative procedures

External drainage

In very complicated cases, particularly where there is obstruction, uncontrolled ascending cholangitis or cyst rupture, it may be preferable to establish some form of temporary external drainage, prior to carrying out definitive surgery.[4] This can be achieved by percutaneous transhepatic cholangiodrainage where appropriate[3] or by open T-tube cholecystotomy. Formal cyst excision and hepaticojejunostomy should be carried out once the general condition of the patient has improved.

Cyst excision and hepaticoduodenostomy

This procedure is somewhat simpler than the conventional operation, as it avoids the need to create a roux loop. It also has the merit of producing a more physiologically 'normal' anatomical result.[51] However, it is believed that these patients are more vulnerable to duodenohepatic reflux, stasis and cholangitis, particularly where the intrahepatic ducts are dilated,[3] and for this reason most authors prefer the roux loop hepaticojejunostomy.

Mucosectomy and hepaticojejunostomy

In longstanding choledochal cysts, the cyst wall may be so thick and adherent that it is very difficult to separate it from adjacent structures such as the hepatic artery and portal vein. In these cases it may be preferable to open the cyst and excise the cyst lining from within, without attempting to excise the cyst itself. Complete removal of the cyst mucosa in this way diminishes the risk of malignancy and allows a hepaticojejunostomy to be carried out in the usual manner.

Choledochocyst-enterostomy

This operation is technically straightforward and may have a role in the acute situation where radical excision is hazardous.[4] However, it is very unsatisfactory in the long run, because of the high incidence of stasis, calculus formation, cholangitis and malignancy. Indeed, most surgeons would suggest that such cases should go on to have a formal cyst excision and hepaticojejunostomy in due course.[53]

'Antireflux valves'

It has been suggested that there might be benefits in creating a drainage limb with an antireflux nipple valve.[54] The reported cases have done satisfactorily, but such operations are considerably more complex, and appear to offer no clear advantages over the more conventional procedure.[55]

Miscellaneous

A variety of other procedures have been described, which generally pertain to the management of specific anatomical variants. Thus:

- Type II cysts may be treated by cyst excision and primary ductal reconstruction. These are rare lesions, of which there are only a handful of reported cases.[56]
- Type III cysts are also very rare and may be removed transduodenally.[57] Small lesions may be treated by sphincteroplasty or possibly by endoscopic sphincterotomy.
- Type V cysts are more difficult to deal with, and may require intrahepatic cystoenterostomy or even hepatic segmentectomy/lobectomy.[23,25,58] Unfortunately, cholangitis and calculus formation can continue to be a problem, even after surgery.[4]

Prognosis

In contrast to choledochocyst-enterostomy, which carries a long-term complication rate in excess of 50%, the results of primary cyst excision and hepaticoenterostomy are very satisfactory. There are many reported series with a long-term survival rate close to 100%, and the incidence of complications varies between 0 and 10%.[2–5,8,49,50,54,59] Possible complications include calculus formation, cholangitis, anastomotic stricture, pancreatitis, anastomotic leak, adhesion obstruction and cholangiocarcinoma in the residual ducts.[60] There is a general consensus that a number of these complications may relate to the quality of the hepato–enteric anastomosis, and in particular to the presence of residual ductal strictures. Because of this, several authors stress the importance of adequate peroperative investigation, and the desirability of a wide anastomosis.[25,49,59] A number of reported series show that cyst excision and hepaticoenterostomy is almost complication-free in children under 5 years of age,[3–5,49] and it is increasingly clear that early diagnosis and cyst excision offers the best hope of trouble free long-term survival. By contrast, the incidence of complications is much higher in older patients in whom the disease process is more advanced.

Conclusions

Congenital choledochal cysts are uncommon anomalies, which have a poor prognosis if left untreated. Early diagnosis followed by cyst excision and hepaticoenterostomy is the management of choice. Patients treated in this way have an excellent chance of complication-free, long-term survival.

Key points

- 60% present before the age of 10 (and may present antenatally on ultrasound).
- Presentation of choledochal cyst:
    Obstructive jaundice (75%)
    Abdominal pain (50%)
    Abdominal mass (30%)
    (All three together in <50% of cases).
- Complications of untreated choledochal cyst:
    Intrahepatic calculi and cholangitis
    Cirrhosis and portal hypertension
    Hepatic abscess
    Haemobilia
    Cholangiocarcinoma.
- Diagnosis:
    Ultrasound
    CT
    Cholangiography:
      ERCP
      PTC
      MRCP
    Scintigraphy (IDA/HIDA).
- Aims of management:
    To allow free hepatico–enteric bile flow
    To remove all cyst mucosa and therefore associated malignant potential
    To exclude any common pancreaticobiliary channel, thereby preventing pancreaticobiliary reflux
    To minimize the subsequent risk of cholangitis.
- Presentation:
    Antenatal ultrasound finding
    Palpable right upper quadrant mass
    Childhood obstructive jaundice
    Cholangitis
    Cholangiocarcinoma (adult).
- Objectives of treatment:
    Facilitate free hepato–enteric bile flow
    Remove all cystic mucosa
    Exclude pancreaticobiliary reflux via common channel
    Minimize subsequent risk of cholangitis.
- Treatment options:
    Excision of cyst with hepaticojejunostomy
    External drainage
    Mucosectomy and hepaticojejunostomy.

REFERENCES

1. Alonzo-Lej F, Revor WB, Pessagno DJ. Congenital choledochal cyst with report of 2 and an analysis of 94 cases. Surg Gynecol Obstet Int Abst Surg 1959; 108: 1–30

2. Stringer MD, Dhawan A, Davenport M et al. Choledochal cysts: lessons from a 20 year experience. Arch Dis Child 1995; 73: 528–31

3. Miyano T, Yamataka A. Choledochal cysts. Curr Opin Pediatr 1997; 9: 283–8

4. Howard ER. Choledochal cysts. In: Howard ER, ed. Surgery of liver disease in children. Oxford: Butterworth-Heinemann, 1991: 78–90

5. Yamataka A, Oshiro K, Okada Y et al. Complications after cyst excision with hepaticoenterostomy for choledochal cysts and their surgical management in children versus adults. J Pediatr Surg 1997; 32: 1097–102

6. Benhidjeb T, Chaoui R, Kalache K et al. Prenatal diagnosis of a choledochal cyst: a case report and review of the literature. Am J Perinatol 1996; 13: 207–10

7. Gallivan EK, Crombleholme TM, D'Alton ME. Early prenatal diagnosis of choledochal cyst. Prenat Diagn 1996; 16: 934–7

8. Rha SY, Stovroff MC, Glick PL et al. Choledochal cysts: a ten year experience. Am Surg 1996; 62: 30–4

9. Vater A. Dissertatio anatomica qua novum bilis diverticulum circa orificum ductus cholidochi. Diputat Anatom Select 1748; 3: 259

10. Douglas. Case of dilatation of the common bile duct. J Med Sci 1852; 14: 97

11. Tsuchida Y, Kawarasaki H, Iwanaka T et al. Antenatal diagnosis of biliary atresia (type I cyst) at 19 weeks gestation: differential diagnosis and etiological implications. J Pediatr Surg 1995; 30: 697–9

12. Babbitt DP. Congenital choledochal cyst: new etiological concept based on anomalous relationships of common bile duct and pancreatic bulb. Ann Radiol 1969; 12: 231–41

13. Gauthier F, Brunelle F, Valayer J. Common channel for bile and pancreatic ducts. Presentation of 12 cases and discussion. Chir Pediatr 1986; 27: 148–52

14. Jesudason SR, Govil S, Mathai V, Kuruvilla R, Muthusami JC. Choledochal cysts in adults. Ann R Coll Surg Engl 1997; 79: 410–3

15. Davenport M, Stringer MD, Howard ER. Biliary amylase and congenital choledochal dilatation. J Pediatr Surg 1995; 30: 474–7

16. Kato T, Asakura Y, Kase M. An attempt to produce choledochal cyst in puppies. J Pediatr Surg 1974; 4: 509–13

17. Wong KC, Lister J. Human fetal development of the hepato-pancreatic duct junction – a possible explanation of congenital dilation of the biliary tract. J Pediatr Surg 1981; 16: 139–45

18. Spitz L. Experimental production of cystic dilatation of the common bile duct in neonatal lambs. J Pediatr Surg 1977; 12: 39–42

19. Petersen C, Biermanns D, Kuske M et al. New aspects in a murine model for extrahepatic biliary atresia. J Pediatr Surg 1997; 32: 1190–5

20. Komi N, Takahara H, Kunitomo K, Miyoshi Y, Yagi T. Does the type of anomalous arrangement of pancreaticobiliary ducts influence the surgery and prognosis of choledochal cyst? J Pediatr Surg 1992; 6: 728–31

21. Todani T, Narusue M, Watanabe Y, Tabuchi K, Okajima K. Management of congenital choledochal cyst with intrahepatic involvement. Ann Surg 1977; 187: 272–80

22. Dhu YC, Lai HS, Chen WJ. Accessory hepatic duct associated with a choledochal cyst. Pediatr Surg Int 1997; 12: 54–6

23. Todani T, Watanabe Y, Toki A et al. Ductoplasty for an aberrant hepatic duct in a choledochal cyst. Pediatr Surg Int 1997; 12: 618–9

24. Jindal RM, Harris N, McDaniel HM, Lehman G, Sherman S. Presentation of choledochal cysts without intrabiliary communication on endoscopic retrograde cholangiopancreatography. Liver Transpl Surg 1996; 2: 468–71

25. Ando H, Kaneko K, Ito F, Seo T, Ito T. Operative treatment of congenital stenoses of the intrahepatic bile ducts in patients with choledochal cysts. Am J Surg 1997; 173: 491–4

26. Komi N, Tamura T, Tsuge S et al. Relation of patient age to premalignant alterations in choledochal cyst epithelium: histochemical and immunohistochemical studies. J Pediatr Surg 1986; 21: 430

27. Shimotake T, Iwai N, Yanagihara J et al. Innervation patterns in congenital biliary dilatation. Eur J Pediatr Surg 1995; 5: 265–70

28. Yamataka A, Kuwatsuru R, Shima H et al. Initial experience with non-breath-hold magnetic resonance cholangiopancreatography: a new noninvasive technique for the diagnosis of choledochal cyst in children. J Pediatr Surg 1997; 32: 1560–2

29. Lugo-Vicente HL. Prenatally diagnosed coledochal cysts: observation or early surgery? J Pediatr Surg 1995; 30: 1288–90

30. Germiller JA, Strouse PJ, Golladay ES, DiPietro MA. Early presentation of choledochal cyst transiently obstructed by an inspissated bile plug. J Pediatr Surg 1997; 32: 1522–5

31. Joseph VT. Surgical techniques and long-term results in the treatment of choledochal cyst. J Pediatr Surg 1990; 25: 782–7

32. Altman RP. Choledochal cyst. Semin Pediatr Surg 1992; 1: 130–3

33. Masetti R, Antinori A, Coppola R et al. Choledochocoele: changing trends in diagnosis and management. Surg Today 1996; 26: 281–5

34. Kaneko K, Ando H, Ito T et al. Protein plugs cause symptoms in patients with choledochal cysts. Am J Gastroenterol 1997; 92: 1018–21

35. Seema, Sharma A, Seth A, Taluja V, Bagga D, Aneja S. Spontaneous rupture of choledochal cyst. Indian J Pediatr 2000; 67: 155–6

36. Ando H, Ito T, Watanabe Y et al. Spontaneous perforation of choledochal cyst. J Am Coll Surg 1995; 181: 125–8

37. Karnak I, Cahit Tanyel F, Buyukpamukcu N, Hicsonmez A. Spontaneous rupture of choledochal cyst: an unusual cause of acute abdomen in children. J Pediatr Surg 1997; 32: 736–8

38. Krepel HP, Siersema PD, Tilanus HW et al. Choledochocoele presenting with anaemia. Eur J Gastroenterol Hepatol 1997; 9: 641–3

39. Tajisi K, Takenawa H, Yamaoka K et al. Choledochal cyst with adenocarcinoma in the cystically dilated intrahepatic bile duct. Abdom Imag 1997; 22: 190–3

40. Miyano T, Yamataka A, Kato Y et al. Choledochal cysts: special emphasis on the usefulness of intraoperative endoscopy. J Pediatr Surg 1995; 30: 482–4

41. Fieber SS, Nance FC. Choledochal cyst and neoplasm: a comprehensive review of 106 cases and presentation of two original cases. Am Surg 1997; 63: 982–7

42. Sanz N, DeMingo L, Florez F, Rollan V. Rhabdomyosarcoma of the biliary tree. Pediatr Surg Int 1997; 12: 200–1

43. Akkiz H, Colokoglu SO, Ergon Y et al. Endoscopic retrograde cholangiopancreatography in the diagnosis and management of choledochal cyst. HPB Surg 1997; 10: 211–18

44. Sharma AK, Wakhlu A, Sharma SS. The role of endoscopic retrograde cholangiopancreatography in the management of choledochal cysts in children. J Pediatr Surg 1995; 30: 65–7

45. Groebli Y, Sarraj A, Pfister L, Lopez J. Spiral-CT cholangiography with 3D reconstruction in the diagnosis of choledochocele. Eur Radiol 2000; 10: 395

46. Dinsmore JE, Murphy JJ, Jamieson D. Pediatric surgical images: MRCP evaluation of choledochal cysts. J Pediatr Surg 2000; 36: 829–30

47. Kim SH, Lim JH, Yoon HK, Han BK, Lee SK, Kim YI. Choledochal cyst: comparison of MR and conventional cholangiography. Clin Radiol 2000; 55: 378–83

48. Sugiyama M, Atomi Y. Endoscopic ultrasonography for diagnosing anomalous pancreaticobiliary junction. Gastroint Endosc 1997; 45: 261–7

49. Miyano T, Yamataka A, Kato Y et al. Hepaticoenterostomy after excision of choledochal cyst in children: a 30-year experience with 180 cases. J Pediatr Surg 1996; 31: 1417–21

50. Saing H, Han H, Chan KL et al. Early and late results of excision of choledochal cysts. J Pediatr Surg 1997; 32: 1563–6

51. Schimpl G, Aigner R, Sorantin E et al. Comparison of hepaticoantrostomy and hepaticojejunostomy for biliary reconstruction after resection of a choledochal cyst. Pediatr Surg Int 1997; 12: 271–5

52. Uno K, Tsuchida Y, Kawarasaki H et al. Development of intrahepatic cholelithiasis long after primary excision of choledochal cysts. J Am Coll Surg 1996; 183: 583–8

53. Chaudhary A, Dhar P, Sachdev A. Reoperative surgery for choledochal cysts. Br J Surg 1997; 84: 781–4

54. Shamberger RC, Lund DP, Lillehei CW, Hendren WH III. Interposed jejunal segment with nipple valve to prevent reflux in biliary reconstruction. J Am Coll Surg 1995; 180: 10–5

55. Raffensperger J. The use of a spur valve in a Roux loop to prevent reflux into the biliary tree. J Pediatr Surg 2000; 35: 1014–15

56. Iuchtman M, Martins MS, Scheidemantel RE. Congenital diverticulum of the choledochus: report of a case. Int Surg 1971; 55: 280–2

57. Powell CS, Sawyers JL, Reynolds VH. Management of adult choledochal cysts. Ann Surg 1981; 193: 666–7

58. Ohmoto K, Shimizu M, Iguchi Y et al. Solitary cystic dilatation of the intrahepatic bile duct. J Clin Pathol 1997; 50: 617–8

59. Todani T, Watanabe Y, Urushihara N et al. Biliary complications after excisional procedure for choledochal cyst. J Pediatr Surg 1995; 30: 478–81

60. Yamamoto J, Shimamura Y, Ohtani I et al. Bile duct carcinoma arising from the anastomotic site of hepaticojejunostomy after the excision of congenital biliary dilatation: a case report. Surgery 1996; 119: 476–9

13 Management of hydatid disease of the liver

Sandro Tagliacozzo

Biological and pathological basis of modern surgery

The echinococcus or hydatid cyst represents the larval stage of *Echinococcus granulosus*, a 2–6 mm long tapeworm. In the adult stage the tapeworm lives in the gut of the dog, the definitive host. The intermediate animal hosts, where the parasite lives and develops at the larval stage, are sheep, cattle, pigs and man (considered an 'accidental' intermediate host). There are also 'sylvatic cycles' of echinococcus which occur in Canada, Alaska, Australia and other countries with different definitive and intermediate hosts according to the local prevalence of animal species.

Human infection is direct or indirect from the dog through the parasite eggs (size 20–25 μm). Once ingested, they hatch and liberate the hexacanth embryo (bearing six hooks). This penetrates the gut wall, enters a mesenteric venule and is transported to the liver, where in most cases it will lodge. However, it may cross the portal network and reach the lung, where it may stop or continue beyond the vascular network, towards the various organs by way of systemic arterial vessels. In the liver the embryo loses its hooks and develops a larval cystic form: the echinococcus cyst or hydatid cyst. If it survives leukocytic response, the cyst grows, reaching 250 μm in diameter after 3 weeks and 1 cm after 5 months.

Structure of the cyst

The echinococcus cyst is composed of the wall and contents. The wall consists of two separate parts: the inner endocyst, namely the wall of the true vesicular metacestode, and the outer connective pericyst or ectocyst, deriving from the host organ, in the case of man the liver, able to ensure nutritional exchanges for a long time (Fig. 13.1). The wall, in

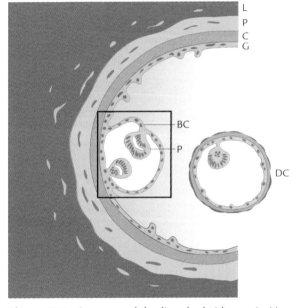

Figure 13.1 Structure of the liver hydatid cyst. L: Liver; P: pericyst; C: chitinous layer; G: germinal layer; BC: brood capsules or vesicles; P: protoscoleces; DC: daughter cysts (similar to mother cyst).

turn, is composed of two layers. The outer layer consists of a cuticle up to, or over 1 mm thick, the chitinous layer, similar to the white of a boiled egg, composed of concentric hyaline laminae. The inner layer consists of a thin (10–25 μm) germinal or parenchymal layer, which represents the living tissue, composed of an outer basal syncitial layer and inner nucleated cells. Its vesiculation perpetuates the parasite life cycle. In a fertile adult cyst, the inner surface of the germinal layer is scattered with innumerable granules, brood vesicles or capsules, 250–500 μm in diameter. They are released into the cystic fluid and, together with the hooks, they form the so-called hydatid sand. Each granule contains 5–30 darker ovoid corpuscles. These are the

A

B

C

D

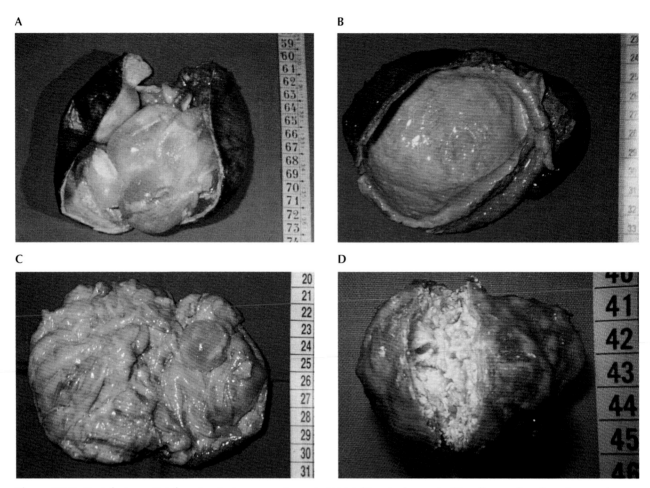

Figure 13.2 Cyst features (total pericystectomy specimens). (A) Multivesicular cyst; (B) yellow-colored cystic membrane for biliary infiltration; (C) calcific cyst of jelly-like necrotic contents and intense biliary infiltration; (D) calcific coarctate cyst of chalk-colored contents and dry clay consistency.

cephalic ends of echinococcus or protoscoleces, invaginated and covered with an anhistic cuticle. Hundreds of thousands of them can be contained in 1 ml of sand! Protoscoleces can produce implantations of cysts in the viscera if there is cystic fluid dissemination.

For a long time, the cyst contents can be composed of hydatid fluid only, a colorless fluid, clear as rock crystal (univesicular cyst), while in the mature cyst there may be a number of cysts similar to the mother cyst, called daughter cysts (multivesicular cysts). The origin and cause of daughter cyst formation is not well known, apart from a non-specific stress of the germinal layer for impaired vital exchanges with the host and decreased endocyst pressure.[1] Among the various causes, pericyst thickening and the penetration of bile between the pericyst and cyst wall and inside it are of concern for the surgeon.

The pericyst, initially composed of very thin connective lamina, subsequently tends to become thicker (up to 1 cm or more), sclerose and calcify. The process of cyst expansion causes compression of hepatic parenchymal structures, in turn engulfed into the pericyst. Large vessels are compressed and displaced while, however, remaining patent for a long time. Similarly, bile ducts remain patent and may open into the pericyst, between it and the parasite wall. This phenomenon is very frequent, unlike the rare frank rupture of the cyst with effusion of the cyst contents into a large duct and the main bile duct. This is of the utmost importance for surgery, since on the one hand its appearance causes major changes in the cyst and pericyst development, and on the other it is a factor in the development of postoperative complications such as biliary fistulas. Bile filtration in the virtual interstitium between the pericyst and chitinous membrane can form a perivesicular biloma with loss of direct contact of the cyst with the pericyst, a decrease in the mother cyst pressure and membrane rupture, all phenomena which from early on can cause endogenous vesiculation. At the same time, the appearance of bile is preliminary to cyst infection.

Endogenous vesiculation indicates an initial positive attempt at survival by the primary parasite, otherwise condemned to death and degeneration.

A

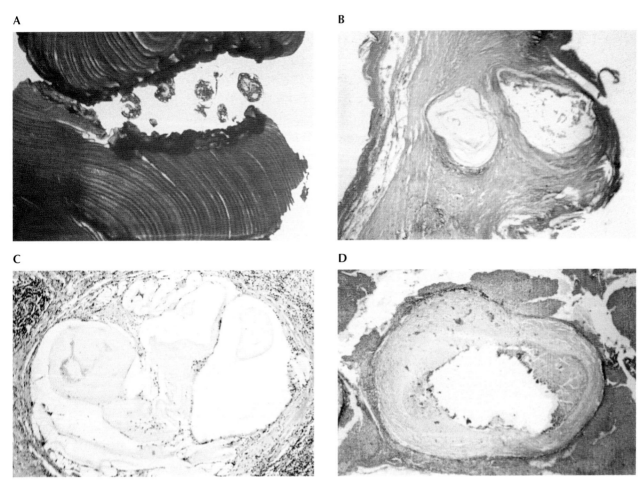

B

C

D

Figure 13.3 Exogenous vesiculation: microscopic appearance. (A) Brood capsules and protoscoleces contained in a protrusion of germinal layer within the cuticle; (B,C) intrapericyst exogenous vesiculation hydatid membranes within the pericyst of primary cyst; (D) extrapericyst exogenous vesiculation encircled by a new pericyst and protruding in the liver parenchyma adjacent to the mother cyst.

Subsequently the neoformed hydatid material packed into the cystic cavity tends to show signs of stress and to degenerate extensively with different aspects of: fruit jelly, putty, plaster, dry clay or pus (Fig. 13.2). At the same time, the fibrous pericyst becomes thicker and calcium deposits appear as increasingly extended and confluent granules and laminae, forming in some cases a continuous thick shell. Some authors consider these degenerative aspects as corresponding to the parasite's death, however this is not so. Except for extreme cases, within the degenerate material, viable hydatids can be found.[2] It is to be stressed that in many cases, the parasite ensures its survival and even favors its expansion in the involved organ by exogenous vesiculation.

Protoscoleces and brood vesicles generated by the germinal layer can penetrate the chitinous membrane through fissures and then tend to advance into the pericyst.[3] Alternatively, there may be germinal islets trapped between the lamellae of the cuticular layer. Once the germinal elements penetrate the pericyst, they may grow inside and

then project towards the liver parenchyma as diverticular protrusions surrounded by their own thin pericyst (Fig. 13.3). In their cavity, they contain cysts that grow favored by easy exchanges through the thin neoformed pericyst and behave as the mother cyst. Because there is no connection with the inner surface of primary pericyst they cannot be detected or even suspected with the most careful examination after emptying (Fig. 13.4). The exogenous cyst, while growing, can pull away from the mother cyst and this results in the commonly observed pattern of two or more adjacent cysts, or 'satellite cysts',[4] separated by a parenchymal septum usually rich in vascular and ductal structures already displaced by the mother cyst. In other frequently observed instances, the exogenous cyst remains in contact with the primary cyst separated by a thin residual septum ('sand-glass-like cyst'), or with the collapse of separating septum, the two cavities communicate through a more or less wide operculum ('sacculations').

As for the presence and frequency of exogenous vesiculation, the phenomenon is either ignored or largely

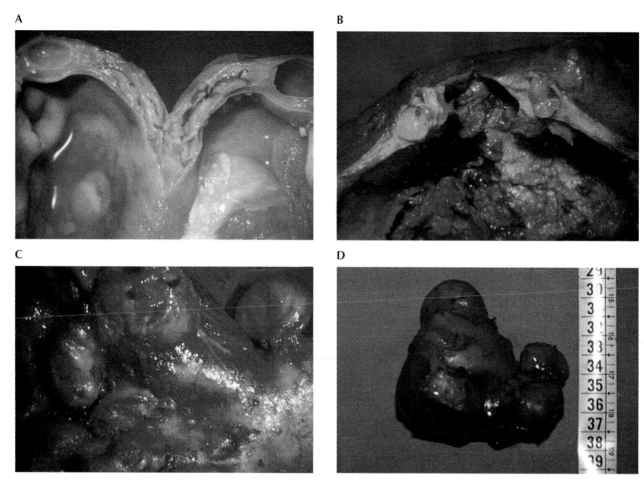

Figure 13.4 Intra- and extrapericyst exogenous vesiculation. Macroscopic appearance in four total pericystectomy specimens. (A,B) Within the pericyst of open cysts viable daughter cysts are observed, separated from the mother cyst cavity; (C,D) clusters of pedunculated pseudodiverticula, non-communicating with the mother cyst cavity, covered with a thin pericyst and containing daughter cysts.

underestimated,[5–9] most likely because of the preference for conservative operations which do not allow its identification. However, it is recognized in about 30% of radical operations for multivesicular cysts.[10,11] This incidence is bound to markedly increase when we accept the hypothesis, mentioned above, that sand-glass-like cysts and dual and multiple adjacent cysts are also an expression of the same event. Once the phenomenon was identified and quantitatively assessed, its importance was recognized beyond biological and pathological interest. Consequently, in a large number of patients where the surgical procedure then performed (and still largely performed) included no removal of the pericyst, this could not be considered effective: actually, only the cyst was resected. Viable, vital parasite foci remained, bound to represent disease progression. This was incorrectly considered a recurrence attributed to implantation from accidental dissemination because of poor protection of the operating field or reinfection. The latter interpretations, already unconvincing, have lost credibility, based on the observation that the findings of exogenous vesiculation and the incidence of recurrence in series of conservative surgery, interestingly

enough, were similar, at about 30%. This was confirmed by the fact that the so-called recurrences were practically absent in series of radical surgery.

Briefly, from the knowledge of the parasite's biology and the pathological relationship between the cyst and liver, stem the criteria of a new, rational surgery of the hydatid disease of the liver. It tends to critically minimize or reduce to nil postoperative biliary complications and the most serious long-term failure, namely recurrence.

Indications for surgery

For the two types of cysts mentioned above, indications for surgery are as follows:

- Univesicular, clear cysts with a thin and elastic pericyst (20% of cases) should be treated by conservative surgery (there is no need for radical surgery);
- Multivesicular, yellow cysts at different developmental stage with fibrous, thick and/or calcific pericyst (80% of cases) should be treated by radical surgery.

For modern rational operative surgery, the choice is not optional but rigorously determined. With the concept of radicality, surgery of liver hydatidosis becomes demanding and therefore selective surgical experience is required as the only means of ensuring a good chance of recovery.

Among radical operations, the choice between anatomical liver resection and total pericystectomy is at the surgeon's discretion; however, it is readily understood that the second operation is undoubtedly more advantageous. In fact, the growth of the cyst is characterized by compression of vascular and ductal structures that supply large, healthy hepatic regions worth preserving, therefore favoring careful pericyst dissection with preservation of structures.

During its development, the hydatid cysts of the liver may undergo a number of complications, some of them clinically dramatic.

Infection of the cavity and its contents is less frequent than was previously thought (2–20%),[12] and was not always clinically manifest. Most likely, it is caused by the penetration of bile into the cavity. Together with the contents, the mother membrane can be destroyed and consequently the altered escavated pericystic wall loses its function of delimiting the infectious process.

Ruptured cyst

Frank rupture into the bile ducts has already been mentioned. This occurrence should be distinguished from biliary communication through ductal fissurations, much more frequent in mature cysts (40–70%).[2,13] Frank rupture, usually into a central bile duct (5–12% of cases),[12] is characterized by the penetration of endocyst material into intra- and extrahepatic bile ducts to the infarction of the common bile duct and gallbladder.[14,15]

The pattern of symptoms usually includes colicky pain accompanied and preceded by jaundice and cholangitic fever.[16] Stenosis of the papilla of Vater and consequent, complete or incomplete, septic or aseptic cholestasis, when lasting 4–6 months, may then cause secondary biliary cirrhosis. In cases with suspected penetration of hydatid material into the bile ducts, intraoperative cholangiography and concomitant surgery with bile duct clearing and external or internal biliary drainage, preferably papillosphincterostomy, is mandatory.

A severe risk in the presence of a huge cyst is its rupture into the peritoneal cavity (5–12% incidence).[17] In most cases, the determining cause is blunt trauma and in children it may occur during play. In children, the cysts may reach huge dimensions and high pressure. At times, rupture into a free cavity may be spontaneous. Another cause of peritoneal effusion of hydatid contents is iatrogenic from percutaneous puncture for diagnosis or emptying, or it may occur during surgery with bad technique and poor isolation of the peritoneal cavity. This complication is very serious. Symptoms are complex, with acute abdominal pain, local signs of peritoneal irritation and anaphylactic reactions of varying degree to severe shock, characterized by intense dyspnea, tachycardia, marked hypotension and urticaria.[18–20] The reaction is due to the abrupt release of allergens reabsorbed from the peritoneal serosa and conveyed to the circulation in a sensitized subject. The cyst rupture may be followed by bile peritonitis with a well-defined or insidious clinical pattern.

Initially, in some cases, rupture may be overlooked and show only long-term manifestations. The most severe manifestation results from the dissemination and implantation of endocyst material on the peritoneal surface shown as innumerable cysts of varying dimensions, often in clusters.[21] Consequences include occupancy, compression and displacement phenomena of organs and structures with extremely severe and complex clinical patterns and corresponding general impairment.

Benzoimidazole therapy has represented a marked improvement in the treatment of rupture of a cyst into the peritoneal cavity. It should be started immediately and given for a prolonged period of time.[22] In cases of manifest, diffuse and inoperable peritoneal hydatidosis, ultrasonography-guided emptying of huge, packed cysts is useful to relieve the most severe clinical patterns of compression and dysfunction.

Rupture of the cyst into the thoracic cavity and bronchobiliary fistula (BBF) are other very severe complications of liver hydatidosis. They are often caused by huge multivesicular cysts of segments VII and VIII, protruding through the diaphragm. Necrosis of the latter from compression, wear and often infection results in cyst communication, exceptionally with the pleural cavity and usually, for previous adhesions, with the pulmonary parenchyma of the lung base, corresponding to the posterior and/or lateral basal segment or medial lobe. Pulmonary inflammation together with the necrotizing action of bile causes erosion into a peripheral bronchus with subsequent passage of hydatid material and bile into the bronchial tree, favored by the differential pressure gradient (Fig. 13.5). Rupture of the cyst into the bronchial tree may be dramatic with abundant expectoration of bile and hydatid material. Daily bile effusion is persistent and increasing, resulting in an extremely severe clinical pattern characterized by cough, abundant expectoration up to 1000 ml of bile and hydatid contents, fever, and very poor general

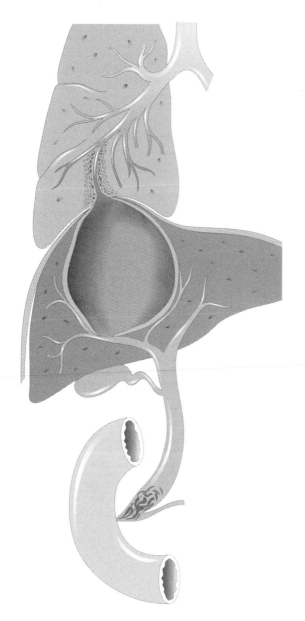

Figure 13.5 Bronchobiliary fistula. Biliary rupture of hepatic cyst, common bile duct obstruction with hydatid material, communication between the cyst cavity and a basal bronchus through an area of attenuated diaphragm are represented.

condition. Bronchopulmonary involvement tends to involve several segments (fatal necrotizing bronchitis) with necrosis and abscess cavities.[23–26] Hydatid BBF is a very severe clinical and pathologic complication requiring early surgery, preferably simultaneously for both the lung and the liver cyst, and is associated with a high mortality.

Diagnosis

Hydatid cyst of the liver may be asymptomatic for years, at times for decades. Diagnosis may be accidental, based on an incidental clinical exam that detects swelling when the cyst is located in a palpable abdominal area or, in the case of a more or less relevant hepatomegaly, subsequently assessed with other exams. Liver hydatidosis may be an incidental finding in a radiograph of the hepatic region when the cyst is calcified, during a chest radiograph for a raised hemidiaphragm or during US exam performed for other reasons such as gallstones. In children, large hepatic swellings from hydatid cysts are accompanied by evident deformations of the chest involving the last ribs and arches. Apart from a sense of pressure, a cyst of the liver may cause boring pain at the basal chest for the diaphragmatic pleural or peritoneal reactive process. Dyspepsia, possibly from reflexes originating in the periductal nervous network, is not unusual. Cholestasis from major bile duct compression may be responsible for fever, also of high grade. Liver function tests remain normal for a long time.

Diagnosis is established using several investigations. Conventional radiology may show a raised hemidiaphragm. In calcific cysts, high density roundish shadows are readily visualized (Fig. 13.6).

Diagnostic imaging

Ultrasonography (US)

At present, this is the most common and useful examination. It is non-invasive, low-cost and reproducible, thus suitable for postoperative follow-up or during medical therapy. US supplies precise information on the size, number, location and vascular and biliary relationships of the cyst as well as on its structure. Images have been described and classified according to types and classes.[27–30]

- Univesicular cysts (type I) are represented by a round anechoic area with posterior enhancement and possible internal echoes due to hydatid sand.
- Images of partial or total detachment of the chitinous layer (type II) show the 'dual wall', 'water-lily', 'water snake' signs.
- Multivesicular cysts (type III) are represented by the typical images of daughter cysts identified by the 'honeycomb', 'rosette', 'spoked-wheel' and 'cluster' sign (Fig. 13.7).
- Semi-solid or pseudotumoral aspects (type IV) are characterized by hypo- and hyperechogenicity.
- Partially or totally calcific cysts (type V) are represented by echoic menisci with posterior shadowing. Calcification is considered pathognomonic especially in endemic areas.

US supplies significant information on biliary involvement of hydatid and parahydatid disease:

A

B

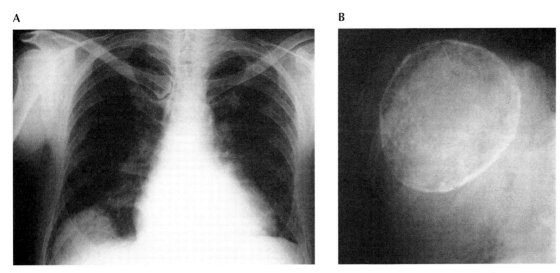

Figure 13.6 Plain radiographs. (A) Partial 'en brioche' image of diaphragm profile; (B) calcific image pathognomonic of hydatid cyst.

A

B

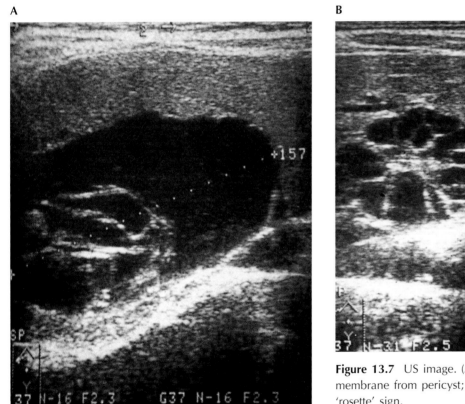

Figure 13.7 US image. (A) Total detachment of parasite membrane from pericyst; (B) multivesicular hydatid cyst: 'rosette' sign.

intra- and extrahepatic bile duct dilation, cholelithiasis or common bile duct lithiasis, and the condition of the hepatic veins, portal system and caval vein. US is also useful in postoperative follow-up.

Computed tomography (CT)
At present, CT is the procedure of choice on which radical surgery is based. Besides precise information on the cyst features, similar to those acquired by US (Fig. 13.8), CT is fundamental in the identification of the vascular relationships, number, site and type of the cysts: dual, sand-glass like, with vesiculations (Fig. 13.9). CT is invaluable for the diagnosis of recurring patterns. Spiral CT is at present the gold standard investigation.

Magnetic resonance imaging (MRI)
This is complementary to CT, especially in the differential diagnosis with hepatocellular carcinoma, organizing hematoma and amebic

A

B

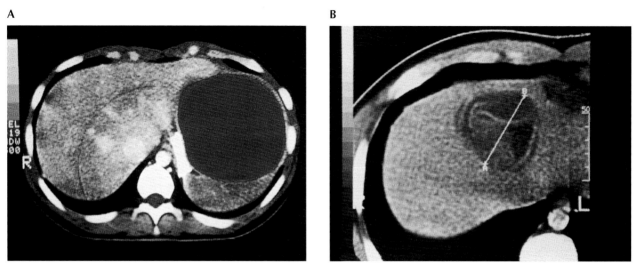

Figure 13.8 CT image. (A) Univesicular cyst; (B) 'water-snake' sign of membrane detachment.

A

B

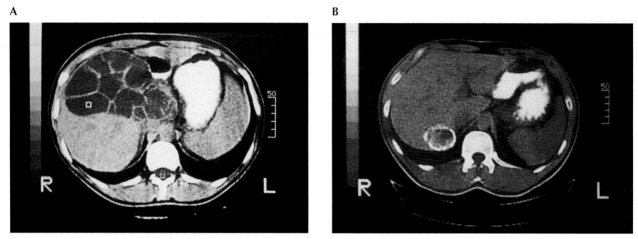

Figure 13.9 CT image. (A) Multivesicular cyst: 'honeycomb' or 'rosette' sign; (B) calcific cyst of segment VII in contact with the caval vein and causing intrahepatic duct dilation stasis.

abscesses.[31–34] The introduction of fast sequences enables the acquisition of images during gadolinium infusion (DTPA). Multiple coronal scans evaluate non-invasively and accurately the relationships with vascular structures: portal vein and inferior caval vein, thus rendering invasive investigations such as venography and arteriography unnecessary (Fig. 13.10). Recently, with MR-cholangiography it has been possible to visualize the intra- and extrahepatic biliary tree with its bile contents.

Angiography

Arterial, parenchymal arteriography, inferior caval vein and hepatic vein venography now play a minor role after the introduction of US and CT-angiography. They are used to detect the relationships with huge or central cysts and in the differential diagnosis with primary liver tumors or metastases.

Preoperative intravenous cholangiography is performed according to the clinical presentation. It may supply information on common bile duct anatomy, but it does not detect the biliary relationship of the cyst. Percutaneous cholangiography is contraindicated in liver hydatidosis for the risk of perforation and dissemination of hydatid contents. Endoscopic retrograde cholangiopancreatography (ERCP) can be considered the most suitable procedure for the characterization of the common bile duct and sometimes of the biliary relationships of the cyst. It allows pre- or postoperative papillotomy with associated bile duct clearing.[35–37] During surgery and after emptying of the cyst in some cases peroperative cholangiography is very useful.

A

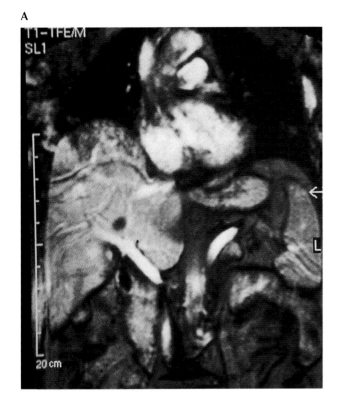

B

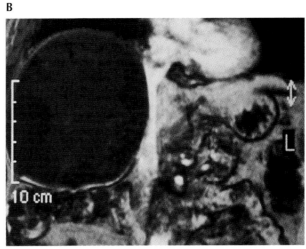

Figure 13.10 (A) MRI coronal T1-weighted sequence after DTPA gadolinium injection with visualization of a cyst, about 2 cm in diameter, of segment IV at the level of portal vein bifurcation (in the same patient a bulky hydatid cyst of segment VII, VIII and V is present); (B) same technique in another patient. Inferior caval vein compression with marked stenosis caused by a bulky cyst of right hemiliver.

Scintography

A common procedure for many years, this has been practically abandoned as a preoperative exam. It is still valid to acquire postoperative anatomic and functional information.

Immunodiagnosis

Immunodiagnosis of hydatidosis now plays a minor role following the progress in diagnostic imaging. In fact, all serum tests are poorly sensitive and/or specific.[38] The concomitant use of several tests is suggested to enhance the specificity when results are concordant and to enhance the sensitivity when there are discrepancies.[39,40] False positives may lead to unnecessary chemotherapy or surgery. False negatives may lead to no treatment at all or to diagnostic puncture, with the consequent risk for anaphylactic shock and dissemination.[41] Tests tend to become negative some time after removal of the cyst, thus they are useless for postoperative control of recurrence.[42] In conclusion, positive and negative tests should be considered respectively reliable only when validated by concomitant findings of other exams.[41] The most common immune tests are the Casoni skin test, the complement fixation test (CFT), the indirect hemagglutination assay (IHA), immuno-electrophoresis (IEP) and the enzyme-linked immunosorbent assay (ELISA). Finally, immunofluorescence (IF) of scoleces should be mentioned. It is a specific and sensitive reaction, but technically difficult to carry out.

Operation

According to location and size, cysts can be divided into parenchymal or superficial and vasculobiliary or deep. In turn the distinction may be based on the predominant vascular relationship. Obviously, the validity of the topographic definition according to hemilivers, sectors, segments or subsegments adopted by the most reliable classifications is confirmed.[43–45] However, because hydatid cysts are spherical and often huge and because they can be removed sparing the healthy tissue then they do not fit properly into the usually adopted anatomical distribution, for cancer surgery in particular. While no intrahepatic expanding neoplasm can be free of vasculobiliary contacts, especially the hepatic veins, superficial cysts have vascular relationships limited to minor peripheral structures. Vasculobiliary or deep cysts represent about 75% of cysts that come to surgery and are those with relationships to first, second and third order branches of hilar elements, the hepatic veins and the inferior caval vein in both its supra-retro and subhepatic segments (Fig. 13.11).[10] First and second order portal branches may be involved with deep cysts located close to the hilum. They are bulky, thus their dissection is difficult both in the case of hemihepatectomy or the more frequent total pericystectomy. Usually, the cysts of segment VII and VIII, on the right, and segment II on the left, have relationships with the major hepatic veins. In these cases dissection of the

A

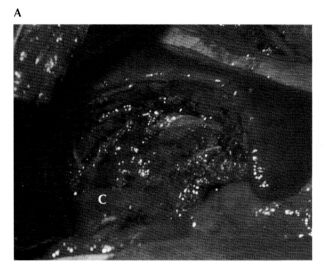

B

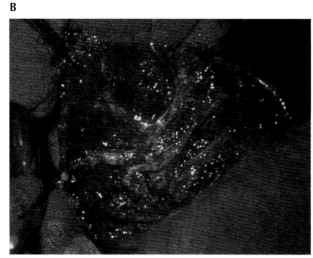

Figure 13.11 Residual surfaces after removal of deep or vasculobiliary cysts: dissected and preserved vascular and biliary elements are indispensable for the survival and function of parenchymal structures adjacent to the cyst. (A) The caval vein (c) and right hepatic vein with branchings are well visualized; (B) vasculobiliary network of hilar origin distribution.

cyst from the cava and involved hepatic vein is mandatory. The latter should be ligated and sectioned or more frequently dissected and preserved with adjacent lateral sutures. As for bile ducts, their adhesion to the pericyst is very dense and dissection is difficult. If there is a communication, this requires very careful dissection for effective repair.

With reference to the hepatic segments of the Couinaud classification, it is suitable to distinguish vasculobiliary or deep cysts according to the topographical denominations immediately indicative of their predominant relationship with hilar vascular and/or hepatic venous or caval vein structures:

- Hepatic venous cysts
- Right or caval intermediate cysts (segments VII, VIII, VI, V)
- Hilar cysts
- Central cysts (interportohepatic) (VIII, IV and V).[46]

In turn, hepatic venous cysts are divided into right (VII and VIII), median (IV), left (II); hilar cysts are divided into right (V), anterior median (IV) and posterior (I), left (II and/or III) (Fig. 13.12).

Evidently, there may be some overlap between locations. For example, right hepatic cysts may extend to the mid right lobe and left hepatic cysts may be located between the two hila. Obviously, these possibilities do not affect the principles on which the classification is based.

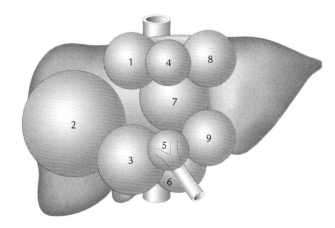

Figure 13.12 Topography of vasculobiliary hydatid cysts. 1, 4, 8: Right, median, left hepatic cysts; 3, 5, 6, 9: right, anterior median, posterior median, left hilar cysts; 2: intermediate cyst; 7: interportohepatic cyst.

Access must be wide for two main reasons: first, because of the frequent presence of adhesions of the protruding cyst to adjacent structures and organs, in particular the diaphragm. Second, because of the need for extended liver mobilization to control the vessels and exploit the liver flexibility to reduce the cavities or residual surfaces after pericyst removal.

Bilateral subcostal incision and right thoracolaparotomy are most commonly performed. The former is definitely suitable for liver surgery, however in hydatidosis because of the very tight adhesions to the right hemidiaphragm in particular, more readily separable only by exposure of the two peritoneal and pleural surfaces, a thoracic approach should be considered. On the other hand, because surgery has become highly specialized, thoracolaparotomy has fallen into disuse by most surgeons expert in liver surgery.

However, thoracolaparotomy increases access during mobilization and dissection of the liver and reduces excessive liver torsion and compression that could cause intraoperative rupture of cysts into the peritoneal cavity or bile ducts. Major steps during right thoracolaparotomy, usually performed on the 8th intercostal space are the oblique patient's position and the splitting of the operating table. The incision starts from the posterior axillary line, follows the space to the costal arch, crosses the abdomen to reach and advance over the median line, 2 cm above the umbilicus. Once the intercostal muscles, the costal arch and the abdominal wall are incised, the incision of the diaphragm follows the course of muscle fibers to the posterior angle of the cut. The incision edges are separated using Finochietto's self-retaining retractor.

In reconstruction, after the retractor is removed and the table split is reduced, the diaphragm edges are sutured with slowly absorbable stitches and then the thoracic and abdominal wall are also sutured. Stitches in the thoracic wall are knotted when all are apposed and adequate resection of the costal arch cartilage is performed. This is mandatory for perfect costal approximation temporarily obtained using a Bernard forceps to grasp the ribs above and below the incision.

Protection of the operating field is mandatory before the planned operation on the cyst or before the cyst is emptied. A cautious approach is to apply protection before liver dissection and when the cyst is protruding from the liver surface and adhering to the adjacent structures and organs. Isolation of the peritoneal and/or pleural cavity to limit the access to the operative field is achieved with dry gauze, preferred by the author, or soaked in a parasiticidal solution or hypertonic saline, however not considered harmless by all. During prior emptying of the cyst the gauze pads should be placed around the site of puncture by the trocar.

Emptying of the cyst is performed with a large caliber trocar, connected with an aspirator by a similarly large non-collapsible tube. As soon as the cyst pressure is relieved and the protruding pericyst tends to collapse, two of its plicae are grasped and raised with Allis or ovum forceps. The amount emptied depends on the contents: it will be practically complete in univesicular cysts, more or less partial if the hydatid material is abundant and dense. When the pericyst wall is opened with electric cautery, direct emptying is completed through a large tube with a frontal opening, connected to a powerful aspirator. If possible, two alternate, separate systems are more suitable because of the inevitable tube blockage. Now and then paraffin oil aspiration is useful to facilitate the flow of material in the tube. Aspiration is easier with a long ovum forceps to mobilize the material attached to the endocyst walls or break big daughter cysts. Clearing of possible communicating sacculations is also necessary. In case of adjacent cysts, separated by a relatively thin septum on indirect palpation, emptying should be performed with the trocar introduced into the cavity through the septum to minimize the risk of dissemination. The breach is widened to complete emptying.

For sterilization of the cyst, performed by injection before emptying, several parasiticidal substances have been used: 2–10% formalin solution, 33% hypertonic saline, 0.5% silver nitrate, 10 vol hydrogen dioxide, 1% iodide alcohol solution and 0.1% cetrimide.[47–50] This method should not be followed for two reasons. First, it appears deceptive to pretend that the entire contents of a multivesicular cyst could be reached by the substance in a few minutes, undergoing the supposed parasiticidal effect.[51] In any case, it would be ineffective against vital elements trapped into the pericyst or developed externally as exogenous vesiculations. Second, practically all solutions markedly damage bile ducts, the cause of severe sclerosing cholangitis, even if in the absence of an open communication.[52–57] Consequently, apart from the actual efficacy, the injection of parasiticidal substances, leaving them in the cavity for some time, should be abandoned.[50] Some, such as iodine solution, can be applied after emptying of the cyst. Benzoimidazole drugs have been used preoperatively for cyst sterilization, however surgery must be delayed and this is not attractive to patients and surgeons because the outcome is not definite.[57–59]

Operations not involving the removal of pericyst adhering to the hepatic parenchyma are considered conservative or non-radical. They were devised many years ago and continued because there were no alternatives, with unsatisfactory results, high morbidity, biliary complications in particular, and a high incidence of recurrence.[2] At present, most conservative operations should be abandoned and replaced by a single updated operation with indications limited to clear univesicular cysts. Their pericyst is thin and elastic, through which the underlying parenchyma is seen. Exogenous vesiculation or biliary fissurations cannot be missed; the latter evidenced by the color of cystic fluid. However, the large size and high pressure typical of

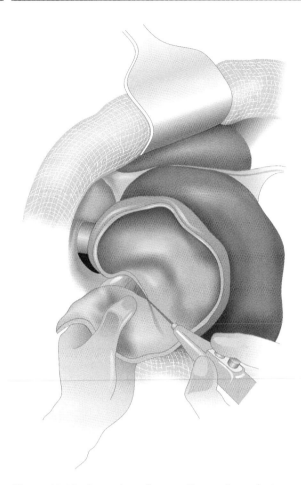

Figure 13.13 Resection of protruding pericyst during conservative surgery. The left hand fingers protect the inferior caval vein.

particular attention should be paid to adjacent structures at risk (Fig. 13.13). The analogy of the method with the 'dôme saillant' resection proposed by Lagrot in the 1950s[60] and still used[61] is only apparent because here it is limited to clear cysts with a thin and soft pericyst after wide field exposure, complete liver mobilization, control of hilar and caval structures. All these measures enable the resection of ample pericyst surfaces up to two-thirds of it, while suturing of residual margins exploits the flexibility of the liver once free of its ligaments.

The control of bile loss is very important. Bile transudation may occur on the resection margins from small orifices, which must be sutured to prevent bile collection within the cavity. As for the search for major communications, the induction of biliary hypertension by compression of the distal hepatic pedicle over the duodenum, squeezing the gallbladder at the same time, may be useful. The possible even minimal communication is evidenced by a drop or flow of bile. In practice, to identify biliary communications injection of dyes is useless since the bile is evident per se and does not soil the surfaces. Peroperative cholangiography is also useless because small dehiscences are not detected, while it is unnecessary in major ones. Cholangiography is useful in the true rupture of the cyst into the common bile duct with effusion of hydatid material. However, these are not typical patterns of univesicular cysts.

Once the residual cystic wall has been controlled, closure is performed by suturing the resection edges. Approximation can be longitudinal, transverse or oblique, but traction should be prevented and circulation in the adjacent parenchyma should not be jeopardized. A double, continuous inverting suture is made with atraumatic mid-sized needles and chromic catgut. In many cases the procedure corresponds to the canalization of the cavity on a rubber tube, advanced outside the cavity in the most suitable position through a counterincision at the level of the hypochondrium or flank. The progress of postoperative cyst collapse until complete obliteration of the cavity can be documented by contrast radiography. Drainage is preferred because in spite of the absence of obvious biliary communications, some days after surgery there may be significant bile leakage which, if drained, heals with no further consequences. In theory, a cavity, reduced as described above, or even left in its original size, could be closed without drainage and heal with no complications. However, the actual possibility of bile collection with the risk of infection and abscess formation, argues in favor of the placement of drains. The use of omentum[62–64] to fill the cavity or cover the residual surface is also unacceptable. In fact, the omentum, an excellent barrier against

these very viable cysts, may be responsible for biliary wall impairment which results, after the cyst is removed, in postoperative bile leakage. In these rare cases, bile is seen through the drainage tube in the residual cavity and is observed for 15–20 days, followed by recovery. Bile leakage following incorrect conservative operations on cysts with thick or calcific pericyst lasts much longer and sometimes causes persistent external biliary fistulas.

After emptying and clearing the cyst cavity, its size and penetration in the depth of liver, especially towards the hilum, the hepatic veins and the retrohepatic caval vein, is assessed. The possible relationships with the hepatic ducts and biliary communication should be carefully evaluated. In fact, it may become evident after emptying and removal of membrane. The extent of pericyst resection is based on how much of it is protruding or how close it is to the hilar and adjacent major vasculobiliary structures. A pericyst margin adequate for subsequent suturing should also be considered. Resection is performed with electric cautery and the help of Allis forceps on the residual margin;

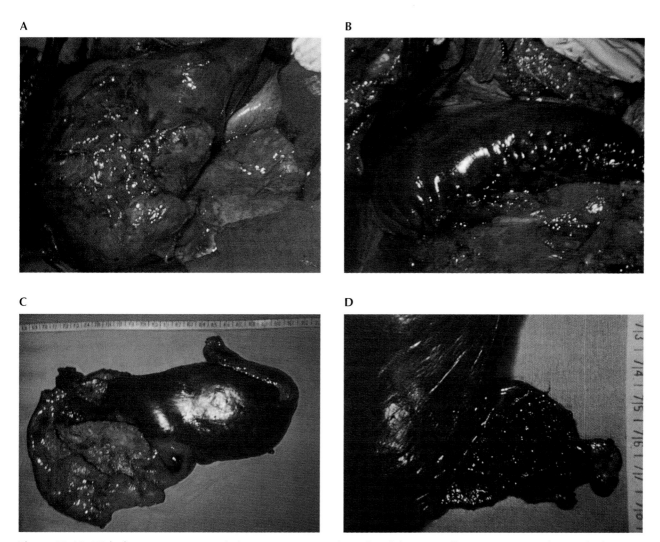

Figure 13.14 Right hepatectomy extended to segment IV and caudate lobe. (A) Bulky cyst mass; (B) the residual surface is sutured; (C) surgical specimen; (D) the gallbladder is packed with hydatid material.

infections, is not equally effective against bile and may even become necrotic. When packed into the cavity, it hinders the interpretation of US or CT images in long-term follow-up to monitor the behavior of the cavity and identify recurrence.[65,66]

Radical operations include anatomical liver resections and total pericystectomy.

Liver resections have been performed for many years for the surgical treatment of liver hydatidosis, and in the majority of cases the indication was of necessity. Giant cysts that occupy an entire hemiliver and beyond; multiple cysts with exclusive or predominant distribution to a lobe; huge cysts occupying completely a hepatic duct so as to hinder its preservation; 'recurring' cysts previously treated with conservative surgery for a huge primary cyst are all rare indications representing approximately 10% in the various series.[7,10] Technically, these anatomical resections are similar to those performed for other

indications, except for the possible extension of the cyst beyond the anatomical limits of the hemiliver or sector to be removed and the biliary relationship on which the indication was probably based (Fig. 13.14). The first occurrence may involve difficult pericyst dissection from vasculobiliary structures supplying territories to be preserved. The techniques to be performed are those of pericystectomy. The biliary relationship may be a result of the rupture of the cyst into a first order duct or by marked displacements, deformations and mural alterations of one or more ducts. Left lateral resection, where parenchymal preservation is unlikely, is usually more frequently required.

Wedge resections should be mentioned in passing. They are still valid in minute marginal anterior cysts.

Total pericystectomy (or cystopericystectomy) is considered to be the ideal radical operation suitable

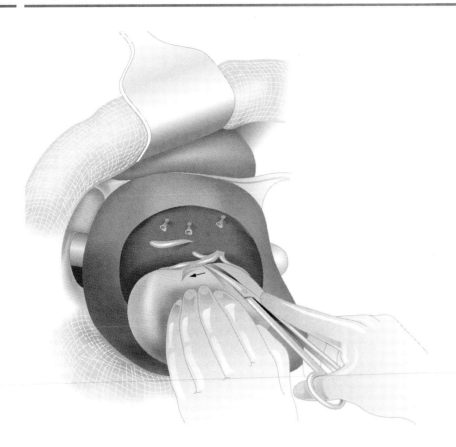

Figure 13.15 Total pericystectomy. Dissection of pericyst from vasculobiliary structures should be along the presumed centriperipheral direction (following the direction of emerging and merging branches).

for the requirements of radicality for the hydatid disease, with maximal preservation of hepatic tissue and complete early recovery. Its feasibility is similar to that of liver resections. The same basic training is required, enhanced by a specific experience. The operation was conceived and proposed by Napalkoff[67] in 1927 and again described in 1936 by Melnikoff.[68] However, in subsequent experiences, results were unsatisfactory and even disastrous due to hemorrhage; thus, following unanimous disapproval, it was practically abandoned. Costantini applied it again in 1950[69] and Yovanovitch in 1959,[70] with indications for peripheral cysts, distant to porta hepatis. Bourgeon, the most convinced supporter, advocated it in 1961, 1964 and 1977, but in practice, in many cases, he favored partial pericystectomy.[5,46,71]

Since the early 1970s it was understood that the persistence of pericyst with its close biliary relationships, more or less wide fissurations and true ruptures, represented the main cause of frequent postoperative complications: abundant, prolonged bile leakage, infections, residual cavities, biliary fistulas.[72,73] The other major reason for the removal of pericyst, exogenous vesiculation and implantation of viable parasites in and out the pericyst, was still overlooked. The correlation of persistent hydatid material with the frequent recurrences with which surgery of hydatidosis seemed to be inevitably burdened, was noted in several series.[11,74] At present, the operation has gained widespread acceptance.[75,76]

Pericystectomy can be performed with the cyst closed or open. In the first case, en bloc removal of the pericyst and its contents is a safe operation with respect to the risk of contamination. In the second case, emptying may favor dissemination, although protection measures make it quite improbable. However, protection measures are necessary also before dissection of a closed cyst. The latter procedure is more elegant, rapid and simpler, but in the case of bulky, deep cysts or those which have ruptured into the common bile duct, the procedure may be risky, thus operations on the open cyst are preferable and necessary. This enables the dissection of pericyst from vasculobiliary structures, even in the most difficult conditions.

When the cyst is protruding from the liver surface at any site, dissection is started in close contact with the pericyst and performed along the transition line between it and the parenchyma sometimes delineated by a groove. This plane is very important, defined according to the features of the cyst and hepatic tissue. Concomitant, chronic, non-parasitic liver disease, or consequent to hepatic vein stasis caused by the cyst, a true Budd–Chiari syndrome, creates major difficulties. The smaller vascular branches entering the pericyst must be electrocoagulated or ligated and dissected. Caution is necessary because consequent bleeding would hinder the field of vision with unnecessary and even considerable blood loss during the procedure. Dissection of large vessels from the

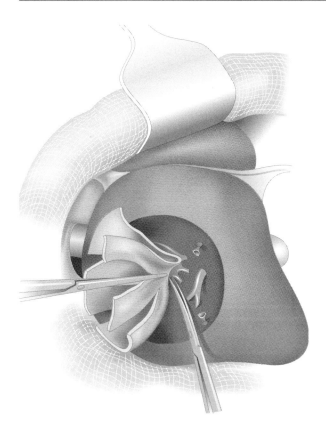

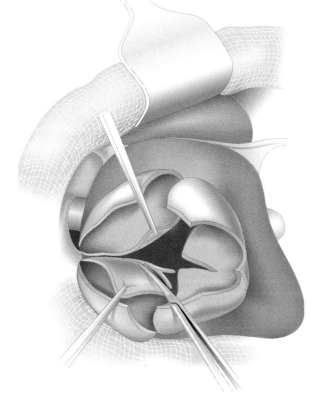

Figure 13.16 Total open pericystectomy. Stripping of pericyst and traction on each strip by folding facilitates deep dissection of vasculobiliary structures also in case of calcific pericyst.

Figure 13.17 Total open pericystectomy. Cautious full depth incision of pericyst with a lancet on the cavity bottom allows access to vessel dissection from several directions, even in the case of very thick cysts.

pericyst should be centriperipheral and along the course of vascular and biliary structures, following the direction of its emerging or confluent branches (Fig. 13.15). In other words, for the dissection around the hepatic veins the direction should be from the apical liver convexity towards the free margin and for hilar elements from the hilum to the periphery. Therefore, in vessel dissection, the surface corresponding to the obtuse angle the branches describe when emerging or merging should be preferred. The large vessel is more readily dissected and longitudinal lacerations are prevented when scissors are trapped into the acute angle between it and its branch. The tight adhesion of large vessels to the pericyst rules out the finger fracture procedure, which might result in pericystectomy as an incorrect, hazardous technique. The use of the ultrasound dissector, which favors the visualization of the vascular network, and hemostasis seems advantageous, while dissection of large vessels from pericyst is still feasible.[51,77]

Dissection is circumferential, according to the cyst location. The dissected parenchyma tends to flatten its spherical hollow surface, leaving the still adhering pericyst area largely uncovered. In very deep cysts and in bulky cysts dissection may become hazardous because the field is no longer under control. For this reason, and to prevent excessive manipulation of the cyst, its emptying is suitable and then open cyst pericystectomy can be performed. The same procedure should be followed in cases of cysts with pedunculated protrusions from exogenous vesiculations. They have a very thin pericyst, which may cause possible lacerations at the level of the pedicle in particular. As a general rule, any risk of cyst rupture should prompt emptying and then operation on the open cyst with a number of advantages, including the possible exploration of the cavity and better handling of the pericyst wall. By folding the pericyst at the level of the dissection plane the procedure is facilitated, especially if the already dissected pericyst is sectioned in strips, subjecting each to tension independently (Fig. 13.16). If the pericyst is not very calcific, another very useful method is to carefully incise it with a scalpel on its internal surface to reach the adhering parenchyma. With a cross- or star-shaped incision, and by lifting backwards each strip with Allis or Kocher forceps and dissecting from different sides, apparently unfavorable situations are resolved and dissection can be completed (Fig. 13.17). Access to mid-sized cysts through a

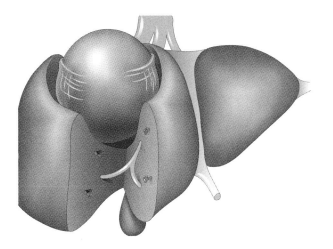

Figure 13.18 Total pericystectomy. In deep, non-emerging cysts, opening of the corresponding fissure is very useful. The cyst becomes accessible from several sides, somewhat similar to more superficial cysts.

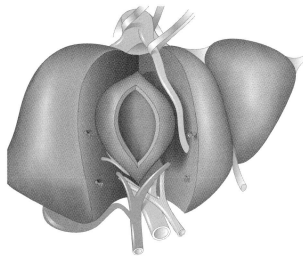

Figure 13.19 Total pericystectomy of deep cysts with multiple vasculobiliary relationships such as interportohepatic cysts is facilitated by opening the median fissure. Venous stasis from compression and compensatory collaterals may be present.

fissure is another very effective and in some cases resolving technique. Once major vasculobiliary structures are reached with dissection, the corresponding fissure is identified, opened and extended to the cyst wall. The cyst is accessible from several sides and seems to become more superficial (Fig. 13.18). Retraction of intersectorial surfaces resolves the problem of the difficult access to the deep hemisphere of the cyst. Therefore, operations on the closed cyst are facilitated with relevant vascular relationships as the interportal liver becomes accessible (Fig. 13.19).

Despite all precautions, during pericystectomy, vascular lacerations may occur, especially the hepatic veins. It is possible to interrupt the dissection on that side of the cyst and compress the parenchyma against the pericyst while the operation is resumed on another side. Direct digital compression of lacerated vascular segment can also allow further dissection and achieve more adequate exposure. The laceration becomes more readily identified and its definitive hemostasis can be performed with a suture which should also maintain vessel patency.

During pericystectomy temporary clamping of the hilum and/or caval vein may be necessary. To prevent bleeding, clamping is limited to 10–15 minutes, a few minutes being usually enough. Pringle's maneuver is not suitable for pericystectomy because of the relatively long time required for pericyst dissection. Clamping of hepatic veins is rarely necessary. Preventive isolation and application of a tape around the subhepatic caval vein and above the confluence of hepatic veins can be a safety precaution. The preparation of the right hepatic vein or the caval surface at the level of its confluence is a valid alternative, especially for cysts of segment VII and VIII. It should be kept in mind that a hepatic vein laceration proximal to the confluence is to be feared more for air embolism than for bleeding.

As for bleeding during total pericystectomy, the aversion shown for a long time by surgeons to this operation was directed against bleeding, at times dramatic, caused by it. This is a possible occurrence, but only when liver surgery is performed by inexperienced surgeons.

As for the amount of blood that should be available for transfusion, within wide variations, 2–4 units are required for peripheral cysts and 6–7 for central ones. Autotransfusion and intraoperative recovery, the latter obviously limited to the sterile phases of the operation, offer great advantage.

Among radical operations, in subtotal pericystectomy one or several areas of the pericyst are not excised; they adhere to vascular structures and their excision would be too hazardous. This fairly common solution is being abandoned because of the growing experience. It may be justified in some crucial areas such as the confluence of hepatic veins into the caval vein and hilar structures, in particular contralateral ones, and in case of cysts extending beyond the involved hemiliver. This is also the case for the retrohepatic caval vein, not rarely protruding in large cystic cavities of the right lobe. The decision whether to leave an area of pericyst in these sites is up to the surgeon alone.

During pericystectomy, a hepatic region may be ischemic because of impairment of blood supply. In this case, the extension of the involved region should be evaluated and identified. In some cases, its removal with pericyst resection is not a problem. Vascular impairment of a wider region is entirely different, but this should not occur.

After pericyst excision, the residual liver surfaces must be treated. They are characterized by a vascular profile of protruding hepatic veins or hilar structures. In general, closure of surfaces with suture of liver margins should not cause any vascular embarrassment. The procedure is simpler after the excision of deep cysts, although closure of external surfaces is very often feasible. In both cases the procedure does not correspond to the closure of a residual cavity but rather to the approximation of involved liver surfaces which then grow and merge through the rapid process of liver regeneration. If approximation is complete and there is no reason to

suggest bile loss, no drainage is necessary in the residual space. With the pericyst completely removed, an omental flap can be used on residual surfaces to prevent adhesion of displaced loops of bowel.

Because of the previously mentioned relationships of the cyst with the intrahepatic bile ducts, during operations on the cyst, complementary surgery on the bile ducts may be necessary. It may be required also for 'parahydatid' biliary pathology, dominated by cholelithiasis which is either consequent, incidental or pre-existing. En bloc cholecystectomy may be necessary for cysts of segments IV and V.

Surgical measures to be taken for intrahepatic bile ducts in case of communication or rupture have already been described. In rupture, peroperative cholangiography can detect bile duct obstruction with clear images of filling defects. Access to the common bile duct is through a choledochotomy or transduodenal papillosphincterostomy with complete clearing of the duct (Fig. 13.20). Bile duct drainage can be external with a T-tube or internal following a papillosphincterostomy or, more rarely, biliary–enteric anastomosis. The author prefers papillosphincterostomy. This can be performed even when pressure increase in the bile ducts secondary to papillitis is suspected, to prevent the appearance or persistence of bile leakage.[78] At present, prophylactic surgical biliary diversion can be replaced by endoscopic papillosphincterotomy, when necessary.[37]

Medical therapy

For over 20 years, benzoimidazole chemotherapy has been used in the treatment of hydatidosis.[79–85] As for liver hydatidosis, it is to be anticipated that results are varying and unpredictable. Biological recovery is rare and limited to young adults affected by univesicular cysts, more often resulting in morphological changes of the cyst, visualized on US or CT exams. The primary parasite can be impaired or even dead, but all proliferation does not cease. This result is achieved after prolonged treatments and is not free of severe side effects due to drug toxicity, and poor absorption and difficult penetration into the cyst, which require high doses. For these reasons, medical therapy is clearly subordinate to surgery. Indications for medical management include inoperable patients, preparation for surgery, patients who could not undergo radical surgery and prophylaxis of postoperative recurrences.[86,87] These indications have subsequently been extended.[58,85]

Benzoimidazole compounds include mebendazole, a well-known antihelminthic used in the treatment of

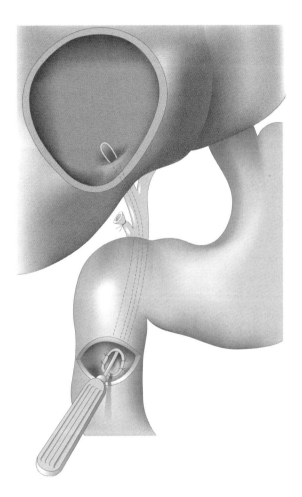

Figure 13.20 Exploration and cleansing of biliary tract. Through papillosphincterostomy the spoon for stones or a probe can be carefully advanced to identify the biliary breach and specify the type of communication, whether lateral or terminal, with the cyst cavity.

intestinal helminthiasis,[88] followed by flubendazole and albendazole. Their mechanism of action involves their interference with the basic structures of the parasite, with the inhibition of absorption mechanisms of glucose in particular, and more generally of nutrition.[89] Absorption following oral administration is low, liver metabolization rapid and clearance is through the urine. Fat intake favors absorption and increases plasma concentration,[90] while it is low inside the cyst and the in vitro proven parasiticidal action is hindered. Doses administered in man are: for mebendazole 4–5 g/day corresponding to 50 mg/kg/day with administration during meals for 3–12 months and for albendazole 10 mg/kg/day in one or two daily administrations in four one-month cycles with 15 days rest, or 10–12 mg/kg/day continuously for 3-month cycles.[58]

In the assessment of results of chemotherapy in man, the definition of death of the parasite and recovery from the disease poses big difficulties and relevant uncertainties. Viability tests on the surgical specimen cannot be considered conclusive as confirmed by the development of parasites from culture of cystic fluid shown to be negative on direct microscopy.[91] More particularly, it is difficult to understand that the drug could overcome the barrier of a dense fibrotic or calcific pericyst, up to 0.5 cm thick, and kill the hydatid material packed into the cavity. It is difficult to believe that exogenous vesiculations within the pericyst can be reached. Recurrence following albendazole therapy occurs in at least 20–30% of responsive cases,[85,92] to which a further 20% of patients, considered negative in whom no change was visualized, should be added.

PAIR (puncture, aspiration, introduction, reaspiration with 95% alcohol or 30% saline solution)[91,93–95] is a non-surgical treatment of hydatid cysts of the liver based on an old method used in inoperable patients with diffuse peritoneal hydatidosis. At present, puncture emptying is proposed again because of the lower risk achieved with benzoimidazole therapy, US guide and use of fine needles. However, the use of this method for all cysts of the liver of any site or type in place of surgery is not acceptable for the same reasons as exploratory punctures for diagnosis or control of the contents viability.

Key points

- Complications of hepatic hydatidosis include:
    Metastatic hydatid
    Secondary bacterial infection
    Intrabiliary rupture
    Intraperitoneal rupture
    Bronchobiliary fistula.
- Diagnosis of hepatic hydatidosis:
    Incidental finding (in patient from endemic region)
    Abdominal mass
    Calcified hepatic cyst on the plain abdominal photograph (AXR)
    Ultrasound/CT/MRI
    Hydatid serology/Casoni skin test.
- Preoperative management:
    Systemic albendazole/mebendazole
    ERCP (exclude cystobiliary fistula)
    Protection of operative field before surgical emptying of cyst contents
    Sterilization of cyst cavity.

REFERENCES

1. Akinoglu A, Arparslan, Kaza K. Hydatid disease of the liver: prevention of postoperative biliary fistula. Arch Hidatid 1991; 30: 649–55
2. Chigot JP, Langlois P, Teboul F, Clot JP, Gentilini M, Mercadier M. Le traitement des kystes hydatiques du foie. Ann Chir 1986; 40: 177–82
3. Euzéby J. L'echinococcose larvaire. Rev Méd Vét 1955; 106: 456–68
4. Kalovidouris A, Voros D, Gouliamos A, Vlachos L. Papavasiliou C. Extracapsular (satellite) hydatid cysts. Gastrointest Radiol 1992; 17: 353–6
5. Bourgeon R, Catalano H, Guntz M. La périkystectomie dans le traitement des kystes hydatiques du foie. J Chir 1961; 81: 153–74
6. Belli L, Del Favero E, Marni A, Romani F. Resection

versus pericystectomy in the treatment of hydatidosis of the liver. Am J Surg 1983; 145: 239–42
7. Moreno Gonzales E, Jovez Navalon JM, Landa Garcia JI et al. Surgical management of liver hydatidosis. 10-year experience with 269 patients. It J Surg Sci 1985; 15: 267–73
8. Debesse B, Dujon A. La périkystectomie au plus près dans le traitement du kyste hydatique du foie. Ann Chir 1987; 41: 646–51
9. Moreno Gonzales E, Rico Selas P, Bercedo Martinez J, Garcia Garcia I, Palma Carazo F, Hidalgo Pascual M. Results of surgical treatment of hepatic hydatidosis: current therapeutic modifications. World J Surg 1991; 15: 254–63
10. Tagliacozzo S, Daniele GM, Pisano G. Pericistectomia

totale per echinococco epatico. Arch Atti Soc It Chir 1979; 1: 657–712

11. Tagliacozzo S, Daniele GM, Pisano G. Total pericystectomy for hydatid disease of the liver. 6° World Congr Coll Int Chir Dig, Lisbona 1980, abst SP5–03

12. Xu Ming-quian. Diagnosis and management of hepatic hydatidosis complicated with biliary fistula. Arch Hidatid 1991; 30: 657–63

13. Assadourian R, Bricot R, Djilalli G et al. Les kystes hydatiques du foie. Table ronde. 84° Congrès de Chirurgie. Rev Ass Fr Chir 1984; 33: 15–39

14. Alper A, Ariogul O, Emre A, Uras A, Okten A. Choledochoduodenostomy for intrabiliary rupture of hydatid cyst of the liver. Br J Surg 1987; 74: 243–5

15. Kattan YB. Intrabiliary rupture of hydatid cysts of the liver into the biliary tracts. Br J Surg 1975; 62: 885–90

16. Lygidakis NJ. Diagnosis and treatment of intrabiliary rupture of hydatid cyst of the liver. Arch Surg 1983; 118: 1186–9

17. Placer C, Martin R, Sanchez E, Soleto E. Rupture of abdominal hydatid cysts. Br J Surg 1988; 75: 157–9

18. Barros JL. Hydatid disease of the liver. Am J Surg 1978; 135: 597–600

19. Marcos Sanchez F, Turabian Fernandez JL, Caballero Gomez F et al. Reacciones alergicas-shock anafilactico como manifestacion de enfermedad hidatica hepatica. Rev Clin Esp 1984; 173: 49–52

20. Giulekas D, Papacosta D, Papacostantinou C, Barbarousis D, Angel J. Recurrent anaphylactic shock as a manifestation of echinococcosis. Scand J Thorac Cardiovasc Surg 1986; 20: 175–7

21. Lewall DB, McCorkell SJ. Rupture of echinococcal cysts: diagnosis, classification and clinical implications. AJR 1986; 146: 391–4

22. Morris DL, Chinnery JB, Hardcaster JD. Can albendazole reduce the risk of implication of spilled protoscolices? An animal study. Trans R Soc Trop Med Hyg 1986; 80: 481–4

23. Tagliacozzo S. Trattamento chirurgico delle fistole bilio-bronchiali nell'idatidosi epatica. Minerva Chir 1973; 28: 732–45

24. Tierris EJ, Angeropoulos K, Kourtis R, Papaevangelou EJ. Bronchobiliary fistula due to echinococcosis of the liver. World J Surg 1977; 1: 99–104

25. Gomez R, Moreno E, Loinaz C et al. Diaphragmatic or transdiaphragmatic thoracic involvement in hepatic disease: surgical trends and classification. World J Surg 1995; 19: 714–9

26. Tagliacozzo S, Daniele GM, Pisano G. Le fistole biliobronchiali nell' idatidosi epatica. Atti Cong Straord Chir Tor, Padova, 1981, I: 221–9

27. Angelini L. Hydatid disease. In: Joseph AEA, Gosgrove DO, eds. Ultrasound in inflammatory disease. New York: Churchill-Livingstone, 1983: 245–55

28. Gharbi HA, Hassine W, Brauner MW, Dupuch K. Ultrasound examination of the hydatic liver. Radiology 1981; 139: 459–63

29. Hassine W, Dupuch K, Gharbi HA. Aspects écho-graphiques de l'hydatidose. J Radiol 1979; 60: 660–6

30. Lewall DB, McCorkell SJ. Hepatic echinococcal cysts: sonographic appearance and classification. Radiology 1985; 155: 773–5

31. Itoh K, Nishimura K, Togashi K et al. Hepatocellular carcinoma MR imaging. Radiology 1987; 164: 21–5

32. Elizondo G, Weissleder R, Stark DD et al. Amebic liver abscess: diagnosis and treatment evaluation with MR imaging. Radiology 1987; 165: 795–800

33. Rummeny E, Weissleder R, Stark DD et al. Primary liver tumors, diagnosis by MR imaging. AJR 1989; 152: 63–72

34. Marani SAD, Canossi GC, Nicoli FA, Albertis GP, Monni SJ, Casolo P. Hydatid disease: MR imaging study. Radiology 1990; 175: 701–6

35. Cottone M, Amuso M, Cotton PB. Endoscopic retrograde cholangiography in hepatic hydatid disease. Br J Surg 1978; 65: 107–8

36. Moreira VF, Merosio E, Simon MA et al. CPRE in echinococcus cysts of the liver. Gastroint Radiol 1985; 10: 124–8

37. Vignote ML, Mino G, De La Mata M, Dios JF, Gomez F. Endoscopic sphincterotomy in hepatic hydatid disease open to the biliary tree. Br J Surg 1990; 77: 30–2

38. Little JM, Hollands MJ, Ekberg H. Recurrence of hydatid disease. World J Surg 1988; 12: 700–4

39. Jiang Ci-Peng. Differential diagnosis between liver echinococcus cyst and non echinococcus cyst. Arch Hidatid 1991; 30: 475–500

40. Baldelli F, Papili R, Francisci D et al. Biological diagnosis of human hydatid disease. Arch Hidatid 1991; 30: 391–400

41. Morris DL. Diagnosis of hydatid disease. In: Morris DL, Richards HS, eds. Hydatid disease. Current medical and surgical management. Philadelphia: Butterworth-Heinemann 1992: 25–56

42. Rickard MD, Honey RD, Brumley JL, Mitchell GF. Serological diagnosis and post-operative surveillance of human hydatid disease. II. The enzyme-linked immunosorbent assay (ELISA) using various antigens. Pathology 1984; 16: 211–5

43. Couinaud C. Le foie. Etudes anatomiques et chirurgicales. Paris: Masson; 1957: 9–33

44. Goldsmith NA, Woodburne RT. Surgical anatomy pertaining to liver resection. Surg Gynecol Obstet 1957; 105: 310–8

45. Tôn Thât Tùng. Chirurgie d'exerese du foie. Paris: Masson, 1962: 5–36

46. Bourgeon R. Les bases physiopathologiques nécessaires à la conduite thérapeutique du kyste hydatique du foie, en particulier par périkystectomie. In: Cirenei A, Hess W, eds. Chirurgie du foie, des voies biliares et du pancreas. Padova: Piccin, 1977: 21–35

47. Meymarian E, Luttermoser GW, Frayha GJ, Schwabe DVM, Prescott B. Host parasite relationship in echinococcosis. Laboratory evaluations of chemical scolicides as adjuncts hydatid surgery. Ann Surg 1963; 158: 211–5

48. Saidi F. A new approach to the surgical treatment of hydatid cyst. Ann R Coll Surg Engl 1977; 59: 115–28

49. Frayha GJ, Bikhazi KJ, Kachachi TA. Treatment of hydatid cysts (*Echinococcus granulosus*) by Cetrimide®. Trans R Soc Trop Med Hyg 1981; 75: 447–50

50. Morris DL. Surgical management of hepatic hydatid cyst. In: Morris DL, Richards KS, eds. Hydatid disease. Current medical and surgical management. Philadelphia: Butterworth-Heinemann 1992: 57–75

51. Little JM. Hydatid disease of the liver. In: Hadfield J, Hobsley M, Tressure T, eds. Current surgical practice, Vol 5. London: Edward Arnold, 1990: 146–61

52. Khodadadi DJ, Kurgan A, Schmidt B. Sclerosing cholangitis following the treatment of echinococcosis of the liver. Int Surg 1981; 66: 361–2

53. Cohen-Solal JL, Eroukmhanoff P, Desoutter P, Loisel JC, Kohlmann G, Flabean F. Cholangite sclerosante survénue après traitement chirurgical d'un kyste hydatique du foie. Sem Hôpitaux Paris 1983; 59: 1623–4

54. Teres J, Gomez-Moli J, Bruguera M, Visa J, Bordas JM, Pera C. Sclerosing cholangitis after surgical treatment of hepatic echinococcal cysts. Report of three cases. Am J Surg 1984; 148: 694–7

55. Belghiti J, Benhamou JP, Houry S, Grenier P, Huguier M, Fékéte F. Caustic sclerosing cholangitis. A complication of the surgical treatment of hydatid disease of the liver. Arch Surg 1986; 121: 1162–5

56. Stubbs RS. Management of hydatid disease: scolicidal agent instillation versus perioperative chemotherapy. HPB Surgery 1990; 2 (suppl): 155

57. Erzurumlu K, Ozdemir M, Mihmanli M, Cevikbas U. The effect of intraoperative mebendazole-albendazole applications on the hepatobiliary system. Eur Surg Res 1995; 27: 340–5

58. Teggi A, Lastilla MG, De Rosa F. Therapy of human hydatid disease with benzoimidazole carbamates. Arch Hidatid 1991; 30: 773–95

59. Tsimoyiannis EC, Siakas Ph, Moutesidou KJ, Karayianni M, Kantoyiannis DS, Gossios KJ. Perioperative benzimidazole therapy in human hydatid liver disease. Int Surg 1995; 80: 131–3

60. Lagrot F, Coriat P. Justification et valeur de la résection du dôme saillant dans les kystes hydatiques du foie. Lyon Chir 1959, 55: 826–37

61. Moumen M, Elalauni ME, Mehane M, Jami D, Mokhtari M, El Fares. La résection du dôme saillant du kyste hydatique du foie. A propos de 360 cas. J Chir 1990; 127: 83–6

62. Goinard P, Note D, Girardot M. IIe: sur le traitement de KHF (kyste hydatique du foie). L'épiploonplastie intracavitaire. Presse Méd 1950; 58: 1203–5

63. Xu Ming-qian. Diagnosis and management of the liver: hydatidosis complicated with biliary fistula. HPB Surgery 1990; 2 (suppl): 153

64. Safioleas M, Misiakos E, Manti, Katsikas D, Skalkeas G. Diagnostic evaluation and surgical management of hydatid disease of the liver. World J Surg 1994; 18: 859–65

65. Chaimoff C, Lubin E, Dintsman M. The postoperative appearance of the liver on scanning following omentopexy of the hydatid cyst. Int Surg 1980; 65: 331–3

66. Beggs I, Walmsley K, Cowie AGA. The radiological appearances of the liver after surgical removal of hydatid cyst. Clin Radiol 1983; 34: 555–63

67. Napalkoff N. A propos de la décortication des Kystes hydatiques. Rev Chir 1927; 65: 524–8

68. Melnikoff AW. Sur la chirurgie des kystes hydatiques. J Chir 1936; 47: 197–219

69. Costantini H, Bourgeon R, Pantin JP, Rives J. Des indications de l'ablation du sac péri parasitaire dans le traitement des kystes hydatiques du foie. La kystectomie de routine des kystes suppurés du foie. J Chir 1936; 66: 177–89

70. Yovanovitch BY. Place de la kystectomie dans le traitement des kystes hydatique du foie. Ann Chir 1959; 13: 31–6

71. Bourgeon R, Guntz M, Catalano H, Alexandre JH, Mouiel J. Incidence de la topographie sur le traitement des kystes hydatiques du foie. J Chir 1964; 88: 375–88

72. Tagliacozzo S. Total pericystectomy and complementary papillostomy in the treatment of hepatic hydatid cyst. Proc XX Biennal World Congr Int Coll Surg, Atene, 1976: 630–1

73. Tagliacozzo S. Typical and atypical (total pericystectomies) resections in the surgical treatment of hydatid disease of the liver. Surg It 1977; 7: 133–42

74. Tagliacozzo S. Exogenous vesiculation and radical treatment of hepatic hydatid cyst. 30th Congr Soc Int Chir, Hamburg, 1983: 51

75. Elhamel A. Pericystectomy for the treatment of hepatic hydatid cysts. Surgery 1990; 107: 316–20

76. Lozano-Montecon R. Cystopericystectomy. In: Symposium: Current treatment of echinococcal disease. International surgical week ISW 95. 36th World Congress of Surgery, Lisbon, 27 August–2 September 1995 (oral communication)

77. Vicente E, Devesa JM, Nuno J, Fernandez JM, Angel V. Progress in the surgical treatment of hepatic hydatid cysts. 34th World Congr ISS/SIC, Stockholm, 1991, A139: 255

78. Tagliacozzo S, Daniele GM. La papillostomie complémentaire dans le traitement chirurgical des kystes hydatiques du foie. Bull Soc Int Chr 1974; 5–6: 493–497

79. Heath DD, Chevis RAF. Mebendazole and hydatid cysts. Lancet 1974; ii: 218–9

80. Muller E, Akobiantz A, Amman RW. Treatment of human echinococcosis with mebendazole. Preliminary observations in 28 patients. Hepatogastroenterology 1982; 29: 236–9

81. Morris DL, Dykes PW, Dickson B, Marriner SE, Bogan JH, Borrows FG. Albendazole in hydatid disease. Br Med J 1983; 286: 103–4

82. De Rosa F, Teggi A. Mebendazole in human hydatidosis. Drugs Exp Clin Res 1985; 11: 875–8

83. Davis A, Pawlowski ZS, Dixon H. Multicentre clinical trials of benzimidazole carbamates in human echinococcosis. Bull WHO 1986; 64: 383–8

84. Todorov T, Vutova K, Mechkov G, Petkov D, Nedelkov G, Tonchev Z. Evaluation of response to chemotherapy of human cystic echinococcosis. Br J Radiol 1990; 63: 523–31

85. De Rosa F, Teggi A. Treatment of echinococcus granulosus hydatid disease with albendazole. Ann Trop Med Parasitol 1990; 84: 467–72

86. World Health Organization. Treatment of human echinococcosis: report of an informal meeting, June 16–July 1, Geneva, 1981

87. World Health Organization. Treatment of human echinococcosis: report of an informal meeting, December 15–16 Geneva, 1983

88. Morris DL. Chemotherapy of hydatid disease in man. In: Morris DL, Richards KS, eds. Hydatid disease. Current medical and surgical management. Philadelphia: Butterworth-Heinemann 1992: 76–93

89. Lacey E. Mode of action of benzoimidazole. Parasitol Today 1990; 6: 112–5

90. Munst GJ, Karlagains G, Bircher J. Concentrations of mebendazole during treatment of echinococcosis. Preliminary results. Eur J Clin Pharmacol 1980; 17: 375–8

91. Filice C, Trosselli M, Brunetti E, Colombo P, Emmi E, D'Andrea F. P.A.I.R. (Puncture, Aspiration, Introduction, Reaspiration) with alcohol under US guidance of hydatid liver cysts. Arch Hidatid 1991; 30: 811–7

92. Morris DL. Albendazole treatment of hydatid disease, follow up at five years. Trop Doc 1989; 19: 179–80

93. Mueller PR, Dawson SL, Ferrucci JT Jr, Nardi GL. Hepatic echinococcal cyst, successful percutaneous drainage. Radiology 1985; 155: 627–8

94. Ben Amor N, Gargouri M, Gharbi HA, Golvan YJ, Dyachi K, Kchouk H. Essai de traitement par ponction des kystes hydatiques abdominaux inopérables. Ann Parasitol Hum Comp 1986; 61: 689–92

95. Bastid C, Hzar C, Doyer M, Sahel J. Percutaneous treatment of hydatid cysts under sonographic guidance. Dig Dis Sci 1994; 37: 1576–80

Further reading

Saidi F. Surgery of hydatid disease. London: WB Saunders, 1976

Morris DL, Richards HS (eds) Hydatid disease. Current medical and surgical management. Philadelphia: Butterworth-Heinemann, 1992

Saidi F. Treatment of echinococcal cysts. In: Nyhus LM, Baker RJ, eds. Mastery of surgery, 3rd edn. Boston: Little, Brown and Co, 1997: 1035–82

Tagliacozzo S. Chirurgia dell' Idatidosi epatica. Rome: EMSI, 1997

14 Management of recurrent pyogenic cholangitis

WY Lau and CK Leow

Introduction

While practising in Hong Kong in 1930, Digby drew attention to a condition which was subsequently known as recurrent pyogenic cholangitis by reporting on eight cases of 'common duct stones of liver origin'.[1] The term recurrent pyogenic cholangitis or RPC was used by Cook et al. in 1954 when they reported their experience with the condition in a series of 90 patients.[2] The synonyms associated with this condition include Asiatic cholangiohepatitis, oriental cholangiohepatitis, Hong Kong Disease,[3] Chinese biliary obstruction syndrome[4] and primary cholangitis.[5] This condition is commonly seen in Chinese living in Canton and Hong Kong but is not restricted to the Chinese in the Orient since it also occurs in Chinese immigrants in Malaysia, Singapore, North America and Australia.[6–8] RPC is also common in Japanese in Japan and Taiwanese in Taiwan. Although rare, RPC has also been reported to afflict occidentals.[9,10]

Pathogenesis

In RPC the gallstones found within the biliary system are calcium bilirubinate stones or pigmented calcium stones. Calcium bilirubinate stones are prevalent in Asia and are very rare in Europe and the United States. In addition to the presence of these friable concretions of various shapes and sizes within the biliary tree, the bile is often muddy in consistency and contains numerous fine particles of calcium bilirubinate. Biochemical analysis of these stones revealed a bilirubin content of 40.2–57.1% and a cholesterol content of 2.9–25.6%. This differs greatly from cholesterol stones, which are common in Europe and the United States, which contain >96% of cholesterol in pure cholesterol stone, and

>71.3% in mixed cholesterol stone but the bilirubin content is only 0.02–5.0%.[11] The peculiarity of the formation of calcium bilirubinate stones in RPC has been ascribed to the high incidence of bile being infected with Escherichia coli (E. coli). In man, the major portion of bilirubin is excreted in bile as bilirubin glucuronide. In the presence of β-glucuronidase, bilirubin glucuronide is hydrolysed into free bilirubin and glucuronic acid. Normally, calcium is secreted into bile and when it combines with the carboxyl radical of free bilirubin, insoluble calcium bilirubinate is formed. Normal bile is free of β-glucuronidase activity, whereas bile infected with E. coli has intense β-glucuronidase activity. Bile calcium content increases in the presence of biliary tract inflammation and this coupled with the increased hydrolysis of bilirubin glucuronide by the β-glucuronidase from E. coli gives rise to the multiple stones formation classically seen in RPC.[11] There are two types of pigmented stones, black and brown. The infected type seen in RPC is the brown pigment stone.

The postulated port of entry for the micro-organisms of bowel origin is via the portal vein from an attack of enteric infection. In the acute stage of RPC, Ong reported that 39.5% of the studied cases had a positive portal blood culture while the positive supraduodenal lymph node culture rate was 38.1%.[12] The rate of infected bile in patients with pigmented stone compared to those with cholesterol stone is correspondingly much higher in the former. In comparing patients with pigmented stones against those with cholesterol stones, Maki demonstrated that 88.3% of the bile in patients with pigmented stone was infected and E. coli was isolated from all cases. This compared to 43.5% in patients with cholesterol stone and of these only 70% of cases had E. coli isolated.[13] However, bacteria excreted into the bile within a non-obstructed biliary system will not usually give rise to infection and an attack of

A

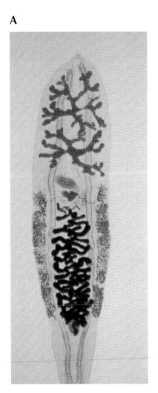

B

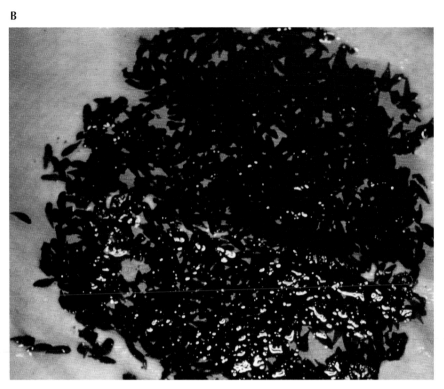

Figure 14.1 (A) Magnified view of *Clonorchis sinensis* (× 12.5). (B) Numerous *Clonorchis* removed from the CBD of one patient.

cholangitis. Thus obstruction by parasites such as *Clonorchis sinensis* (Fig. 14.1) and *Ascaris lumbricoides* can initiate the sequence of events which eventually lead to the formation of intrahepatic pigment stones.[2] Furthermore, the egg or carcass of the parasite can act as a nidus for the deposition of calcium bilirubinate.[13] However, only a proportion of patients with RPC have positive ova in stools indicating parasitic infestation, while in some patients the remains of parasites can be identified within the stones recovered.[12,13] *Clonorchis* infection does not occur in the Sarawak state of West Malaysia due to the absence of the snail, Bithynia, which is the first intermediate host in the life cycle of *Clonorchis sinensis.*[12] Yet RPC is common among the Chinese and the indigenous race, the Dyaks. Thus parasitic infestation is only one of the aetiological factors for RPC. Maki suggested that the migration of roundworms through the ampulla of Vater leads to papillitis and secondary dyskinesia of the common bile duct (CBD). This leads to increased intrahepatic ductal pressure, dilatation of the CBD and poor drainage of the biliary system.[13] A poorly draining biliary system contributing to the formation of intrahepatic stones and colonization of the bile by bacteria was experimentally shown in rabbits by Ong in 1962. Rabbits who had the CBD constricted by a linen thread prior to a single intraportal injection of an *E. coli* suspension developed ductal dilatation and stone formation in the CBD and

intrahepatic ducts. On culture, the bile from the gallbladder and bile ducts was positive for *E. coli.*[12]

In the mid 1950s in Japan, the proportion of pigmented to cholesterol stones found in professionals was almost equal. However, almost 90% of the gallstones found in farmers were of pigmented calcium stone. As the farmers were economically less well off, they could only afford a diet which was deficient in fat and protein. It was postulated that the deficient diet may be a factor for the development of pigmented stone.[13] Matsushiro et al. have demonstrated that a diet low in protein and fat leads to lower levels of glucaro-1:4-lactone, a powerful inhibitor of β-glucuronidase, in bile.[14] The reduced level of glucaro-1:4-lactone in bile thus permits increased hydrolysis of bilirubin glucuronide to free bilirubin and glucuronic acid by the bacterial β-glucuronidase present in infected bile. The free bilirubin then conjugates with calcium in the bile to form the typical calcium bilirubinate stones of RPC. In Hong Kong, RPC is no longer seen in the younger generation born and bred in modern-day Hong Kong. Young patients, in their 30s, who present to our institution with RPC are invariably immigrants from China. We suspect that the much better social and economic conditions of modern-day Hong Kong have played a role in eradicating the condition.[15] The reduced incidence of gastroenteritis, the inabilility of the enteric organism, which gained

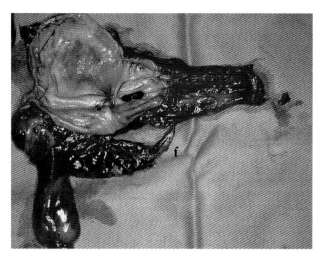

Figure 14.2 A totally destroyed left liver lobe consisting of a cavernous biliary sac with negligible liver parenchymal tissue. (f = falciform ligament).

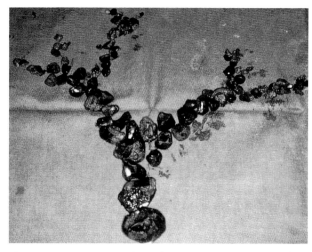

Figure 14.3 Large number of pigment stones removed from one patient with RPC.

entry via the portal blood, to establish itself within the liver parenchyma due to better host defence from an improved high protein, low carbohydrate diet and possibly the fact that less Chinese herbal medicine is being consumed by the modern generation of youngsters may all have contributed to the demise of this condition.

Pathology

Macroscopically, due to the repeated attacks of biliary sepsis, it is common to find adhesions between the liver surface and the surrounding parietal peritoneum, especially the diaphragmatic surface, at operation. The liver surface is scarred and prominent dilated ducts may be obvious. The affected lobe of the liver, usually the left, is normally atrophic with compensatory hypertrophy of the remaining lobe. On palpation, the stones within the dilated biliary ducts are easily palpable. Occasionally, the underlying lobe can be so destroyed by the repeated attacks of cholangiohepatitis that what remains is a cavernous biliary sac with minimal surrounding liver parenchyma (Fig. 14.2). Within the sac is a soup of biliary mud and stones. The brown pigment stones are soft stones which crumble when squeezed between fingers or forceps. The size variation goes from fine grains to stones of 4–5 cm in diameter. The stones are irregular, can take up the shape of the biliary duct or become faceted when the stones are packed (Fig. 14.3). Apart from the stones, the bile duct is filled with biliary mud. This is a broth of mucus, altered bile products, microcalculi, desquamated epithelium, parasites and pus.

The pathological hallmark of RPC is the steadily progressive, recurrent cholangiohepatitis with periportal fibrosis. Histologically, in the the early acute stage of an attack of cholangiohepatitis, it is similar to that of bacterial cholangitis associated with cholecystitis and calculus obstruction seen in the Western world,[16] while the histological picture of the acute, chronic and advanced stage of the disease is not dissimilar to that seen in sclerosing cholangitis.[17] In the early lesions the lumen of the small biliary ducts is filled with pus, with rapid extension into the surrounding tissue. There is marked dissociation of the liver cells by polymorphonuclear infiltration of the sinusoids together with Kupffer cell hyperplasia. In the lobules around the affected duct there is a varying degree of cellular necrosis. Resolution of the underlying inflammation leads to dense round-cell infiltration which is then replaced by fibrous tissue. In the larger intrahepatic ducts, the duct wall becomes inflamed, ulcerated and destroyed together with the formation of cholangitic abscesses. Resolution results in intense fibrosis which accounts for the undue prominence of the duct wall seen on sectioning a liver affected by RPC. During the acute episode, these larger ducts can become irregular in calibre and short segments of relative stricture can occur at intervals along the duct. The duct proximal to the stenosis dilates. Recurrent attacks of infection and resolution lead to permanent damage of the duct wall and the ducts remain dilated. The relative stricture then becomes a true localized stricture. These strictures are most frequently encountered at the site of ductal confluence. One of the main concerns of these inflammatory strictures is malignant transformation into cholangiocarcinoma. Ohta et al., from their autopsy studies, suggested that repeated inflammatory damage to the ductal epithelium from the attacks of cholangitis can lead to atypical epithelial hyperplasia, dysplasia and eventually cholangiocarcinoma.[18]

The left lobe of the liver is preferentially affected. The exact reason for this is unknown. One possible explanation may be the selective distribution of portal blood within the liver. Two studies suggested that the left lobe of the liver receives blood from the colon and the left lobe will be the first port of call for enteric organisms such as E. coli which have entered the portal venous system.[19,20] Colonization of the bile with E. coli will lead to the production of β-glucuronidase in the biliary system. Another explanation is that the more oblique course of the left hepatic duct results in poorer drainage of the left ductal system as compared to the right hepatic duct, thus leading to increased incidence of stone formation. If stones are found in the right hepatic duct, almost invariably stones are found in the left duct. In one study of 115 patients with hepatolithiasis, the ratio of stones found in the left and right hepatic ducts was 6:1.[5] The stones form in the dilated ducts proximal to the stricture site. These strictures can be multiple and bilobar in distribution and commonly occur at the origin of the right and left hepatic ducts. Stones within the common bile duct are usually lodged at the supraduodenal portion of the duct or at the ampulla. At ERCP, a patulous ampulla of Vater (probably a result of repeated passage of stones) is not an uncommon finding in patients with RPC.

The bile in patients with hepatolithiasis is usually infected with enteric organisms. The two most common organisms isolated are E. coli and Klebsiella species. The overall positive bile culture rate has been reported to be as high as 87% and the incidence of positive culture in patients requiring surgical intervention and those which settled on conservative measures is similar (90% versus 85%).[21]

The gallbladders in these patients are usually thin-walled, large and distended. The majority of them do not contain gallstones. While the incidence of CBD stones and biliary mud varied from 60 to 90%, the incidence of associated gallstones in the gallbladder was only 15 to 40%.[4,7] Macroscopically, the gallbladder looks normal but histological examination invariably shows features compatible with low grade chronic cholecystitis. Along the gastro-hepatic omentum gross lymphadenitis with enlarged lymph nodes is commonly encountered.

Clinical presentation

Patients with RPC tend to be younger (third and fourth decade) than those affected by cholesterol stone disease, which is much more prevalent in older women, in the Western world. Although the condition does not have a particular sex prevalence, those afflicted are almost invariably from the lower socio-economic classes. The usual presentation consists of the classical Charcot's triad of abdominal pain, fever (with or without chills and rigors) and jaundice which signifies an attack of cholangitis. The patient may not notice the jaundice but a history of tea-coloured urine is usual. The jaundice is usually not severe since cholangitis secondary to a completely obstructed biliary system will rapidly progress to acute suppurative obstructive cholangitis with septicaemia. In addition to the triad of symptoms, these patients also develop mental confusion and shock, which is referred to as Reynaud's pentad. The epigastric/right upper quadrant pain is usually described as a constant and gnawing/cutting[12] pain, which may radiate to the back. Vomiting is not a constant feature. Patients have spiking fever, not unlike that seen with an underlying abscess or collection, which normally resolves rapidly when the conservative treatment has been effective.

On examination, the patient looks unwell and restless with a tinge of jaundice. The associated jaundice is typically mild and clinically can be just discernible. Abdominal examination may reveal the telltale signs of surgical scars from previous operations. Tenderness with varying degree of guarding is noted in the epigastrium or right upper quadrant. A tender hepatomegaly may be present. Marked tenderness may imply the presence of an underlying abscess. Deterioration in the abdominal signs (increasing and generalized tenderness) and/or the development of worsening haemodynamic parameters (persistent hypotension, tachycardia, poor urine output despite adequate resuscitation) argues for emergency surgical intervention to decompress the biliary system.

Those patients who present or develop shock have a flushed facie, warm periphery, bounding peripheral pulse and hypotension. The massive vasodilatation and reduced cardiac contractility secondary to the endotoxaemia adequately explain the state of shock.

Investigations

Both the haematological and biochemical tests do not differentiate patients with RPC from those with other causes of biliary obstruction and infection. Full blood count will reveal an underlying leucocytosis with neutrophilia and mild thrombocytopaenia in some patients. A number of patients will also have a concomitant mild derangement of the clotting profile with a prolonged prothrombin time. The deranged liver function test is compatible with an obstructive picture with a moderately raised level of bilirubin and a high serum alkaline phosphatase level. The level of γ-glutamyltranspeptidase is elevated. The slightly elevated alanine transaminase level in some patients is a reflection of the parenchymal damage secondary to the underlying infection within the biliary system.

Other than showing the presence of pneumobilia in some cases, a plain abdominal radiograph is not helpful. The calcium bilirubinate stones are radiolucent because of the low calcium and high bilirubin content. The least expensive and most helpful investigation is ultrasonography (USG). It can demonstrate the presence of stones within the dilated intrahepatic and common bile ducts, the presence or absence of an underlying liver abscess and occasionally the presence of a solid liver mass secondary to malignancy complicating a benign stricture. Also it can reveal the presence or absence of gallstone(s) within the gallbladder. Intra- and extrahepatic ductal stones are present in the majority of patients, but cholelithiasis is much less common and is seen in the minority of cases. Although intrahepatic stones normally cast sonic shadows on USG, the presence of air within the bile ducts (either spontaneously or secondary to previous biliary drainage procedures) can give rise to highly reflective echoes with posterior shadows, thus confusing and misleading the radiologist in diagnosing the presence of stones within the bile ducts. In about 3% of RPC, pneumobilia is present.[22] In some cases the amorphous and small stones can form a cast of the biliary tree and, under such circumstances, highly reflective echoes and posterior acoustic shadowing on USG may be absent. It may then be difficult to identify dilated bile ducts and the ducts can appear as soft tissue masses on USG.[7]

USG images and their interpretation are operator dependent. Computed tomography (CT) removes this bias and can provide images of the dilated intra- and extrahepatic ducts, even if they are filled with sludge or pus. On CT scanning these filling defects are of higher attenuation than bile, but have a lower attenuation than contrast-enhanced liver parenchyma.[23] Although uncommon, the amorphous stones which completely fill the ducts and are isodense with the hepatic parenchyma could be missed on CT. Unlike USG, there is no difficulty in distinguishing pneumobilia from stones on CT and visualization of the extrahepatic ducts is not limited by overlying bowel gas.

USG and CT do not provide sufficient details of the ductal anatomy. Cholangiography, in the form of

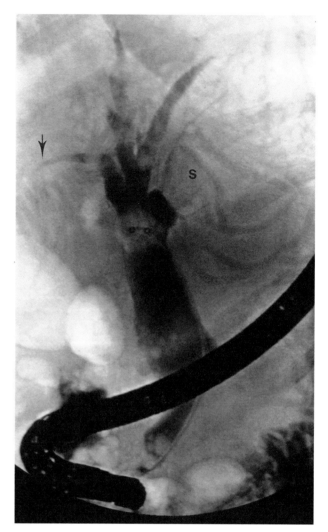

Figure 14.4 Typical truncated biliary tree appearance together with the arrow or spear head sign (arrow) on ERCP. A large stone(s) in the left duct.

endoscopic retrograde cholangiopancreatography (ERCP) and/or percutaneous transhepatic cholangiography (PTC), is essential for the detail delineation of the entire biliary tract. Older methods of delineating the biliary tracts such as oral cholecystography and intravenous cholangiography are no longer used because they provide suboptimal visualization of the ductal system. In addition to the potential complication of allergic reaction to the contrast injected, there is no place for intravenous cholangiography in the presence of biliary obstruction or cholangitis. Our first line of investigation is ERCP since it is both diagnostic and therapeutic. The typical cholangiogram will show dilated extrahepatic ducts in more than half the cases. The intrahepatic ducts have the classical 'truncated tree' pattern where the 'tree' has been trimmed back to its 'main branches'. The terminal end of these 'branches' are tapered, resembling an arrow or a spear head (Fig. 14.4). It is more common to see a dilated left ductal system containing calculi than an

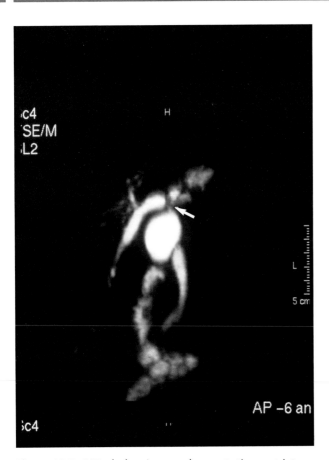

Figure 14.5 MR cholangiogram demonstrating a stricture (arrow) at the confluence of the right and left hepatic ducts.

affected right system. There may be an accompanying relative or true stricture distal to the dilated ducts. When a stone or stricture prevents the filling of the intrahepatic ducts, or when it is technically impossible to perform an ERCP due to previous biliary–enteric bypass surgery, PTC under USG guidance is performed. As a result of the stones and stricture(s), the biliary anatomy can be very complicated. Once an obstructed biliary duct is punctured during PTC, the obstructed system must be drained to avoid cholangitis and/or bile leak. Underfilling during cholangiography can lead to missed segmental ducts. More importantly, the paucity of intrahepatic ducts shown on cholangiograms should prompt the surgeon to count the number of segmental ducts present in order not to miss the diagnosis of undrained segment(s). Cholangiography complements USG and CT and their findings should be considered as a whole and not in isolation.

We have shown that magnetic resonance (MR) cholangiography is comparable to ERCP in diagnosing choledocholithiasis.[24] Apart from being non-invasive, MR cholangiography can delineate biliary strictures which may be difficult to show or missed on ERCP due to technical reasons (Fig. 14.5). In a recent study by Park

et al. MR cholangiography has been shown to be better than ERCP/PTC.[25] Occasionally, a radioisotope scan is performed to demonstrate the presence of undrained or hypo-functioning liver segments.

The radiographic features of certain conditions can simulate RPC. Sclerosing cholangitis can lead to biliary tract strictures. However, these are usually more peripherally located and there is a lack of the marked proximal dilatation and stones seen in RPC. Although the common bile duct is massively dilated in choledochal cysts, in most cases, there is an abrupt transition to normal or slightly dilated proximal ducts.[26] Patients with Caroli disease (cavernous ectasia of the biliary tract) have dilated intrahepatic ducts and calculi but the extrahepatic ducts are disproportionately small.[27] The condition is often associated with renal cystic disease[28] which, on CT, helps to distinguish it from RPC.

In almost all cases, given the clinical and investigation findings, the diagnosis of RPC is seldom in doubt. The investigations merely help to define the extent and severity of the underlying disease and guide the management plan.

Acute management

RPC patients have repeated attacks of acute cholangitis which would settle on conservative measures in the majority of cases. The need for urgent therapeutic interventional procedures only applies to a minority of cases such as those with signs of peritonitis secondary to perforated gangrenous gallbladder, ruptured liver abscess or those with septicaemic shock despite conservative measures. The role of definitive procedures for most patients who settled on conservative measures depends on the frequency and severity of each attack, presence of biliary strictures (which may be malignant) and the presence of any existing co-morbid medical conditions.

The initial approach to any acute attack is to control the underlying infection with the commencement of intravenous fluid infusion, antibiotic treatment after blood culture, prescription of adequate analgesia and keeping the patient nil per oral. Our standard first line antibiotic regimen is cefuroxime. Metronidazole is sometimes prescribed to cover the anaerobe *Bacteroides fragilis*, which is present in a minor proportion of patients who have had previous biliary tract surgery and/or complicated anatomy due to stones and strictures. An urgent ultrasound scan of the liver is performed to identify the extent of lithiasis within the biliary tree, the presence of a liver mass which can be an abscess or an underlying cholangiocarcinoma. Those patients who fail to respond or have evidence of a severe attack of cholangitis with or without shock undergo an urgent ERCP. The smallest amount of contrast feasible is used during ERCP as increased biliary pressure from excessive contrast injection will result in cholangiovenous reflux, which can lead to septicaemia. No attempt is made to perform a full cholangiogram or to remove all calculi from the biliary system. In the procedure, the system is decompressed with a nasobiliary drain. Only when the patient's condition has improved and stabilized would a check cholangiogram with endoscopic removal of stones be performed. If part of the biliary tree cannot be decompressed adequately because of an obstructing distal stone or stricture, then endoscopic drainage alone may not be adequate and successful. As such, percutaneous transhepatic biliary drainage of the obstructed biliary ducts will be of use. However, these drainage tubes are small and can be easily blocked by the tenacious biliary mud. If a liver abscess is present, the abscess is drained percutaneously under ultrasound guidance.

The patient is monitored closely after admission for signs of deterioration. Those responding to the conservative treatment will have a reduction in abdominal pain, a fall in temperature towards normal and the disappearance of tachycardia over the first 24–48 hours. If there is no obvious improvement after 48 hours, the possibility of undrained biliary system or individual liver segments due to impacted stones or underlying strictures must be considered and the need for urgent surgical intervention entertained. At any time during conservative management, the presence of increasing abdominal pain coupled with shock and peritoneal signs mandates urgent surgical treatment.

Those patients who present in shock must be actively resuscitated. Those who respond quickly can be treated conservatively, while those who fail must undergo therapeutic intervention. It is unclear why conservative measures work for some but not others. In a series of 88 RPC patients presenting with acute cholangitis, 17% required therapeutic intervention for septicaemic shock. A pulse rate greater than 100/min and a platelet count of more than 150 × 10⁹/l within 24 hours of presentation were the only two independent factors which predicted the need for therapeutic intervention.[21]

The sole aim of an urgent therapeutic intervention during an acute attack is to decompress the obstructed biliary system. Non-operative interventional procedures using the endoscopic or percutaneous routes are preferred to open surgical route.[29] Occasionally, open surgery is required to deal with peritonitis as a result of gangrenous cholecystitis or ruptured liver abscess. The most expedient means to

decompress the CBD is insertion of a large T-tube. No attempt is made to perform definitive surgery. When the usually enlarged and thick walled CBD is opened, thick infected biliary mud and bile will gushed out. The biliary mud and friable bilirubinate stones are scooped out. Following a gentle saline flush of the CBD, a bougie is passed down the CBD into the duodenum to check for patency of the lower end of the CBD. The way an impacted stone in the lower end, which cannot be removed during CBD exploration, is dealt with depends on whether there is a concomitant attack of pancreatitis. In the absence of acute pancreatitis, the stone can be dealt with percutaneously via the T-tube tract when the acute episode is over. In the presence of acute pancreatitis, a transduodenal sphincteroplasty is performed to remove the stone. An alternative is the use of electrohydraulic lithotripsy to fragment the impacted stone, thus avoiding a transduodenal sphincteroplasty.[30]

The patency of the right and left hepatic ducts is checked to ensure there is free flow of bile into the CHD and CBD. Any strictures found are dilated with graduated sounds to release the infected bile and mud dammed up behind the stricture(s). Gentle irrigation of the hepatic ducts with saline is performed. Irrigation or flushing at high pressure via a syringe must be resisted as this can initiate or aggravate a septicaemic state. When bile flow from both hepatic ducts is established, a large bore T-tube is placed, the choledochotomy closed with catgut and the operation terminated. The T-tube not only decompresses the system but also affords a percutaneous route for endoscopic intervention when the patient has recovered.

Large palpable liver abscesses are drained intra-operatively. Multiple small abscesses will respond to appropriate antibiotics after the biliary system is decompressed. A cholecystectomy is performed only when it is grossly distended or there is evidence of cystic duct obstruction, empyema or gangrene of the gallbladder. During the emergency CBD exploration, an otherwise non-inflamed gallbladder, with or without stone(s) in situ, is left behind because of the added risk of performing a cholecystectomy in an ill patient.

Definitive management

The definitive management of RPC is to use a multidisciplinary approach,[31] aiming to remove all biliary stones, to establish adequate drainage to the biliary system, and to resect non-functioning liver segments which harbour bacteria and serve as foci of infection. If properly performed, definitive interventional procedures decrease the episodes and the severity of future attacks of cholangitis. In some patients cure is possible.

A

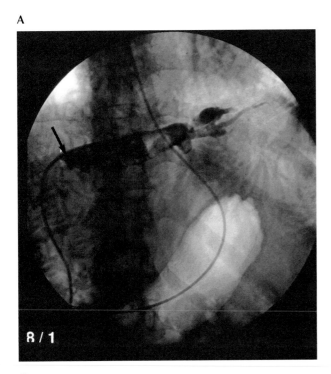

B

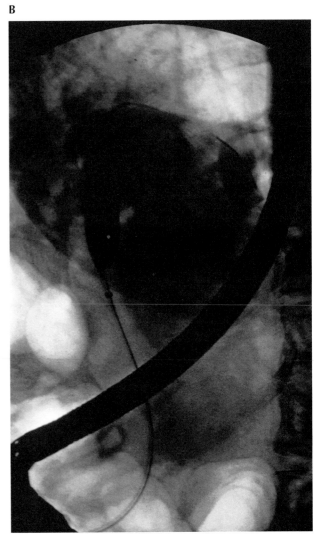

C

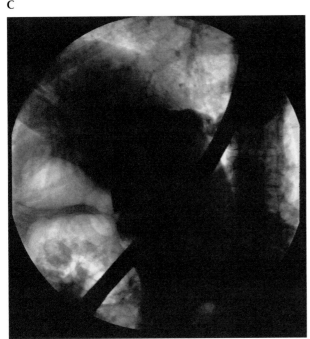

Figure 14.6 (A) ERCP demonstrating the presence of stones proximal to a relative stricture (arrow) in the left hepatic duct, (B) the stricture is dilated with a balloon prior to stone retrieval and (C) the dilated left duct is cleared of stones.

Minimal access approach

Once the acute episode has settled, more definitive treatment via the endoscope or under radiological guidance can be performed. Those treated initially by nasobiliary drainage have a check cholangiogram to delineate the extent of lithiasis and the existence of ductal stricture(s). Stones within the CBD and CHD can be removed with a dormia basket and large stones can be crushed with the mechanical lithotripter or fragmented by laser prior to their removal. For those RPC patients with stones confined to the CBD, endoscopic sphincterotomy with stone extraction only is safe and effective. The medium-term result of endoscopic sphincterotomy is comparable to surgical sphincteroplasty. In 118 patients who underwent endoscopic treatment, 95.8% remained symptom free after a median follow-up of 2.3 years,[8] compared to 83.4% who had a good outcome after surgical sphincteroplasty at a mean follow-up of 7.3 years.[32] In the absence of ductal strictures, small intrahepatic calculi not retrieved by ERCP can be shattered by extracorporeal shock wave lithotripsy (ESWL) and the fragments allowed to fall into the bowel through a widely patent sphincteroplasty.

Intrahepatic calculi within dilated biliary ducts usually lie proximal to a site of relative or true stricture. The stricture can be dilated sufficiently to allow complete removal of the stones endoscopically (Fig. 14.6). When the stricture is confined to one lobe of the liver which is atrophic, and the contralateral liver lobe is normal or relatively unaffected, hepatic resection should be performed unless the patient is medically unfit to undergo liver resection. In the presence of multiple strictures, a more conservative approach with repeated dilatation can be successful in achieving stone clearance and control of disease. Balloon dilatation of intrahepatic biliary strictures prior to stone removal has been reported to be highly successful. The immediate overall success rate of complete stone clearance with balloon dilatation in 57 patients was 94.5%.[33] Long segmental strictures which are likely to restenose can be stented successfully. The main complications of dilatation therapy include septicaemia, haemobilia, mild diarrhoea and restenosis. The cumulative probability of stricture recurrence after dilatation is 4% at 2 years and 8% at 3 years.[33] The true long-term patency rate following dilatation alone is still unknown since benign strictures treated surgically can recur 10 or more years later, as partial obstructions can remain completely asymptomatic for long periods. Apart from the problem of restricturing, it is difficult to rule out the presence of a malignant stricture with certainty.

In patients with a percutaneous transhepatic biliary drainage (PTBD) catheter in situ, the tract can be dilated to allow dormia basket stone retrieval under fluoroscopic screening or to allow passage of a flexible twin channel choledochoscope. Under direct vision the stone(s) can be fragmented with the electrohydraulic lithotripter and the fragments removed with a basket. Intrahepatic strictures can be dilated or stented. Instillation of stone dissolving agents directly into the affected biliary duct has been advocated by some, but we do not practise this approach as it is often painful, time-consuming, ineffective and can lead to ascending cholangitis and sepsis. In patients where the initial endoscopic approach has failed, the established percutaneous route can be combined with endoscopy subsequently to achieve stone clearance or stricture dilatation.

In those patients who received acute surgical intervention and T-tube decompression of the biliary system, the tract is allowed to mature. After 6 weeks, any stones present can be removed through the tract with a choledochoscope or under radiological control.

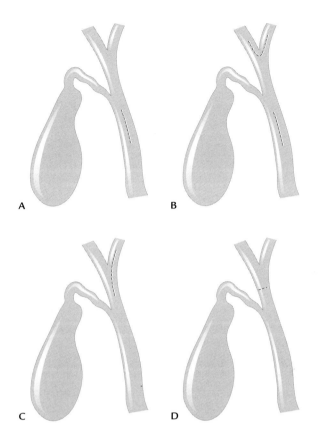

Figure 14.7 (A) Longitudinal incision for the exploration of CBD only, (B) separate incisions for exploration of the CBD and the hepatic ducts, (C) incision for the combined exploration of the CBD and one of the hepatic ducts (left side is shown), (D) horizontal incision over the CHD for CBD exploration and subsequent formation of hepaticojejunostomy (---- = incision).

Definitive surgery

Since RPC can and does affect the biliary tract at different sites with varying degrees of severity, the aim of the surgery is to provide adequate biliary drainage for bile and debris. This encompasses stone extraction, stricturoplasty or excision of stricture, resecting non-functioning liver segments and creating a bilio–enteric bypass with a permanent percutaneous access loop to the biliary tract to allow subsequent access to the biliary system for stone extraction and dilatation of stricture(s). Before embarking on definitive surgery, it is mandatory to have a complete knowledge of the location of calculi and stricture(s), and the uni- or bilobar extent of disease with or without concomitant liver atrophy.

In the presence of predominantly extrahepatic disease, simple exploration of the common bile duct with intra-operative choledochoscopy will suffice. In the absence of extrahepatic ductal stricture, the incisions used for the exploration of the CBD and hepatic ducts will depend on the location of the stones (Fig. 14.7A–D).

We routinely remove the gallbladder in these patients since, histologically, it shows underlying evidence of low grade inflammation. Furthermore, if the sphincter of Oddi has been previously destroyed, the gallbladder will be permanently in a collapsed state. The placement of a large T-tube following the exploration will allow post-operative imaging of the biliary tracts and any residual stones found can be easily removed under radiological control or with a flexible choledochoscope. When there is stenosis of the ampulla of Vater or distal CBD, or impacted stone(s) in the lower CBD, a transduodenal sphincteroplasty is performed. In patients who have had multiple operations on the CBD, the standard approach can be difficult. Under such circumstances, Ong et al. have described an extraperitoneal approach to the duodenum, which is located by its anterior position to the right kidney. A transduodenal sphincteroplasty is performed and the CBD explored from below.[34,35] However, this approach is seldom necessary as the result of endoscopic sphincterotomy has been shown to be comparable.[8]

In the presence of extra- and intrahepatic calculi, stone extraction can be difficult if they are impacted, situated behind relative or true ductal strictures or present within angulated ducts such as the right posterior or left medial segmental ducts. Although direct hepatotomy can be performed to remove the stones, it can be very bloody if the stones are deep-seated. Following the removal of all the stones within the CBD and CHD, after a choledochoscopic examination to rule out any strictures in the right and left hepatic ducts, the right and left ducts are flushed with saline. The right and left lobes of the liver are gently massaged in between the flushing. This manoeuvre normally helps to discharge more biliary mud and small stones from the intrahepatic ducts. Once the effluent is relatively clear, a repeat choledochoscopy is performed. Any residual stones can be retrieved with a dormia basket. Segmental ductal stricture is dilated prior to stone retrieval. Any impacted or large stones can be shattered with the electrohydraulic lithotripter introduced through the working channel of the flexible choledochoscope. It is not always possible to clear the intrahepatic ducts of stones completely. Once the large stones and strictures are dealt with, small stones or fragments can be left to 'fall out', provided an adequate biliary drainage procedure has been performed.

The thick, dilated CBD/CHD with an inelastic wall behaves more like a cavernous sac which does not drain adequately, even in the presence of a sphincteroplasty. Although it is reasonable to perform a supraduodenal choledochoduodenostomy as a biliary drainage procedure, this has the disadvantage that patients may develop 'sump syndrome', developing symptoms of pain and fever, which is thought to be a result of debris being lodged in the diseased distal CBD. While the sump syndrome can be treated by performing an endoscopic sphincterotomy, supraduodenal choledochoduodenostomy is contra-indicated in the presence of a proximal biliary tract stricture or when the CBD is not wide enough. Under such circumstances, we routinely perform an end to side hepaticojejunostomy with a retrocolic Roux-en-Y loop. This provides a widely patent anastomosis for biliary drainage and for small stones to fall freely into the loop of bowel. Furthermore, the closed end of the Roux loop can provide a permanent access route to the biliary tract.

With the hepaticojejunostomy it is crucial that the access loop is short and has a straight course from the anterolateral abdominal wall to the anastomosis. A poorly constructed jejunal loop with redundant length makes subsequent choledochoscopy and access to the intrahepatic ducts difficult. The access loop can either be placed intraperitoneally, to be accessed percutaneously under ultrasound guidance, or it can be placed under the skin as a hepaticocutaneous jejunostomy. We prefer to leave the loop intraperitoneally. In those cases where immediate access to the biliary tract is not necessary, the end of the loop is tacked to the peritoneal surface of the anterolateral abdominal wall with catgut. The staples from the GIA stapler used to transect the jejunum during Roux loop formation or the ligaclips placed around the blind end of the loop at the end of the operation allow the interventional radiologist subsequently to identify and access the loop percutaneously. Once the loop is punctured, the tract can be gradually dilated to admit a twin channel choledochoscope for endoscopic manipulation.[15] For those cases where access to the biliary tract is required soon after the operation, a 24 Fr catheter is introduced through the anterolateral abdominal wall into the access loop at the end of the operation. The tract is allowed to mature for 4–6 weeks before instrumentation.

Hepaticocutaneous jejunostomy has been used by others.[36] Although the biliary tract can be accessed sooner through the cutaneous stoma compared to our technique, the cutaneous stoma is not without its complication. Fifteen per cent of patients with hepaticocutaneous jejunostomy, performed either with the cutaneous stoma formed at the initial operation or subsequently created from its subcutaneous site, did experience complications. These complications include wound infection of the closed stoma wound, development of cutaneous fistula after stoma closure, difficulty in reconstructing the stoma for subsequent use and development of parajejunostomy hernia. Repeated therapeutic intervention of the biliary tract is inevitable due to the chronic relapsing nature of the condition. The formation of a hepaticojejunostomy with an access loop is a satisfactory and adequate way to manage further attacks of stones, strictures and cholangitic attacks. On a median follow-up time of 27 months, symptoms recurred only in 12 patients (29%). Only one patient required a reoperation for stricture while the others were adequately treated through the access jejunal loop.[36]

RPC predisposes to the formation of inflammatory, non-iatrogenic strictures in the biliary tract. Strictures in the subsegmental and peripheral ducts are difficult to treat. Fortunately, obstruction of these minor ducts does not produce jaundice and the cholangitic attacks may pass unnoticed and the infection subsides without any intervention. However, strictures in the major bile ducts do lead to unrelenting cholangitis, stones and liver abscess formation, septicaemic episodes and death. Over a 10-year period, we treated 57 patients with major bile duct strictures.[37] Forty-four of the 60 strictures involved the left hepatic duct (23) or the left lateral segmental ducts (21). Strictures in the CBD/CHD can be treated by the formation of a choledochojejunostomy or a hepaticojejunostomy. Stricture involving the confluence of the hepatic ducts can be treated by hepatotomy and Y-V plasty, but the procedure is technically difficult and bleeding, bile leakage and restenosis are potential serious complications.[5,38] We have stopped performing Y-V plasty for such strictures due to our poor results. Instead, we treat such strictures by performing bilateral hepaticojejunostomy. In a relatively normal left lobe of the liver with a left duct stricture at its origin, a left duct approach as described by Hepp and Couinaud[39] for a side-to-side anastomosis between the left duct and a Roux loop can be performed without the need for a left hepatectomy. The biliary drainage procedures performed for these inflammatory strictures are occasionally combined with liver resection, or liver resection alone is performed to deal with these strictures.

Before embarking on hepatic resection, the severity of symptoms, status of the remaining biliary tract, parenchymal functional reserve and alternative procedures have to be considered. Hepatic resection is only performed for those with recurrent, troublesome and localized severe disease. Disease can be confined to the left lateral segment which is atrophic and contains large number of calculi within cavernous bile ducts. In more extensive disease, the medial segment of the left lobe can also be affected due to a tight stricture in the left hepatic duct. Hepatectomy is performed not only to remove the source of symptoms and sepsis, but also to remove the underlying stricture which has the potential to turn malignant. Liver resection for right-sided disease is unusual. By the time resection is necessary, the right lobe is usually destroyed, with compensatory left lobe hypertrophy. Consequently, a right hepatectomy should lead to little functional disturbance. In one series of 172 patients with hepatolithiasis, liver resection was necessary in 37% of patients, of which left lateral segmentectomy and left hepatectomy accounted for most of the resections (90.5%). Right hepatectomy was only performed in one patient.[40] Troublesome adhesions between the diseased liver and the diaphragm and adjacent viscera can make liver resection difficult. Severe adhesions and fibrosis around the left hepatic vein and the inferior vena cava can make dissection in the region difficult and severe bleeding from these structures due to injudicious dissection can be a problem. The overall operative mortality in hepatic resection for hepatolithiasis is low (≤2%), but the morbidity, such as wound infection, subphrenic collections and biliary fistulae, from operating on an underlying septic condition is correspondingly high (approximately 30%).

Complications

In RPC the biliary mud and stones within the common bile duct can lead to acute pancreatitis. In 1971, Ong et al. reported that approximately half of all patients with acute pancreatitis, in Hong Kong, were associated with RPC.[41] Another report claims that about 20% of RPC patients had high serum amylase levels but were clinically asymptomatic.[42] In some patients, the big common bile duct stones can lead to the formation of a choledochoduodenal fistula.

Liver abscesses complicating RPC can present with rupture into the peritoneal cavity or adjacent viscera. A left lobe liver abscess can rupture into the pericardial cavity and cause cardiac tamponade,[43] while a right lobe abscess can lead to the formation of a pleurobiliary or bronchobiliary fistula.[44] A chronic abscess can, on clinical and radiological grounds, be indistinguishable from an underlying cholangiocarcinoma. The final diagnosis can only be certain after histological examination of the resected specimen.

Cholangiocarcinoma complicating RPC has been reported. The higher incidence of cholangiocarcinoma in areas where RPC is also prevalent has been attributed to the presence of *Clonorchis sinensis* infestation.[45] In a necropsy study of 50 cases of cholangiocarcinoma, 92% of the cases were associated with clonorchiasis and intrahepatic stones were found in 20% of the cases.[45] In a huge series of 1105 cases of hepatolithiasis studied over the period 1978–90, Chen et al.[46] reported that the incidence of cholangiocarcinoma in these patients increased from

2.4% (between 1978 and 1987) to 13.7% (between 1988 and 1990), despite a decreasing incidence of clonorchiasis in the population.

Thrombophlebitis of the branches of the portal vein due to the underlying periductal inflammation can lead to portal venous thrombosis with an enlarged spleen.[6] Occasionally, septic emboli to the pulmonary tree can lead to the development of lung abscesses and significant pulmonary hypertension.[6,47]

Despite multiple operations, RPC patients with long-standing severe disease can develop secondary biliary cirrhosis and liver failure.[48] When cirrhosis sets in, portal hypertension and bleeding oesophageal varices ensue, thus making further corrective surgery for the underlying stricture(s) more hazardous. In these patients the only available option is liver transplantation.

Conclusions

As the name implies, RPC runs a recurrent and unrelenting course with variable frequencies of attacks of cholangitis. Medical therapy is ineffective and surgical treatment is not entirely satisfactory. Despite surgery, stones and strictures can return. In Hong Kong and Taiwan, the peak age incidence of RPC has changed over the years from the third to the fifth decade in the 1950s and 1970s to the seventh decade in the early 1990s.[49] This is due to an increasing proportion of patients who have survived previous surgery, only to have RPC recur again in later life. In Hong Kong, young patients in their third

and fourth decade of life who present to us with RPC are invariably immigrants from mainland China. RPC is a dying disease in Hong Kong, but is still common in China. Although there are various theories on the pathogenesis of RPC, we believe the condition is closely linked to the level of social and economic conditions of a community. Surgery merely deals with the consequences of the condition, but does not address its roots. With better living conditions and public hygiene, perhaps RPC can be eradicated in this millennium. Until then, a judicious choice of a mixture of treatment, both medical and surgical, is necessary to achieve a satisfactory and long-lasting solution to a recurrent inflammatory condition.

Key points

- Calculi are predominantly calcium bilirubinate.
- Probably secondary to *E. coli* infection of bile.
- Presentation:
  - Third and fourth decade
  - Recurrent attacks of cholangitis
  - Obstructive jaundice
  - Preferentially affects left lobe.
- Investigations:
  - Plain abdominal radiography (AXR)
  - CT
  - ERCP ± PTC.
- Complications:
  - Acute pancreatitis
  - Liver abscess
  - Cholangiocarcinoma
  - Portal thrombophlebitis
  - Secondary biliary cirrhosis.

REFERENCES

1. Digby KH. Common-duct stones of liver origin. Br J Surg 1930; 17: 578–91
2. Cook J, Hou PC, Ho HC et al. Recurrent pyogenic cholangitis. Br J Surg 1954; 42: 188–203
3. Mage S, Morel AS. Surgical experience with cholangiohepatitis (Hong Kong Disease) in Canton Chinese. Ann Surg 1965; 162: 187–90
4. Harrison-Levy A. The biliary obstruction syndrome of the Chinese. Br J Surg 1962; 49: 674–85
5. Choi TK, Wong J, Ong GB. The surgical management of primary intrahepatic stones. Br J Surg 1982; 69: 86–90
6. Chou ST, Chan CW. Recurrent pyogenic cholangitis: a necropsy study. Pathology 1980; 12: 415–28
7. Federle MP, Cello JP, Laing FC et al. Recurrent pyogenic cholangitis in Asian immigrants. Use of ultrasonography, computed tomography, and cholangiography. Radiology 1982; 143: 151–6
8. Lam SK. A study of endoscopic sphincterotomy in recurrent pyogenic cholangitis. Br J Surg 1984; 71: 262–6
9. Wilson MK, Stephen MS, Mathur M et al. Recurrent pyogenic cholangitis or 'oriental cholangiohepatitis' in occidentals: case reports of four patients. Aust N Z J Surg 1996; 66: 649–52
10. Menu Y, Lorphelin JM, Scherrer A et al. Sonographic and computed tomographic evaluation of intrahepatic calculi. AJR 1985; 145: 579–83

11. Maki T. Pathogenesis of calcium bilirubinate gallstone: role of *E. coli*, β-glucuronidase and coagulation by inorganic ions, polyelectrolytes and agitation. Ann Surg 1966; 164: 90–100

12. Ong GB. A study of recurrent pyogenic cholangitis. Arch Surg 1962; 84: 63–89

13. Maki T. Cholelithiasis in the Japanese. Arch Surg 1961; 82: 599–612

14. Matsushiro T, Suzuki N, Sato T et al. Effects of diet on glucaric acid concentration in bile and the formation of calcium bilirubinate gallstones. Gastroenterology 1977; 72: 630–3

15. Leow CK, Lau WY. Biliary access procedure in the management of oriental cholangiohepatitis. Am Surg 1998; 64: 99

16. Flinn WR, Olson DF, Oyasu R et al. Biliary bacteria and hepatic histologic changes in gallstone disease. Ann Surg 1977; 185: 593–7

17. Thorpe MEC, Scheuer PJ, Sherlock S. Primary sclerosing cholangitis, the biliary tree and ulcerative cholangitis. Gut 1967; 8: 435–48

18. Ohta G, Nakanuma Y, Terada T. Pathology of hepatolithiasis: cholangitis and cholangiocarcinoma. Prog Clin Biol Res 1984; 152: 91–113

19. Copher GH, Dick BM. 'Streamline' phenomena in portal vein and selective distribution of portal blood in liver. Arch Surg 1928; 17: 408–19

20. Hahn PF, Donald WD, Grier RC Jr. Physiological bilaterality of the portal circulation; streamline flow of blood into liver as shown by radioactive phosphorus. Am J Physiol 1945; 143: 105–7

21. Fan ST, Lai ECS, Mok FPT et al. Acute cholangitis secondary to hepatolithiasis. Arch Surg 1991; 126: 1027–31

22. Wastie ML, Cunningham IGE. Roentgenologic findings in recurrent pyogenic cholangitis. AJR 1973; 119: 71–7

23. Itai Y, Araki T, Furui S et al. Computed tomography and ultrasound in the diagnosis of intrahepatic calculi. Radiology 1980; 136: 399–405

24. Chan YL, Chan ACW, Lam WWM et al. Choledocholithiasis: comparison of MR cholangiography and endoscopic retrograde cholangiography. Radiology 1996; 200: 85–9

25. Park MS, Yu JS, Kim KW et al. Recurrent pyogenic cholangitis: comparison between MR cholangiography and direct cholangiography. Radiology 2001; 220: 677–82

26. Araki T, Itai Y, Tasaka A. CT of choledochal cyst. AJR 1980; 135: 729–34

27. Kaiser JA, Mall JC, Salmen BJ et al. Diagnosis of Caroli disease by computed tomography: report of two cases. Radiology 1979; 132: 661–4

28. Mujahed Z, Glenn F, Evans JA. Communicating cavernous ectasia of the intrahepatic ducts (Caroli's disease). AJR 1971; 113: 21–6

29. Lillemoe KD. Surgical treatment of biliary tract infection. Am Surg 2000; 66: 138–44

30. Fan ST. Transduodenal sphincteroplasty for impacted stone made unnecessary by electrohydraulic lithotripsy. Surg Gynecol Obstet 1989; 169: 363–4

31. Cosenza CA, Durazo F, Stain SC et al. Current management of recurrent pyogenic cholangitis. Am Surg 1999; 68: 939–43

32. Choi TK, Wong J, Lam KH et al. Late result of sphincteroplasty in the treatment of primary cholangitis. Arch Surg 1981; 116: 1173–5

33. Jeng KS, Yang FS, Ohta I et al. Dilatation of intrahepatic biliary strictures in patients with hepatolithiasis. World J Surg 1990; 14: 587–93

34. Ong GB, Kwong KH, Cheng FCY. Extraperitoneal transduodenal choledocho-duodenostomy for removal of overlooked common bile duct stones. Aust N Z J Surg 1970; 40: 166–70

35. Choi TK, Lee NW, Wong J et al. Extraperitoneal sphincteroplasty for residual stones: an update. Ann Surg 1982; 196: 26–9

36. Fan ST, Mok F, Zheng SS et al. Appraisal of hepaticocutaneous jejunostomy in the management of hepatolithiasis. Am J Surg 1993; 165: 332–5

37. Lau WY, Chan KL, Li AKC. Surgical treatment of inflammatory strictures of the major bile ducts. Asian J Surg 1990; 13: 51–4

38. Lau WY, Fan ST, Yip WC et al. Surgical management of strictures of the major bile ducts in recurrent pyogenic cholangitis. Br J Surg 1987; 74: 1100–2

39. Hepp J, Couinaud C. L'abord et l'utilisation du canal hepatique gauche dans les reparations de la voie biliaire principale. Presse Med 1956; 64: 947–8

40. Fan ST, Lai ECS, Wong J. Hepatic resection for hepatolithiasis. Arch Surg 1993; 128: 1070–4

41. Ong GB, Adiseshiah M, Leong CH. Acute pancreatitis associated with recurrent pyogenic cholangitis. Br J Surg 1971; 58: 891–4

42. Wong J, Choi TK. Recurrent pyogenic cholangitis. Prog Clin Biol Res 1984; 152: 175–92

43. Choi TK, Wong J. Recurrent pyogenic cholangitis. In: Schwartz SI, Ellis H, Husser WC, eds. Maingot's abdominal operations. Volume 2, 9th edn. New Jersey: Prentice-Hall International, 1990: 1519–31

44. Wei WI, Choi TK, Wong J et al. Bronchobiliary fistula due to stones in the biliary tree: report of two cases. World J Surg 1982; 6: 782–5

45. Chou ST, Chan CW. Mucin-producing cholangiocarcinoma: an autopsy study in Hong Kong. Pathology 1976; 8: 321–8

46. Chen MF, Jan YY, Wang CS et al. A reappraisal of cholangiocarcinoma in patient with hepatolithiasis. Cancer 1993; 71: 2461–5

47. Lai KS, McFadzean AJS, Young RTT. Microemboli pulmonary hypertension in pyogenic cholangitis. Br Med J 1968; 1: 22–4

48. Jeng KS, Shih SC, Chiang HJ et al. Secondary biliary cirrhosis. A limiting factor in the treatment of hepatolithiasis. Arch Surg 1989; 124: 1301–5

49. Fan ST, Choi TK, Lo CM et al. Treatment of hepatolithiasis: improvement of result by a systemic approach. Surgery 1991; 109: 474–80

15 Management of liver abscess

Justin Geoghegan, Dermot Malone and Oscar Traynor

Introduction

Liver abscess was recognized in the time of Hippocrates, but was first recorded in modern medical literature during the first part of the nineteenth century.[1,2] These early observations noted that this condition was almost invariably fatal, a viewpoint supported by several reports that appeared around the beginning of the 1900s.[3,4] The landmark description by Oschner in 1938 of a 62% survival rate in a patient series treated by surgical drainage was the first report to demonstrate any real progress in the treatment of liver abscess.[5] Combined with the rapid developments in antibiotic therapy, surgical drainage remained the mainstay of treatment for the next two decades. Percutaneous drainage was first reported in 1953.[6] More recently, in parallel with other developments in minimal access techniques, radiologically-guided non-operative drainage has effectively replaced surgical drainage in all but a few circumstances.[7]

Improvements in diagnostic imaging, antibiotic therapy and the adoption of percutaneous drainage techniques have all contributed to improved outcomes in the management of liver abscess.[8] Nevertheless, this condition still frequently results in severe illness with an associated mortality in some series as high as 35%.[9] The reasons for this lie in important changes which have occurred in the demographics and aetiology of liver abscess. Increasingly, this disease occurs in an older population, many of whom have serious underlying disease, so that usually it is the underlying condition which determines the outcome rather than the liver abscess itself.[9–11]

Successful management requires a multidisciplinary team approach. Patients remain under the primary care of the surgical service but, in most cases, the majority of interventions are performed by the radiologist. Therefore, close communication between these two teams is essential if good outcomes are to be achieved. Major input from gastroenterology, microbiology and intensive care specialists may also be needed. Radiology training authorities in both the United Kingdom and United States recommend that catheter drainage of easily accessible intra-abdominal abscesses, including liver abscesses, should be within the capability of a fully trained general radiologist.[12] However, for liver abscesses that are not easily accessible the patient should be referred to a specialist hepatobiliary team which includes an interventional radiologist. Delay in referring appropriate patients may result in unnecessarily prolonged hospitalization and jeopardize outcome.

Liver abscess may be categorized as being pyogenic or amoebic depending on the causative organism. Pyogenic abscess is due to bacterial or occasionally fungal infection, whereas amoebic abscess is due to infection with the protozoon *Entamoeba histolytica*. These two entities can overlap considerably in their clinical presentation and appearances on imaging. However, because there are major differences in pathogenesis, clinical course, complications and management they are considered separately in this chapter.

Pyogenic liver abscess

Aetiology and pathogenesis

The incidence of liver abscess in autopsy series has remained fairly constant over the last 50 years at between 0.01% and 0.59%.[5,11,13,14] However, there have been important shifts in aetiological patterns with an increasing proportion occurring as complications of other hepatobiliary disorders or of their treatment (Fig. 15.1).[10,11,15] Ascending cholangitis has replaced portal pyaemia due to intra-abdominal infection as the commonest cause of liver abscess. An increasing percentage of patients with liver abscess due to ascending cholangitis have underlying malignant disease, with the remainder due to

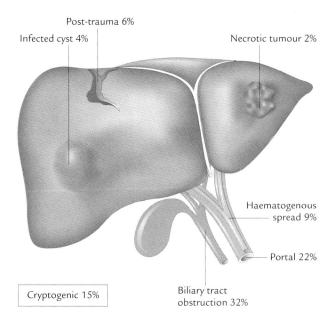

Post-trauma 6%

Infected cyst 4%

Necrotic tumour 2%

Haematogenous spread 9%

Portal 22%

Cryptogenic 15%

Biliary tract obstruction 32%

Figure 15.1 Aetiology of liver abscess.

choledocholithiasis or biliary stricture.[8,9,16] Endoscopic or percutaneous stenting or instrumentation of the obstructed biliary tree is an important progenitor of biliary sepsis. Eventual stent occlusion sets the scene for cholangitis and possibly liver abscess formation. Portal pyaemia is classically associated with appendicitis or other colonic conditions such as complicated diverticulitis or perforated carcinoma, but may also be caused by necrotizing pancreatitis.[5] Complication of these conditions by liver abscess has become increasingly unusual because of earlier presentation and diagnosis, and improvements in management of the primary pathology. Around 15–25% of cases are classified as cryptogenic with no underlying cause identifiable.[8–10,17–19] Liver abscess may also occur due to direct extension into the liver parenchyma of a localized perforation of an adjacent viscus, particularly the gallbladder, colon, stomach or duodenum.

Haematogenous spread from non-gastrointestinal sources accounts for 10–20% of liver abscesses and has been reported most typically in association with bacterial endocarditis and in intravenous drug abusers. This scenario is also being seen with increasing frequency in immunocompromised patients, many of whom have underlying haematological or other malignancy, or AIDS.[10,19] Opportunistic pathogens, such as *Pseudomonas* species or *Candida*, are more frequently isolated in these patients.

An increasing proportion of liver abscesses occur as complications of therapy of other hepatobiliary disorders.[20,21] Liver abscess formation may occur as

a complication of arterial chemoembolization of hepatocellular carcinoma.[22] Risk factors for abscess formation include advanced age, tumour size greater than 5 cm, and gas forming in the embolized tumour. Interstitial tumour therapy by cryoablation or percutaneous injection of alcohol have also been reported to be associated with liver abscess formation in a small percentage of patients.[23] A high index of suspicion with early recourse to diagnostic aspiration is needed in patients with liver tumours who develop clinical evidence of sepsis following interstitial lytic therapy.

Immunosuppression following liver transplantation may also predispose to liver abscess formation. Biliary reconstruction by Roux-en-Y hepaticojejunostomy is cited as a predisposing factor in some case reports. A range of causative organisms have been reported including *Haemophilus parainfluenzae*, *Pseudomonas* and *Candida*.[24–26]

Morphology and microbiology

The site, distribution and bacteriology may give important clues about the underlying aetiology. Liver abscess may be single or multiple. The majority of cases of single abscess occur in the right liver and isolated left-sided abscess occurs in 10% or less.[11,18] Multiple abscesses usually involve both sides or the right side alone, and the left side is rarely affected in isolation. Whether or not this apparent predilection for the right side simply reflects the greater parenchymal mass of the right liver remains unclear. It has been postulated that it reflects preferential distribution of portal inflow from the superior mesenteric vein territory to the right liver.[27] However, this theory is difficult to sustain given that appendicitis is now rarely the primary septic source yet the right-sided preponderance of liver abscesses persists. Single abscesses are more likely to be cryptogenic, in contrast to multiple abscesses.[10,17–19] The latter are more likely to be due to uncontrolled sepsis in the biliary tree or haematogenous dissemination from a remote septic focus and are more frequently associated with a profound systemic septic response.

The commonest organisms responsible for pyogenic liver abscess are Gram-negative aerobes with *E. coli* and *Klebsiella* being the commonest isolates, reflecting the gastrointestinal origin of these infections in the majority of cases. In one large series from Taiwan, *Klebsiella* species were found more frequently in single abscesses and *E. coli* was more commonly isolated from multiple abscesses, although most other series are too small to reproduce this finding.[18] Abscesses arising from a gastrointestinal source are usually polymicrobial.

Table 15.1 **Clinical features of liver abscess**

	Percentage
Fever	83
Abdominal pain	63
Jaundice	50
Anorexia	77
Nausea	27
Vomiting	27
Hepatomegaly	67
Septic shock	10
Diabetes	15

The proportion of cases in which anaerobic organisms are identified has increased as a result of improvements in culture techniques, so that in recent series these organisms account for up to 30% of isolates.[16-19] Liver abscess occurring as a consequence of bacteraemia arising from a non-gastrointestinal focus is more likely to be monomicrobial, most frequently due to staphylococci or streptococci.

Clinical features

The average age of affected patients has increased over the last 30 years and, in recent series, the mean age of patients with liver abscess lies within the sixth decade, with approximately equal incidence in both sexes. The clinical features may be relatively non-specific. The commonest symptoms are fever, abdominal pain and jaundice (Table 15.1). Nausea, anorexia and vomiting are common. Localized tenderness and hepatomegaly may also be present. Septic shock requiring aggressive intensive care management is present in up to 20% of patients. The proportion of patients with diabetes mellitus varies in reported series from 15 to 45%.[18] Approximately 10% of patients present with signs of generalized peritonitis due to intraperitoneal rupture of the abscess.

Laboratory findings

In most instances the white cell count is elevated. Up to two-thirds of patients are anaemic, reflecting the chronicity of the clinical presentation. More than 50% of patients have abnormal liver function tests. Alkaline phosphatase and transaminases are elevated in 60–80% of patients, while serum bilirubin is increased in 30%. Serum albumin may be lowered as a non-specific response to inflammation.

Similarly, prothrombin time and other coagulation parameters may be grossly abnormal in patients with severe sepsis. Blood cultures are positive in 30–50% of all patients. The causative organism can be grown from aspirated pus in approximately 85–90% of cases.[15,17,18,28] Sterile culture may be due to improper handling of specimens or prior antibiotic administration.

Diagnosis

Improvements in imaging techniques have led to earlier diagnosis of liver abscess and more accurate differentiation from other conditions.

Chest radiograph shows an elevated right hemidiaphragm or pleural effusion in 50% of cases (Fig. 15.2A). This is typically so non-specific as to be unhelpful. The plain film of the abdomen has no significant role in diagnosis. Angiography and especially scintigraphy were previously widely used diagnostic tools in this situation.[29,30] Indium-labelled leucocyte scanning has a sensitivity greater than 95%, but the additional information given by cross-sectional imaging has meant that isotope scanning and angiography have become redundant in diagnosis of liver abscess.

Initial evaluation of the liver is usually by ultrasound, which has a sensitivity of 75–90%. The sonographic appearances of liver abscess varies as the disease progresses.[31-33] Early on, the lesion tends to be less distinct and hyperechoic (Fig. 15.3B). This is a non-specific finding which may also be produced by unrelated conditions such as focal fatty change. As the abscess matures, the margins become better demarcated and the contents typically become hypoechoic (Fig. 15.3A). There are usually some internal echoes and, because fluid attenuates ultrasound less than the surrounding solid liver, increased through-transmission of sound is usually seen. This shows as a hyperechoic (bright) shadow behind the lesion. This sign is very useful in differentiating solid from fluid-containing liver lesions. It may occasionally be absent when pus is very thick—its absence does not exclude the diagnosis of liver abscess. Ultrasound may fail to detect multiple small abscesses or a single abscess high in the right liver.

CT scanning has a sensitivity of 97% or greater and is more accurate than ultrasound in differentiating liver abscess from other lesions.[34,35] A typical protocol would be to scan the liver in 8–10 mm slices with helical CT, beginning the scan 60–70 s after a pump injection of iodinated contrast medium. The aim is to scan the liver during the portal venous phase of enhancement, which provides maximum

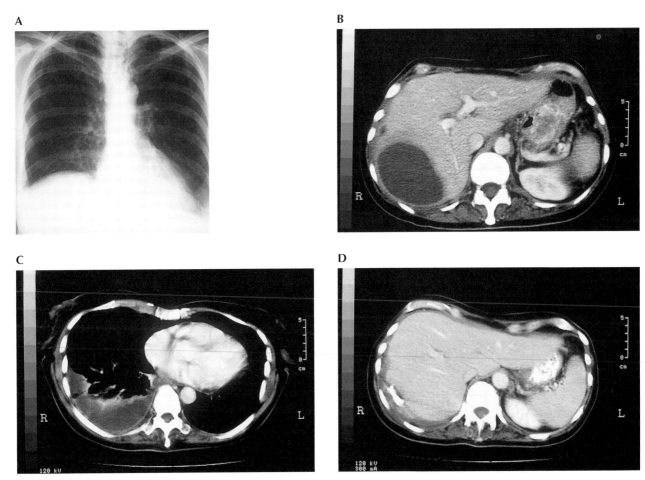

Figure 15.2 Management of liver abscess. Case history: A 56-year-old woman underwent a laparoscopic division of pelvic adhesions and re-presented one week later with abdominal pain and peritonitis due to a distal ileal laceration. She underwent a modified right hemicolectomy. Postoperatively she remained febrile. An abdominal ultrasound (not shown) demonstrated a liver abscess. She was referred to a hepatobiliary unit for percutaneous drainage. (A) Chest radiograph on admission: the right hemidiaphragm is slightly elevated. (B) CT liver on admission: the liver abscess is shown as a large hypodense (dark) lesion in the right liver. The patient proceeded to have the abscess drained by a low intercostal access route under ultrasound and screening guidance. The initial clinical improvement was less than expected. Anaerobic streptococci and *Candida albicans* were cultured from the pus. Further clinical improvement followed the optimization of antimicrobial therapy. A low-grade fever persisted and she complained of pain around the catheter entry site. (C,D) CT thorax and abdomen one week after drainage: there is now a moderate-sized right pleural effusion and basal pulmonary atelectasis. The liver abscess has been adequately drained. The catheter is well shown in the subcapsular right lobe of the liver. There is a little subphrenic fluid.

continued

liver-to-lesion attenuation differences. Typically, the lesion itself does not enhance on contrast injection (Fig. 15.3D,E). It may be surrounded by a peripheral rim of contrast enhancement (Fig. 15.3E). The outline may be highly variable. Some appear round or oval but many have an irregular or lobulated margin (Fig. 15.3A). Gas bubbles or an air-fluid level are diagnostic of liver abscess, but are present in only 20% of cases.[36]

In its current state of development, magnetic resonance imaging does not appear to offer any great advantage over CT in the characterization of infective focal lesions in the liver.[35,37] It may have a role if associated

biliary pathology is suspected as MR cholangiography can non-invasively confirm or exclude this and facilitate planning of subsequent intervention.[38]

Differential diagnosis of pyogenic liver abscess includes amoebic abscess and other parasitic liver cysts, particularly hydatid disease, necrotic or infected primary or metastatic tumour, and coincidental simple liver cysts and other benign solid liver lesions (Table 15.2).

Amoebic abscess is considered separately later in this chapter. Hydatid disease should be suspected in endemic areas or in immigrants from or travellers to

E F G

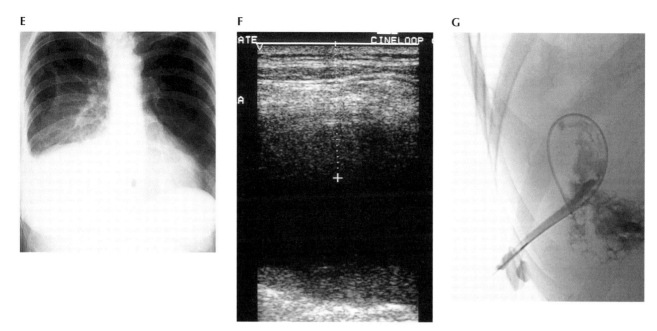

Figure 15.2 continued (E) Chest radiograph one week after drainage: the pleural effusion and right basal atelectasis are evident and were not present predrainage. The low-grade pyrexia was considered either due to right basal pneumonia or pleural contamination from the catheter access tract. (F) Ultrasound of chest: the pleural effusion has been identified and marked for aspiration. Twenty ml of turbid serous fluid were aspirated and sent for microbiological examination. There were no pus cells or micro-organisms. The effusion was considered most likely reactive. (G) 'Tractogram' 10 days after catheter insertion: the catheter has been removed over a guidewire. A vascular sheath, with a side-port, is being used to inject the (dark) contrast along the tract as the sheath is withdrawn. There is no evidence of any pleural or peritoneal connection along the tract. Pleural transgression had been excluded. The patient's condition had improved. The abscess drainage tube was uneventfully removed.

Table 15.2 **Differential diagnosis of liver abscess**
Pyogenic liver abscess
Amoebic abscess
Entamoeba histolytica
Parasitic liver cysts
Echinococcus granulosus
Ascaris lumbricoides
Clonorchis sinensis
Tumour
Simple liver cyst

these regions. Serological testing is positive in 80% of cases. The classical radiological findings include calcification in the cyst wall in 20–30% of instances, the presence of daughter cysts which may float freely within the lumen of the primary cyst and a floating detached inner membrane.[36] Identification of hydatid disease is critical as it has generally been considered that percutaneous puncture should be avoided because it may lead to widespread intraperitoneal dissemination of the infection. Some

authors, however, suggest that this may be overcautious and that percutaneous drainage of hydatid cysts can be performed safely provided a sufficiently long track through normal hepatic parenchyma is used.[39] Percutaneous sclerotherapy of hydatid cysts has also been reported.[40] Hydatid cyst disease is dealt with in more detail in Chapter 13.

Management

The fundamental aims of management are the complete drainage of pus, treatment with antibiotics and identification and elimination of the primary source of infection (if any). The introduction of percutaneous drainage techniques marked the beginning of the shift in management from major open surgery to minimally invasive therapy involving close teamwork between the surgeon, gastroenterologist and interventional radiologist. Percutaneous drainage has, combined with appropriate antibiotic therapy, become the mainstay of treatment.[8–10,17,18,41–44] Once the diagnosis is likely based on clinical and/or radiological information, management comprises planning, performing and following-up a percutaneous drainage procedure.

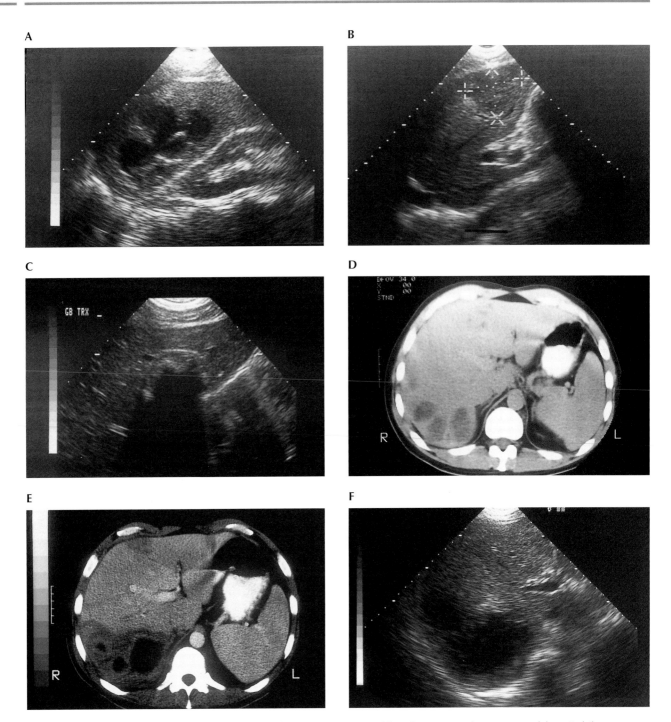

Figure 15.3 Management of liver abscess. Case history: A 37-year-old male presented to a general hospital for investigation of fever and abdominal pain. A diagnosis of liver abscess was made after an ultrasound of the abdomen. He was admitted and commenced on antibiotic therapy. (A) Ultrasound on admission: the abscess in the right liver shows as a lobulated, hypoechoic lesion. The margins of the abscess are very sharply delineated. The right kidney is shown behind the right liver. (B) Ultrasound on admission: there is a second lesion in the left lobe of the liver (cursors). This is more echogenic and less well-defined than the large right lobe lesion. (C) Ultrasound on admission: the gallbladder is contracted and contains many stones. These cast a dense, dark acoustic shadow. (D) CT on admission: axial enhanced scan. At this axial level, the lobulated abscess deep in the right lobe of the liver appears as three separate, moderately hypodense cavities. The left lobe lesion is less clearly shown. The patient's condition had not improved significantly after 10 days of antibiotic therapy. The local radiologists did not consider the abscess suitable for percutaneous drainage. He was transferred to a hepatobiliary unit. (E) CT after 10 days of antibiotic therapy: the abscess deep in the right lobe now contains less fluid and has a very thick rim of inflammatory tissue. The left lobe abscess has a more homogeneous inflammatory appearance—there is no evidence of any cavity or fluid in the left lobe of the liver. (F) Ultrasound after 10 days of antibiotic therapy: a thick inflammatory rim of moderately hypoechoic (dark) tissue can now be seen around the the more hypoechoic (darker) central cavity deep in the right lobe of the liver. The pus contains more echoes than on the scan performed 10 days earlier. Percutaneous drainage was requested as the patient's clinical condition had not improved significantly. *continued*

G

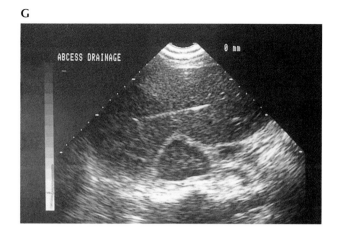

H

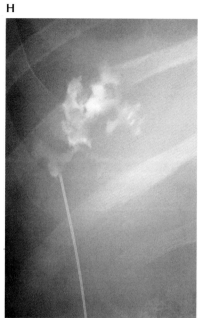

I

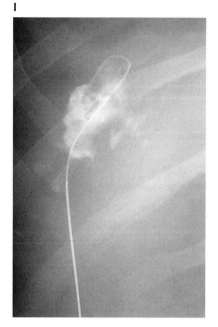

J

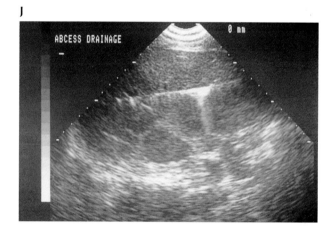

K

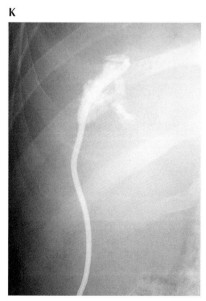

Figure 15.3 continued (G) Abscess drainage—ultrasound-guided needle puncture: this oblique intercostal scan shows the hyperechoic (bright) needle entering the hypoechoic (dark) inflammatory area deep in the right lobe of the liver. The bevelled tip of the 22 g needle shows as a bright terminal echo. (H) Abscess drainage—cavity opacification under fluoroscopic guidance: after withdrawal of some pus to confirm needle tip position and obtain a sample for culture and sensitivity a few ml of contrast were injected to identify the dependent portion of the cavity. (I) Abscess drainage—guidewire placement under fluoroscopic guidance: a stiff interventional guidewire with a floppy 'J' tip, which will coil in the cavity (and not penetrate the back wall), is introduced. (J) Abscess drainage—guidewire visualization with ultrasound: the guidewire is very hyperechoic (bright) and its introduction and position can be monitored with ultrasound also. (K) Abscess drainage—tract dilatation under fluoroscopic guidance: serial dilators (8, 10, 12 Fr) are passed over the guidewire to prepare the tract for catheter placement. This is an important step of the procedure which reduces the risk of unwanted hepatic trauma. *continued*

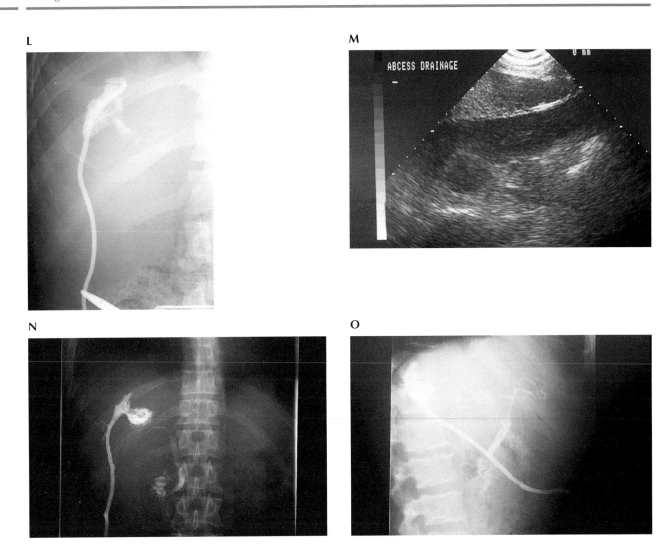

Figure 15.3 continued (L) Abscess drainage—catheter placement under fluoroscopic guidance: a 12 Fr catheter with an end-hole, multiple distal side-holes and a separate 'sump' lumen to improve drainage and allow irrigation (Ring-McLean catheter, Cook, Bloomington, Indiana, USA) has been placed over the guidewire. (M) Ultrasound scan after catheter placement: there is no evidence of any haematoma/complication despite the long catheter tract. The two walls of the catheter are seen as hyperechoic (bright) 'tram tracks'. (N) Sinogram 10 days postdrainage: the patient's pyrexia has resolved, he feels better, the white cell count has fallen and there is no drainage from the catheter. The sinogram shows a small cavity at the tip of the catheter. Forceps mark the skin entry site. (O) The depth of the abscess cavity can be best appreciated on the lateral view. The catheter tract communicates with the biliary tree. There is no evidence of any stones in the extrahepatic bile ducts, which drain freely. This communication was presumably iatrogenic and was of no clinical importance in the absence of stones, strictures etc. The catheter was uneventfully removed.

Planning the procedure involves patient preparation and sometimes includes further imaging to select a safe access route. Proper preparation should minimize the risk of haemorrhagic and septic complications. Informed consent should be obtained by a person qualified to perform the procedure. The patient should be adequately hydrated and any coagulopathy corrected. The initial choice of antibiotics should provide broad spectrum cover against Gram-positive and negative organisms and include agents effective against anaerobic infection. The combination of a second or third generation cephalosporin with metronidazole or alternatively ampicillin, with an aminoglycoside and metronidazole, gives reasonable cover against the commonly isolated organisms, although alternative choices may be dictated by local antimicrobial treatment policy. Subsequently, the antibiotics given can be modified based on bacteriological information gained from the initial percutaneous aspirate.

Percutaneous drainage can be performed under ultrasound or CT guidance. Patients require sedation and analgesia with a combination of anxiolytic and opiate drugs. Fentanyl (Sublimaze) and midazolam (Versed, Hypnovel) are widely used. Appropriate monitoring (pulse oximeter, ECG, automatic BP monitor) is recommended. In the authors' unit the preferred technique for catheter drainage is to perform the procedure on a fluoroscopic table, using ultrasound guidance for the initial puncture and radiographic guidance for guidewire and catheter manipulations (Fig. 15.3G–L). Ultrasound guidance enables the operator to scan obliquely and parasagittally during puncture and facilitates subcostal and low intercostal access.[41] (Fig. 15.3G). It is suggested that diagnostic aspiration under ultrasound or CT guidance to confirm the diagnosis and obtain material for bacteriological examination should not be performed unless a therapeutic aspiration/drainage is carried out at the same session. The abscess is punctured under ultrasound guidance and 5–10 ml of pus is aspirated for microbiological culture. Iodinated contrast (half the aspirated volume) is injected to identify the cavity on fluoroscopy (Fig. 15.3H) and then, under fluoroscopic or ultrasound guidance, a stiff interventional guide wire is placed (Fig. 15.3I,J), the tract is dilated (Seldinger technique, Fig. 15.3K) and a drain up to 12 Fr in calibre is inserted (Fig. 15.3L). It is important to minimize contrast injection and guidewire/catheter manipulation before the pressure in the abscess has been relieved by aspiration/drainage. Septicaemia can occur if this principle is ignored. The contents of the cavity are aspirated and the catheter is secured.

The clinical assessment determines the timing of follow-up imaging. Rapid resolution of fever, a fall in the white cell count (WCC) and little drainage from the cavity indicate a satisfactory result. Imaging may be 'electively' scheduled for these patients. Ultrasound should suffice (Fig. 15.3M). Injection of contrast through the catheter is performed to assess the cavity size and evaluate for biliary connections (Fig. 15.3N). The catheter is removed when ultrasound shows no residual pus, the daily drainage is minimal (<10 ml, excluding irrigant) and the patient is well. In most series the duration of catheter drainage required for resolution ranges from 2 to 14 days.

The patient who is not responding immediately requires more aggressive management, including urgent imaging and intervention. The common reasons for failure to respond quickly are inadequate drainage of pus, inadequate antimicrobial therapy, associated pneumonia, pleural transgression by the drainage catheter or, rarely, antibiotic allergy.

Inadequately drained abscesses are usually loculated and another interventional procedure will be needed. The authors prefer to use enhanced CT scanning rather than ultrasound to evaluate patients in these circumstances as dressings securing the catheter and gas in the drained cavity hamper visualization with ultrasound (Fig. 15.2C,D). If there are no apparent undrained loculi, contrast should be injected under fluoroscopic guidance to confirm catheter patency and position. Repositioning of the catheter side-holes in the cavity may be needed, although this is less likely if a pigtail catheter has been used. Pus may be quite viscous. Regular irrigation of the catheter and connecting tubing may be advisable to prevent catheter occlusion.

Although empyema is rare, pleural contamination should be considered and a chest radiograph performed if a catheter has been placed intercostally (Fig. 15.2E).[45] If a pleural effusion is present, a pleural tap and 'tractogram' will confirm or exclude the diagnosis. If significant pleural contamination is confirmed, a pleural drainage catheter can be inserted with its tip near the abscess drain. This may be removed when the effusion and liver abscess are both drained. The abscess catheter should stay in until a tract has formed around it (Fig. 15.2G).

The presence of multiple abscess cavities does not contraindicate percutaneous catheter drainage, although multiple catheters may need to be introduced to achieve satisfactory resolution.[46,47] The appearance of septation or loculation may be misleading on CT scan as, frequently, apparently loculated areas in an abscess cavity are interconnected, allowing successful drainage by a single catheter (Fig. 15.3D). Antibiotic therapy may be the principal therapy in some instances of multiple abscess formation, in which the abscesses are too small and numerous to be drained. Mortality in this situation is high and special efforts must be made to identify a distant septic focus or biliary abnormality that is the underlying cause of the problem.[10,18] In a severely ill patient biliary decompression with an endoscopic nasobiliary drain or percutaneous biliary drain may be necessary.

The original description of percutaneous treatment of liver abscesses by McFadzean described simple needle aspiration with intracavitary antibiotic instillation.[6] Percutaneous needle aspiration without catheter placement is still favoured in several institutions on the basis that a single aspiration will be adequate in 50% of patients and that an indwelling catheter requires considerable maintenance and may cause significant discomfort or complications.[42–44] Catheter drainage is reserved for patients who fail to respond to simple aspiration alone. A number of clinical series demonstrate complete resolution after a single aspiration in up to 50% of patients, with the remaining patients requiring two or three aspirations in approximately equal proportion.[42–44] Up to eight sessions of treatment have rarely been required. In a randomized comparison of the two approaches catheter drainage resulted in resolution in all patients so treated, whereas needle aspiration was associated with a 40% failure rate. Catheter drainage also shortened the time spent in hospital compared to treatment by aspiration (11 versus 5 days).[48] Needle aspiration alone is more likely to be successful if the abscess is unilocular, less than 5 cm in diameter and there is no suggestion of chronicity. A long established cavity may have a thick, fibrotic wall that does not collapse down when its contents are evacuated (Fig. 15.3E). Needle aspiration will also fail if there is a fistulous communication with the gut or biliary tree.[36]

These apparently conflicting viewpoints may be reconciled by treating abscesses less than 4 cm in diameter with needle aspiration and reserving catheter drainage for larger lesions. It seems sensible to proceed to catheter insertion in patients not cured by two needle aspirations. Smaller abscesses need no percutaneous intervention. There is no evidence to suggest that the aggressive approach to follow-up outlined above should be modified in patients treated with needle aspiration rather than catheter drainage. The authors suggest that there is no place for a single diagnostic, 'quasi-therapeutic' needle aspiration in the management of liver abscess.

After the acute episode, the duration of antibiotic therapy is usually 3–6 weeks in total. Further investigation should be directed to identify any underlying septic source. Based on the clinical features and ultrasound and CT appearances, specific evaluation of the biliary tree by ERCP or MR cholangiography may be appropriate. Obstruction of the biliary tree by stones or tumour may be responsible for formation of multiple abscesses. Depending on the clinical scenario, evaluation of the colon may be considered by contrast enema, although modern CT techniques give quite a good evaluation of the colon and can show large tumours, diverticular disease and their complications. For this reason, the initial diagnostic CT scans should cover the abdomen and pelvis.

Close co-operation is needed between interventional radiologist and surgeon in the selection of patients for percutaneous drainage rather than surgical treatment. In approximately 10% of patients surgical intervention is required.[49] Table 15.3 shows the indications for surgery. Incomplete or unsuccessful percutaneous drainage in the presence of severe sepsis may jeopardize the patient's chances of survival, particularly as it may take a considerable length of time before it becomes clear that the percutaneous approach is not going to be effective. Failure of percutaneous drainage may occur because the cavity is multiloculated, the catheter is too small

Table 15.3 **Indications for surgical treatment**
Failure/complication of percutaneous drainage
Multiloculation
Intraperitoneal rupture/signs of peritonitis
Co-existing pathology requiring surgical treatment
Hepatolithiasis

(typically 10–12Fr catheters are needed), a fistula to the biliary tract is present or because the abscess is actually a necrotic tumour. The specific procedure performed must be individualized, based on the particular circumstances at hand, but the simplest procedure is external drainage. This may be all that is required if the abscess contents are too viscid to drain satisfactorily through percutaneous drains or if an abscess cavity is multiloculated. A surgical approach is clearly indicated in certain circumstances such as free intraperitoneal rupture of the abscess and to deal with complications of catheter insertion such as bleeding (Fig. 15.4) or intraperitoneal leakage of the abscess contents.

Surgical intervention may also be needed to deal with the underlying cause of liver abscess. Failure to identify and treat surgically an intra-abdominal septic focus is one of the major contributors to the consistently elevated mortality associated with this condition. The most likely source of sepsis is in the biliary tract, with an increasing proportion due to malignant disease. Complicated gallstone disease still accounts for about 14% of these cases, but in most instances biliary obstruction due to choledocholithiasis can be decompressed endoscopically or by percutaneous drain placement in the acute setting, reducing the need for emergency operative exploration of the common bile duct. Appendicitis has virtually disappeared as a cause of liver abscess because of earlier recognition and treatment, but benign conditions of the colon, particularly diverticulitis and inflammatory bowel disease, remain important causes, as does colonic malignancy.

Surgical drainage can be performed by a transperitoneal or an extraperitoneal approach. In earlier series, the extraperitoneal approach through the bed of the 12th rib or by an anterior subcostal incision was popular because it eliminated the possibility of peritoneal contamination associated with abscess drainage. However, because of improvements in antibiotic therapy this advantage has become of less significance and is outweighed by the additional benefit of being able to perform a thorough search for a primary focus and the improved access afforded by a transperitoneal exploration.[49] A midline incision

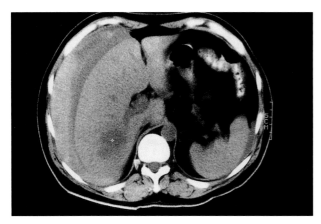

Figure 15.4 Massive subcapsular haematoma due to right hepatic vein injury by a percutaneous catheter. The abscess cavity is seen in segment VII. Treated by right hepatectomy.

gives good exposure of the entire peritoneal cavity. Intraoperative ultrasound greatly assists localization of the abscess cavity and may identify additional abscesses not seen on preoperative imaging. Needle aspiration can be performed to confirm the diagnosis before blunt puncture of the abscess cavity. Any loculations should be broken down and pus collected for microbiological examination along with a biopsy of the cavity wall. Dependent drainage is encouraged by appropriate selection of the puncture site and drain positioning. Large bore tube drains are preferable to corrugated or soft rubber drains as they allow postoperative contrast studies and/or irrigation of any residual cavity.

There are a number of reports of laparoscopic as opposed to open drainage of liver abscesses, including cases of ruptured liver abscess.[50,51] Accurate localization of the collection may be difficult at laparoscopy without the help of laparoscopic ultrasound. Certainly in patients with ruptured abscess the aims of surgical treatment including placement of drains and peritoneal lavage, and biopsy of the abscess cavity should be attainable by laparoscopy.

Hepatic resection may be necessary in patients with failure to control sepsis due to true multiloculation, when there is extensive associated parenchymal destruction, or long standing biliary obstruction causing parenchymal atrophy in addition to abscess formation.[15,49,52,53] Certainly, formal hepatic resection can produce dramatic improvement in appropriately selected patients. Any lingering suspicion that the lesion may be a necrotic tumour is sufficient grounds for performing an anatomical hepatic resection rather than external drainage. In one series from Hong Kong the presence of hepatolithiasis was the most important indicator of the likelihood of requiring hepatic resection, with the left liver being more frequently involved than the right.[15]

Outcome and prognosis

A number of reports have analysed risk factors for mortality associated with liver abscess. The factors that most consistently appear to be predictive of poor outcome include preoperative shock, hyperbilirubinaemia, hypoalbuminaemia, coagulopathy, diabetes, leucocytosis and the presence of malignancy.[15,54] As drainage techniques, antibiotic therapy and supportive treatment for organ failure syndromes become progressively more effective, the underlying causative pathology increasingly determines the outcome. Overall mortality figures in series over the last 10 years range from 2 to 35%. It is of relevance to note that in the series with the highest mortality, 30% of patients had malignant disease (Table 15.4).

Table 15.4 Recent series of pyogenic liver abscess comparing incidence of cryptogenic aetiology and malignancy with mortality

Reference	Year	No of patients	Cryptogenic (%)	Malignancy (%)	Mortality (%)
Miedema and Dineen[11]	1984	106	13.2	2.8	53
Farges et al.[8]	1988	46	15.2	ns	24
Wong[41]	1990	21	19	9.5	10
Bowers et al.[17]	1990	34	26	ns	12
Branum et al.[10]	1990	73	27	13	19
Stain et al.[19]	1991	54	36	4	2
Mischinger et al.[54]	1994	46	20	6.5	17.4
Chu et al.[15]	1996	83	45	6	18
Rintoul et al.[9]	1996	23	13	30	34.7
Chou et al.[18]	1997	483	54	4.5	12.8

Amoebic abscess

Amoebic abscess is worthy of separate consideration as there are important differences in the target population and management compared with pyogenic abscess. Amoebic dysentery was recognized in most ancient civilizations and observations of associated abdominal masses almost certainly refer to hepatic amoebic abscess formation. It was not until 1891 that the precise role of *Entamoeba histolytica* in this disorder was confirmed.[55]

Epidemiology and pathogenesis

An estimated 10% of the world's population are infected with *Entamoeba histolytica* although less than 10% of individuals are symptomatic.[56] Amoebic dysentery is the commonest clinical manifestation and between 3 and 7% develop amoebic hepatic abscess.[57] In non-endemic regions, amoebic liver abscess is limited to immigrants from or patients with a history of travel in an endemic area, and chronically institutionalized patients. In approximately 30% of sexually active homosexual males *Entamoeba histolytica* is detectable on stool culture and these form another high risk group.[56]

The organism is ingested orally in cystic form and released in the small intestine as trophozoites. These invade the colonic mucosa and enter mesenteric venules, through which they are carried to the liver. Direct invasion of mesenteric lymphatics may lead to pulmonary involvement. The organism causes local tissue destruction as a result of tissue infarction due to hepatic venular obstruction and, probably more importantly, adhesion to hepatocytes and release of cytolytic toxins. This process results in liquefaction necrosis and abscess formation. The pus contained in the cavity, which is composed of a mixture of blood and necrotic hepatic tissue, is typically described as resembling 'anchovy sauce'.[58]

Clinical features

In most series of amoebic liver abscess there is a marked male predominance. The clinical features are broadly similar to those seen with pyogenic abscess, except that tender hepatomegaly and diarrhoea are more likely and jaundice and severe systemic sepsis are less common compared to pyogenic abscess.[59] Intraperitoneal rupture presents with signs of peritonitis.[60] Pericardial rupture may cause cardiac tamponade. Intrapleural rupture produces sudden-onset dyspnoea with the signs of a pleural effusion. Rupture into the bronchial tree produces a cough productive of large volumes of brown sputum. Because this produces drainage of the underlying liver abscess it may be associated with significant improvement in the patient's overall condition.[61]

Diagnosis

Antiamoebic antibodies are present in 90–95% of patients with amoebic abscess and are detectable by haemagglutination or enzyme-linked immunoabsorbent assay (ELISA).[56,62] However, the organism is commonly not detectable in the stool of these patients. Chest radiograph is abnormal in 50% of patients. Ultrasound demonstrates a clearly defined round or oval hypoechoic cavity, usually situated peripherally in a subcapsular position.[63] An echogenic rim may be seen on CT, which enhances further on contrast administration.[64] Amoebic abscess is single in over 80% of cases and shows a marked predilection for the right liver, reflecting the fact that the primary site of access to the portal system is usually in the right colon.[65]

Management

In general terms amoebic abscess responds well to antiamoebicidal drug treatment and, unlike pyogenic abscess, drainage is normally not necessary.[56,66] Metronidazole is firmly established as the first-choice drug. Usually, obvious clinical improvement occurs within 72 hours of commencing treatment. For non-responders, chloroquine or emetine are alternative choices.[67] Emetine was widely used prior to the introduction of metronidazole. It must be given by intramuscular injection and may cause cardiac side effects. Newer agents such as secnidazole offer alternatives for patients not responding to metronidazole.[68]

Because of the accuracy of serological testing, needle aspiration is usually not necessary for diagnosis and there is good evidence that it does not accelerate resolution compared to treatment with amoebicidal drugs alone.[69] In the rare case in which serology is negative, aspiration may be necessary to differentiate amoebic from pyogenic abscess. Other indications for percutaneous drainage include (a) large symptomatic abscess, particularly if rupture is imminent because of subcapsular position, (b) to exclude secondary bacterial infection, (c) poor response to medical treatment, and (d) if there is a contraindication to medical therapy, such as pregnancy.[36]

Complications

The ability of the *Entamoeba* organism to destroy surrounding tissues occasionally produces some dramatic complications. Free intraperitoneal rupture occurs more commonly than in pyogenic abscess. Rupture into the pericardium, the pleural cavity or into the bronchial tree with formation of a biliary–bronchial fistula may also occur. Intraperitoneal or intrapericardial rupture is much more likely to occur if the abscess is situated in the left liver. Indeed, the presence of a large amoebic abscess in this site is an indication for percutaneous drainage to avoid the risk of rupture.[60,61]

Outcome

Complete resolution is the norm with treatment, although it may typically take 6 months or longer for complete disappearance of the cavity. The mortality associated with amoebic liver abscess is less than 3%.[56] Recurrence of amoebic abscess is extremely rare because the host develops immunity following the first episode.[58]

Conclusions

Liver abscess continues to pose significant diagnostic and management challenges. The mortality associated with this condition has not been dramatically reduced despite improvements in treatment strategies, mainly because of changes in the patient population and the underlying aetiology. The use of a minimal access approach by a multidisciplinary team consisting of surgeon, interventional radiologist, microbiologist and endoscopist is important to ensure a satisfactory outcome. With optimal management the outcome appears largely to be determined by the underlying disease (Table 15.4).

Key points

- Aetiology:
    Bacterial (pyogenic):
        Ascending cholangitis
        Portal pyaemia
        Haematogenous from non-GI source (10–20%)
        Hepatic embolization
    Amoebic.
- Diagnosis:
    Clinical history of aetiologic factors
    Blood cultures
    US
    CT (97% sensitivity)
    MRC (for associated biliary pathology)
    Amoebic/hydatid serology.
- Pyogenic abscess:
    Main objective is to drain pus and locate origin of sepsis
    Attempt percutaneous drainage.
- Amoebic abscess:
    Drainage not normally necessary
    First-line therapy: metronidazole
    Second-line therapy: secnidazole.

REFERENCES

1. Frey CF, Zhu Y, Suzuki S. Liver abscess. Surg Clin North Am 1989; 69: 259–71

2. Bright R. Observations on jaundice: more particularly on that form of the disease which accompanies diffused inflammation of the liver. Guys Hospital Report 1836; 1: 604–37

3. Kobler G. Zur aetiologie vier Leberabscesse. Arch Pathol Anat Physiol Klin Med 1901; 1963: 134–6

4. Gerster AG. On septic thrombosis of the roots of the portal vein in appendicitis, together with some remarks on peritoneal sepsis. Med Rec 1903; 63: 1005–15

5. Oschner A, DeBakey M, Murray S. Pyogenic abscesses of the liver. II. An analysis of forty-seven cases with review of the literature. Am J Surg 1938; 40: 292–19

6. McFadzean AJ, Chang KP, Wong CL. Solitary pyogenic abscess of the liver treated by closed aspiration and antibiotics. A report of 14 consecutive cases of recovery. Br J Surg 1953; 41: 141–52

7. Seeto RK, Rockey DC. Pyogenic liver abscess: changes in aetiology, management and outcome. Medicine 1996; 75: 99

8. Farges O, Leese T, Bismuth H. Pyogenic liver abscess: an improvement in prognosis. Br J Surg 1988; 75: 862–5

9. Rintoul R, O'Riordain MG, Laurenson IF, Crosbie JL, Allan PL, Garden OJ. Changing management of pyogenic liver abscess. Br J Surg 1996; 83: 1215–8

10. Branum GD, Tyson GS, Branum MA, Meyers WC. Hepatic abscess. Changes in etiology, diagnosis, and management. Ann Surg 1990; 212: 655–62

11. Miedema BW, Dineen P. The diagnosis and treatment of pyogenic liver abscess. Ann Surg 1984; 200: 328–35

12. Royal College of Radiologists. Training and practice in interventional radiology. Clinical Radiology Reports and Guidelines 1997 (http:\\www5.rea.net/enquiries/publications/tpir.html)

13. Sherman JD, Robbins SL. Changing trends in the casuistics of hepatic abscess. Am J Med 1960; 28: 943–50

14. Pitt HA, Zuidema GD. Factors influencing mortality in the treatment of pyogenic hepatic abscess. Surg Gynecol Obstet 1975; 140: 228–34

15. Chu K-M, Fan S-T, Lai EC, Lo C-M, Wong J. Pyogenic liver abscess. An audit of experience over the past decade. Arch Surg 1996; 131: 148–52

16. Gyorffy EJ, Frey CF, Silva J, McGahan J. Pyogenic liver abscess. Diagnostic and therapeutic strategies. Ann Surg 1987; 206: 699–705

17. Bowers ED, Robison DJ, Doberneck RC. Pyogenic liver abscess. World J Surg 1990; 14: 128–32

18. Chou FF, Sheen-Chen SM, Chen YS, Chen MC. Single and multiple pyogenic liver abscesses: clinical course, etiology, and results of treatment. World J Surg 1997; 21: 384–8

19. Stain SC, Yellin AE, Donovan AJ, Brien HW. Pyogenic liver abscess. Modern treatment. Arch Surg 1991; 126: 991–6

20. Carrel T, Lerut J, Baer H, Blumgart LH. Hepatic abscess following biliary tract surgery. Eur J Surg 1991; 157: 209–13

21. Marcus SG, Walsh TJ, Pizzo PA, Danforth DN Jr. Hepatic abscess in cancer patients. Characterization and management. Rch Surg 1993; 128: 1358–64

22. Chen C, Chen PJ, Yang PM et al. Clinical and microbiological features of liver abscess after transarterial embolization for hepatocellular carcinoma. Am J Gastroenterol 1997; 92: 2257–9

23. De Baere T, Roche A, Amenabar JM et al. Liver abscess formation after local treatment of liver tumours. Hepatology 1996; 23: 1436–40

24. Friedl J, Stift A, Berlakovitch GA et al. Haemophilus parainfluenzae liver abscess after successful liver transplantation. J Clin Microbiol 1998; 36: 818–9

25. Korvick JA, Marsh JW, Starzl TE, Yu VL. *Pseudomonas aeruginosa* bacteremia in patients undergoing liver transplanation: an emerging problem. Surgery 1991; 109: 62–8

26. Annunziata GM, Blackstone M, Hart J, Piper J, Baker Al. Candida (*Torulopsis glabrata*) liver abscesses eight years after orthotopic liver transplantation. J Clin Gastroenterol 1997; 24: 176–9

27. Kinney TD, Ferrebee JW. Hepatic abscess. Factors determining its localization. Arch Pathol 1948; 45: 41–7

28. Hansen PS, Schondeyer HC. Pyogenic hepatic abscess. A 10-year population-based retrospective study. APMIS 1998; 106: 396–402

29. Northover JMA, Jones BJ, Dawson JL, Williams R. Difficulties in diagnosis and management of pyogenic liver abscess. Br J Surg 1982; 69: 48–51

30. Fawcett HD, Lantieri RL, Frankel A et al. Differentiating hepatic abscess from tumor: combined 111In white blood cell and 99mTc liver scans. AJR 1980: 135: 53–6

31. Newlin N, Silver TM, Stuck KJ et al. Ultrasonic features of pyogenic liver abscess. Radiology 1991; 139: 155–9

32. Kugligowska E, Connors SK, Shapiro JH. Liver abscess: sonography in diagnosis and treatment. AJR 1982; 138: 253–7

33. Halvorsen RA, Korobkin M, Foster WI et al. The variable appearance of hepatic abscess. AJR 1984; 141: 941–4

34. Baron RL, Freeny PC, Moss AA. The liver. In: Moss AA, Gamsu G, Genant HK, eds. Computed tomography of the body: with magnetic resonance imaging, 2nd edn. Philadelphia: WB Saunders, 1992: 735–822

35. Saini S. Imaging of the hepatobiliary tract. N Engl J Med 1997; 336: 1889–94

36. Ros PR, Barreda P, Gore RM. Focal hepatic infections. In: Gore RM, Levine MS, Laufer I, eds. Textbook of gastrointestinal radiology. Philadelphia: WB Saunders, 1994: 1947–67

37. Mergo PJ, Ros PR. MR imaging of inflammatory disease of the liver. Magn Reson Imag Clin N Am 1997; 5: 367–76

38. Reinhold C, Bret PM. Current status of MR cholangiopancreatography. AJR 1996; 166: 1285–95

39. Mueller PR, Dawson SL, Ferrucci JT, Nardi GL. Hepatic echinococcal cyst: successful percutaneous drainage. Radiology 1985; 155: 627–8

40. Kabaaloiglu A, Apaydin A, Sindel T, Arslan G, Özkaynak C, Lüleci E. Hydatid liver cysts: mid-term results of percutaneous image-guided sclerotherapy. J Intervent Radiol 1998; 13: 59–62

41. Wong KP. Percutaneous drainage of pyogenic liver abscess. World J Surg 1990; 14: 492–7

42. Giorgio A, Tarantino L, Mariniello N et al. Pyogenic liver abscess: 13 years of experience in percutaneous nedle aspiration with US guidance. Radiology 1995; 195: 122–4

43. Ch Yu S, Hg Lo R, Kan PS, Metreweli C. Pyogenic liver abscess: treatment with needle aspiration. Clin Radiol 1997; 52: 912–6

44. Miller FJ, Ahola DT, Bretzman PA, Fillmore DJ. Percutaneous management of hepatic abscess: a perspective by interventional radiologists. J Vasc Interv Radiol 1997; 8: 241–7

45. McNicholas M, Mueller P, Lee M et al. Percutaneous drainage of subphrenic fluid collections that occur after splenectomy: Efficacy and safety of transpleural versus extrapleural appraoch. AJR 1995; 165: 355–9

46. Bernadino ME, Berkman WA, Plemmons M et al. Percutaneous drainage of multiseptated hepatic abscess. J Comp Assist Tomogr 1984; 8: 38–41

47. Tazawa J, Sakai Y, Maekawa S et al. Solitary and multiple pyogenic liver abscesses: characteristics of the patients and efficacy of percutaneous drainage. Am J Gastroenterol 1997; 92: 271–4

48. Rajak CL, Gupta S, Jain S, Chawla Y, Gulati M, Suri S. Percutaneous treatment of liver abscess: needle aspiration versus catheter drainage. AJR 1998; 170: 1035–9

49. Pitt HA. Surgical management of hepatic abscess. World J Surg 1990; 14: 498–504

50. Tay KH, Ravintharan T, Moe MN, See AC, Chng HC. Laparoscopic drainage of liver abscess. Br J Surg 1998; 85: 330–2

51. Siu WT, Chan WC, Hou SM, Li MK. Laparoscopic management of ruptured pyogenic liver abscess. Surg Laparosc Endosc 1997; 7: 426–8

52. Knoop M, Kling N, Langrehr JM et al. Is liver abscess still an indication for liver resection? Zentralbl Chir 1995; 120: 461–6

53. Kurosaki I, Takagi K, Hatakeyama S et al. Right hepatectomy for pyogenic liver abscess with true multiloculation. J Gastroenterol 1997; 32: 105–9

54. Mischinger HJ, Hauser H, Rabl H et al. Pyogenic liver abscess: studies of therapy and analysis of risk factors. World J Surg 1994; 18: 852–8

55. Martinez-Baez M. Historical introduction. In: Martinez-Palomo A, ed. Amebiasis. Human parasitic diseases, Vol 2. Amsterdam: Elsevier, 1986: 1–9

56. Reed Sl. Amebiasis: an update. Clin Infect Dis 1992; 14: 385–93

57. Chuah SK, Changchien CS, Sheen IS et al. The prognostic factors of severe amoebic liver disease – a retrospective study of 125 cases. Am J Trop Med 1992; 46: 398–402

58. Ravdin JI, Guerrant RL. A review of the parasite cellular mechanisms involved in the pathogenesis of amebiasis. Rev Infect Dis 1982; 4: 1185–207

59. Sepulveda B, Manzo NT. Clinical manifestations and diagnosis of amebiasis. In: Martinez-Palomo A, ed. Amebiasis. Human parasitic diseases, Vol 2. Amsterdam: Elsevier, 1986: 169–87

60. Sarda AK, Bal S, Sharma AK, Kapur MM. Intraperitoneal rupture of amoebic liver abscess. Br J Surg 1989; 76: 202–3

61. Greaney GC, Reynolds TB, Donovan AJ. Ruptured amebic liver abscess. Arch Surg 1985; 120: 555–61

62. Sharma M, Saxena A, Ghosh S, Samantarary JC, Talwar GP. A simple and rapid Dot-ELISA dipstick technique for detection of antibodies to *Entamoeba histolytica* in amebic liver abscess. Ind J Med Res 1988; 88: 409–15

63. Ralls PW, Colletti PM, Quinn MF, Halls JM. Sonographic findings in hepatic amebic abscess. Radiology 1982; 145: 123–6

64. Radin DR, Ralls PW, Colletti PM et al. CT of amebic liver abscess. AJR 1988; 150: 1297–301

65. Cevallos AM, Farthing MJ. Parasitic infections of the gastrointestinal tract. Curr Opin Gastroenterol 1993; 9: 96–102

66. Ralls PW, Barnes PF, Johnson MB et al. Medical treatment of hepatic amoebic abscess: rare need for percutaneous drainage. Radiology 1987; 165: 805–7

67. Thompson JE, Forlenza S, Verma R. Amebic liver abscess: a therapeutic approach. Rev Infect Dis 1985; 7: 171–9

68. Bhatia S, Karnad DR, Oak JL. Randomized double-blind trial of metronidazole versus secnidazole in amebic liver abscess. Ind J Gastroenterol 1998; 17: 53–4

69. Sharma MP, Rai RR, Acharya SK, Ray JC, Tandon BN. Needle aspiration of amoebic liver abscess. Br Med J 1989; 299: 1308–9

16 Cirrhotic portal hypertension

Robert Sutton and David Marcus Gore

What are the key pathophysiological changes that influence management?

Chronic, chemical, metabolic, virological or immunological injury leads to hepatocyte necrosis, causing sustained inflammation, as well as cytokine-mediated activation and transformation of fat-storing Ito cells.[1] These cells subsequently act as a major source of liver fibrogenesis.[2] Sinusoidal basement membrane thickening is an early change in the microvasculature, followed by collagen deposition in the space of Disse and, later, fibrosis in and around the portal tracts.[3] The sinusoidal spaces are narrowed, and despite a relative increase of spontaneous intrahepatic shunting, portal venous resistance increases, whilst the remaining hepatocyte mass becomes more and more removed from direct splanchnic circulatory access. There is upregulation of intrahepatic vasomotor tone, although the exact role of endothelins, nitric oxide and their receptors remains to be determined.[4] Regenerative nodules also contribute to the architectural distortion resulting from liver fibrosis. The principal impact of these changes is a reduction in the capacity of all hepatic synthetic, metabolic and detoxifying functions. Most noticeable amongst many are the nutritional and neurological effects, particularly hepatic encephalopathy, which is more likely at times of increased demand on the liver.

A decrease in both systemic and splanchnic arteriolar resistance occurs early in the course of chronic liver disease, candidate factors for which include increased production or decreased elimination of circulating levels of glucagon, prostacyclin or bile acids, increased nitric oxide production and/or altered receptor sensitivity controlling vasomotor tone.[5] The sympathetic nervous system, renin–angiotensin system and antidiuretic hormone are all activated to retain sodium and water, expand plasma volume and increase cardiac index, so as to

---

Table 16.1 Key pathophysiological changes in cirrhotic portal hypertension

- Liver fibrosis and architectural distortion
- Decreased hepatocyte mass and function
- Decreased systemic vascular resistance
- Decreased splanchnic arteriolar resistance
- Increased sodium and water retention
- Increased intrahepatic vascular resistance
- Portosystemic collaterals and hypersplenism

---

maintain tissue perfusion pressure, even though arterial blood pressure tends to run at relatively low levels in these patients.[6] As sodium retention is upregulated, sodium should be administered sparingly, otherwise further fluid retention will occur (Table 16.1). Splanchnic inflow, pooling and congestion are increased by similar mechanisms, exacerbating any portal hypertension, that in turn is associated with the development of portosystemic collaterals, notably in the submucosal layers of the oesophagus and upper stomach. The spleen is a particular focus of congestion, that induces enlargement and hypersplenism. Variceal haemorrhage or ascites are likely to occur once the portal venous pressure gradient (portal vein pressure minus inferior vena cava pressure) is above 12 mmHg.[7]

How should suspected cirrhotic portal hypertension be investigated?

Routine haematology with full blood count and clotting studies, especially of the extrinsic pathway by prothrombin time, and biochemistry with electrolytes, urea, creatinine, bilirubin, albumin and liver enzymes are all mandatory. This may be extended with assay of several plasma proteins,

Table 16.2 Outline of investigation of cirrhotic portal hypertension

- Full blood count
- Clotting screen (especially prothrombin time for extrinsic pathway)
- Urea and electrolytes
- Liver function tests (bilirubin, albumin, liver enzymes)
- Hepatitis screen (A, B and C)
- Autoantibodies
- Immunoglobulins
- α_1-Antitrypsin
- Iron studies
- Copper studies
- Liver biopsy
- Endoscopy
- Ultrasound
- Wedged hepatic vein pressure
- Mesenteric angiography
- CT/MR scan

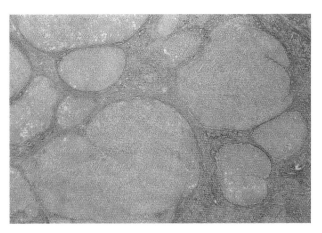

Figure 16.1 Liver biopsy of a patient with alcoholic cirrhosis (courtesy of Dr F Campbell).

Table 16.3 Child–Pugh classification of chronic liver disease: grade A, total of 5–6 points; B, 7–9 points; C, 10–15 points

Clinical or biochemical measures	Points scored for increasing abnormality		
	1	2	3
Encephalopathy (grade[a])	None	I, II	III, IV
Ascites	Absent	Slight	Moderate
Bilirubin (μmol/l)	<34	34–51	>51
For PBC[b] bilirubin (μmol/l)	<68	68–170	>170
Albumin (g/l)	>35	28–35	<28
Prothrombin (s prolonged)	1–4	4–6	>6

[a]Clinical grade in the table after Trey et al.;[8] Number Connection Test ≤ 30 s 1 point, 31–50 s 2 points, >50 s 3 points.
[b]Primary biliary cirrhosis.

including α_1-antitrypsin, caeruloplasmin and transferrin, supplemented with further copper and iron studies to obtain pointers to a cause for cirrhosis. Serum immunoglobulins and autoantibodies may help further in this regard. Liver biopsy conducted at an appropriate stage will complement tests to establish a cause for cirrhosis (Table 16.2 and Fig. 16.1). Quantitative tests of liver function are not recommended for routine clinical use; Child–Pugh grading is by far the most powerful prognostic indicator (Table 16.3).[8,9] It is important to appreciate the effect of timing on the use of the Child–Pugh system: on admission for an acute variceal haemorrhage Child–Pugh grading is a powerful predictor of short-term, but not long-term survival. However, following recovery, Child–Pugh grading is a powerful predictor of long-term survival.[9] Child–Pugh grading may be made more accurate by the addition of the Number Connection Test (Child–Pugh–NCT),[9] a standardized test of the presence and severity of hepatic encephalopathy that is far simpler than electroencephalography or visual evoked potential recording. In patients with unexplained encephalopathy or abdominal pain an ascitic tap may identify spontaneous bacterial peritonitis, whereas further microbiological assessment must at an early stage include tests for hepatitis virus infection (at least hepatitis A, B and C).

Upper and, less usually, lower gastrointestinal endoscopy is also mandatory, and that during the initial stage following an acute bleed. The size of the varices (less or more than half the radius of the open oesophageal lumen) contribute to the likelihood of a first (index) or recurrent bleed, as do red vascular markings on their surface.[10] Further haemodynamic evaluation can be undertaken radiologically, which will also identify abnormal morphology, using ultrasound, computerized axial tomography or magnetic resonance imaging. Duplex ultrasonography cannot only determine patency but also direction of flow in the portal and splenic veins, although the optimal method is venous phase angiography via the coeliac and superior mesenteric arteries (Fig. 16.2). Systemic venography via the right internal jugular or femoral vein is particularly useful in the measurement of hepatic vein pressure gradient (wedged minus free hepatic vein pressure). The hepatic vein pressure gradient closely parallels the portal venous pressure gradient, and when over 12 mmHg identifies sinusoidal portal hypertension indicative of a likely cirrhotic aetiology. This technique may be coupled with transjugular liver

A

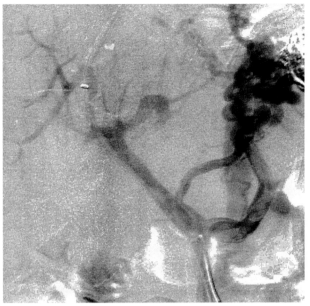

B

Oesophageal lumen
Mucosa
Varices
Submucosa
Muscularis

Oesophagus

Perioesophageal plexus

Azygos vein
Short gastric veins

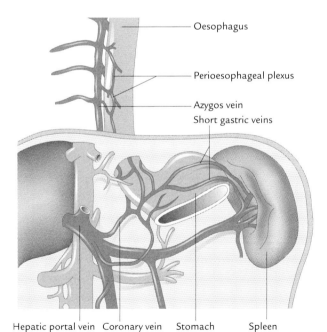

Hepatic portal vein   Coronary vein   Stomach   Spleen

Figure 16.2 (A) Venous phase mesenteric angiogram showing dilated vessels and portosystemic collaterals characteristic of portal hypertension (courtesy of Dr P Rowlands). (B) Diagrammatic representation of portal venous system and its collaterals.

biopsy, appropriate in patients with significant clotting abnormalities that render percutaneous biopsy unsafe.

The use of various diagnostic tests depends on the clinical scenario; under emergency circumstances, some must be omitted. If surgery is considered and time allows, standard tests of cardiac and respiratory function should also be undertaken.

What is first-line management for cirrhotic portal hypertension?

Acute variceal haemorrhage

A patient who presents with haematemesis or melaena may have clinical features that are suspicious of chronic liver disease, or be known to have cirrhosis. Usually within 4 hours of admission and resuscitation an early upper gastrointestinal endoscopy must be performed, to identify and characterize the presence of varices in the oesophagus and/or stomach (Table 16.4). Any varices seen must be assumed to be the source of bleeding; even in the rare circumstance of an actively bleeding additional lesion, management must include control of the portal hypertension. Portal hypertensive gastropathy, where the lining of the stomach is visually altered with multiple red markings, may be the source of some bleeding, but in the presence of varices, the latter are more likely to be, and should

Table 16.4 **First-line management of cirrhotic portal hypertension**
Acute variceal haemorrhage • Vasoactive drug when suspected or confirmed (5 days) • Upper gastrointestinal endoscopy • Sclerotherapy or variceal banding (2 sessions) • ± Sengstaken–Blakemore or Minnesota tube (24 hours) • Broad-spectrum antibiotics • Lactulose orally and magnesium sulphate enemas • HDU/ITU care Recurrent variceal haemorrhage • As for acute variceal haemorrhage • Consider shunt at an early stage (after 10 units) Diuretic resistant ascites • Salt and fluid restriction (<20 mmol and <1.5 l per day) • Paracentesis with IV albumin replacement • Consider peritoneovenous or portosystemic shunt Advanced cirrhosis • Continuing supportive management • Appropriate specific therapies • Consider liver transplantation

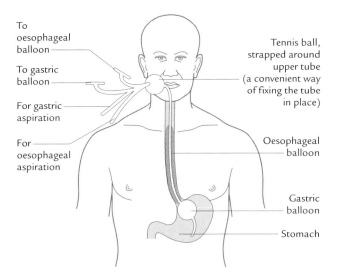

To oesophageal balloon

To gastric balloon

For gastric aspiration

For oesophageal aspiration

Tennis ball, strapped around upper tube (a convenient way of fixing the tube in place)

Oesophageal balloon

Gastric balloon

Stomach

Figure 16.3 Sengstaken–Blakemore tube with 10 point protocol for placement:

1. Concise explanation to patient, and anaesthetic throat spray.
2. Test 4 channels of tube, 2 balloons, and exclude leaks.
3. Expeditious passage with lubricant (patient may need restraining).
4. 300 ml air into gastric balloon (stop if significant pain/difficulty).
5. Draw tube back to about 40 cm mark and apply traction.
6. Fill oesophageal balloon with radiopaque dye to 40 mmHg.
7. Apply continuous low-grade suction to both aspiration ports.
8. Check position (radiograph), then check oesophageal balloon every hour.
9. Deflate oesophageal balloon at 12 hours, later gastric balloon.
10. Apply tamponade for no longer than 24 hours for continued bleeding.

be assumed to be the source. The endoscopy requires an experienced operator, with the full support of experienced nurses and technicians; it is no place for the overenthusiastic novice. Additionally, when bleeding has been severe and is continuing, an experienced anaesthetist is needed, not only to assist with resuscitation, but also to intubate the patient and guard the airway. Although general anaesthesia may impair liver perfusion and metabolism further, the primary objective is complete control of haemorrhage, since survival is much less likely in any patient continuing to bleed. To achieve this, endoscopic therapy should be administered at the earliest opportunity. In the demanding scenario of an acute bleed, injection sclerotherapy is preferred over banding ligation, as a general rule. If such therapy cannot be given, a Sengstaken–Blakemore or Minnesota quadruple

lumen tube should be correctly and safely inserted (Fig. 16.3), and the patient transferred to a specialist unit, which is in any case preferable.[11]

An intravenous infusion of somatostatin (250 μg/h) or octreotide (50 μg/h) or intermittent intravenous boluses of terlipressin (1–2 mg every 4–6 h) should be started as soon as the diagnosis of variceal haemorrhage is suspected, and continued for up to 5 days as adjuvant to endoscopic therapy.[12] Broad-spectrum prophylactic antibiotics should also be administered, as these patients have depressed immunity, and ascitic, chest, urinary or other infections are thereby rendered less likely.[13] A second session of endoscopic therapy, usually by banding ligation, should be undertaken within 2 to 3 days, and conversion to beta blockade and/or vasodilators is recommended before discharge. Programmed variceal obliteration, principally by banding, should then be undertaken, as far as possible on an outpatient basis, but allowing for all the investigations necessary, some of which may require inpatient care.

Recurrent variceal haemorrhage

Recurrent haemorrhage may occur following initial control, during the same admission. Following any variceal haemorrhage the very high risk of recurrent haemorrhage falls with time; more rebleeds occur in the first 6 weeks than in any subsequent period, although some risk of rebleeding remains.[14] Thus recurrent haemorrhage may precipitate a subsequent inpatient admission. Although definitions vary, there is consensus that a clinically significant recurrent haemorrhage is one that induces a fall in systolic blood pressure to below 100 mmHg, or >20 mmHg; or an increase in pulse rate to above 100/min, or >20/min; or a need for 2 or more units of blood to maintain haemoglobin levels, or a fall in haemoglobin of >2 g/dl.[15] If a recurrent haemorrhage occurs following initial control, the severity of the bleed will determine whether a Sengstaken–Blakemore or Minnesota quadruple lumen tube is required. An additional session of endoscopic therapy may be added, or the second session hastened; any adjuvant vasoactive agent should be increased to maximum dosage. Management of hepatic encephalopathy is likely to require particular care with lactulose, neomycin (both may be given via nasogastric tube) and magnesium sulphate enemas, where possible avoiding analgesics, sedatives and hypnotics.

Management of a second or subsequent admission for recurrent variceal haemorrhage falls into the same pathway as above, but more major interventions must be considered at an earlier rather than later stage (Table 16.4).

Diuretic resistant ascites

If salt restriction <20 mmol/day and fluid restriction to 1.5 l/day, as well as potassium-sparing together with other diuretics fail to reduce and control ascites, paracentesis with intravenous albumin replacement is appropriate. However, diuretic therapy should not be too aggressive, since when continued, the patient may develop hepatorenal syndrome, with oliguria, low urinary sodium and renal failure. This may respond to ornipressin at a dose of 1 U/h, which can be continued for several days to maintain urine output, with fluid supplementation as necessary.[16] If paracentesis has to be repeated frequently, peritoneal–venous shunting with a Denver or LeVeen shunt may be considered, or some form of portal decompression (Table 16.4).[17]

Advanced cirrhosis

As outlined above, Child–Pugh grading is the most effective predictor of long-term survival in cirrhotic portal hypertension. Some insight into prognosis can also be gained by determination of the patient's general health status, energy and activity, as well as the presence and severity of hepatic encephalopathy. Usually the presence of this last complication is attendant upon another compromising event: it may for example be drug induced, relate to infection, acute variceal haemorrhage or follow non-specific deterioration; correction should be directed to the cause. Age, renal function and, for those patients with an alcoholic aetiology, abstinence or otherwise, are also relevant. Much of the management is supportive, with continuation of specific therapies if still appropriate (e.g. interferon regimes for viral hepatitis, venesection for haemochromatosis). A key consideration is candidature for liver transplantation, likely for those patients under 65 with advanced cirrhosis but no intercurrent malignancy or other condition that would severely compromise likely success (Table 16.4).[18] Alcoholic patients usually have to be abstinent for at least 6 months, with programmes conducting thorough interviewing of close family members, not only to confirm abstinence, but also to determine suitability for transplantation with prolonged immunosuppression and review.

How is treatment chosen after failure of endoscopic management?

It is widely agreed that two clinically significant rebleeds from oesophageal varices, or one significant

Table 16.5 **Options in the treatment of variceal haemorrhage in cirrhotic portal hypertension after failure of endoscopic management**
• Dependent on status of patient • Dependent on regional availability • Narrow diameter H-graft portocaval shunt • Distal splenorenal shunt • Devascularization • Transjugular intrahepatic portosystemic shunt

rebleed from gastric varices, constitute strong indications for further intervention during or after failure of the endoscopic plus pharmacological management described above.[11,14,15] This should be the case whether the rebleeds are during a single admission or during recurrent admissions. A few units specializing in this area are more interventionist, conducting portal decompressive procedures earlier in the pathway; however, this approach must be regarded as experimental, as it has not gained wide acceptance. However, there are more who would support more major intervention after 10 or more units of blood have had to be given during a single admission, as beyond this point patients tend to deteriorate rapidly; control of haemorrhage is the first aim of therapy (Table 16.5).

The next consideration is the choice of major intervention; this will depend partly on regional availability and partly on the status of the patient. Diversion of all portal blood from the portal vein

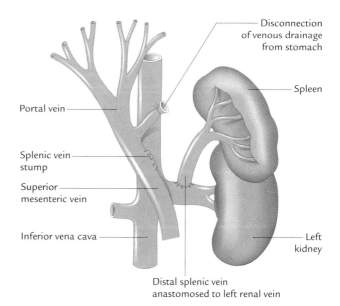

Figure 16.4 Distal splenorenal selective portosystemic shunt.

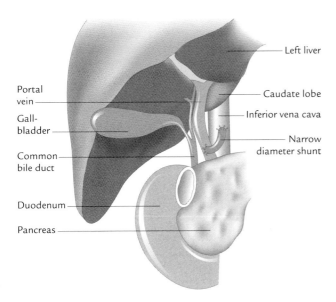

Figure 16.5   Narrow diameter H-graft portocaval shunt.

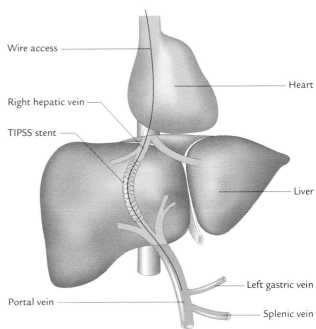

Figure 16.6   Transjugular intrahepatic portosystemic shunt.

into the inferior vena cava by surgical *total* portosystemic shunting was first popularized by Whipple in the 1940s, and maintained a major role for at least 20 years.[11] The high incidence of new or worsened hepatic encephalopathy attendant upon this form of shunting led to the development by Warren of the *selective* distal splenorenal shunt (Fig. 16.4).[19] In this form of shunt the azygos venous circulation draining the oesophagus, stomach, pancreas and spleen is separated from the portal venous drainage (which is maintained via the portal vein) and decompressed via the distal splenic vein into the left renal vein. This procedure remains an important alternative today, although it is less applicable to emergency scenarios, because preoperative angiographic evaluation should be detailed, and it is technically more difficult than alternatives. More recently the *partial* or narrow-diameter portocaval shunt has been developed by Sarfeh and colleagues,[20] as well as Bismuth and colleagues (Fig. 16.5).[21] In this procedure an externally ringed PTFE (polytetrafluoroethylene) graft of 2 to 3 cm is placed between the portal vein and inferior vena cava; the narrow diameter of 8 or 10 mm ensures that, although the portal pressure gradient is reduced to below 12 mmHg, a gradient remains, sufficient to maintain nutrient portal vein flow to the liver. This procedure usually requires less dissection than other forms of shunt, can be undertaken more readily during emergency scenarios and reduces the incidence of encephalopathy attendant upon total shunting.[22]

Devascularization procedures have been popular in a number of centres, the minimum being an oesophageal transection.[23] Despite apparent simplicity, considerable dissection within the abdominal cavity including gastrotomy with likely peritoneal contamination is necessary, and control of gastric varices with plication may be particularly awkward. In the emergency scenario a Sengstaken–Blakemore or Minnesota quadruple lumen tube is likely to be in place; this must be removed before adequate access to the stomach and oesophagus can be obtained, during which time further haemorrhage may occur. Additionally, recurrent haemorrhage during prolonged follow-up is more likely after devascularization than after surgical shunting. The addition of splenectomy and gastric devascularization may make this less likely, but entrains other complications.

Currently the most popular major intervention is TIPSS, transjugular intrahepatic portosystemic shunt (Fig. 16.6).[24,25] Accomplished radiologically, access is usually obtained via the right internal jugular vein and right hepatic vein to the right portal vein, a track dilated, and a stent inserted to reduce the portal venous pressure gradient. Correctly, the gradient should be less than 12 mmHg, but stenosis and occlusion are common, so repeated shunt gradient measurements are necessary to determine the need for further intervention.[26] Adequate patency may be maintained by dilation techniques, or insertion of another TIPSS through or beside the first. The appeal of this technique is the minimal access required, and although general anaesthesia is usually given, it can be performed with sedation and local anaesthesia. However, following a first TIPSS, reintervention is necessary in 70–80% of cases within a year as well as recurrently, to maintain a gradient less than 12 mmHg.[26] Furthermore, liver haemodynamics are impaired significantly more following TIPSS than following partial or selective surgical shunting, presumably because TIPSS steals more portal blood from the liver (flow in the distal right portal vein is likely to be minimal following TIPSS).[27] Thus hepatic encephalopathy may be more likely following TIPSS, if fully patent, than following partial or selective surgical shunting. Nevertheless, for the patient in a more adverse state because of age over 65, more advanced cirrhosis, or other intercurrent condition, or for the patient soon to be a candidate for liver transplantation, TIPSS is likely to be preferable.

What factors are integral to the success of surgical shunting?

Status of patient

Patient selection must be undertaken carefully, for although cirrhotic patients are in general a high risk group, some patients are likely to fare particularly poorly with surgery (Table 16.6). Thus patients

---

Table 16.6 Factors integral to the success of surgical shunting

Status of patient
- Child–Pugh grade A or B
- Under 65 with minimal intercurrent disease

Status of hospital team
- Specialist tertiary hepatobiliary unit

Patient preparation
- Complete investigations (as far as possible)
- Correction of clotting abnormalities
- Antibiotic prophylaxis
- Anti-liver failure regime

Operative technique
- Extreme care in securing haemostasis
- Vascular surgical technique
- Measurement of portal pressures

Postoperative care
- Sodium restriction
- Prophylactic antibiotics
- Antiliver failure regime
- Ornipressin renal support
- Nutritional support
- Shuntogram at 5–7 days

Follow-up
- Monitor shunt function
- Treat underlying disease

---

known to have been Child–Pugh grade C status before the onset of acute variceal haemorrhage, or those remaining Child–Pugh grade C status between separate inpatient episodes of acute variceal haemorrhage, may have insufficient hepatic reserve to fare well with surgery. Patients over the age of 65, or with significant intercurrent disease, may be considered less likely to fare well with surgery. TIPSS would be preferable in these patients, as it is in patients who are candidates for liver transplantation, where the risks of surgery, as well as hilar dissection and adhesion formation, may compromise future success.

There are, however, a number of patients who are Child–Pugh grade C on admission with acute variceal haemorrhage, but whose grading improves to A or B on recovery.[9] Thus Child–Pugh grade C status on admission with acute variceal haemorrhage is not per se a contraindication to surgery, although the severity of any progression in liver failure may suggest that significant improvement is less likely.

Status of hospital team

Portal hypertension accounts for no more than 10% of all hospital admissions for gastrointestinal bleeding in most Western countries; higher incidences are found where viral hepatitis is commoner, as in the Far East. The nature and severity of the complications of portal hypertension are such that specialist hepatobiliary expertise is required; tertiary referral units offering a comprehensive range of treatments are the preferred service providers. Complementary medical, radiological, surgical and pathological services are essential components; the surgical component is probably best maintained in the hands of one or two committed and experienced individuals; more surgeons are needed in transplant units (Table 16.6).

Patient preparation

A small stock of requisite grafting materials must be continually maintained in the hospital, as the intermittent need for this type of surgery tends to result in neglect of this aspect. The investigations outlined above will assist in the evaluation prior to surgery; radiological investigations are particularly important. How far investigations are extended will depend on the urgency; these must address the nature and severity of varices, liver function, the underlying aetiology and vascular anatomy. As far as possible, clotting abnormalities should be corrected; acutely, this may require fresh frozen plasma and platelet transfusions, as well as vitamin K (Table 16.6). Antibiotic prophylaxis must be started, if not already begun. Magnesium sulphate enemas, together with oral neomycin and lactulose (via nasogastric tube if necessary) are administered to minimize hepatic encephalopathy. Obtaining consent may necessarily be brief; under these circumstances, co-operation from relatives is desirable.

Operative technique

Key points are outlined; details of technique should be learnt with an experienced surgeon. Central venous access if essential; an arterial line and urinary catheter should also be placed. The use of barbiturates, certain inhalational anaesthetics (especially halothane) and sedatives is avoided. In the approach to the hepatic hilum for narrow-diameter portocaval grafting, sandbag tilting to the left with split table angulation (head down) at the costal margin is desirable; for distal splenorenal shunting sandbag tilting to the right is preferred, but with similar angulation at the costal margin. However, if urgency dictates, and a decision as to the type of shunt cannot be made before surgery, tilting is not essential. By placing each arm in 90° abduction, a later change in operative strategy remains readily possible, for which an alteration in sandbag support, if used, would have to be made. Extended right or extended left subcostal incisions are required for each form of these two leading types of shunt, respectively.

Essential to all surgery in patients with portal hypertension is extreme care at all times in securing haemostasis, much of which must be done with ligation prior to division in places and planes where simple division with or without diathermy haemostasis is otherwise adequate. Reduction of blood loss to a minimum is vital to help secure a successful outcome; correction of abnormal haemostasis is sometimes necessary before, during and/or after surgery. A Sengstaken–Blakemore or Minnesota quadruple lumen tube may be kept in place throughout, and if considered necessary, for several hours after the procedure. At operation, the abdominal cavity should be completely explored; liver inspection, palpation, ultrasound and biopsy are useful in assessment, including in the identification of a hepatocellular carcinoma. Key principles of vascular surgery must be adhered to (Table 16.6); intimal damage must be minimal, anastomoses must be accomplished gently but securely with fine (5/0 prolene) everting sutures and all knots on the outside, vessels and grafts must lie naturally to minimize turbulence, and any compromise of patency must be avoided, with frequent flushes of heparinized saline throughout. Ligation of collaterals will assist towards a lastingly successful outcome, particularly the right and left gastric veins.

Drains are not placed as this would allow for persistent leakage of ascites.

Integral to formation of a narrow-diameter shunt is exposure of the anterior two-thirds of the inferior vena cava, from the renal vessels to beneath the caudate lobe, a portion of which may require resection to ensure direct angled entry of the graft from the portal vein.[27] The portal vein is exposed from the duodenum/neck of the pancreas to its bifurcation over sufficient distance to permit application of a small Satinsky clamp. Direct puncture of either vessel with a fine 23G needle connected to a pressure gauge, previously zeroed at the level of the right atrium, is used to measure the portal pressure gradient (portal venous minus inferior vena caval pressure). As mentioned previously, after shunting this gradient should be less than 12 mmHg to minimize the risk of recurrent haemorrhage; with severe portal hypertensive gradients over 20 mmHg, this is likely to require a 10 mm diameter ringed PTFE graft, rather than the more usual 8 mm graft. The graft is flushed with heparinized saline to remove air from the interstices. Satinsky clamps may then be alternately placed on each vessel, without complete occlusion, whilst allowing formation of the anastomoses. The cava is opened longitudinally anterolaterally 20–30° to the left, for up to 2 cm without excision; a right sided stay suture is useful to hold the cut open. Horizontal 5/0 prolene everting mattress sutures are used to place a bevelled graft coming into the vena cava at an angle to minimize turbulence. The anastomosis is then tested, and if necessary further sutures placed, to ensure haemostasis. The graft is again bevelled and trimmed by careful judgement to allow accurate alignment from the portal vein, over as short a length (2–4 cm) to the cava as possible, and a similar anastomotic technique with angulation to minimize turbulence again used. The posterior row can be partly placed without apposition, to allow subsequent approximation, although too long a row of sutures of this kind is difficult to tighten without tearing the vein. Once fashioned, the shunt should sit neatly and comfortably in place, and a thrill should be palpable in the cava near the caval anastomosis. The portal pressure gradient is measured again; if below 12 mmHg, this indicates a satisfactorily functioning shunt, which must otherwise be cleared with a Fogarty balloon inserted through the side wall of the shunt, or the shunt must be refashioned.

Distal splenorenal shunting requires access to the lesser sac by careful taking down of the gastroepiploic arcade and splenocolic ligament, ligation and division of the inferior mesenteric vein, and dissection of the splenic, superior mesenteric and portal veins.[28] The splenic vein is first approached posteriorly, and after mobilization of the portal vein at the neck of the pancreas, a key step is meticulously careful anterior and superior mobilization of the splenic vein from the pancreas. The splenic vein is divided proximally, with complete splenopancreatic disconnection of the distal portion, which is of proven benefit in preventing late recurrent haemorrhage in alcoholic cirrhosis. This is, however, more difficult once the vein is occluded, as it exacerbates congestion and the likelihood of bleeding during dissection. Division of the retroperitoneum to expose the left renal vein should be accompanied by ligation, to prevent chylous ascites from lymphatic leaks, and by division of the left suprarenal vein, to permit mobilization. As with all surgical shunts, the alignment of apposed venous conduits can be difficult to judge, but a Satinsky is used to partially occlude the renal vein, a longitudinal venotomy made, and the distal splenic vein trimmed and anastomosed to lie comfortably, at an angle to the renal vein, so reducing turbulence. Everting 5/0 prolene horizontal mattress sutures are recommended, which may be placed in an interrupted fashion anteriorly to prevent purse-stringing. Measurement of pressures is less useful in distal splenorenal shunting, but may be used to confirm a significant drop associated with a patent shunt.

Postoperative care

Colloid and crystalloid replacement should include 5% or 10% dextrose with minimal saline, and broad-spectrum antibiotics continued for at least 48 hours. Every effort should be made to prevent or identify and treat specific infections early. If urine output falls in the presence of adequate cardiac filling pressures, and arterial pressures are low, vasoconstrictive inotropes are unlikely to assist, as cirrhotic patients tend to run low systemic blood pressures from widespread vasodilatation, and such medication may reduce liver perfusion. A preferable alternative is the administration of 1 U/h ornipressin IV, which reduces intrarenal and intrahepatic shunting, whilst inducing modest systemic vasoconstriction; administration may be continued for several days, even though this is an unlicensed indication.[16] Improvement in renal function frequently ensues, as may occur with hepatic function, even though there had been a substantial diversion of portal blood flow. Magnesium sulphate enemas, with lactulose and neomycin via the nasogastric tube, should be continued until it is evident that any encephalopathy has resolved. Upon resumption of oral intake, sodium intake must be restricted to less than 20 mmol/day to control ascites, and fat to less than 30 g/day (for 4 weeks) to prevent chylous ascites. Attention to nutritional requirements is most important in cirrhotic patients (Table 16.6). A modest dose of a potassium-sparing diuretic is likely to be helpful after distal

splenorenal shunting, as portal vein pressure remains high despite portal–azygos disconnection.

If rebleeding occurs after surgery, endoscopic investigation should be pursued, since further endoscopic variceal therapy may be helpful. Although the uncommon event of recurrent variceal haemorrhage after a shunt is likely to indicate shunt dysfunction, patients may have sclerotherapy or banding induced ulcers, peptic ulcers or even patent but decompressed varices in the presence of functioning shunts. Nevertheless, such bleeding will hasten the need for radiological assessment.

Radiological shunt assessment is routine at 5 to 7 days after surgery; for narrow-diameter portocaval shunts, a transfemoral approach is taken, a shuntogram performed to confirm patency as well as the direction of portal vein flow and pressures across the shunt measured. If thrombosis is identified, balloon dilatation can be undertaken and thrombolysis instituted from the portal vein side for 24 hours, followed by repeat angiography. Following distal splenorenal shunting similar investigation should determine an absence of a gradient across the anastomosis, but a gradient of up to 10 mmHg between the left renal vein and cava may persist for several weeks. Portal vein flow and adequate portal–azygos disconnection should be confirmed with superior mesenteric angiography.

Follow-up

Initial follow-up should focus on recovery from surgery, some 4 to 6 weeks after discharge, or earlier if indicated. General status, liver function and the presence as well as severity of any hepatic encephalopathy should be evaluated. Sodium restriction and oral lactulose are continued; the continued input of a knowledgeable dietician will help to ensure effective nutrition. Subsequent follow-up should focus on the underlying condition, together with hepatological physicians, whilst monitoring shunt function (Table 16.6). Duplex ultrasound is a useful screening tool, whilst shuntography is recommended at one year or if there is evidence of recurrent portal hypertension. Consideration of the need and suitability for liver transplantation is made at each visit.

When should liver transplantation be considered?

The principal indications for liver transplantation in patients with chronic liver disease who present with

Table 16.7 **Indications for liver transplantation**[18,29]
• Intolerable quality of life because of liver disease
• Anticipated survival less than 1 year from liver failure
• Absence of contraindications e.g. AIDS, extrahepatic malignancy
• Detailed guidelines for specific liver diseases

complications from portal hypertension are an estimated survival (from liver disease) of less than 1 year and/or quality of life (because of liver disease) intolerable to the patient (Table 16.7).[18,29] Of all prognostic systems, the Child–Pugh grading is the most accurate in predicting survival from cirrhosis (but not liver transplantation), having been the focus of many prospective studies; the Number Connection Test is a simple bedside addition that renders assessment of hepatic encephalopathy more objective.

Patients who were Child–Pugh grade C before, or who remain grade C at least 3 weeks following recovery from variceal haemorrhage, or who remain grade C between separate inpatient admissions, are at particularly high risk of an early death.[9] Indeed, consideration may be precipitated by any complication indicative of poor hepatic reserve; this is less likely to be appropriate for Child–Pugh A or B patients. Contraindications include advanced age, unfitness from significant intercurrent disease of other systems, extrahepatic malignancy or psychological unsuitability, including ongoing alcohol abuse. The evaluation is difficult and has both objective and subjective components. In those centres without liver transplantation services, well maintained and effective dialogues with such a centre is essential.

What is the evidence base for the management strategy outlined?

The Cochrane HepatoBiliary Review Group

There have been at least 200 randomized controlled trials in the field of portal hypertension, and many more in the management of cirrhosis.[30] To attempt to provide a systematic review of all components addressed in this chapter would not be productive. Nevertheless, leading components must be highlighted, to support the overall approach. The reader is referred to the ongoing work of the Cochrane HepatoBiliary Group (CHBG), which has the objective

of conducting systematic reviews across the whole field of hepatobiliary surgery and medicine,[31] as part of the published work of the worldwide Cochrane Collaboration.[32] This is available on CD-ROM and is updated regularly. The task is so large that it is appropriate to invite contributions from all interested parties who may be able to contribute!

Prognosis

The continued primacy of Child–Pugh grading has been discussed; this is apparent from all prospective studies, and from retrospective studies. Serum creatinine is the next best independent candidate prognostic marker.[9] Quantitative tests of liver function have, as yet, not gained wide acceptance in routine use for the evaluation of patients with cirrhotic portal hypertension.

Endoscopic therapy

Endoscopic therapy has been compared to drug therapy and found to be equally or more efficacious in stopping acute variceal haemorrhage in the short term.[33] Drug therapies have unpredictable effects on hepatic haemodynamics, in many cases cannot be continued long term and, when continued long term, have been associated with higher rates of rebleeding than associated with endoscopic therapy.[34] However, significant advantages have been demonstrated for the combination of drug and endoscopic therapies, both acutely[35] and long-term.[36]

Endoscopic therapy has been compared to distal splenorenal shunts[37] and TIPSS.[38] In all comparisons there was a higher rate of rebleeding associated with endoscopic therapy, but a lower rate of new or worsened hepatic encephalopathy. Providing endoscopic therapy is expertly administered, and adjuvant pharmacological therapy is added, most centres would prefer to avoid the major intervention of a shunt as first-line therapy, whatever the type, to reduce the likelihood of hepatic encephalopathy and any accelerated deterioration in liver function.[11] However, in view of the effectiveness of shunts in controlling bleeding, the indications of two clinically significant rebleeds from oesophageal varices, one from gastric varices, or a transfusion requirement of 10 or more units of blood during a single admission, should be adhered to in the majority of cases.[11,14,15]

Partial or selective versus total shunt

Randomized trials have demonstrated selective shunts to be as effective in controlling bleeding, with recurrence rates below 5%, but to result in significantly less new or worsened hepatic encephalopathy, compared to total shunts.[39] Similarly, a randomized trial of partial versus total shunts demonstrated the same.[22] Expertly constructed shunts of principal types have long-term patency rates exceeding 90%. Thus where a surgical shunt has been chosen for treatment, the choice should be made between a partial or selective shunt; in the emergency scenario, the former is preferred. Total shunts should be avoided, because of the higher incidence of hepatic encephalopathy, that has no attendant benefit.

Surgical versus TIPS shunt

A single trial has compared narrow-diameter portocaval versus TIPS shunts.[27,40] Overall, surgical shunts resulted in significantly fewer treatment failures and were shown to maintain hepatic parenchymal perfusion more effectively. A further trial comparing distal splenorenal versus TIPSS is underway in the USA, supported by NIH funding, with recruitment over halfway (MJ Henderson, personal communication). The high rates of TIPSS stenosis and occlusion discussed above must be borne in mind when choosing between shunts, as must the status of the patient and the likelihood of future liver transplantation. Additionally, when the decision is taken by physicians managing cirrhotic patients that a shunt is required, considering the outcome of either form of shunt in dedicated hands, surgeons should not be allowed to become deskilled nor disinterested.

On whom should the management of cirrhotic portal hypertension depend?

The strategies discussed depend on a high level of expertise that must be maintained across a range of interdependent specialties. This range cannot be maintained in all acute hospitals, particularly in those countries where the incidence of cirrhosis is less than 25 per 100 000 per annum, as in most countries of the Western world. Thus it is recommended that patients with significant complications of cirrhosis and portal hypertension, particularly acute variceal haemorrhage, are referred to units specializing in their care—the earlier, the better.

Investigation of suspected cirrhotic portal hypertension

- Routine haematology and clotting.
- Full biochemistry.

- Special plasma proteins:
  α_1-antitrypsin
  Caeruloplasmin
  Transferrin.
- Copper and iron studies.
- Autoantibodies.
- Viral studies (hepatitis A, B and C).
- Liver biopsy.
- Upper and lower GI endoscopy.

Risk factors for variceal haemorrhage

- Varices greater than half radius of open oesophageal lumen.
- Red vascular markings on mucosal surface.
- Hepatic vein pressure gradient >12 mmHg.

Management pathway for acute variceal haemorrhage

Haematemesis and/or melaena with/without clinical features of liver disease

- Resuscitate and endoscope within 4 hours of admission.
- If varices identified, injection sclerotherapy and/or banding.
- Administer IV terlipressin boluses or octreotide infusion.
- Administer IV broad-spectrum antibiotics.
- If bleeding uncontrolled, Sengstaken–Blakemore tube, maximum 24 hours.

Transfer patient with variceal haemorrhage to specialist unit

- Continue vasoactive and antibiotic drugs for 5 days.
- Administer anti-liver failure regime with lactulose and $MgSO_4$ enemata.
- Second session of endoscopic therapy.
- Conversion to β-blockade prior to discharge.
- Subsequent programmed variceal obliteration.

Definition of uncontrollable or recurrent variceal haemorrhage

- On same admission defined by fall in systolic BP of 20 mmHg or <100 mmHg.
- On same admission defined by rise in pulse of 20/min or >100/min.
- On same admission defined by fall in Hb by 2 g/dl or need for >2 units in 6 h.

- On subsequent admission defined by further haematemesis/melaena.
- If subsequent admission requires repeat endoscopy again within 4 hours.

Management of uncontrollable or recurrent variceal haemorrhage

- Passage of Sengstaken–Blakemore tube.
- Maximum vasoactive medication.
- Repeat endoscopic therapy if 2 or more days since last attempted.
- Radiological or surgical shunting if 2 or more oesophageal variceal rebleeds.
- Radiological or surgical shunting if 1 or more gastric variceal rebleeds.

Criteria for partial or selective surgical shunt

- Child–Pugh grade A or B status, less likely to be considered for liver transplant.
- Recurrent oesophageal variceal bleeding despite endoscopic treatment.
- Early gastric variceal rebleeding despite endoscopic treatment.
- Transfusion requirement of 10 or more units of blood.
- Both short-term and long-term control of bleeding important objectives.

Criteria for TIPS radiological shunt

- Child–Pugh grade C status, less liver reserve, potential liver transplant candidate.

- Recurrent oesophageal variceal bleeding despite endoscopic treatment.
- Early gastric variceal rebleeding despite endoscopic treatment.
- Transfusion requirement of 10 or more units of blood.
- Short-term control of greater importance than long-term control.

Criteria for subsequent liver transplant

- Child–Pugh grade C status.
- Estimated survival <1 year.
- Poor quality of life.
- Suitable age group (<70) with absence of major intercurrent disease.
- Psychological suitability without ongoing alcohol abuse.

Key points

- Management of portal hypertension should be in specialist units.
- Early endoscopy and endoscopic therapy should follow resuscitation.
- Vasoactive drugs, antibiotics and anti-liver failure treatment mandatory.
- Balloon tamponade, then surgical or radiological shunt for failure of endoscopic treatment.
- Careful assessment for liver transplantation.

REFERENCES

1. Sprenger H, Kaufmann A, Garn H, Lahme B, Gemsa D, Gressner AM. Induction of neutrophil-attracting chemokines in transforming rat hepatic stellate cells. Gastroenterology 1997; 113: 277–85
2. Friedman SL. Cytokines and fibrogenesis. Semin Liver Dis 1999; 19: 129–40
3. Goddard CJ, Smith A, Hoyland JA et al. Localisation and semiquantitative assessment of hepatic procollagen mRNA in primary biliary cirrhosis. Gut 1998; 43: 433–40
4. Farzaneh-Far R, Moore K. Nitric oxide and the liver. Liver 2000; 21: 161–74
5. Lebrec D, Morequ R. Pathogenesis of portal hypertension. Eur J Gastroenterol Hepatol 2001; 13: 309–11
6. Groszmann RJ. Hyperdynamic state in chronic liver diseases. J Hepatol 1993; 17 (Suppl 2): S38–40
7. Feu F, Garcia-Pagan JC, Bosch J et al. Relation between portal pressure response to pharmacotherapy and risk of recurrent variceal haemorrhage in patients with cirrhosis. Lancet 1995; 346: 1056–9
8. Trey C, Burns DG, Saunders SJ. Treatment of hepatic coma by exchange blood transfusion. N Engl J Med 1966; 274: 473–81
9. Khan S, Jenkins SA, Williamson P et al. Long-term prognostic study of prognostic factors in cirrhotic portal hypertension. Gut 1999; 44 (Suppl 1): A56
10. North Italian Endoscopic Club. Prediction of the first variceal hemorrhage in patients with cirrhosis of the liver and esophageal varices. A prospective multicentre study. N Engl J Med 1988; 319: 983–9
11. Sutton R, Shields R. The place of portal-systemic shunting. In: Blumgart LH, ed. Surgery of the liver and biliary

tract, 2nd edn. London: Churchill Livingstone, 1994

12. Boyer TD. Pharmacologic treatment of portal hypertension: past, present and future. Hepatology 2001; 34: 834–9

13. Bernard B, Grange JD, Khac EN, Amiot X, Opolon P, Poynard T. Antibiotic prophylaxis for the prevention of bacterial infections in cirrhotic patients with gastrointestinal bleeding: a meta-analysis. Hepatology 1999; 29: 1655–61

14. McCormack G, McCormick PA. A practical guide to the management of oesophageal varices. Drugs 1999; 57: 327–35

15. de Franchis R, Pascal JP, Ancona E et al. Definitions, methodology and therapeutic strategies in portal hypertension. A Consensus Development Workshop, Baveno, Lake Maggiore, Italy, 5–6 April 1990. J Hepatol 1992; 15: 256–61

16. Guevara M, Gines P, Fernandez-Esparrach G et al. Reversibility of hepatorenal syndrome by prolonged administration of ornipressin and plasma volume expansion. Hepatology 1998; 27: 35–41

17. Rodes J. Intractable ascites management: the role of side-to-side portacaval shunt. HPB Surg 1999; 11: 200–4

18. Neuberger J, James O. Guidelines for selection of patients for liver transplantation in the era of donor-organ shortage. Lancet 1999; 354: 1636–9

19. Warren WD, Zeppa R, Fomon JJ. Selective trans-splenic decompression of gastroesophageal varices by distal splenorenal shunt. Ann Surg 1967; 166: 437–55

20. Sarfeh IJ, Rypins EB, Mason GR. A systematic appraisal of portacaval H-graft diameters. Clinical and hemo-dynamic perspectives. Ann Surg 1986; 204: 356–63

21. Adam R, Diamond T, Bismuth H. Partial portacaval shunt: renaissance of an old concept. Surgery 1992; 111: 610–6

22. Sarfeh IJ, Rypins EB. Partial versus total portacaval shunt in alcoholic cirrhosis. Results of a prospective, randomized clinical trial. Ann Surg 1994; 219: 353–61

23. Rikkers LF, Jin G. Surgical management of acute variceal hemorrhage. World J Surg 1994; 18: 193–9

24. Zemel G, Katzen BT, Becker GJ, Benenati JF, Sallee DS. Percutaneous transjugular portosystemic shunt. J Am Med Assoc 1991; 266: 390–3

25. Rossle M, Siegerstetter V, Huber M, Ochs A. The first decade of the transjugular intrahepatic portosystemic shunt (TIPS): state of the art. Liver 1998; 18: 73–89

26. Casado M, Bosch J, Garcia-Pagan JC et al. Clinical events after transjugular intrahepatic portosystemic shunt: correlation with hemodynamic findings. Gastroenterology 1998; 114: 1296–303

27. Rosemurgy AS, Goode SE, Zwiebel BR, Black TJ, Brady PG. A prospective trial of transjugular intrahepatic portasystemic stent shunt versus small-diameter prosthetic H-graft portacaval shunts in the treatment of bleeding varices. Ann Surg 1996; 224: 378–84

28. Henderson JM. Distal splenorenal shunt. In: Blumgart LH, ed. Surgery of the liver and biliary tract, 2nd edn. London: Churchill Livingstone, 1994

29. British Society of Gastroenterology. Indications for referral and assessment in adult liver transplantation: a clinical guideline. Gut 1999; 45 (Suppl 6) VI1–VI22

30. Kjaergard LL, Nikolova D, Gluud C. Randomised clinical trials in HEPATOLOGY: predictors of quality. Hepatology 1999; 30: 1134–8

31. Gluud C, Jorgensen T, Morabito A, Pagliaro L, Poynard T, Sutton R. The Cochrane Hepatobiliary Group. In: Bircher J, Benhamou J-P, McIntyre N, Rizzetto M, Rodes J, eds. Oxford textbook of clinical hepatology, 2nd edn. Oxford: Oxford University Press, 1999

32. Cochrane Collaboration. Cochrane Library. Issue 4. Oxford: Update Software, 1999

33. Jenkins SA, Shields R, Davies M et al. A multicentre randomised trial comparing octreotide and injection sclerotherapy in the management and outcome of acute variceal haemorrhage. Gut 1997; 41: 526–33

34. Teres J, Bosch J, Bordas JM et al. Propranolol versus sclerotherapy in preventing variceal rebleeding: a randomized controlled trial. Gastroenterology 1993; 105(5): 1508–14

35. Avgerinos A, Nevens F, Raptis S, Fevery J. Early administration of somatostatin and efficacy of sclerotherapy in acute oesophageal variceal bleeds: the European Acute Bleeding Oesophageal Variceal Episodes (ABOVE) randomised trial. Lancet 1997; 350(9090): 1495–9

36. Jenkins SA, Baxter JN, Critchley M et al. Randomised trial of octreotide in the long-term management of cirrhotic patients after variceal haemorrhage. Br Med J 1997; 315: 1338–42

37. Spina GP, Henderson JM, Rikkers LF et al. Distal spleno-renal shunt versus endoscopic sclerotherapy in the prevention of variceal rebleeding. A meta-analysis of 4 randomized clinical trials. J Hepatol 1992; 16: 338–45

38. Papatheodoridis GV, Goulis J, Leandro G, Patch D, Burroughs AK. Transjugular intrahepatic portosystemic shunt compared with endoscopic treatment for prevention of variceal rebleeding: a meta-analysis. Hepatology 1999; 30: 612–22

39. Langer B, Taylor BR, Mackenzie DR, Gilas T, Stone RM, Blendis L. Further report of a prospective randomized trial comparing distal splenorenal shunt with end-to-side portacaval shunt. An analysis of encephalopathy, survival, and quality of life. Gastroenterology 1985; 88: 424–9

40. Rosemurgy AS, Serafini M, Zweibel BR et al. Transjugular intrahepatic portosystemic shunt vs. small diameter prosthetic H-graft portacaval shunt; extended follow-up of an expanded randomized prospective trial. J Gastrointest Surg 2000; 4: 589–97

17 Management of hilar cholangiocarcinoma

Pierre F Saldinger, William R Jarnagin and Leslie H Blumgart

Introduction

Hilar cholangiocarcinoma remains a challenging disease for both doctor and patient. Of all tumors arising in the biliary tree it is the most difficult to manage. The majority of patients will die within 6 months to a year of diagnosis if not treated; death is usually related to local tumor spread and the effects of biliary obstruction and cholangitis leading to liver failure.[1,2]

The purpose of this chapter is to define a systematic approach to diagnosis, work-up and treatment of hilar cholangiocarcinoma based on the following premises:

1. Preoperative diagnosis of cholangiocarcinoma is almost always possible without the need for tissue diagnosis. The possibility of a benign localized stricture mimicking a malignant one has to be considered.[3]
2. Preoperative imaging including magnetic resonance cholangiopancreatography (MRCP) and duplex sonography provides an excellent guide to the extent of the tumor and its resectability.[4,5]

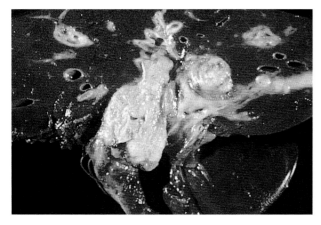

Figure 17.1 Specimen after extended left hepatectomy and caudate lobectomy for papillary cholangiocarcinoma. Note the intraductal growth pattern of the tumor.

3. Invasive studies such as angiography and cholangiography (percutaneous or endoscopic) should be used in selected cases and not as routine investigations.
4. Resection with negative margins is the goal of every exploration. This can be accomplished with a low mortality and gives excellent relief of symptoms and long-term survival.[4,5]

In a more recent analysis of 225 patients with hilar cholangiocarcinoma, the authors found the proposed T-staging (see Table 17.3) to correlate with resectability and survival (see Table 17.4).

Pathology

Hilar cholangiocarcinoma is a primary adenocarcinoma of the extrahepatic biliary system located within the confluence of the hepatic ducts or arising from the common hepatic duct and extending to the confluence.

Special characteristics of cholangiocarcinoma include invasive spread with neural, perineural and lymphatic involvement. Recognition of the well-described subepithelial spread of tumor cells[6] is of special surgical importance in obtaining a tumor-free margin. In 1957, Sako first introduced the idea of classifying cholangiocarcinoma based on macroscopic appearance.[7] There are three morphologically distinct types of bile duct cancer: nodular-sclerosing, papillary and diffuse. Nodular-sclerosing cholangiocarcinoma is the most common and represents approximately 70% of all bile duct cancers whereas papillary cholangiocarcinoma is less common and represents about 25%. The papillary variant appears to be more common in the lower bile duct. The diffuse type remains quite rare.[6] Papillary cholangiocarcinoma (Fig. 17.1), which grows within the lumen of the bile duct, has a better prognosis than the other types.[8]

Presentation and symptoms

Most patients with hilar cholangiocarcinoma present with obstructive jaundice. However, jaundice may not be present in some cases where there is incomplete biliary obstruction (i.e. right or left hepatic duct) or segmental biliary obstruction. Segmental obstruction may go unrecognized for months, resulting in ipsilateral lobar atrophy without overt jaundice. These patients will usually be diagnosed secondary to an elevated alkaline phosphatase found during routine examination.

Infection

Bacterial contamination of the bile (bacterbilia) is relatively common in patients with hilar cholangiocarcinoma.[9] However, in the absence of prior biliary intubation, frank cholangitis is uncommon at initial presentation. Endoscopic or percutaneous instrumentation as well as previous operation significantly increase the incidence of bacterial contamination and the risk of infection. Bacterial contamination of the biliary tract in partial obstruction is not always clinically apparent. The presence of overt or subclinical infection at the time of surgery is a major source of postoperative morbidity and mortality. *Escherichia coli, Klebsiella* and *Enterococcus* are the most common pathogens identified. However, this spectrum of organisms may change after endoscopic or percutaneous intubation, both of which are associated with greater morbidity and mortality following surgical resection or palliative bypass for hilar cholangiocarcinoma. We have analyzed 71 patients who underwent either a curative resection or palliative biliary bypass for proximal cholangiocarcinoma.

All patients who were stented endoscopically and 62% of the patients who were stented percutaneously had bacterobilia. Postoperative infectious complications were increased two-fold in those patients stented before surgery compared to non-stented patients. Non-infectious complications were equal in both groups.[10] *Enterococcus, Klebsiella, Streptococcus viridans* and *Enterobacter aerogenes* were the most common organisms isolated from intraoperative bile cultures. This spectrum of bacteria must be considered when administrating perioperative antibiotics. It is imperative to take intraoperative bile specimens for culture in order to adjust the antibiotics postoperatively.

Atrophy

Portal venous inflow and bile flow are important in maintenance of liver cell size and mass.[11] Segmental or lobar atrophy may result from a portal venous occlusion or biliary obstruction. Either or both of these findings are often present in patients with hilar cholangiocarcinoma and arise through a gradual process of involvement of the lobar hepatic ducts and portal vessels. Longstanding biliary obstruction may cause moderate atrophy while concomitant portal venous compromise results in rapid and severe atrophy of the involved segments. Appreciation of gross atrophy on preoperative imaging is important since it often influences therapy.[11] We consider atrophy to be present if cross-sectional imaging demonstrates a small, often hypoperfused lobe (Fig. 17.2) with crowding of the dilated intrahepatic ducts (Fig. 17.3). Tumor involvement of the portal vein is usually present if there is compression/narrowing, encasement or occlusion seen on imaging studies.

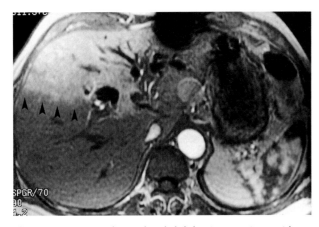

Figure 17.2 MRI of atrophic left lobe in a patient with hilar cholangiocarcinoma and obstructed left portal vein. Note the demarcation of the parenchyma between the normal right lobe and the atrophic left lobe (arrowheads).

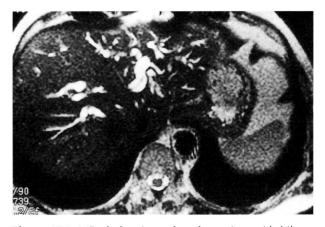

Figure 17.3 MR cholangiography of a patient with hilar cholangiocarcinoma and left lobe atrophy. Note the close proximity of the bile ducts in the atrophic left lobe compared to the right lobe.

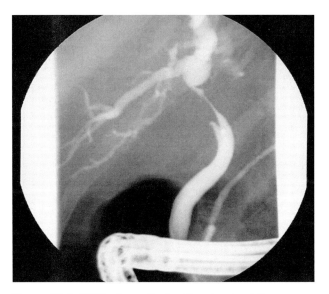

Figure 17.4 ERCP of a patient with a benign hilar stricture mimicking a hilar cholangiocarcinoma. Also known as malignant masquerade.

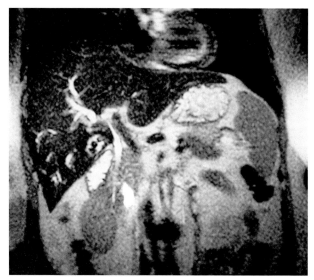

Figure 17.5 MR cholangiography of the same patient as in Fig. 17.4. Again, there is a benign stricture with malignant appearance. Perifocal inflammation is seen, suggestive of a mass.

Diagnosis

The diagnosis of hilar cholangiocarcinoma is usually made on evaluation of obstructive jaundice or elevated liver enzymes. Most patients are referred after having had some studies done elsewhere, usually a computed tomography (CT) scan and some form of direct cholangiography (percutaneous transhepatic cholangiography (PTC) or ERCP). These studies are often inadequate for full assessment of the tumor extent. We have found that the combination of duplex ultrasound and magnetic resonance cholangiopancreatography (MRCP) provides significantly more information than any other combination of studies. Many patients will have been surgically explored prior to referral, often without reaching a definitive diagnosis.[12] In our view, histologic confirmation of malignancy is not mandatory prior to exploration. The vast majority of hilar strictures are the result of cholangiocarcinoma. Alternative diagnoses (gallbladder carcinoma, benign strictures) are possible; however, these are best assessed and treated at operation (resection or bypass).

Distinguishing hilar cholangiocarcinoma from a gallbladder carcinoma may be difficult. Tumor infiltrating segment IV and the right liver is frequently seen in gallbladder cancer but is less common with cholangiocarcinoma. In addition, selective involvement of the segment V duct and the common hepatic duct is highly suggestive of gallbladder carcinoma. Differentiating the diffuse form of cholangiocarcinoma and sclerosing cholangitis represents another potential diagnostic dilemma.

Although uncommon, localized strictures of the biliary confluence may be of benign origin. Histologic examination of these strictures reveals a benign sclerosing pattern originally reported by us[3] and subsequently by others.[13,14] This diagnosis usually cannot be made without radical resection of the lesion. While certain radiographic features might suggest a benign stricture, cholangiocarcinoma must remain the leading diagnosis until definitively disproven (Figs 17.4 and 17.5). Excessive reliance on percutaneous needle biopsy or biliary brush cytology is dangerous, since they are often misleading and one may miss the opportunity to resect an early cholangiocarcinoma. We firmly believe that all suspicious hilar lesions, especially in the absence of portal vein involvement and/or lobar atrophy, should be considered for resection. Palliative biliary intubation should be reserved for patients unfit for surgery or those with clearly irresectable disease. Likewise, radiation therapy and chemotherapy should be used only in cases where surgery is not feasible and a diagnosis of malignancy has been unambiguously established.

Duplex sonography

Ultrasonography is a non-invasive but operator dependent study that often precisely delineates tumor extent. Ultrasonography may not only demonstrate the level of biliary ductal obstruction but can also provide information regarding tumor extension within the bile duct and in the periductal tissues

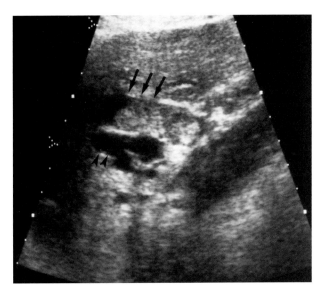

Figure 17.6 Ultrasound of a patient with a papillary cholangiocarcinoma growing down the common hepatic duct (black arrows). The portal vein is seen behind the bile duct (black arrowheads).

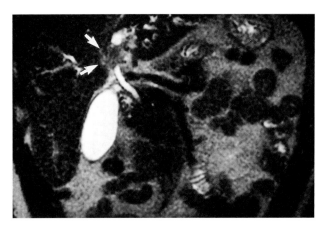

Figure 17.7 MR cholangiography of a patient with a hilar cholangiocarcinoma obstructing the left duct. In addition to the biliary anatomy the MRCP offers information on tumor extension (arrows).

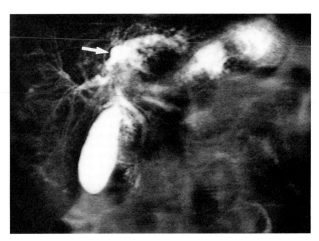

Figure 17.8 Three-dimensional reconstruction of the MR cholangiogram seen in Fig. 17.7. The dilated left bile duct (arrow) is seen as well as the normal sized right bile ducts.

(Fig. 17.6).[15–17] Duplex ultrasonography is firmly established as a highly accurate predictor of vascular involvement and resectability. In a series of 19 consecutive patients with malignant hilar obstruction, ultrasonography with color spectral Doppler technique was equivalent to angiography and CT portography in diagnosing lobar atrophy, level of biliary obstruction, hepatic parenchymal involvement, and venous invasion.[18] Duplex ultrasonography is particularly useful for assessing portal venous invasion. In a series of 63 consecutive patients from MSKCC, duplex ultrasonography predicted portal vein involvement in 93% of the cases with a specificity of 99% and a 97% positive predictive value. In the same series angiography with CT angioportograpy had a 90% sensitivity, 99% specificity and a 95% positive predictive value.[19]

Magnetic resonance cholangiopancreatography (MRCP)

In our practice MRCP has almost replaced endoscopic and percutaneous cholangiography for the preoperative assessment of hilar cholangiocarcinoma. Several studies have demonstrated its utility in evaluating patients with biliary obstruction.[20–23] MRCP may not only identify the tumor and the level of biliary obstruction but may also reveal obstructed and isolated ducts not appreciated at endoscopic or percutaneous study (Figs 17.7 and

17.8). Furthermore, unlike other modalities, MRCP does not require biliary intubation. Potential infectious complications, which may increase operative morbidity, are thus avoided.[24]

Staging and assessment for resectability

While it has been recognized that hilar cholangiocarcinomata are small and apparently well localized, few authors have remarked on the relationship between adjacent vascular involvement and the extent of spread along the bile ducts into the hepatic parenchyma. These factors may compromise complete excision of the tumor unless partial hepatectomy is performed, occasionally with reconstruction

Table 17.1 **Criteria for irresectability**

- Hepatic duct involvement up to secondary radicles bilaterally
- Encasement or occlusion of the main portal vein proximal to its bifurcation
- Atrophy of one liver lobe with encasement of contralateral portal vein branch
- Atrophy of one liver lobe with contralateral secondary biliary radicle involvement
- Metastatic disease to liver or lung

Table 17.2 **Current AJCC primary tumor stage (T stage)**

Tx   Primary tumor cannot be assessed
T0   No evidence of primary tumor
Tis Carcinoma in situ
T1   Tumor invades the mucosa (T1a) or muscle layer (T1b)
T2   Tumor invades the perimuscular connective tissue
T3   Tumor invades adjacent structures: liver, pancreas, duodenum, gallbladder, colon, stomach
N0   No nodal involvement
N1   Metastases to periductal, cystic duct and/or hilar lymph nodes
N2   Metastases to periportal, periduodenal, or retroperitoneal nodes
M1   Distant metastases

Stage groupings

Stage	T	N	M
Stage 0	Tis	N0	M0
Stage I	T1	N0	M0
Stage II	T2	N0	M0
Stage III	T1–2	N1–2	M0
Stage IVA	T3	AnyN	M0
Stage IVB	AnyT	AnyN	M1

of the blood supply to the liver remnant. Adequate intraoperative assessment of vascular involvement requires extensive hilar dissection and may be technically difficult, especially if there has been prior biliary intervention. Therefore, an approach aimed at full radiological diagnosis has been made, leading to a synthesis of all the available preoperative data. This allows preoperative staging and decision as to whether the patient is a potential candidate for curative resection. Previously, longitudinal ductal tumor extension has been assessed by either endoscopic retrograde cholangiopancreatography (ERCP) or percutaneous transhepatic cholangiography (PTC). Hepatic angiography with late phase portography combined with CT portography was previously used by us and others to assess radial spread of the tumor.[12] At MSKCC, we favor duplex ultrasound and MRCP to stage patients before surgery.[17,18,25] The radiological criteria used to define irresectability are listed in Table 17.1.

Currently, there is no clinical staging system available that stratifies patients preoperatively into subgroups based on potential for resection. The modified Bismuth–Corlette classification stratifies patients based on the extent of biliary duct involvement by tumor.[26] Although useful to some extent it is not indicative of resectability or survival. The current AJCC T stage system (Table 17.2) is based largely on pathological criteria and has little applicability for preoperative staging. The ideal staging system should accurately predict resectability, the need for hepatic resection and correlate with survival. Such a system would assist the surgeon in formulating a treatment plan and help the patient understand the treatment options and outcome.

We have proposed a preoperative staging system using preoperative imaging, taking into account the extent of biliary ductal involvement, vascular involvement and lobar atrophy.[4,5] This T staging system is based on the extent of local disease irrespective of N or M status (Table 17.3).

Table 17.3 **Modified preoperative T staging for cholangiocarcinoma (after Burke et al.[4,5])**

T1 Tumor confined to confluence and/or right or left hepatic duct without vascular involvement

T2 Tumor confined to confluence and/or right or left hepatic duct with ipsilateral liver atrophy. No vascular involvement demonstrated

T3 Tumor confined to confluence and/or right or left hepatic duct with ipsilateral portal venous branch involvement with/without associated ipsilateral lobar atrophy. No main portal vein involvement (occlusion, invasion or encasement)

T4 Either of the following:
Tumor involving both right and left hepatic ducts up to secondary radicles bilaterally
Main portal vein encasement

We have compared this system to the AJCC classification in a series of 87 patients with cholangiocarcinoma. There was no correlation between stage and resectability or median survival using the AJCC system (Table 17.4). In the proposed staging system, resectability was highest in the T1 group (48%), and decreased progressively to 0 in the T4 group

Table 17.4 **Resectability and median survival in patients with hilar cholangiocarcinoma staged according to AJCC criteria**

Stage	N	Curative resection (%)	Median survival (months)
I	0	—	—
II	68	34	16
III	0	—	—
IV a	11	73	46
IV b	8	0	9
Total	87		

Table 17.5 **Percentage of patients able to undergo curative resection and requiring hepatectomy stratified by proposed T staging criteria (after Burke et al.[4,5])**

T stage	N	Resected N (%)	Hepatectomy N (%)
1	40	19 (48)	11 (58)
2	7	3 (43)	3 (100)
3	32	8 (25)	8 (100)
4	8	0	0
Total	87	30 (35)	22 (73)

Table 17.6 **Percentage of patients with distant or nodal metastases found on preoperative scan or at operation and survival stratified by proposed T stage (after Burke et al.[4,5])**

T stage	N	Metastases N (%)	Median survival (months)	5-year survival (%)
1	40	12 (30)	21 ± 3	20
2	7	1 (14)	35 ± 21	29
3	32	17 (52)	10 ± 2	16
4	8	1 (13)	14 ± 12	0
Total	87			

(irresectable due to extent of local disease). The percentage of patients requiring partial hepatectomy for complete resection also increased with T stage (Table 17.5). The proposed staging system does not consider the presence of nodal or distant metastases, nevertheless the incidence of these findings on preoperative imaging and at laparotomy increased with increasing T stage (Table 17.6).

Portal vein involvement was the only independent predictor of resectability while portal vein involvement, hepatic lobar atrophy and hepatic ductal extension were independent predictors of the need for hepatectomy.[4,5] In this context the importance of portal vein involvement and liver atrophy in relation to the extent of ductal cancer spread becomes evident. Thus ipsilateral involvement of vessels and bile ducts is usually amenable to resection while contralateral involvement is not.

These results emphasize the need for a more reliable preoperative system for selecting patients who are candidates for a potentially curative resection. The role of laparoscopy in the staging of cholangiocarcinoma remains to be defined. A recent study which examined the role of laparoscopy combined with laparoscopic ultrasound in a mixture of hepatobiliary and pancreatic malignancies detected radiological occult metastases in 30% of the patients.[27] However, there was no mention of the number of patients with hilar cholangiocarcinoma. Hilar cholangiocarcinoma is often considered slow to metastasize. In our experience, however, many patients have radiographically occult peritoneal or nodal metastases. Preoperative imaging predicts irresectability based on local extension but is poor for assessing nodal or peritoneal metastases. In our recent series, 23 of 39 patients irresectable at laparotomy were found to have metastatic disease. Fourteen had gross metastatic disease to periportal or retroperitoneal lymph nodes (Table 17.7). CT scan only indicated lymphadenopathy in four of these patients. Nine patients had unsuspected metastatic disease found on exploration: four had omental and/or peritoneal metastases, three had liver metastases, and two had both liver and peritoneal disease.[4,5] Further studies will define whether laparoscopy contributes to diagnosis in some such patients without the need for laparotomy.

Treatment options

There are two objectives in the therapy of hilar cholangiocarcinoma: complete tumor excision with negative margins if possible, and restoration of biliary–enteric continuity. Patients should be fully evaluated for possible curative resection before any

Table 17.7 Summary of factors precluding a curative resection in patients at initial evaluation or at exploratory laparotomy

Group	N	Local extension	Nodal metastases	Distant metastases	Other[a]
Unresectable at presentation	21	9	0	8	4
Unresectable at laparotomy	39	8	14	9	8
Total	60	17 (28%)	14 (23%)	17 (28%)	12(20%)

[a] Age, comorbidity, sepsis.

intervention is performed, since stent-associated infection and inflammation renders assessment and exploration difficult. If resection is clearly not feasible, then transtumoral drainage or paratumoral surgical bypass offer satisfactory palliation and could be combined with radiotherapy (vide infra).

Orthotopic liver transplantation has been attempted for unresectable hilar tumors. Klempnauer and colleagues reported four long-term survivors out of 32 patients submitted to transplantation for hilar cholangiocarcinoma.[28] The same group also reported a 17.1% 5-year survival for their overall transplant group.[29] Presently most centers do not perform liver transplantation for cholangiocarcinoma. The high incidence of lymph node metastases is of concern and larger series taking this into account with long term follow-up will be required before liver transplantation can be recommended for unresectable disease.[30]

Resection

The goal of any surgical exploration in patients with hilar cholangiocarcinoma is to perform a complete resection with intent to cure. Our criterion for curative resection is an R0 resection (negative margins and no residual tumor). However, this definition is not applied as stringently by all investigators and reported results are often not comparable.

We have performed an analysis of patients treated during a 20-year period under the direction of one surgeon (LHB) using precise preoperative assessment and patient selection, allowing an aggressive approach to resection with the intent to cure.[8] From 1977 to 1985, of the 131 patients who were assessed, 27 were resected with curative intent. Local bile duct excision was performed in 11 patients while 16 underwent a bile duct excision combined with hepatectomy. Twelve (44%) who underwent resection had positive margins. The perioperative mortality was 7.4%. The median survival after resection was 22 months.[31]

In the period from 1986 to 1990, 29 of 41 patients assessed were explored for possible curative resection. Eight of these patients were found to have unresectable disease and underwent a biliary–enteric bypass. A local tumor excision was performed in 12 patients and concomitant hepatic resection in nine. Seven patients (33%) had positive margins after resection. Operative mortality was 5%. The median survival for resected patients was 36 months (range 10–58 months).[32]

More recently, at MSKCC, 90 patients with hilar cholangiocarcinoma were assessed over a 5-year period (1992–97). Sixty-nine patients were explored for possible resection and 30 were resected. Thirty-nine of these patients were found to be unresectable at laparotomy. Local tumor resection was performed in eight patients and bile duct/tumor excision with concomitant hepatic resection in 22 patients. Four patients (17%) had positive margins after resection. The perioperative mortality was 6%. The median survival for all resected patients was 40 months. Histologically positive margins significantly shortened survival (22 months). On the other hand, median survival in patients with negative margins was greater than 60 months. The 5-year survival for the latter group was 56 months.[4,5] The summary of this analysis is shown in Table 17.8 and reflects the current trend in the state-of-the-art treatment of hilar cholangiocarcinoma. Comparing the results from these three time periods, there is a progressive increase in the percentage of R0 resections and partial hepatectomy. We firmly believe that these two factors are intimately related and are responsible for the improved survival.

Table 17.8 Summary of experience with the treatment of 269 patients with hilar cholangiocarcinoma over 20 years

	1977–1985	1986–1990	1991–1997
Reference	30	31	4
Patients evaluated	131	48	90
Patients resected	27	21	30
Negative margin	15 (56%)	14 (67%)	25 (83%)
Hepatectomy	16 (60%)	9 (43%)	22 (73%)
Operative mortality	7.4%	5%	6%
Median survival	25 months	36 months	40 months
5-year survival	22%	NA	56%

NA, not available.

Concomitant hepatectomy including caudate lobectomy[33] is often necessary to achieve negative margins. Indeed, several recent studies show a parallel between the number of patients undergoing partial hepatectomy and negative margins (Table 17.9). We perform caudate resection in all cases with suggested tumor extension into the caudate lobe. The principal caudate lobe duct drains into the left hepatic duct. Tumors extending into the left hepatic duct almost always involve the caudate duct and usually require caudate resection.[34] A dilated caudate duct, suggesting tumor involvement, may occasionally be visualized on preoperative imaging (Fig. 17.9). In some cases intraoperative frozen section of the caudate duct margin may help the decision to proceed to caudate resection. The importance of negative resection margins for long-term survival is confirmed by the results of our study.[4,5] Of the 90 patients evaluated for resection, 69 underwent exploration and 30 had a potentially curative resection (removal of all gross disease), 22 (73%) of which required partial hepatectomy. Of these 30 patients, 25 (83%) had a negative histologic margins

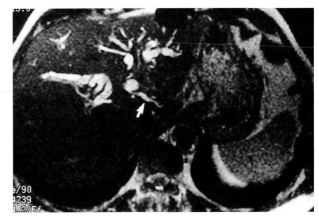

Figure 17.9 MR cholangiography showing a dilated caudate duct (arrow) in a patient with hilar cholangiocarcinoma extending into the left duct.

(R0) and a significantly better survival than patients with positive margins (Table 17.10). It is of interest that in this resected group 15 patients had involvement of secondary biliary radicles by tumor, 11 had

Table 17.9 Influence of partial hepatectomy on histological margins in patients who underwent a potentially curative resection for hilar cholangiocarcinoma: summary of recent studies

Author	Potential curative resection (N)	Hepatectomy (%)	Negative margins (%)
Cameron et al[64]	39	20	15
Hadjis et al[31]	27	60	56
Klempnauer et al[28]	147	79	79
Burke et al[4,5]	30	73	83
Nimura et al[33]	55	98	83

Table 17.10 **Influence of histologic margins on survival (from Burke et al.[4,5])**

Resection	N	Hepatic resection (%)	30-day mortality (%)	Median survival (months)	5-year survival (%)
PCR[a]	30	22 (73)	2 (6)	40 ± 10	45
Negative margins	25	20 (80)	2 (6)	not reached	56
Positive margins	5	2 (40)	0 (0)	22 ± 10[b]	0

[a] Potentially curative resection.
[b] $P \leq 0.01$.

unilateral lobar liver atrophy and eight had encasement or occlusion of a major portal vein branch. All these features are considered ominous signs of irresectability. There can be no doubt that a negative margin (R0) is necessary to call a resection 'potentially' curative.

Technique

Invasion of the main portal vein or its branches by tumor is a major determinant of resectability. Such vascular involvement may be documented on preoperative duplex sonography or MRCP. The preoperative analysis of vascular involvement and ductal extension of tumor is an essential part of operative planning and gives valuable information to the surgeon with respect to the extent of operation and operative strategy. Several technical steps during the exploration and the resection of hilar cholangiocarcinoma are crucial to the success of the operation.[35-37] Local resection for small tumors not extending beyond second order intrahepatic bile ducts and not involving the major vessels may be possible. In this situation, resection must include removal of the entire supraduodenal bile duct, gallbladder, cystic duct, and extrahepatic hepatic ducts, together with clearance of the supraduodenal tissues including the related lymph nodes. In most patients, however, there is intrahepatic extension of the tumor, and right or left portal vein involvement or both. In these cases, en bloc liver resection, often with caudate lobectomy, is necessary to achieve tumor clearance. This can only be done if intraoperative assessment shows that a tumor-free remnant with intact biliary drainage and blood supply can be left in situ.

Hepatic resection can be limited to removal of segments IV and V including the caudate lobe.[33] This technique allows resection of some centrally located tumors while preserving a substantial amount of liver tissue. In our experience this is not often applicable since many patients have a degree of lobar atrophy warranting extended resection.[4,5]

The general preparation for surgery includes suitable intraoperative monitoring and the possibility for rapid transfusion. The patient's central venous pressure is kept below 5 mmHg during the operation so as to keep blood loss low during retrohepatic dissection, dissection of the hepatic veins and parenchymal transection.[38] The patient is positioned in 15° Trendelenburg in order to avoid air embolism.

The following description emphasizes the initial steps of dissection, the initial stages of exposure of the hilar structures, their dissection, en bloc liver resection and subsequent biliary–enteric reconstruction. The specifics of caudate lobectomy are discussed in Chapter 3.

Incision and exploration

The abdomen is entered through a bilateral subcostal incision with proximal extension to the xiphoid if necessary. Careful bimanual palpation of the liver is performed to rule out unsuspected masses in the liver. Palpation of the caudate lobe is performed after incision of the lesser omentum, allowing access to the lesser sac. A Kocher maneuver is performed to allow access to the retroduodenal lymph nodes. The ligamentum teres is elevated exposing the undersurface of the liver and allowing thorough examination of the subhilar and retroduodenal area. Precise assessment of tumor extension and biopsy of any suspicious lesions or lymph nodes with frozen section analysis should be performed. Evidence of multicentricity within the liver, intrahepatic metastases, spread to distant sites or N2 level lymph nodes precludes resection. With any of these findings, the patient should be considered for appropriate biliary–enteric bypass.

Excision of the bile duct and partial hepatectomy

In order to reach the confluence of the bile ducts and assess its relation to the portal vein, the common bile duct must first be transected above the duodenum and turned upwards (Fig. 17.10).[35] The liver hilum is then fully exposed anteriorly by lowering the hilar plate after incision of Glisson's capsule along the base of segment IV. Exposure may be improved by dividing the bridge of liver tissue between the base of segment IV and the left lateral segment (Fig. 17.11). A plane can easily be developed between the posterior aspect of the bile duct tumor and the portal vein, provided there is no tumor invasion into the vessels. The gallbladder is also mobilized so that the entire extrahepatic biliary apparatus is turned forward and upwards (Figs 17.12 and 17.13).

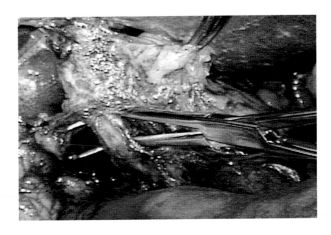

Figure 17.10 Dissected distal common bile duct displayed by the right angle clamp. The next step involves transection of the duct and oversewing of the stump on the duodenal side. The other end is secured by stay sutures and elevated so as to allow access to the portal vein. A rim of tissue is sent for frozen section to confirm tumor clearance.

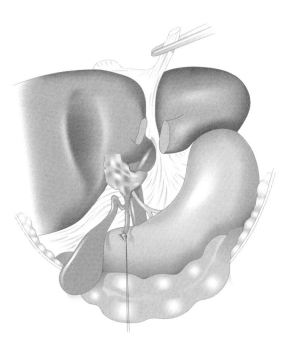

Figure 17.11 The bridge of liver tissue at the base of the umbilical fissure has been divided. This is readily done by fracturing it between finger and thumb or by dividing it with diathermy. The gallbladder has been mobilized together with the common bile duct. The biliary confluence and left hepatic duct together with the tumor have been lowered from beneath the overhanging quadrate lobe. (After Blumgart LH, ed. Surgery of the liver and biliary tract, 2nd edn, 1994. With permission from Churchill Livingstone, London.)

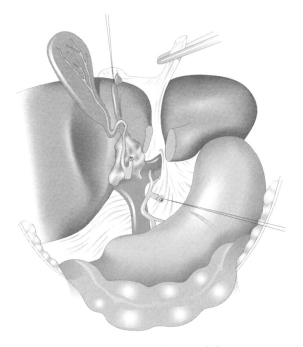

Figure 17.12 The entire extrahepatic biliary apparatus is elevated together with associated connective tissues and nodes so as to allow dissection anterior to the bifurcation of the portal vein. The hepatic artery and portal vein are skeletonized. Here the right hepatic artery has already been divided and is retracted to the left improving exposure to the portal vein branches. (After Blumgart LH, ed. Surgery of the liver and biliary tract, 2nd edn, 1994. With permission from Churchill Livingstone, London.)

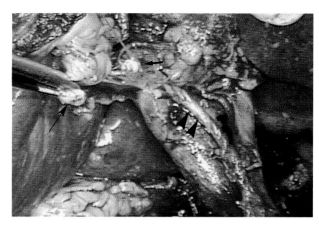

Figure 17.13 Operative view of situation depicted in Fig. 17.12. Portal vein and hepatic arteries have been completely skeletonized. The right hepatic artery (arrowheads) has not been divided yet. The arrow points at the transfixed distal end of the bile duct, which is being retracted upwards and to the right.

At this point, the surgeon should assess the proximal extent of tumor by palpation and, if necessary, by biopsy. The caudate ducts deserve particular attention since en bloc removal of the caudate lobe is frequently necessary and is recommended as a routine by some authors.[11,34,39] Resection is then performed. It is important to obtain frozen section of the bile duct margin in order to ascertain tumor clearance. This portion of the operation is illustrated in Figs 17.14 and 17.15.

If hepatectomy is performed, inflow control is obtained by ligation and transection of the ipsilateral branch of the portal vein and hepatic artery. Extrahepatic control and division of the ipsilateral hepatic vein is performed prior to parenchymal transection. Parenchymal transection is then proceeded with (Figs 17.16 and 17.17).

Biliary–enteric continuity is reconstructed by hepaticojejunostomy to a Roux-en-Y loop of jejunum. After removal of the tumor there may be two or more exposed ducts. Adjacent ducts are brought together and it is usually possible to create a situation where there are no more than three separate orifices to be anastomosed. A Roux-en-Y loop of jejunum is prepared and brought up, usually in a retrocolic fashion. Anastomosis is now carried out in an end-to-side fashion between the exposed ducts and the side of the jejunal loop (Fig. 17.18) close to its termination using a single layer of 4/0 interrupted Vicryl sutures employing the techniques described by Blumgart and Kelley[40] and by Voyles and Blumgart.[41] Details of the anastomotic technique

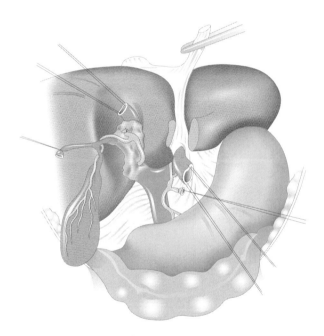

Figure 17.14 The left hepatic duct has been divided clear of tumor and is held on stay sutures. Its distal end, together with the tumor, common hepatic duct and gallbladder, is turned to the right. Note that after transection of the left hepatic duct and during dissection behind the confluence towards the right, one may encounter bile ducts issuing from the caudate lobe. In this instance each duct encountered is individually marked with stay sutures for subsequent anastomosis. A rim of tissue is sent from the left duct and eventual caudate ducts for frozen section to ascertain tumor clearance. (After Blumgart LH, ed. Surgery of the liver and biliary tract, 2nd edn, 1994. With permission from Churchill Livingstone, London.)

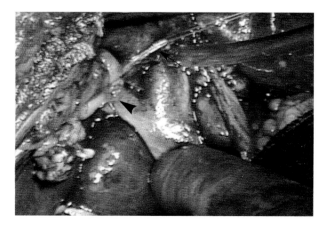

Figure 17.15 Operative view illustrating the situation in Fig. 17.14. The surgeon's finger is on the main portal vein. The left hepatic duct has been transected and secured with sutures (arrow). The distal end of the left hepatic duct together with the tumor, common hepatic, common bile duct and gallbladder is turned to the right (arrowhead).

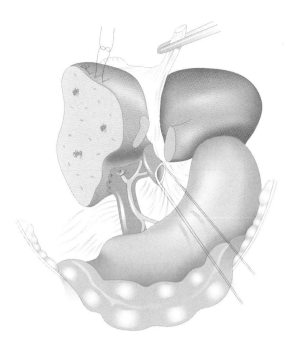

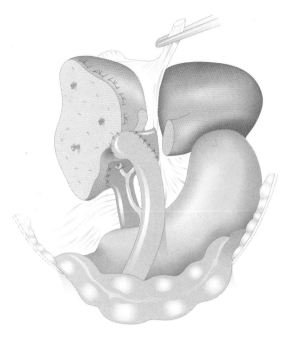

Figure 17.16 The right branch of the portal vein has been divided and oversewn using a 3/0 vascular suture. A vascular stapler may also be used. Portal vein resection and reconstruction is necessary if the tumor encroaches on the portal vein bifurcation or involves the bifurcation directly. Resection of that segment is performed after transection of the ipsilateral bile duct and hepatic artery. Reconstruction is then performed between the main portal trunk and the preserved branch. The right liver has been removed, together with the attached biliary structures containing the tumor, using a simple crushing technique. The left hepatic duct is held on stay sutures ready for subsequent anastomosis. (After Blumgart LH, ed. Surgery of the liver and biliary tract, 2nd edn, 1994. With permission from Churchill Livingstone, London.)

Figure 17.18 Completed biliary reconstruction to liver remnant with a retrocolic Roux-en-Y loop. (After Blumgart LH, ed. Surgery of the liver and biliary tract, 2nd edn, 1994. With permission from Churchill Livingstone, London.)

are illustrated in Figs 17.19–17.25. It is important to state that such high anastomoses to multiple ducts should not be done to a single duct at a time and working sequentially. Such an approach is difficult at best and may be impossible. The best method is to place the entire anterior set of sutures to all exposed ducts and then separately place the entire posterior row of sutures. The jejunum is then railroaded up on the posterior sutures. The posterior layer of sutures to all exposed ducts is tied first and the individual anterior layers then completed sequentially. We routinely employ closed suction drainage of the anastomosis.

Palliative options

The majority of patients with hilar cholangiocarcinoma are not suitable for resection. In this setting, the management options include some form of biliary decompression or supportive care. Jaundice alone is not necessarily an indication for biliary decompression, given the associated morbidity and mortality. Our current indications for biliary decompression in inoperable patients are intractable pruritus, cholangitis, the need for access for intraluminal radiotherapy and to allow recovery of hepatic parenchymal function in patients receiving chemotherapeutic agents. Supportive care alone is

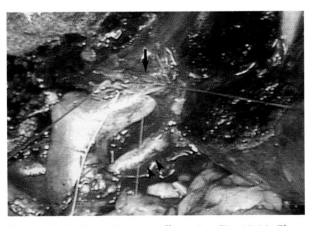

Figure 17.17 Operative view illustrating Fig. 17.16. The arrowhead points to the right portal vein stump. The left hepatic duct (arrow) and a caudate duct are held with stay sutures. The two arrowheads delineate the left hepatic artery.

A B

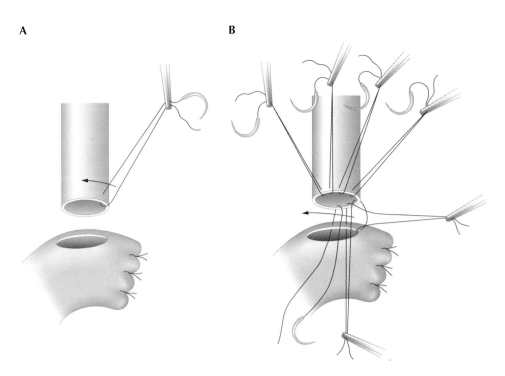

Figure 17.19 Placement of anterior sutures outside in. The needles are kept in place and the sutures held up so as to expose the posterior aspect of the bile duct (A). The posterior row is then placed (B). The posterior sutures are then held up and the jejunum 'railroaded' upwards to meet the bile duct (see Fig. 17.20). (After Blumgart LH, Fong Y, eds. Surgery of the liver and biliary tract, CD-ROM, 1997. With permission from Churchill Livingstone, New York.)

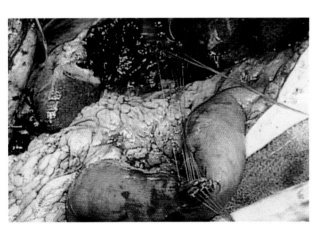

Figure 17.20 Operative view illustrating the posterior sutures just prior to 'railroading'.

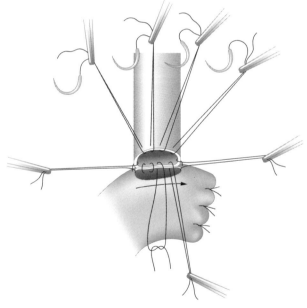

Figure 17.21 Tying of the posterior sutures. (After Blumgart LH, Fong Y, eds. Surgery of the liver and biliary tract, CD-ROM, 1997. With permission from Churchill Livingstone, New York.)

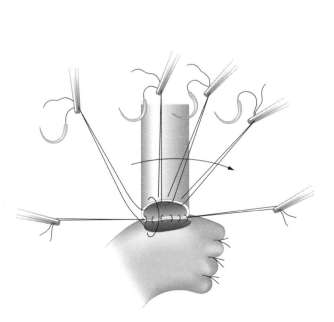

Figure 17.22 Sutures from the previously placed anterior row are now passed through the jejunum. (After Blumgart LH, Fong Y, eds. Surgery of the liver and biliary tract, CD-ROM, 1997. With permission from Churchill Livingstone, New York.)

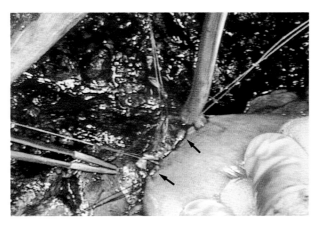

Figure 17.23 Operative view of half completed hepaticojejunostomy. Two individual bile ducts can be seen (arrows).

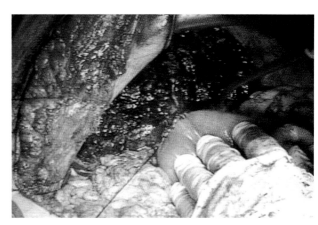

Figure 17.25 Operative view of a completed hepaticojejunostomy after excision of the bile duct, extended left hepatectomy and caudate lobectomy for a papillary bile duct cancer.

A

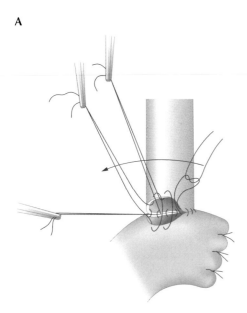

B

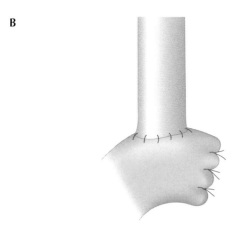

Figure 17.24 Tying of the anterior row (A) and completed anastomosis (B). (After Blumgart LH, Fong Y, eds. Surgery of the liver and biliary tract, CD-ROM, 1997. With permission from Churchill Livingstone, New York.)

probably the best approach for elderly patients with significant co-morbid conditions, provided that pruritis is not a major feature. Patients who are found to be unresectable at operation represent a different group and operative biliary decompression is usually performed successfully[4,5] and can be so constructed as to provide access to the biliary tree for postoperative irradiation.[42]

Assessment of palliative biliary drainage procedures is difficult since the spectrum of patients ranges from the critically ill and irresectable to those in relatively good health with potentially resectable tumors. All patients should be properly assessed by experienced personnel with a view toward possible resection. This point cannot be overemphasized. If the patient is deemed unresectable, the diagnosis should be confirmed with a biopsy. Biliary decompression can be obtained either by percutaneous transhepatic puncture or by endoscopic stent placement. It is important to realize that these patients have a short life expectancy and periprocedural complications extend hospital stay and consume time. Hilar tumors are more difficult to transverse with the endoscopic technique. The failure rates and incidence of subsequent cholangitis are high,[43] and for this reason we avoid this method whenever possible.

Percutaneous biliary drainage (PBD)

Percutaneous transhepatic biliary drainage can be performed in most patients with biliary obstruction, with some exceptions. Jaundice in the setting of portal vein occlusion, without intrahepatic biliary dilatation, usually is not correctable by biliary intubation and should not be performed. It is critical to consider the presence of lobar atrophy prior to percutaneous stenting, since drainage of an atrophic lobe will not relieve jaundice. Uncorrectable coagulopathy increases the risk of bleeding, and temporary control with fresh frozen plasma should be achieved. Hepatic metastasis and massive ascites can cause technical difficulties, but in expert hands safe and successful PBD can usually be achieved.

Biliary drainage is usually performed in several steps including initial access, temporary internal/external drainage and final internalization. Drainage of one liver lobe is usually sufficient to achieve decrease in serum bilirubin and relieve pruritus. In some cases, however, drainage of the contralateral biliary tree might be necessary. The sequence of events in such a case is illustrated in Figs 17.26–17.29. All manipulations should be done under broad antibiotic coverage since transient bacteremia or even sepsis can follow. We favor the placement of expandable metallic Wallstents for palliation of high malignant strictures. Metallic stents are permanent and can only be removed surgically, often with difficulty. They should not be placed in *any* patient unless resection has been definitively excluded as an option. Resection can be performed in the presence of multiple indwelling

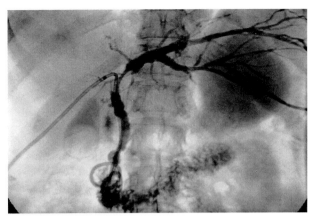

Figure 17.27 Puncture of the left system. The previously placed internal/external drain (see Fig. 17.26) is seen coming from the right. Note this time the right hepatic duct is not seen, clearly indicating separation of the right and left system by the tumor. Drainage of the contralateral system is indicated if the bilirubin is not decreasing or if there is persistent cholangitis.

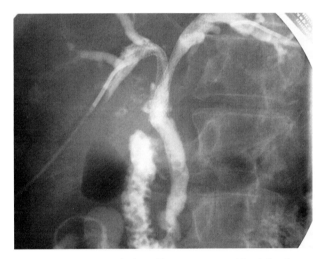

Figure 17.28 Expanded Wallstents in situ. The bile ducts are seen bilaterally and there is free flow of contrast into the duodenum.

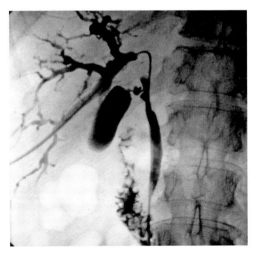

Figure 17.26 Puncture of the right biliary system showing the drain bridging the stricture at the hilum. Note the absence of the left hepatic duct and its branches. This first step establishes access to the biliary tree and decompresses the biliary tree via external or internal/external drainage. Internal/external drains are catheters which extend from the intrahepatic biliary tree to the duodenum, with sideholes both above and below the obstruction. They offer the possibility of complete internal biliary drainage as a trial prior to internalization. Once the drainage has proven to efficiently decompress the biliary tree and infection is controlled, internalization is performed by placement of an endoprosthesis.

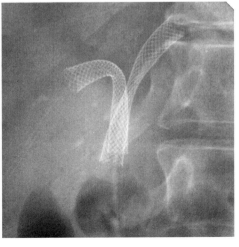

Figure 17.29 Fully expanded Wallstents on a plain film.

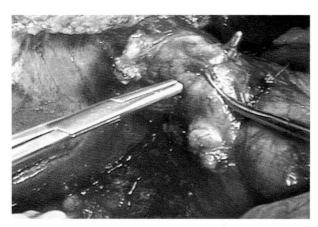

Figure 17.30 Encircled common bile duct containing three Wallstents. Note the inflamed and thickened aspect of the duct.

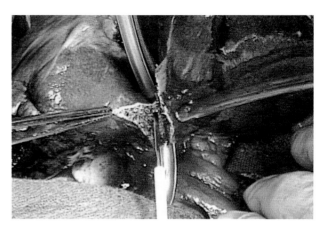

Figure 17.32 The bridge of tissue between segment IV and segment III is transected, facilitating access to the umbilical fissure.

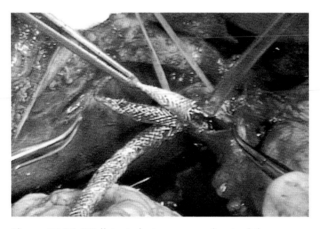

Figure 17.31 Wallstents being removed out of the common duct (Fig. 17.30).

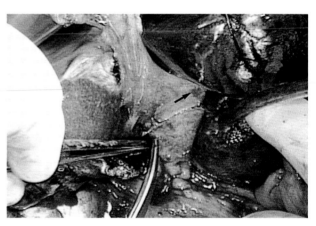

Figure 17.33 Display of the segment III pedicle (arrow) in the umbilical fissure.

stents, but it is preferable to avoid this situation (Figs 17.30 and 17.31). The reported patency rate for metallic stents is 6–8 months,[44–47] which concurs with our findings of a mean patency of 6.1 months in 35 patients palliated for malignant high biliary obstruction by placement of expandable metallic endoprostheses. The periprocedural mortality was 14% at 30 days and seven patients (24%) had documented stent occlusion requiring repeated intervention.[48]

Segment III bypass

Patients who are found to be unresectable at the time of exploration are candidates for a biliary–enteric bypass. We favor an intrahepatic bypass to the segment III duct. This method is not often chosen primarily, since PBD is suitable in most irresectable cases. However, this approach has several advantages over PBD, provides excellent

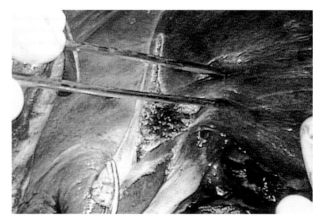

Figure 17.34 A hepatotomy is made to allow access to the superior aspect of the segment III pedicle.

palliation and should be considered once the patient has been submitted to operation. The technical aspects of this procedure are illustrated in Figs 17.32–17.36. This method carried an 11% mortality

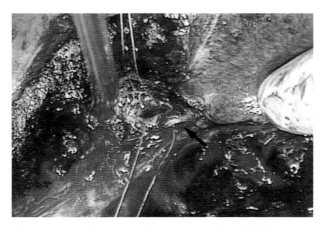

Figure 17.35 The exposed segment III duct held by stay sutures is seen at the bottom of the hepatotomy (arrow).

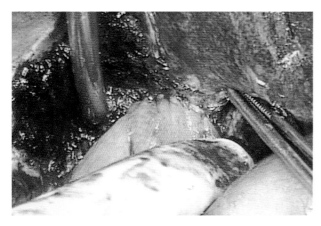

Figure 17.36 Completed anastomosis to the segment III bile duct.

in the senior author's (LHB) initial experience with 20 patients.[49] In a later series of 20 patients managed at Memorial Sloan–Kettering Cancer Center there was no operative mortality and the 1-year bypass patency was 80%.[50]

Radiotherapy

A number of authors advocate a combination of internal and external irradiation.[51–60] We advocate access to the biliary tree by either percutaneous route or by means of an operative biliary bypass whereby a jejunal limb is delivered to the subcutaneous tissue providing percutaneous access.[42] In a next step Wallstents are placed through the stricture. Brachytherapy is delivered by iridium-192 seeds placed in brachytherapy catheters through the stented area. It is our practice to administer 2000 cGy at 1.0 cm over 48 hours. The catheters are then removed and 5000 cGy of external beam radiation is

delivered over 5–6 weeks. Twelve patients were treated in that fashion with a median survival of 14.5 months. All patients survived at least 6 months. Cholangitis and transient hemobilia were the only complications, none of them severe.[42] Others have documented the safety of this approach.[51–60] There may be a survival benefit as well as increased stent patency; some long-term survivors have been reported. However none of the studies are randomized and only a few compare a treated to an untreated group. Further study of this promising modality is certainly warranted.

Photodynamic therapy

Ortner and colleagues have recently evaluated the efficacy of photodynamic therapy in unresectable hilar cholangiocarcinoma.[60] This method has previously been used in the treatment of tumors of the esophagus, colon, stomach, bronchus, bladder and brain. It is a two-step procedure. First a photosensitizer is injected then direct illumination via cholangioscopy activates the compound, causing tumor cell death. The authors treated nine patients in this fashion who had failed endoscopic stenting. They report a 0% mortality for the procedure, however there was a 25% mortality related to the initial endoscopic stenting, which must be considered. The authors do not mention their indication for biliary drainage. This information is important in order to assess the extent of disease prior to therapy. Detailed reasons for irresectability are not discussed, and the reported median survival of 439 days is therefore difficult to interpret. The data presented in this report, including decrease in bilirubin and some improved quality of life, do not suffice to advocate routine use of this method. Comparison in a randomized controlled fashion to other palliative modalities will be needed to define its real value.

Chemotherapy

Chemotherapy has been investigated in uncontrolled studies. No benefit has been demonstrated in the uncontrolled series published to date. Two phase II studies analyzing the effect of 5-FU combined with interferon alpha-2b and the effect of paclitaxel failed to show any benefit.[62,63]

Conclusions

The treatment of hilar cholangiocarcinoma continues to evolve. Judicious use of preoperative investigations using duplex ultrasound, CT scan and especially MRCP and improvements in surgical techniques have allowed better patient selection and the performance of appropriately radical operations with an acceptable mortality. Long-term survival and possible cure, rather than palliation, is now the primary aim. Results presented in this chapter justify an aggressive approach in attempting resection with negative margins. It should be recognized that partial hepatectomy is usually necessary to achieve this goal.

All methods of biliary–enteric decompression, whether surgical or intubational, have considerable morbidity but allow reasonable palliation in some patients. Radiotherapy and photodynamic therapy may have a role in increasing stent patency and possibly survival. However, further study is required to establish their position within the current armamentarium.

Hilar cholangiocarcinoma should not be approached with therapeutic nihilism. Diagnostic and therapeutic approaches to these lesions require special expertise and patients should be referred to centers where adequately trained teams are available.

Key points

- Preoperative diagnosis is almost always possible without the need for tissue diagnosis.
- Exclude rare benign strictures mimicking malignant obstruction.
- Preoperative imaging of extent and resectability:
  MRCP
  Duplex US.
- Angiography and cholangiography need not be used routinely and only in selected cases.
- Resection with negative margins is the goal of treatment.

REFERENCES

1. Farley DR, Weaver AL, Nagorney DM. 'Natural history' of unresected cholangiocarcinoma: patient outcome after noncurative intervention. Mayo Clin Proc 1995; 70: 425–9

2. Okuda K, Kubo Y, Okazaki N, Arishima T, Hashimoto M. Clinical aspects of intrahepatic bile duct carcinoma including hilar carcinoma: a study of 57 autopsy-proven cases. Cancer 1977; 39: 232–46

3. Hadjis NS, Collier NA, Blumgart LH. Malignant masquerade at the hilum of the liver. Br J Surg 1985; 72: 659–61

4. Burke EC, Jarnagin WR, Hochwald SN, Pisters PWT, Fong Y, Blumgart LH. Hilar cholangiocarcinoma: patterns of spread, the importance of hepatic resection for curative operation and a presurgical clinical staging system. Ann Surg 1998; 228: 385–94

5. Jarnagin WR, Fong Y, DeMatteo RP et al. Staging, resectability and outcome in 225 patients with hilar cholangiocarcinoma. Ann Surg 2001; 4: 507–17

6. Weinbren K, Mutum SS. Pathological aspects of cholangiocarcinoma. J Pathol 1983; 139: 217–38

7. Sako K, Seitzinger GL, Garside E. Carcinoma of the extra-hepatic bile ducts: review of the literature and report of six cases. Surgery 1957; 41: 416–37

8. Saldinger PF, Cvetkowski B, Spivack J et al. Outcome of patients with hilar cholangiocarcinoma: importance of histological subtypes. Manuscript in preparation

9. McPherson GA, Benjamin IS, Hodgson HJ, Bowley NB, Allison DJ, Blumgart LH. Pre-operative percutaneous transhepatic biliary drainage: the results of a controlled trial. Br J Surg 1984; 71: 371–5

10. Hochwald SN, Burke EC, Jarnagin WR, Fong Y, Blumgart LH. Association of preoperative biliary stenting with increased postoperative infectious complications in proximal cholangiocarcinoma. Arch Surg 1999; 134 (3): 261–6

11. Hadjis NS, Blumgart LH. Role of liver atrophy, hepatic resection and hepatocyte hyperplasia in the development of portal hypertension in biliary disease. Gut 1987; 28: 1022–8

12. Voyles CR, Bowley NJ, Allison DJ, Benjamin IS, Blumgart LH. Carcinoma of the proximal extrahepatic biliary tree: radiologic assessment and therapeutic alternatives. Ann Surg 1983; 197: 188–94

13. Verbeek PC, van Leeuwen DJ, de Wit LT et al. Benign fibrosing disease at the hepatic confluence mimicking Klatskin tumors. Surgery 1992; 112: 866–71

14. Wetter LA, Ring EJ, Pellegrini CA, Way LW. Differential diagnosis of sclerosing cholangiocarcinomas of the common hepatic duct (Klatskin tumors). Am J Surg 1991; 161: 57–62

15. Gibson RN, Yeung E, Thompson JN et al. Bile duct obstruction: radiologic evaluation of level, cause, and tumor resectability. Radiology 1986; 160: 43–7

16. Okuda K, Ohto M, Tsuchiya Y. The role of ultrasound, percutaneous transhepatic cholangiography, computed tomographic scanning, and magnetic resonance imaging in the preoperative assessment of bile duct cancer. World J Surg 1988; 12: 18–26

17. Hann LE, Greatrex KV, Bach AM, Fong Y, Blumgart LH. Cholangiocarcinoma at the hepatic hilus: sonographic findings. AJR 1997; 168 (4): 985–9

18. Hann LE, Fong Y, Shriver CD et al. Malignant hepatic hilar tumors: can ultrasonography be used as an alternative to angiography with CT arterial portography for determination of resectability? J Ultrasound Med 1996; 15: 37–45

19. Bach AM, Hann LE, Brown KT et al. Portal vein evaluation with US: comparison to angiography combined with CT arterial portography. Radiology 1996; 201: 149–54

20. Itoh K, Fujita N, Kubo K et al. MR imaging of hilar cholangiocarcinoma—comparative study with CT. Nippon Igaku Hoshasen Gakkai Zasshi – Nippon Acta Radiol 1992; 52: 443–51

21. Guthrie JA, Ward J, Robinson PJ. Hilar cholangio-carcinomas: T2–weighted spin-echo and gadolinium-enhanced FLASH MR imaging. Radiology 1996; 201: 347–51

22. Lee MG, Lee HJ, Kim MH et al. Extrahepatic biliary diseases: 3D MR cholangiopancreatography compared with endoscopic retrograde cholangiopancreatography. Radiology 1997; 202: 663–9

23. Schwartz LH, Coakley FV, Sun Y, Blumgart LH, Fong Y, Panicek DM. Neoplastic pancreaticobiliary duct obstruction: evaluation with breath-hold MR cholangiopancreatography. AJR 1998; 170: 1491–5

24. Heslin MJ, Brooks AD, Hochwald SN et al. A preoperative biliary stent is associated with increased complications after pancreatoduodenectomy. Arch Surg 1998; 133: 149–54

25. Hann LE, Schwartz LH, Panicek DM, Bach AM, Fong Y, Blumgart LH. Tumor involvement in hepatic veins: comparison of MR imaging and US for preoperative assessment. Radiology 1998; 206: 651–6

26. Bismuth H, Nakache R, Diamond T. Management strategies in resection for hilar cholangiocarcinoma. Ann Surg 1992; 215: 31–8.

27. Callery MP, Strasberg SM, Doherty GM, Soper NJ, Norton JA. Staging laparoscopy with laparoscopic ultrasonography: optimizing resectability in hepatobiliary and pancreatic malignancy. J Am Coll Surg 1997; 185: 33–9

28. Klempnauer J, Ridder GJ, Werner M, Weimann A, Pichlmayr R. What constitutes long-term survival after surgery for hilar cholangiocarcinoma? Cancer 1997; 79: 26–34

29. Pichlmayr R, Weimann A, Klempnauer J et al. Surgical treatment in proximal bile duct cancer. A single-center experience. Ann Surg 1996; 224: 628–38

30. Pichlmayr R, Weimann A, Oldhafer KJ et al. Role of liver transplantation in the treatment of unresectable liver cancer. World J Surg 1995; 19: 807–13

31. Hadjis NS, Blenkharn JI, Alexander N, Benjamin IS, Blumgart LH. Outcome of radical surgery in hilar cholangiocarcinoma. Surgery 1990; 107: 597–604

32. Baer HU, Stain SC, Dennison AR, Eggers B, Blumgart LH. Improvements in survival by aggressive resections of hilar cholangiocarcinoma. Ann Surg 1993; 217: 20–7

33. Nimura Y, Hayakawa N, Kamiya J, Kondo S, Shionoya S. Hepatic segmentectomy with caudate lobe resection for bile duct carcinoma of the hepatic hilus. World J Surg 1990; 14: 535–43

34. Mizumoto R, Suzuki H. Surgical anatomy of the hepatic hilum with special reference to the caudate lobe. World J Surg 1988; 12: 2–10

35. Blumgart LH, Benjamin IS. Cancer of the bile ducts. In: Blumgart LH, ed. Surgery of the liver and the biliary tract, 2nd edn. London: Churchill Livingstone, 1994: 967–96

36. Blumgart LH. Liver resection – liver and biliary tumors. In: Blumgart LH, ed. Surgery of the liver and the biliary tract, 2nd edn. London: Churchill Livingstone, 1994: 1495–538

37. Blumgart LH, Baer HU. Hilar and intrahepatic biliary-enteric anastomosis. In: Blumgart LH, ed. Surgery of the liver and biliary tract, 2nd edn. London: Churchill Livingstone, 1994: 1051–67

38. Cunningham JD, Fong Y, Shriver C, Melendez J, Marx WL, Blumgart LH. One hundred consecutive hepatic resections. Blood loss, transfusion, and operative technique. Arch Surg 1994; 129: 1050–6

39. Mizumoto R, Kawarada Y, Suzuki H. Surgical treatment of hilar carcinoma of the bile duct. Surg Gynecol Obstet 1986; 162: 153–8

40. Blumgart LH, Kelley CJ. Hepaticojejunostomy in benign and malignant high bile duct stricture: approaches to the left hepatic ducts. Br J Surg 1984; 71: 257–61

41. Voyles CR, Blumgart LH. A technique for the construction of high biliary–enteric anastomoses. Surg Gynecol Obstet 1982; 154: 885–7

42. Kuvshinoff BW, Armstrong JG, Fong Y et al. Palliation of irresectable hilar cholangiocarcinoma with biliary drainage and radiotherapy. Br J Surg 1995; 82: 1522–5

43. Liu CL, Lo CM, Lai EC, Fan ST. Endoscopic retrograde cholangiopancreatography and endoscopic endoprosthesis insertion in patients with Klatskin tumors. Arch Surg 1998; 133: 293–6

44. Tsai CC, Mo LR, Lin RC et al. Self-expandable metallic stents in the management of malignant biliary obstruction. J Form Med Assoc 1996; 95: 298–302

45. Roeren T, Tonn W, Richter GM, Brambs HJ, Kauffmann G. Percutaneous therapy of malignant obstructive jaundice using expandable metal stents: a prospective study of 92 patients. Rofo 1996; 165 (2): 181–7

46. Shapiro MJ. Management of malignant biliary obstruction: nonoperative and palliative techniques. Oncology 1949; 9: 493–6

47. Schmassmann A, von Gunten E, Knuchel J et al. Wallstents versus plastic stents in malignant biliary obstruction: effects of stent patency of the first and second stent on patient compliance and survival. Am J Gastroenterol 1996; 91: 654–9

48. Glattli A, Stain SC, Baer HU, Schweizer W, Triller J, Blumgart LH. Unresectable malignant biliary obstruction: treatment by self-expandable biliary endoprostheses. HPB Surgery 1993; 6: 175–84

49. Baer HU, Rhyner M, Stain SC et al. The effect of communication between the right and left liver on the outcome of surgical drainage for jaundice due to malignant obstruction at the hilus of the liver. HPB Surgery 1994; 8: 27–31

50. Jarnagin WR, Burke EC, Powers C, Fong Y, Blumgart LH. Intrahepatic biliary enteric bypass provides effective palliation in selected patients with malignant obstruction at the hepatic duct confluence. Am J Surg 1998; 175: 453–60

51. Karani J, Fletcher M, Brinkley D, Dawson JL, Williams R, Nunnerley H. Internal biliary drainage and local radiotherapy with iridium-192 wire in treatment of hilar cholangiocarcinoma. Clin Radiol 1985; 36: 603–6

52. Fletcher MS, Brinkley D, Dawson JL, Nunnerley H, Williams R. Treatment of hilar carcinoma by bile drainage combined with internal radiotherapy using 192iridium wire. Br J Surg 1983; 70: 733–5

53. Leung JT, Kuan R. Intraluminal brachytherapy in the treatment of bile duct carcinomas. Australas Radiol 1997; 41: 151–4

54. Vallis KA, Benjamin IS, Munro A et al. External beam and intraluminal radiotherapy for locally advanced bile duct cancer: role and tolerability. Radiother Oncol 1996; 41: 61–6

55. Bowling TE, Galbraith SM, Hatfield AR, Solano J, Spittle MF. A retrospective comparison of endoscopic stenting alone with stenting and radiotherapy in non-resectable cholangiocarcinoma. Gut 1996; 39: 852–5

56. Eschelman DJ, Shapiro MJ, Bonn J et al. Malignant biliary duct obstruction: long-term experience with Gianturco stents and combined-modality radiation therapy. Radiology 1996; 200: 717–24

57. Leung J, Guiney M, Das R. Intraluminal brachytherapy in bile duct carcinomas. Austr NZ J Surg 1996; 66: 74–7

58. Kamada T, Saitou H, Takamura A, Nojima T, Okushiba SI. The role of radiotherapy in the management of extrahepatic bile duct cancer: an analysis of 145 consecutive patients treated with intraluminal and/or external beam radiotherapy. Int J Rad Oncol Biol Phys 1996; 34: 767–74

59. Alden ME, Mohiuddin M. The impact of radiation dose in combined external beam and intraluminal Ir-192 brachytherapy for bile duct cancer. Int J Rad Oncol Biol Phys 1994; 28: 945–51

60. Foo ML, Gunderson LL, Bender CE, Buskirk SJ. External radiation therapy and transcatheter iridium in the treatment of extrahepatic bile duct carcinoma. Int J Rad Oncol Biol Phys 1997; 39: 929–35

61. Ortner MA, Liebetruth J, Schreiber S et al. Photodynamic therapy of nonresectable cholangiocarcinoma. Gastroenterology 1998; 114: 536–42

62. Patt YZ, Jones DV Jr, Hoque A et al. Phase II trial of intravenous flourouracil and subcutaneous interferon alfa-2b for biliary tract cancer. J Clin Oncol 1996; 14: 2311–5

63. Jones DV Jr, Lozano R, Hoque A, Markowitz A, Patt YZ. Phase II study of paclitaxel therapy for unresectable biliary tree carcinomas. J Clin Oncol 1996; 14: 2306–10

64. Cameron JL, Pitt HA, Zinner MJ, Kaufman SL, Coleman J. Management of proximal cholangiocarcinomas by surgical resection and radiotherapy. Am J Surg 1990; 159: 91–7

18 Pitfalls in cholecystectomy

Ali W Majeed and Alan G Johnson

Introduction

Cholecystectomy is one of the commonest elective surgical procedures performed today, with over 500 000 operations being performed annually in the United States alone.[1] In the UK, the cholecystectomy rate is approximately 70 per 100 000 population per year.[2] Evidence is accumulating that the cholecystectomy rate has risen markedly following the introduction of laparoscopic cholecystectomy. This unexplained increase in rate may reflect surgical enthusiasm for a new procedure with consequent alteration of operative indications, rather than a true increase in the incidence of symptomatic gallbladder stones.[3,4]

Standard ('open') cholecystectomy

The first successful cholecystectomy in a human was performed by Karl Langenbuch in 1882 who used a T-shaped incision in the right upper quadrant of the abdomen. Theodor Kocher (1841–1917) is generally credited with the long right subcostal incision which has been used as a 'standard' approach to cholecystectomy for most of the previous century.[5] Cholecystectomy through any upper abdominal incision has been the accepted treatment for symptomatic gallstones for over a century.[6]

Mortality

Several large studies of patients of all ages and with a variety of gallbladder stone disease indicate that the mortality associated with cholecystectomy in all types of patients (including those at very high risk) with or without common bile duct exploration has remained at approximately 1%.[6–8] A number of large studies of elective cholecystectomy without common bile duct exploration have been associated with no deaths; these are summarized in Table 18.1.

Table 18.1 **Major series of elective open cholecystectomy with no mortality**

Author/year	No. of patients
Ganey et al. 1986[8]	1024
McSherry 1989[6]	1693
Gilliland and Traverso 1990[9]	671
Pickleman 1986[10]	389
Fowkes and Gunn 1980[11]	274

In patients below 50 years of age the mortality of 'open' cholecystectomy alone is under 1 in 1000.

The mortality for common duct exploration ranges from 0% in young fit (<50 years) patients to 5.8% in elderly (>70 years) patients. The majority of deaths occur in elderly patients, particularly when common bile duct exploration is undertaken because there may be jaundice and cholangitis in addition to respiratory and cardiovascular problems. Moreover, the proportion of elderly patients coming to surgery for gallstone disease is significantly higher than 50 years ago.[12]

Morbidity

Intraoperative complications
The major intraoperative complications of cholecystectomy are injury to the bile ducts or the hepatic artery and frequent anatomical variations in these structures make them particularly liable to accidental injury (see Chapter 1).

The prognosis of hepatic artery injury depends on the site of injury, the extent of the collateral circulation and the state of the portal circulation, in addition to co-existing sepsis and hypoxia.[13]

A

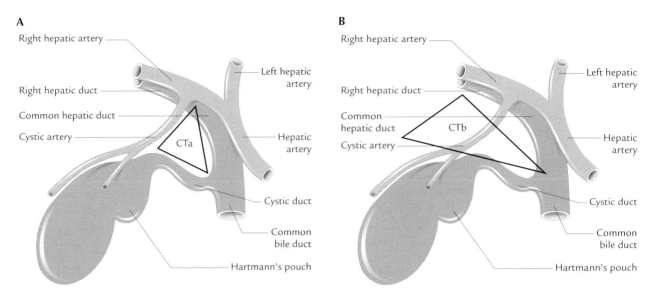

B

Figure 18.1 (A) Calot's original description of his triangle (CTa). (B) Modern understanding of Calot's triangle (CTb).

Collaterals have been shown arteriographically to develop rapidly after hepatic artery ligation and hepatic oxygenation is usually preserved. These collaterals continue to increase in size and number over the ensuing period and liver function is usually not affected.[14]

The triangle bounded by the liver, common hepatic duct and cystic duct is called Calot's triangle after Jean Francois Calot, 1861–1944, a Parisian surgeon who described the triangle in his doctorate thesis 'De la cholecystectomie'. His original description of the triangle describes the cystic artery as the superior boundary, cystic duct as the inferior boundary and common hepatic duct as the medial boundary.[15] The superior boundary is now commonly regarded as the edge of the liver (Fig. 18.1). Clear dissection and display of structures of this triangle are vital if injury to the common bile duct is to be avoided. A common pitfall is traction on the cystic duct which 'tents' the common bile duct and exposes it to injury, and this is especially likely in patients with a foreshortened cystic duct due to severe fibrosis of the gallbladder. Inflammation and oedema in this region make dissection more difficult and hazardous (Fig. 18.2).

The incidence of bile duct stricture following open cholecystectomy has been reported to be approximately 0.05%.[16] Iatrogenic bile duct injury is the commonest cause of benign stricture of the extrahepatic bile ducts and it is said that three major factors contribute to this complication: 'dangerous anatomy; dangerous disease and dangerous surgery'.[17] Biliary ductal injury may go unrecognized at operation and become manifest days or weeks later

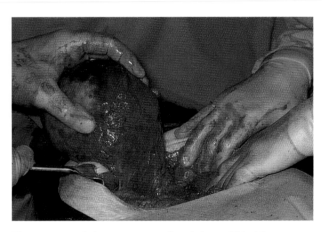

Figure 18.2 A large mucocoele of the gallbladder showing gross inflammation and oedema in the region of Calot's triangle.

with obstructive jaundice, bile peritonitis or an external biliary fistula. The blood supply to the bile duct is axial and even partial transection may result in ischaemia of either end with subsequent stricturing.[18]

Postoperative complications

The wound infection rate after elective open cholecystectomy without common duct exploration was around 2–5%,[19,20] and has fallen dramatically since the introduction of perioperative single-dose antibiotic prophylaxis and this is now routinely recommended.

Accumulation of bile or blood within the subhepatic space is a common postcholecystectomy complication and may occur in up to 20% of patients.[21,22] In many instances, the subhepatic collections originate from minor operative injury to the liver and its biliary ductules. This complication often follows the resection of gallbladders that are intrahepatic in position or tightly adherent to the liver due to chronic cholecystitis. These collections may become infected and remain localized to the subhepatic space or may follow anatomic pathways to involve other peritoneal compartments. In one early series, biliary surgery accounted for 23% of the subphrenic abscesses which presented to the authors.[23] These collections can be identified and drained under ultrasound or CT control and the need for reoperation is often avoided.[24] The sensitivity of ultrasound in detecting minor fluid collections after surgery is high and the vast majority do not need intervention unless signs of systemic sepsis are manifest.

Small-incision ('mini') cholecystectomy

Before the advent of laparoscopic cholecystectomy, surgeons were beginning to realize that a large incision was not required for the safe conduct of an open cholecystectomy, partly due to the introduction of sophisticated imaging which obviated the need for a thorough 'exploratory laparotomy'. Dubois and Berthelot[25] published a large series of 1500 patients who underwent cholecystectomy through a 3–5 cm incision with minimal morbidity and short hospital stay. Merrill[26] reported a consecutive series of 82 unselected patients (15 of whom were 100 kg or or more in weight) with a variety of gallbladder disease. The average length of his incisions was 5.5 cm. The median postoperative hospital stay was 2 days and there was no mortality or major morbidity. O'Dwyer et al.[27] reported a series of 55 patients undergoing the procedure, with the important difference that junior trainee surgeons (albeit under supervision) performed 40% of the procedures. Despite this, the average operating time was 61 minutes with an average hospital stay of 3.9 days. There were no major complications. Goco and Chambers[28] reported a similar study of 50 patients and the hospital stay in their study was reduced to 1.5 days. Moss[29] reported his first 100 patients who were discharged from hospital within 24 hours of elective small-incision cholecystectomy, with no ill-effects. Ledet[30] has considerable experience with minicholecystectomy and published a series of 1207 patients who underwent minicholecystectomy.[31] Of the 1207 patients, 74% were admitted for day surgery, 88% of whom were discharged in less than 12 hours, 9.3% in 24 hours or less and 1.7% in greater than 24 hours; 0.3% were readmitted within 2 weeks. The complication rate was 0.2%; two cases required laparotomy, with no common duct injuries.

The cost of the procedure was US$435; the average time it took working patients to return to work was 11.4 days.

Assalia et al.[32] published a randomized study comparing 'standard' with 'mini' cholecystectomy and showed that mean operative time was 60 and 59 minutes, respectively. Mean operative difficulty, estimated on a 1–10 scale, was 3.4 and 5.6, respectively (P = 0.05). Mean postoperative analgesia requirements (number of doses of 10 mg morphine sulphate) were 5.8 and 4.0, respectively (P = 0.002). Mean duration of hospitalization was 4.7 and 3.0 days, respectively (P = 0.001). Mean 'overall patient satisfaction', estimated on a 1–10 scale, was 6 and 8.3, respectively (P = 0.002) and the authors concluded that minicholecystectomy offers less pain, earlier recovery and better cosmetic results than the conventional 'open' procedure.

Small-incision cholecystectomy performed by an experienced surgeon under optimum conditions is a safe and quick procedure and the results in terms of morbidity and hospital stay are excellent.[25] The procedure is applicable to all patients with all forms of gallbladder disease providing they are fit to undergo general anaesthesia.

Choice of incision

There is considerable misunderstanding about what is meant by a small incision, resulting in anxiety about the adequacy of exposure (Fig. 18.3). Anatomically, the common bile duct (and the cystic duct–common duct junction) lie close to the midline. The positioning of the incision is critical. Some descriptions of minicholecystectomy require the incision to be made over the surface marking of the gallbladder fundus,[33] an area which is of least concern during a cholecystectomy. Access to the cystic duct–common duct junction (Calot's triangle) is difficult with these approaches and a small laterally placed subcostal incision is probably the worst option. Others have described the operation through the midline[29] or low transverse[30] incisions. The gallbladder neck lies close to the right extremity of the porta hepatis[35] and is therefore higher in the abdomen than is commonly perceived. A lateral subcostal incision exposes the fundus of the gallbladder but requires a long medial extension to expose the cystic–common hepatic duct junction adequately. The lateral part of such an incision serves little purpose. Other descriptions of transverse incisions suggest that these should be sited midway between the umbilicus and the xiphisternum; in our experience this required strong upward retraction to expose the cystic duct–common duct junction adequately. Tyagi et al.[34] have described a

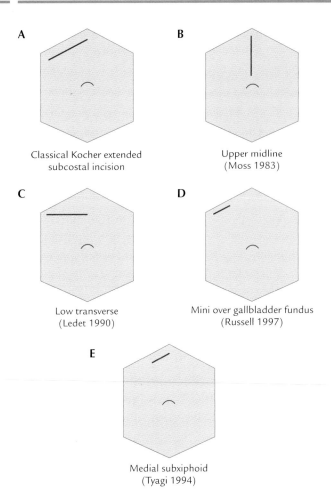

Figure 18.3 Incisions for 'open' cholecystectomy. (A) Classical Kocher extended subcostal incision (1888). (B) Upper midline.[29] (C) Low transverse.[30] (D) Mini over gallbladder fundus.[33] (E) Medial subxiphoid.[34]

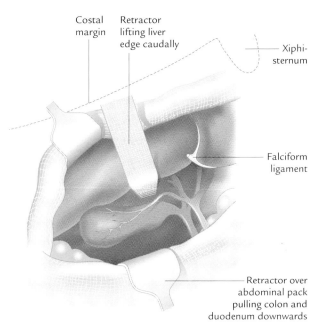

Figure 18.4 Exposure of Calot's triangle during mini-cholecystectomy using the subxiphoid approach.[34]

similar 'subxiphoid' approach and our experience confirms the suitability of this approach. The incision also provides ready access to the common bile duct if the need to explore it arises and we have performed many choledochoduodenostomies through this incision easily and without the need for extension. The small size of the incision does not allow a hand to be inserted into the abdomen, making suture ligation of the cystic duct and artery difficult in obese patients and ligating clips greatly facilitate the procedure.

Procedure of small-incision cholecystectomy

The patient is placed prone on the operating table and prepared and draped as for a standard open cholecystectomy. It is preferable to extend the right arm as this allows the surgeon to stand closer to the patient and view the operative field directly from above. An operating headlight may be used, but has not proved to be necessary in our experience.

Incision

The positioning of the incision is critical to the operation. It is a transverse 5 cm (± 2 cm, depending on the size of the patient) skin incision which extends from the midline across to the right costal margin (Fig. 18.4). The incision should commence approximately two fingerbreadths below the tip of the xiphisternum. This incision is much higher than described in standard texts and has the advantage of being directly over the junction of the cystic and common bile ducts. On the other hand, subcostal or laparoscopic approaches view the cystic duct–common duct junction obliquely from below.

The skin edges are retracted with angled retractors and the anterior rectus sheath divided. The rectus muscle may be divided with diathermy in the line of the skin incision. Alternatively, the rectus muscle may be split or retracted laterally. There is some evidence that splitting the rectus may have an advantage in terms of postoperative recovery.[36] The combined posterior rectus sheath and peritoneum are next picked up with haemostats and incised. These structures are divided to the full extent of the skin incision.

An abdominal retractor (standard or narrow) is used to retract the liver edge and an abdominal gauze pack is then inserted over the surface of this retractor into the peritoneal cavity. A second retractor is placed over the gauze pack (which may need to be adjusted) to retract the colon and duodenum. It may be helpful to deflate a distended stomach with the temporary insertion of a nasogastric tube (removed at the end of the operation). The gallbladder neck is identified and grasped with forceps. Retraction of the gallbladder neck to the patient's right stretches the peritoneal covering over the cystic–common hepatic duct junction, which is carefully cleared. Pledget dissection reveals the cystic duct, which is cleared anteriorly and posteriorly with the help of a Lahey dissector. A medium-large Liga-Clip™ on a clip applier (reloadable laparoscopic clip appliers may be used, but are expensive) is used to place a clip on the cystic duct–gallbladder junction. It is helpful if the clip appliers are angled at the tip to allow the clips to be applied at right angles to the cystic duct and artery. If a cholangiogram is to be performed (we perform operative cholangiography routinely) the cystic duct can be cannulated at this stage. If not, two further clips are applied to the cystic duct, which is then divided. Further blunt dissection reveals the cystic artery which is similarly clipped. The gallbladder is usually removed from the liver bed with diathermy as in the laparoscopic approach. The abdominal packs must be removed carefully to avoid entangling the metal clips on the cystic duct and artery. An abdominal retractor is positioned to protect these clips and the pack can be gently removed over its surface. The rectus sheath is closed in two layers with a continuous running monofilament suture.

Comparison of small-incision and laparoscopic cholecystectomy

Soon after its introduction, laparoscopic cholecystectomy was hailed as 'the biggest advance in surgery since the introduction of general anaesthesia' and in an attempt to prove the superiority of laparoscopic cholecystectomy over existing techniques, proponents of this new technique attempted comparisons with 'historical controls' of open cholecystectomy.[5,37,38] Such comparisons may be inappropriate and misleading, especially in series where the open operation was performed by inexperienced trainees and the laparoscopic procedure by trained consultants. The conviction that laparoscopic cholecystectomy is better than open cholecystectomy permeated into the lay public through the popular press,[38–40] aided by strong commercial pressures from laparoscopic instrument manufacturers.[41] Similarly, reports of increased risk of bile duct injury led to 'bad press' for laparoscopic cholecystectomy.[42] These swings of popular opinion for and against laparoscopic cholecystectomy pointed to the need for a properly randomized comparative trial in which these biases were eliminated and the advantages and disadvantages of laparoscopic access

were quantified. Barkun reported a small prospective randomized trial comparing laparoscopic versus open cholecystectomy,[43] in which patients were randomized before surgery, but the trial may have been influenced by a bias towards laparoscopic cholecystectomy. This is evidenced by patient-assessed outcomes and objective assessments being neutral or in favour of 'mini' open cholecystectomy and outcomes assessed by unblinded carers usually being in favour of laparoscopic cholecystectomy.[44] The Glasgow trial comparing laparoscopic and minilaparotomy cholecystectomy, where patients were randomized in the outpatient clinic,[45] is open to the same criticisms as the Barkun study (the assessors being unblinded to the interventions). This trial, however, did not show a significant difference in the final patient outcome between the two procedures, although laparoscopic cholecystectomy showed an early advantage in terms of hospital stay and postoperative pain. However, the operating time was higher than that for small-incision cholecystectomy and it was calculated that the laparoscopic procedure cost UK£400 more per operation.

In 1996, we published a prospective randomized comparison between laparoscopic and small-incision cholecystectomy in 200 patients which was designed to eliminate bias for or against either technique.[46] Patients were randomized in the operating theatre and anaesthetic technique and pain-control methods were standardized. Four experienced surgeons did both types of procedure after having spent a year of training in each procedure. Identical wound dressings were applied in both groups so that carers could be kept blind to the type of operation. We found there was no significant difference between the groups for age, sex, body mass index and American Society of Anesthesiologists grade. Laparoscopic cholecystectomy took significantly longer than small-incision cholecystectomy (median 65 (range 27–140) minutes versus 40 [18–142] minutes, $P = 0.001$). The operating times included operative cholangiography, which was attempted in all patients. We found no significant difference between the groups for hospital stay (postoperative nights in hospital, median 3.0 (1–17) nights for laparoscopic versus 3.0 (1–14) nights; actual stay 2.5 days due to surgery conducted on afternoon operating lists) for small-incision cholecystectomy ($P = 0.74$), time back to work for employed persons (median 5.0 weeks versus 4.0 weeks; $P = 0.39$) and time to full activity (median 3.0 weeks versus 3.0 weeks; $P = 0.15$).

There is no doubt that after an uncomplicated cholecystectomy (whether through a small incision or laparoscopically) recovery is quick and patient satisfaction is high. If patient selection is good, adequate long-term symptom relief can be expected.

Unfortunately, cholecystectomy is also one of the most unforgiving of surgical procedures if complications arise. Common bile duct damage is one of the most disastrous complications of cholecystectomy and is not feared without reason (see Chapter 19). Injured common ducts are a source of prolonged morbidity and recurrent hospital admissions in patients (who are often young and otherwise fit) and are a potent cause of litigation.[47] Depending on the nature of the injury to the duct, recurrent stricturing, cholangitis and secondary biliary cirrhosis may ensue, occasionally requiring liver transplantation: a high price to pay for an otherwise 'routine' surgical procedure.[48] McMahon (personal communication) has calculated that £500 need to be added to the cost of every cholecystectomy in Britain to cover the cost of further treatment and litigation if the rate of bile duct damage continues.

The difficult cholecystectomy (or 'when to convert a laparoscopic cholecystectomy')

Converting a laparoscopic cholecystectomy to an open procedure is sometimes perceived as a 'failure' of the laparoscopic procedure and enthusiasts strive to keep the conversion rate as low as possible. Indeed, a major criticism of our randomized trial was our conversion rate of 20% (which included conversions for common duct stones because of our protocol of routine cholangiography—the actual conversion rate was 12%). Large series from Nottingham[49] and Scotland[50] reported conversion rates of 15–20% and this is probably a closer reflection of general surgical practice. While it has been suggested that conversion rates may fall with increasing experience,[51] there are plenty of anecdotal reports where surgeons have struggled for many hours to complete an operation laparoscopically. Rationalization of resources requires the surgeon to carry out an initial dissection and, if no progress is being made after a reasonable amount of time (20 minutes or so) to define the anatomical structures of Calot's triangle, then the operation should be converted. Attempts have been made to predict a difficult cholecystectomy where an open approach would be better from the start. Significant preoperative predictors of conversion in one study[52] were acute cholecystitis, increasing age, male sex, obesity and thickened gallbladder wall found by ultrasound. In another study of 1300 patients undergoing laparoscopic cholecystectomy,[53] causes of 56 conversions were described and analysed. Logistic regression analysis of 23 parameters identified the following data as associated with a higher risk for conversion: pain or rigidity in the right upper abdomen ($P = $

0.01), thickening of the gallbladder wall on preoperative ultrasound ($P = 0.05$), intraoperatively found dense adhesions to the gallbladder or in Calot's triangle ($P = 0.001$) and intraoperatively found acute inflammation of the gallbladder ($P = 0.01$). Clinical findings of an acute cholecystitis associated with intraoperative dense scarring in Calot's triangle were the best factors predicting conversion from laparoscopic to open cholecystectomy.

A difficult cholecystectomy may therefore relate to access, anatomy, disease states of the gallbladder and bile ducts or to operative technique.

Difficult access

Complications during *access* for cholecystectomy were not common before the era of laparoscopic cholecystectomy. However, the requirement for creating a pneumoperitoneum has introduced a new range of complications and this is considered one of the most dangerous phases of a laparoscopic cholecystectomy. Many surgeons favour the use of the Veress needle, the main advantage of using this technique being a reduction of 'gas leak' around the subumbilical port. In inexperienced hands, the use of the Veress needle is associated with a higher incidence of visceral perforation and emphasis should be placed on using an 'open' technique for creation of a pneumoperitoneum. This technique involves opening the peritoneal cavity under vision before a port is introduced. If there has been a previous incision in the area, it is likely that the small bowel may be adherent to the posterior aspect of this incision and care needs to be taken to avoid damaging it. Some surgeons prefer a 'stab' approach for initial entry into the peritoneum. This is a particularly dangerous technique if the abdominal wall is not adequately separated from the underlying viscera because the knife can easily penetrate bowel and sometimes the abdominal aorta, especially in very thin patients. A useful method is to apply a towel clip to the umbilicus after making a skin incision below the umbilicus. Traction on this clip allows the abdominal wall to be lifted away from underlying viscera. Occasionally, obesity can cause problems with open insertion of the subumbilical cannula, but if there is any difficulty, the incision should be extended and safety must not be compromised on this account. In obese people gas leaks can occasionally occur and can be annoying and disruptive. Various techniques have been employed to avoid it; these include flanged ports or ports with a built-in inflatable balloon or those with a tapering screw (Hasson cannula). Probably the simplest and most effective method of securing a gas leak is to insert a purse-string suture around the incision in the linea alba. This can be tied around the cannula and should effectively prevent a gas leak. A useful tip is to examine the abdominal cavity carefully with the laparoscope to ensure no damage has occurred at entry.

Triangulation and exposure

Working ports need to be separated spatially enough to allow good triangulation and enhanced leverage to allow safe dissection to be carried out. This prevents the problem of instruments 'fighting' each other in a cramped area. During a laparoscopic cholecystectomy, tilting the head end of the patient up and the left side down (i.e. towards the surgeon) helps displace abdominal viscera away from the liver and allows a better view of Calot's triangle. Occasionally, an additional fan retractor will be required, especially in obese patients, if there is a very floppy caudate lobe of the liver that obstructs view.

Difficult anatomy

A knowledge of all anatomical variations in biliary structures is essential for anyone undertaking biliary surgery (see Chapter 1). 'Inadvertant' division of structures which have not been recognized is a leading source of litigation. It is vital that a clear and unambiguous definition of anatomy should be obtained before any structure is ligated or divided, and the importance of this step is becoming clear with increasing experience with laparoscopic cholecystectomy. If there is any doubt about structures in Calot's triangle, a very safe rule is to stay very close to the gallbladder wall (the 'safety zone'[54,55]) or perform a fundus-first dissection.

Major anomalies (gallbladder agenesis, gallbladder duplication, double cystic duct) are very rare and must not be assumed to occur if the anatomy of the area is unclear. A tented common bile duct can look suspiciously like a double cystic duct (Fig. 18.5)! Minor anomalies relate to the relationship of the cystic duct and artery to each other and to the common bile duct and careful dissection and identification of structures will normally display them. Occasionally, the cystic duct enters the right hepatic duct rather than the common bile duct (see Chapter 1). The important junction to identify clearly in a laparoscopic operation is between the cystic duct and the gallbladder and *not* the cystic duct with the common bile duct (i.e. staying close to the gallbladder). Occasionally, the cystic duct arises from the left side of the common duct and crosses the common bile duct either anteriorly or posteriorly. Attempts to dissect it to its origin must not be made and, contrary to previous opinion, leaving a long cystic duct stump is of no consequence in comparison to the complications associated with common bile duct injury.

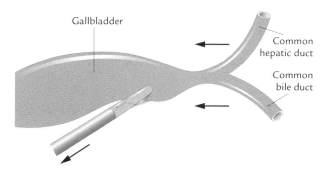

Figure 18.5 Too much lateral retraction of the gallbladder results in tenting of the extrahepatic bile ducts, which may then be inadvertently clipped or damaged.

Unfortunately, most instances of common bile duct damage occur when there is no evidence of a biliary anomaly and it is for this reason that it cannot be overstated that there should be a clear and unequivocal identification of biliary anatomy before ligating or dividing any structure.

Dangerous pathology

Acute inflammation

Cholecystectomy is feasible both laparoscopically and through a 'mini' incision in acute inflammation of the gallbladder. A plane of oedema that exists between the liver and the gallbladder often helps the dissection. However, this area may be hyperaemic and thus bleed more than normal tissue. Current evidence suggests that early and delayed cholecystectomy in acute cholecystitis gives the same results if carried out within 72 hours of the acute attack.[56] Organizing fibrosis may make the procedure extremely difficult if carried out soon after this 'window' of opportunity.[57] There has always been a transatlantic difference in attitudes to the treatment of acute cholecystitis, with Americans recommending early operation and Europeans relying on conservative treatment followed by 'interval' cholecystectomy. This is largely due to the methods of payment and delivery of health care, rather than the difference in the pathology or natural history of the disease. More than 20 years ago, a prospective randomized trial had shown that open operation performed within 7 days of the start of the acute attack was quicker and safer than delayed operation at 2–3 months. Similarly, a randomized trial of early (less than 72 hours) versus delayed (8–12 weeks) laparoscopic cholecystectomy found a better outcome in those having early operation.[58] In the delayed group, eight patients (20%) had to undergo urgent operation for spreading peritonitis and the laparoscopic conversion rate was actually higher in the delayed group (although other studies have shown a lower rate). In a small study comparing laparoscopic versus large-incision open cholecystectomy for acute cholecystitis,[59] the stay was shorter after laparoscopic cholecystectomy (4 versus 6 days). However, the groups were not comparable in that operative cholangiograms were only done in the open group, and most of the operations in the open group were done by junior surgeons, whereas the laparoscopic operations were performed by more experienced surgeons. A prospective study of a small-incision (mini) cholecystectomy for acute cholecystitis has shown results which are comparable to those from the laparoscopic series.[33]

From the available evidence, acute cholecystectomy is a safe procedure and the total hospital stay and recovery period would be less than two-stage treatment. As with all laparoscopic operations, the surgeon must be prepared to convert to open operation if there is any doubt about the anatomy, and operative cholangiography is an important method of confirming this.

Chronic inflammation/fibrosis

Chronic inflammation can sometimes lead to a shrunken fibrosed gallbladder and it can be very difficult in these patients to delineate anatomy clearly.[60] If the operation is being attempted laparoscopically and if there is any doubt about the safety of dissection, the operation must be converted to an open approach. At open cholecystectomy, a fundus-first dissection in these situations is advised, and if the cystic duct cannot be dissected safely because of dense fibrosis in Calot's triangle, a subtotal cholecystectomy is a very safe option. The gallbladder can be amputated and its interior washed out. The stump can be oversewn with absorbable suture. The 'Mirizzi syndrome' (large stone in gallbladder neck causing jaundice by extrinsic compression of the common bile duct) can be approached in the same manner (Fig. 18.6). The gallbladder neck is amputated, the large stone obstructing the common bile duct can be removed and the gallbladder stump oversewn, without the need for any dissection, close the common bile duct. This procedure is hazardous

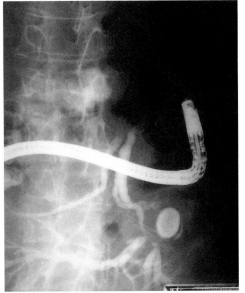

A

Figure 18.6 (A) ERCP demonstrating the Mirizzi syndrome. A large solitary calculus impacted in Hartmann's pouch, causing inflammatory reaction which has resulted in a biliary stricture. (B) CT scan of the liver of the same patient, showing the calculus impacted in Hartmann's pouch. (C) Visceral angiogram of the same patient, demonstrating a completely normal vascular anatomy with no evidence of tumour neovasculature.

B

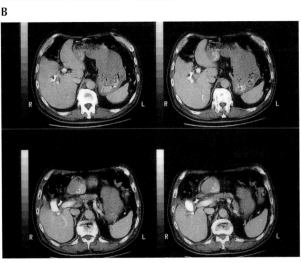

C

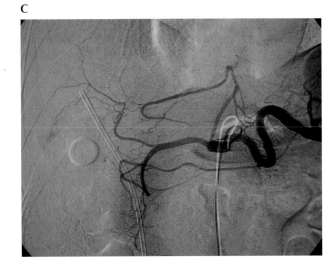

at best when contemplated laparoscopically[61] and an open approach is recommended.

If there is inflammation or fistula formation in the fundus of the gallbladder into the colon or duodenum it is much safer to leave behind a cuff of gallbladder, which is oversewn in two layers with absorbable suture.

Tense gallbladder

The gallbladder may be difficult to grasp if it is very tense due to either an empyaema or a mucocoele, or occasionally if it is packed with calculi. In these cases, insertion of a long spinal needle through the skin into the gallbladder with aspiration of bile, pus or mucus can relax the gallbladder wall and allow it to be grasped. Normally a 5 mm instrument is used for cephalad retraction of the gallbladder fundus, but if the gallbladder wall is very thickened, it may have to be replaced by a 10 mm grasper. In patients with an empyaema or mucocoele, a stone impacted in Hartmann's pouch may make dissection of Calot's triangle difficult. Aspirating the gallbladder may reduce the pressure on the fundus, allowing dislodgement of such a stone. If this is not possible, the 10 mm grasper can be used to grasp the stone and retract Hartmann's pouch in order to display the cystic duct. During an open cholecystectomy, simple aspiration of the gallbladder with proximal dislodgement of the stone facilitates dissection of the cystic–hepatic duct junction.

Abnormal cystic duct

The cystic duct may be short or wide or both. Extreme care should be exercised in these situations as the risk of causing common duct damage is high. During an open cholecystectomy, a fundus-first dissection is strongly recommended and the cystic duct stump can then be divided and oversewn with a fine absorbable suture. During a laparoscopic operation the cystic duct–gallbladder junction must be clearly identified. Occasionally, the cystic duct stump is too wide to accept laparoscopic clips. Inadequate closure of the cystic duct will lead to postoperative bile leakage. It is recommended that such patients should have their cystic stump ligated either with a preformed endo-loop suture or using a laparoscopic suturing technique.

Xanthogranulomatous cholecystitis

This is a severe form of cholecystitis and can be macroscopically indistinguishable from gallbladder cancer and laparoscopic treatment is therefore hazardous.[62] Unfortunately, the xanthogranulomatous process continues unless completely excised. Probably the best option in difficult cases is to biopsy the gallbladder and drain it and refer the patient on to a specialist hepatobiliary surgeon.

Dangerous techniques

Diathermy

Injudicious use of diathermy around the cystic duct–common hepatic duct junction is potentially hazardous because this can lead to stricturing of the common bile duct and subsequent jaundice.[63] An understanding of the physics of electrosurgery is vital for the safe use of surgical diathermy, which relies on the principle that high frequency current can pass through the body with no effects other than the production of heat.[64,65] The amount of heat produced by the current is inversely proportional to the electrode area. Two types of diathermy electrode are commonly used: monopolar and bipolar. 'Polarity' refers to the number of electrical poles at the site of application, the main difference being the distance between the poles. For monopolar diathermy, the second pole is the dispersive electrode plate, usually attached to the patient's thigh. Bipolar electrodes are only a few millimetres apart and only the tissue located between these poles is affected. Much more power is required in monopolar mode because the body is a poor electrical conductor. Power density is the key element that determines the thermodynamic effect on tissue and a concentrated electrical field leads to vaporization (cutting) of tissue and a more dispersed field results in coagulation. Monopolar electrical energy is the most frequently used method of dissection in laparoscopic surgery today.

Potential problems associated with the laparoscopic use of monopolar electrocoagulation relate to unrecognized energy transfer ('stray current') outside the view of the laparoscope. During laparoscopic surgery electrical energy is passed through the abdominal wall via cannulae (which may be conductors) or by instruments to tissues being dissected. The only part of this circuit that is visible is the tissue being dissected. Potentially dangerous factors[66,67] are listed in Table 18.2.

Table 18.2 Problems using diathermy during laparoscopic cholecystectomy

- *Insulation defects*: particularly with non-metal cannulae
- *Capacitative coupling*: may discharge current to adjacent bone, causing full thickness burn
- *Arcing*: particularly with older machines
- *Residual heat*: especially with monopolar electrocoagulation

Insulation defects, although frequently not directly visible, may lead to delivery of electrical energy at a site beyond the view of the laparoscope. The hazard of insulation failure depends on the location of the point of failure along the length of the instrument. Outside the view of the camera, thermal injury may occur to any viscus in contact with the defective instrument. If it occurs within the metal cannula, the only evidence may be interference with the electrosurgical generator, jerking of the abdominal wall, or interference with the video monitor. This may be harmless as the current is dissipated by broad contact at the abdominal wall. If, however, the defective instrument is within a plastic cannula, there may be no clue to insulation failure. It is important that single-use instruments are not resterilized as this can lead to insulation breaks and inadvertent direct coupling.

Capacitative coupling can lead to laparoscopic complications.[68] A capacitor exists wherever an insulating material separates two conductors that have a potential difference between them. With monopolar diathermy, up to 70% of the active electrode current is induced in the cannula wall. With non-conductive cannulae, the only outlet for this stored charge may be a nearby bowel loop resulting in a full-thickness burn. For this reason, all-metal cannulae are recommended to allow safe dissipation at the abdominal wall. Electrical energy dissipated through tissue has the ability to cause distant necrosis that may become apparent only some time after surgery. The temperature generated by an electrical current is inversely proportional to the fourth power of the diameter of the body along which it is conducted. Structures of small diameter are, therefore, at risk of necrosis and subsequent perforation or stricture if they are in the line of current dispersion.[69]

Arcing occurs when a high-voltage current jumps the distance between the electrode and nearest body tissue. This sparking discharge may occur if the electrode is left active but not in contact with the point of dissection and is proportional to voltage. Although considerable variation exists, diathermy machines that are more than 5 years old may be able to generate a peak-to-peak potential difference of 6000 V. Such a discharge can produce necrosis at the contact point of the spark.

Residual heat: in addition to the hazards of electrical current in diathermy dissection, the tip of an activated electrode generates substantial heat energy. If the active electrode is not in contact with tissue, a temperature of over 500°C can be generated and a thermal burn may result even after the diathermy has been made inactive. If monopolar electrocoagulation is to continue as the preferred mode of dissection in laparoscopic surgery it is essential that surgeons understand its method of action and potential pitfalls.

Lasers have been readily adapted to laparoscopic surgery but have no proven safety benefit over the less expensive and more freely available electrocautery systems.[70] Laser dissection methods rely on the ability of light energy to excite molecules sufficiently to cause heating of the recipient tissue and disruption of structural proteins.[71] Carbon dioxide laser dissection, in particular, has an inherent 'backstop effect' that is difficult to control and may lead to inadvertent damage of structures adjacent to the area of intended coagulation. Deflection of a free laser beam by collision of the probe against another instrument or hand tremors may cause damage to adjacent structures. Newer technology using the neodymium–yttrium–aluminium–garnet laser with contact tips has eliminated the danger of a free beam loose in a body cavity, but energy penetrates deeply (3–4 mm) and may injure adjacent tissue inadvertently. Laser energy is highly absorbed by dark pigments, thus coagulated superficial layers tend to inhibit further penetration of energy.

High-frequency ultrasonic coagulation is an alternative to electrosurgery as a cutting and coagulating energy source adapted for laparoscopic use.[72,73] A piezoelectric transducer is housed in a handpiece, causing a blade tip to vibrate at high frequencies. The mechanical energy causes cutting and coagulation by vibrational forces; this cavitational effect vaporizes intracellular water and disrupts cell walls. Maximum blade temperatures do not normally exceed 80°C and the spread of necrosis from the point of contact (in the epidermis) is less than 0.05 mm, compared with up to 0.35 mm for electrothermal necrosis.[74] Water jet dissection[75] facilitates liver surgery, but its role in laparoscopic surgery remains to be established. It is possible that electrosurgery will be replaced by these newer methods but, until then, a full understanding of monopolar electrocoagulation should be an integral part of training programmes in laparoscopic surgery.

Guidelines for the safe use of diathermy are listed in Table 18.3. Bipolar methods are safer in principle and should be used in preference to monopolar electrodes, particularly when the anatomical field is crowded. However, bipolar diathermy is very limited at performing dissection due to the instrument 'sticking' to the coagulated tissue and currently most surgeons prefer monopolar techniques.

Retraction

Traction on the gallbladder in a laparoscopic operation is in its long axis. This has the potential to

Table 18.3 **Guidelines for the safe use of diathermy**
1. Excessive use of diathermy should be avoided because cleavage planes can be obscured by the heat-induced contraction of tissues. 2. Before applying the electrode to vital structures, the intensity of the coagulation current should be tested to ensure the desired tissue effect. 3. Diathermy should never be used blindly to control bleeding. The surgeon should be willing to convert to an open operation when the dissection becomes bloody or otherwise difficult.

cause 'tenting' of the common bile duct, which then appears to be continuous with the cystic duct (being in the same axis) and can be accidentally divided. Such injuries can be quite severe if a segment of the common duct is removed. The key to avoidance of common bile duct injury is to apply additional lateral traction with the grasper in the surgeon's left hand. This pulls the gallbladder neck away from the liver and a window can be created between it and the liver. If there is tenting of the common bile duct, it will take the shape of a 'V' and can be recognized more easily.

Previous abdominal surgery

Previous upper abdominal surgery is not considered a contraindication to laparoscopic cholecystectomy. If the midline scar extends to the umbilicus, care must be taken when the initial pneumoperitoneum is created. Careful clearance of these adhesions can often be accomplished to allow the cholecystectomy to proceed. However, if there is any doubt, it is preferable to convert to an open operation with the high right transverse incision described previously.

Non-retractile liver

The liver can be difficult to retract if it is fibrosed as in chronic hepatitis or cirrhosis. Occasionally, very fatty livers can be difficult to retract. In these situations (as with a prominent floppy caudate lobe)

it is advisable to insert an extra retractor. An atraumatic fan retractor can be a very useful instrument to allow a good view of the gallbladder and cystic duct in these situations.

The role of cholangiography

Operative cholangiography during cholecystectomy has two roles, one is to identify common bile duct stones and the other is to define biliary anatomy and thus avoid injury to the bile duct. The management of common duct stones is discussed elsewhere. Whether cholangiography reduces the incidence of common duct injury is contentious,[76,77] and detractors point to the possibility of ductal injury already having been committed at the time of insertion of the cholangiography catheter. There is no doubt however, that if cholangiography with intraoperative screening is routinely conducted before division of structures, these injuries can be recognized at the time of surgery and can limit damage, especially if the cholangiogram catheter is introduced via a small cut and held by a loosely placed clip.

Key points

- Bile duct injury may well go unrecognized at operation and then become manifest days or weeks later as obstructive jaundice, bile peritonitis or external biliary fistula.
- There is little or no difference in operating time, in hospital stay and time to full recovery between laparoscopic and minicholecystectomy.
- Indications to convert to open cholecystectomy:
    Inability to define Calot's triangle after 20 minutes of dissection
    Acute cholecystitis
    Preoperative and operative suspicion of gallbladder cancer
    Previous abdominal surgery with dense adhesions.
- Role of cholangiography:
    Identify stones in the biliary tract
    Define biliary anatomy, and to reduce the risk of bile duct injury.

REFERENCES

1. Freiherr G. Gallstones: Statistical considerations. In: Ferruci JT, Delius M, Burhenne HJ, eds. Biliary Lithotripsy. Chicago: Year Book Medical Publishers, 1989; 139–40

2. Holland C, Heaton KW. Increasing frequency of gallbladder operations in the Bristol clinical area. Br Med J 1972; 3: 672–5

3. Bernard HR, Hartman TW. Complications after laparoscopic cholecystectomy. Am J Surgery 1993; 165: 533–5

4. Bateson M. Second opinions in laparoscopic cholecystectomy [see comments]. Lancet 1994; 344: 76

5. Hardy KJ, Miller H et al. An evaluation of laparoscopic versus open cholecystectomy. Med J Aust 1994; 160 (2): 58–62

6. McSherry C. Cholecystectomy: the gold standard. Am J Surg 1989; 158: 174–8

7. Doyle PJ, Ward-McQuaid JN, McEwen Smith A. The value of routine peroperative cholangiography—a report of 4000 cholecystectomies. Br J Surg 1982; 69: 617–9

8. Ganey JB, Johnson PA, Prillaman PE, McSwain GR. Cholecystectomy: clinical experience with a large series. Am J Surg 1986; 151: 352–7

9. Gilliland TM, Traverso LW. Modern standards for comparison of cholecystectomy with alternative treatments for symptomatic cholelithiasis with emphasis on long-term relief of symptoms. Surg Gynecol Obstet 1990; 170: 39–44

10. Pickleman J, Gonzalez RP. The improving results of cholecystectomy. Arch Surg 1986; 121 (8): 930–4

11. Fowkes FGR, Gunn AA. The management of acute cholecystitis and its hospital cost. Br J Surg 1980; 67: 613–7

12. Bates T, Harrison M, Lowe D, Lawson C, Padley N. Longitudinal study of gallstone prevalence at necropsy. Gut 1992; 33: 103–7

13. Brittain RS, Marchioro TL, Hermann G, Waddell WR, Starzl TE. Accidental hepatic artery ligation in humans. Am J Surg 1964; 107: 822–32

14. Koehler RE, Korobkin M, Lewis F. Arteriographic demonstration of collateral arterial supply to the liver after hepatic artery ligation. Radiology 1975; 117: 49–54

15. Wood M. Presidential address: eponyms in biliary tract surgery. Am J Surg 1979; 138 (6): 746–54

16. Andren-Sandberg A, Alinder G, Bengmark S. Accidental lesions of the common bile duct at cholecystectomy. Ann Surg 1985; 201: 328–32

17. Johnston GW. Iatrogenic bile duct stricture: an avoidable surgical hazard? Br J Surg 1986; 73: 245–7

18. Northover JMA, Terblanche J. A new look at the arterial blood supply of the bile duct in man and its surgical implications. Br J Surg 1979; 66: 161–7

19. Coles B, van Heerden JA, Keys TF. Incidence of wound infection for common general surgical procedures. Surg Gynecol Obstet 1982; 154: 557–60

20. Fyfe AHB, Mohammed R, Dougall AJ. The infective complications of elective cholecystectomy. J R Coll Surg Edin 1983; 28: 90–5

21. Neff CC, Simeone JF, Ferruci JT, Mueller PR, Wittenberg J. The occurence of fluid collections following routine abdominal surgical procedures: sonographic survey in asymptomatic postoperative patients. Radiology 1983; 146: 463–6

22. Ghahremani GG. Postcholecystectomy complications. CRC Crit Rev Diag Imag 1984; 23: 119–49

23. Wang SMS, Wilson SE. Subphrenic abscess: the new epidemiology. Arch Surg 1977; 112: 934–6

24. Palestrant AM, Vine HS, Sacks BA, Weinstein M, Ellison H. Nonoperative drainage of fluid collections following operations on the biliary tract. Surg Gynecol Obstet 1983; 156: 305–9

25. Dubois F, Berthelot B. Cholecystectomie par mini-laparotomie. Nouv Presse Med 1982; 11: 1139–41

26. Merrill J. Minimal trauma cholecystectomy (a no-touch procedure in a well). Am J Surg 1988; 54: 256–61

27. O'Dwyer PJ, Murphy JJ, O'Higgins NJ. Cholecystectomy through a 5 cm subcostal incision. Br J Surg 1990; 77: 1189–90

28. Goco IR, Chambers LG. 'Mini-cholecystectomy' and operative cholangiography. A means of cost containment. Am Surg 1983; 49: 143–5

29. Moss G. Mini-trauma cholecystectomy. J Abdom Surg 1983; 25: 66–74

30. Ledet WP. Ambulatory cholecystectomy without disability. Arch Surg 1990; 125: 1434–5

31. Seale AK, Ledet WP Jr. Minicholecystectomy: a safe, cost-effective day surgery procedure. Arch Surg 1999; 134 (3): 308–10

32. Assalia A, Schein M, Kopelman D, Hashmonai M. Minicholecystectomy vs conventional cholecystectomy: a prospective randomized trial—implications in the laparoscopic era. World J Surg 1993; 17: 755–9

33. Russell RCG. Minimally invasive surgery for gallstone disease: mini-cholecystectomy. In: Carter, Russell, Pitt, Bismuth, eds. Rob and Smith's operative surgery, 5th edn. London: Chapman and Hall Medical Publishers, 1997: 295–9

34. Tyagi NS, Meredith MC, Lumb JC et al. A new minimally invasive technique for cholecystectomy. Ann Surg 1994; 220: 617–25

35. Launois B, Jamieson GG. In: Modern operative techniques in liver surgery. Churchill Livingstone, 1993: 14–5

36. Baguley PE, de Gara CJ, Gagic N. Open cholecystectomy: muscle splitting versus muscle dividing incision: a randomized study. J R Coll Surg Edin 1995; 40: 230–2

37. Grace PA, Quereshi A, Coleman J et al. Reduced postoperative hospitalisation after laparoscopic cholecystectomy. Br J Surg 1991; 78: 160–2

38. Williams LF, Chapman WC, Bonau RA, McGee EC, Boyd RW, Jacobs JK. Comparison of laparoscopic

cholecystectomy and open cholecystectomy in a single center. Am J Surg 1993; 165: 459–65

39. Kingman S. Simple way to lose a stone. The Independent on Sunday News magazine, 2 June 1991

40. Macintyre IMC, Wilson RG. Laparoscopic cholecystectomy. Br J Surg 1993; 80: 552–9

41. Emberton M, Howerton R. Laparoscopic cholecystectomy (letter). Br Med J 1992; 304: 777

42. Altman LK. Surgical injuries lead to new rule. New York Times; 1992: 4

43. Barkun JS, Barkun AN, Sampalis JS et al. Randomised controlled trial of laparoscopic versus mini cholecystectomy. The McGill Gallstone Treatment Group. Lancet 1992; 340: 1116–9

44. Nicholl JP, Brazier JE. Laparoscopic versus mini-incision cholecystectomy (letter). Lancet 1993; 341: 47

45. McMahon AJ, Russell IT, Baxter JN et al. Laparoscopic versus minilaparotomy cholecystectomy: a randomised trial [see comments]. Lancet 1994; 343: 135–8

46. Majeed AW, Troy G, Nicholl JP et al. Randomised, prospective, single-blind comparison of laparoscopic and small-incision cholecystectomy. Lancet 1996; 347: 989–94

47. Cates JA, Tompkins RK, Zinner MJ et al. Biliary complications of laparoscopic cholecystectomy. Am Surg 1993; 59: 243–7

48. Gigot J, Etienne J, Aerts R et al. The dramatic reality of biliary tract injury during laparoscopic cholecystectomy. An anonymous multicenter Belgian survey of 65 patients. Surg Endosc 1997; 11: 1171–8

49. Steele RJC, Marshall K, Lang M, Doran J. Introduction of laparoscopic cholecystectomy in a large teaching hospital: independant audit of the first 3 years. Br J Surg 1995; 82: 968–71

50. Fullarton GM, Bell G and the West of Scotland Laparoscopic Cholecystectomy Audit Group. Prospective audit of the introduction of laparoscopic cholecystectomy in the west of Scotland. Gut 1994; 35 (8): 1121–6

51. Cagir B, Rangraj M, Maffuci L et al. The learning curve for laparoscopic cholecystectomy. J Laparoendosc Surg 1994; 4: 419–27

52. Fried GM, Barkun JS, Sigman HH et al. Factors determining conversion to laparotomy in patients undergoing laparoscopic cholecystectomy. Am J Surg 1994; 167: 35–39; discussion 39–41

53. Schrenk P, Woisetschlager R, Wayand WU. Laparoscopic cholecystectomy. Cause of conversions in 1300 patients and analysis of risk factors. Surg Endosc 1995; 9: 25–8

54. Espiner HJ, Rowe A, Eltringham WK, Miller R. Laparoscopic cholecystectomy (letter). Br Med J 1991; 302: 847

55. Taniguchi Y, Ido K, Kimura K et al. Introduction of a 'safety zone' for the safety of laparoscopic cholecystectomy. Am J Gastroenterol 1993; 88: 1258–61

56. Lujan JA, Parrilla P, Robles R et al. Laparoscopic cholecystectomy vs open cholecystectomy in the treatment of acute cholecystitis: a prospective study. Arch Surg 1998; 133: 173–5

57. Koperna T, Kisser M, Schulz F. Laparoscopic versus open treatment of patients with acute cholecystitis. Hepatogastroenterology 1999; 46: 753–7

58. Lo C-M, Liu C-L, Fan S-T, Lai ECS, Wong J. Prospective randomised study of early versus delayed laparoscopic cholecystectomy for acute cholecystitis. Ann Surg 1998; 227: 461–7

59. Kiviluoto T, Siren J, Luukonen P, Kivilaakso E. Randomised trial of laparoscopic versus open cholecystectomy for acute and gangrenous cholecystitis [see comments]. Lancet 1998; 351: 321–5

60. Molloy M, Sorrell MJ, Bower RH et al. Patterns of morbidity and resource consumption associated with laparoscopic cholecystectomy in a VA medical center. J Surg Res 1999; 81: 15–20

61. Contini S, Dalla Valle R, Zinicola R, Botta GC. Undiagnosed Mirizzi's syndrome: a word of caution for laparoscopic surgeons—a report of three cases and review of the literature. J Laparoendosc Adv Surg Tech A 1999; 9: 197–203

62. Balague C, Targarona EM, Sugranes G et al. Xanthogranulomatous cholecystitis simulating gallbladder neoplasm: therapeutic implications. Gastroenterol Hepatol 1996; 19: 503–6

63. Moosa AR, Easter DW, van Sonnenberg E, Casola G, D'Agostino H. Laparoscopic injuries to the bile duct: a cause for concern. Ann Surg 1992; 164: 57–62

64. Nduka CC, Super PA, Monson JR, Darzi AW. Cause and prevention of electrosurgical injuries in laparoscopy [see comments]. J Am Coll Surg 1994; 179: 161–70

65. Soderstrom RM. Electrosurgical injuries during laparoscopy: prevention and management. Curr Opin Obstet Gynecol 1994; 6: 248–50

66. Hunter JG. Laser use in laparoscopic surgery. Surg Clin North Am 1992; 72: 655–64

67. Voyles CR, Tucker RD. Education and engineering solutions for potential problems with laparoscopic monopolar electrosurgery. Am J Surg 1992; 164: 57–62

68. Willson PD, van der Walt JD, Moxon D, Rogers J. Port site electrosurgical (diathermy) burns during surgical laparoscopy. Surg Endosc 1997; 11: 653–4

69. McAnena OJ, Willson PD. Diathermy in laparoscopic surgery. Br J Surg 1993; 80: 1094–6

70. Corbitt JD. Laparoscopic cholecystectomy: laser versus electrosurgery. Surg Laparosc Endosc 1991; 1: 85–8

71. Dretler SP. Laser lithotripsy: a review of 20 years of research and clinical applications. Lasers Surg Med 1988; 8: 341–56

72. Amaral JF. Laparoscopic application of an ultrasonically activated scalpel. Gastrointest Endosc Clin North Am 1993; 3: 381–91

73. Murai R, Ando H, Hirohara S et al. Laparoscopic cholecystectomy with an ultrasound surgical aspirator. Surg Endosc 1995; 9: 88–90

74. Hambley R, Hebda PA, Abell E, Cohen BA, Jegasothy BV. Wound healing of skin incisions produced by ultrasonically vibrating knife, scalpel, electrosurgery, and carbon dioxide laser. J Dermatol Surg Oncol 1988; 14: 1213–7

75. Baer HU, Maddern GJ, Blumgart LH. New water-jet dissector: initial experience in hepatic surgery. Br J Surg 1991; 78: 502–3

76. Adamsen S, Hansen OH, Funch–Jensen P et al. Bile duct injury during laparoscopic cholecystectomy: a prospective nationwide series. J Am Coll Surg 1997; 184: 571–8

77. Flowers JL, Zucker KA, Graham SM et al. Laparoscopic cholangiography. Results and indications. Ann Surg 1992; 215: 209–16

19 Treatment strategies for benign bile duct injury and biliary stricture

Lygia Stewart

There are many factors to consider when treating a patient with a bile duct injury or benign biliary stricture. There are many causes of biliary stricture (Table 19.1), but most bile duct injuries or strictures occur as a result of cholecystectomy for symptomatic gallstone disease. The majority of these patients are young (40–50 years), female, have a long

Table 19.1 Causes of biliary stricture

Postoperative bile duct injury or stricture
- Biliary surgical procedures:
  Cholecystectomy
  Common bile duct exploration
  Biliary–enteric anastomoses (especially with normal-sized ducts)
- Other abdominal procedures:
  Gastrectomy
  Pancreatic operations
  Hepatectomy
  Portacaval shunt or other portal vein procedures

Traumatic bile duct injury
- Following blunt penetrating trauma

Inflammatory
- Chronic pancreatitis
- Gallstones and recurrent cholangitis
- Subhepatic abscess, liver abscess
- Parasitic infections

Other
- Primary sclerosing cholangitis
- Radiation fibrosis
- Duodenal diverticulum
- Papillary stenosis
- Chronic duodenal ulcer

life expectancy, and are in the most productive years of their life. Because of this, it is essential that these patients have prompt recognition of their problem and a reliable treatment with a long-term success rate. Unlike malignant strictures, treatment durability is an essential factor in determining treatment success for benign biliary strictures.

The changing pattern of the surgical management of gallstone disease is also an important factor. Laparoscopic cholecystectomy has largely replaced open cholecystectomy for the management of gallstone disease. In addition, not only are bile duct injuries following laparoscopic cholecystectomy more prevalent than following open cholecystectomy,[1] but their clinical presentation is different. The symptoms of patients with laparoscopic bile duct injuries are usually more vague than those following open cholecystectomy. Thus, it is important to be able to recognize these symptoms and initiate an appropriate evaluation and treatment plan. Three factors increase the morbidity associated with the treatment of these injuries: delay in diagnoses, extended length of treatment, and treatment failure.

Laparoscopic bile duct injuries

Injury classification (Figs 19.1 and 19.2)

Traditionally, biliary strictures have been classified using the Bismuth classification. This system relates to the level of the stricture and is shown in Fig. 19.1. As can be seen, Bismuth type I is a stricture in the common duct >2 cm from the hepatic bifurcation, a type II is a stricture in the common hepatic duct

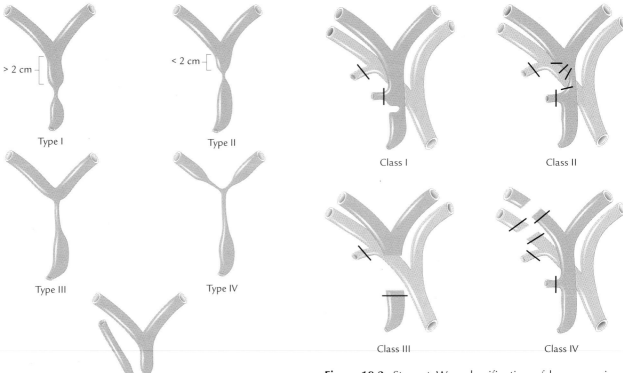

> 2 cm

Type I

< 2 cm

Type II

Type III

Type IV

Type V

Figure 19.1 Classification of biliary injuries and stricture based on the Bismuth classification of malignant biliary strictures.

Class I

Class II

Class III

Class IV

Figure 19.2 Stewart–Way classification of laparoscopic bile duct injuries.

<2 cm from the bifurcation, a type III is at the bifurcation, a type IV is above the bifurcation of the right and left hepatic ducts, and a type V is a stricture of a right sectorial duct that comes off the common hepatic duct before the main hepatic duct bifurcation. This classification has proven useful in determining the difficulty of the reconstruction and comparing surgical results.

Because laparoscopic cholecystectomy has become the standard of treatment for symptomatic gallstones, laparoscopic bile duct injuries now comprise the majority of biliary injuries. We have analyzed a large number of these laparoscopic bile duct injuries and note that these injuries present in a different manner than injuries associated with open cholecystectomy, the mechanism of injury is different, and classification of these injuries can aid in their diagnoses and treatment. We have found that there are four patterns of laparoscopic bile duct injuries, and these are shown in Fig. 19.2. Class I injuries involve incision of the common bile duct with no loss of duct; class II injuries consist of a stenosis of the duct with or without an associated fistula; class III injuries involve transection and excision of a large, variable portion of the common bile duct, common hepatic duct, or right and left hepatic ducts; and class IV injuries involve damage (partial excision or incision) to the right hepatic duct (or a right sectorial duct) plus, often (65–70%), injury to or ligation of the right hepatic artery. Division or injury of the right or common hepatic artery can also be seen in association with about 20% of class II and 20–25% of class III injuries.

This laparoscopic bile duct injury classification complements the Bismuth classification, which would further identify the level of a class II or III injury for example. Unlike the type V stricture of the Bismuth classification, we noted that the majority of injuries to the right ductal system involved the main right hepatic duct rather than a sectorial duct. The other difference between this classification system and the Bismuth system is that it corresponds to the mechanism of the injury, which can aid in efforts to prevent these injuries.

In addition to injuries of the main bile ducts, cystic duct leaks can occur, as well as complex bile leaks from right-sided biliary radicles in the gallbladder bed that are injured when the dissection is carried too deep into the hepatic parenchyma.

Table 19.2 **Mechanism of laparoscopic bile duct injury**	
Class I	CBD mistaken for cystic duct, but recognized
	Cholangiogram incision in cystic duct extended into CBD
Class II	Bleeding, poor visibility
	Multiple clips placed on CBD/CHD
Class III	CBD mistaken for cystic duct, not recognized
	CBD/Hepatic ducts transected and/or resected
Class IV	RHD (or R sectorial duct) mistaken for cystic duct
	R hepatic artery mistaken for cystic artery
	RHD (or R sectorial duct) and R hepatic artery transected

Mechanism of injury (Table 19.2)

An understanding of the mechanism of these injuries can not only help prevent their occurrence, but also aid in their identification. Table 19.2 lists the mechanism of injury for laparoscopic bile duct injuries.

Class I injuries occur in two ways. First, when the common bile duct is mistaken for the cystic duct, but the mistake is identified with an operative cholangiogram. Second, when the cystic duct incision for the cholangiogram catheter is inadvertently extended into the common bile duct. Class II injuries result when clips are mistakenly applied to the bile duct during attempts to control bleeding. The surgeon's view of the structures in this area invariably has been compromised by the bleeding when this injury occurs. We noted that some patients with class II injuries had a right hepatic artery that originated from the superior mesenteric artery, which probably contributed to the injury. Class Ill injuries, the most common, occur when the common bile duct is confused with the cystic duct and subsequently transected. This is a deliberate action because the surgeon thinks that it is the cystic duct. Generally, a portion of the common bile duct and part of the common hepatic duct are removed during the gallbladder dissection. In some cases, the resection can follow the biliary radicles into the porta and involve resection to the level of the right and left hepatic ducts, or even higher into the right and left sectorial ducts. Class IV injuries are caused by misidentifying the right hepatic duct (or a right sectorial duct) for the cystic duct, and the right hepatic artery for the cystic artery (often thought to be a second cystic artery).

Cystic duct leaks occur when clips on the cystic duct either become dislodged or do not encompass the entire duct. Complex leaks from the gallbladder bed can occur when the dissection is carried too deep into the hepatic parenchyma, injuring small biliary radicles.

Clinical presentation (Table 19.3)

Class I injuries

The clinical and radiographic findings according to class of injury are listed in Table 19.3. Most class I injuries are recognized intraoperatively (about 60–70%) either when an intraoperative cholangiogram demonstrates the injury or when bile is observed draining from the injured (but not transected) common bile duct. About 30% of class I injuries are not recognized intraoperatively. These patients present with mild abdominal pain, abdominal distention, ileus, with mild elevations in alkaline phosphatase (average 250 U/l) and bilirubin (average 2.3 mg/dl). In the group we analyzed, none of these patients were clinically jaundiced. Ultrasound and CT scans demonstrate an abdominal fluid collection without dilated bile ducts. ERCP reveals an intact biliary tree with a fistula.

Class II injuries

Patients with this class of injury present with the signs and symptoms classically associated with bile duct injuries. The majority of these patients (60–70%) present with obstructive jaundice, pruritus, and occasionally cholangitis, with elevated bilirubin and alkaline phosphatase levels. The remainder of the patients, who have associated biliary fistulas, present similar to class I injuries with mild abdominal pain, abdominal distention, ileus, with mild elevations in alkaline phosphatase and none to mild (2.4 mg/dl) elevations in bilirubin. Some patients may have a prolonged bile leak from a surgically placed drain that then closes, with the subsequent development of a biliary stricture and jaundice. CT and ultrasound scans demonstrate dilated bile ducts in patients without biliary fistulas, or non-dilated ducts and abdominal fluid collections in patients with associated biliary fistulas. ERCP shows the lesion, invariably with multiple clips overlying it (Fig. 19.3), with or without a fistula.

Table 19.3 Clinical and radiologic presentation of laparoscopic bile duct injuries

	Clinical presentation	Imaging studies
Cystic duct leak	Abdominal pain, distention	CT/US: non-dilated ducts, fluid collection ERCP: intact ducts, fistula at cystic duct stump
Class I	Abdominal pain, distention, Cholangiogram ID injury	CT/US: non-dilated ducts, fluid collection ERCP: intact ducts, fistula
Class II	Jaundice, pruritus, abdominal pain, with fistula: distention	CT/US: dilated ducts or non-dilated ducts, ± fluid ERCP: multiple clips CBD/CHD, stricture, ± fistula
Class III	Abdominal pain, distention, fever, leukocytosis	CT/US: non-dilated ducts, fluid collection ERCP: truncated CBD with clip, non-filling hepatic ducts PTC: hepatic ducts separate from CBD, with fistula HIDA: tracer into abdomen, not CBD or duodenum
Class IV	Hemorrhage, distention, abdominal pain, fever, leukocytosis	CT/US: non-dilated ducts, fluid collection ERCP: non-filling right hepatic duct, clip right hepatic duct PTC: right hepatic duct separate from CHD, with fistula HIDA: tracer into CBD, duodenum, and abdomen

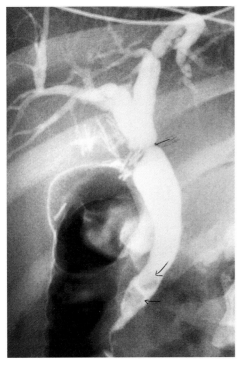

Figure 19.3 Cholangiogram of a class II bile duct injury. Note clips causing biliary stricture.

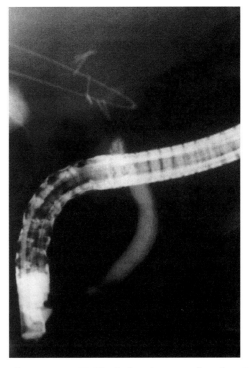

Figure 19.4 ERCP cholangiogram of a class III injury. Note truncated common duct and clip occluding it. This cholangiogram demonstrates only the distal extent of the injury and is therefore incomplete; PTC is needed to delineate the proximal extent of the injury.

Class III injuries

Patients with class III injuries present like class I injuries, only they can have a more toxic illness. About 25% of these injuries are recognized during the index operation when bile is seen to drain from the common (or hepatic) duct. The remainder of patients present later with abdominal pain, abdominal distention, ileus, and cholangitis. Laboratory abnormalities are highly variable in these patients. Total bilirubin can be normal or elevated (average of 4–5 mg/dl), alkaline phosphatase can be normal to elevated (average of 225 U/l), and white blood cell count similarly can be normal to mildly elevated (average 13 000/cm²). CT and ultrasound scans demonstrate an abdominal fluid collection and non-dilated bile ducts. ERCP distinguishes class III from other bile duct injuries involving a biliary fistula. The findings in class III injuries consist of a truncated common bile duct that is occluded with a clip, and non-filling of the biliary radicles (Fig. 19.4). PTC demonstrates the proximal extent of these injuries.

Class IV injuries

These patients present with abdominal pain, abdominal distention, ileus, cholangitis, hepatic abscess (20–25%), and, unlike the other injuries, many (45%) of these patients can have associated severe hemorrhage requiring large blood transfusions. On evaluation, CT and ultrasound demonstrate non-dilated ducts and fluid collections. ERCP demonstrates injury to or occlusion of the right hepatic duct (or a right sectorial duct) by a clip, and PTC demonstrates a fistula from the right hepatic ductal system.

Cystic duct leaks and complex bile leaks

Patients with cystic duct leaks present similar to those with class I injuries and are differentiated from major biliary injuries with cholangiography. Complex bile leaks from small peripheral branches of the right hepatic duct can also occur due to dissection into the liver during removal of the gallbladder from the hepatic bed. These patients present with abdominal pain, distention, ileus, fever, and because the site of the leak is often not appreciated early, can often develop sepsis, jaundice, and abdominal abscess. The diagnoses can be difficult. On evaluation, CT demonstrates non-dilated ducts and fluid collections. ERCP shows an intact common bile duct and sometimes demonstrates the biliary fistula from a branch of the right hepatic duct, but not always. HIDA scans, which are generally not useful in major biliary injuries, can be helpful in these leaks and will demonstrate bile flow into the common bile duct as well as the abdomen. Unlike cystic duct leaks, which are easily managed, these patients can have a severe clinical course with the development of abdominal abscess, yeast infections, sepsis, and ARDS.

Diagnoses, evaluation and initial management

Intraoperative diagnoses (Table 19.4)

Several features of the gallbladder dissection might indicate a possible bile duct injury. These are summarized in Table 19.4. Routine cholangiography, if used, can often prevent a serious injury to the common bile duct, that is, it can limit the injury to a class I injury rather than class III injury. Abnormalities of the routine cholangiogram that indicate that the common duct has been mistaken for the cystic duct include failure to opacify the

---

Table 19.4 Intraoperative clues to a bile duct injury

- Cholangiogram abnormalities:
    - Failure to opacify the proximal hepatic ducts
    - Narrowing of the CBD at the site of cholangiogram catheter insertion
- Bile drainage:
    - Drainage of bile from any location other than a lacerated gallbladder
    - Bile draining from a tubular structure
- Atypical features of cystic duct:
    - A 'cystic duct' that is not completely encompassed by the standard M/L clip, which measures 9 mm in the closed position, the structure may be the common duct
    - A 'cystic duct' that can be traced without interruption behind the duodenum, that will prove to be the common duct, not the cystic duct
- Anomalous anatomy:
    - Second cystic duct, aberrant duct, accessory duct, or suspected duct of Lushka, these are generally the common duct or a hepatic duct
    - Second cystic artery, this may be the right hepatic artery
    - Lymphatics surrounding the 'cystic duct' or more tissue around the cystic duct than is usually encountered, this indicates that the dissection is in the porta
    - Fibrous tissue in the gallbladder bed, indicates transection of the proximal hepatic ducts

proximal hepatic ducts, and narrowing of the common bile duct at the insertion site of the cholangiogram catheter. If the proximal hepatic ducts do not fill during cholangiography, the patient should be positioned in Trendelenburg, the bile aspirated from the duct, morphine sulphate given to cause spasm of the sphincter of Oddi, and the study repeated using fluoroscopy if possible. Failure to opacify the proximal ducts after these measures generally indicates that the cholangiocatheter is in the common bile duct (rather than the cystic duct), and there is a class I bile duct injury. Failure to recognize it at this point would result in transection of the common duct and transformation of the injury into a more serious, class III injury.

The finding of what appears to be atypical or unusual anatomy during the gallbladder dissection might also indicate that the common duct is being dissected rather than the cystic duct. Bile drainage from any location other than a lacerated gallbladder generally indicates a bile duct injury, especially if the bile is draining from a tubular structure. Certain features of what is thought to be the cystic duct might also indicate that the common duct, rather than the cystic duct, is being dissected. These include a duct that is not completely encompassed by the standard M/L clip (which is 9 mm in the closed position), and a duct that can be traced without interruption behind the duodenum. Finally, any suspicion that there is anomalous anatomy should raise the suspicion that the common duct is being dissected rather than the cystic duct. Examples of anomalous anatomy include a second cystic duct, aberrant duct, accessory duct, or suspected duct of Lushka, these are generally the common duct or a hepatic duct; a second cystic artery, this may be the right hepatic artery; lymphatics surrounding the 'cystic duct' or more tissue around the cystic duct than is usually encountered, which indicates that the dissection is in the porta; and fibrous tissue in the gallbladder bed, which can indicate transection of the proximal hepatic duct.

If any of these features are present, the surgeon should re-examine the area and re-identify the anatomy. Ultrasound can be used to aid in identification of ductal structures, and a cholangiogram should be obtained to document the anatomy. If an anomalous duct, or bile draining from a tubular structure is seen, a cholangiogram of this duct needs to be obtained. If the anatomy cannot be reliably sorted out, the procedure should be converted to an open operation, and this should be the default unless the anatomy is clearly identified. It is important to remember that any potential morbidity from a laparotomy is minor compared to a bile duct injury.

Postoperative diagnosis

As noted above, laparoscopic bile duct injuries present in a more occult manner than biliary injuries associated with open cholecystectomy. Most patients (70–80%) have an associated biliary fistula and present with abdominal pain, distention, ileus, nausea, with occasional fever and leukocytosis. Also, despite large amounts of bilious ascites, patients with a biliary fistula are often (40–50%) not jaundiced or severely ill, and laboratory data can be normal or minimally abnormal. Any patient who presents with these findings, or persistent biliary drainage from a surgical drain, either during their initial hospitalization, at a follow-up visit, or in the emergency room, should be considered to have a bile duct injury until proven otherwise. In addition, a complication should also be suspected in patients who require a prolonged (>3 days) postoperative hospital stay after a laparoscopic cholecystectomy.

Patients with evidence of a biliary fistula or jaundice should have an imaging study to look for fluid in the abdomen, either an ultrasound or preferably an abdominal CT scan. We do not recommend the use of an HIDA scan in this situation, since we have noted several instances where this test has been misleading or uninterpretable. If a fluid collection is found, it should be percutaneously drained. *The surgeon should not take the patient to the operating room for an exploratory laparotomy at this point.* If the fluid is bile, an ERCP should be obtained to delineate the anatomy. If the entire biliary tree is not imaged on ERCP, a PTC should be obtained to image the proximal biliary tree.

If a bile duct injury is found, there is no need to rush to the operating room. The patient should be stabilized first, bilious ascites drained, any infections controlled, and the anatomy of the injury clearly delineated prior to any consideration of repair.

Errors in diagnoses

In studying a large cohort of these patients we noted several errors that led to diagnostic delay. Failure to appreciate an abnormal postoperative course following laparoscopic cholecystectomy is the main cause of diagnostic delay. Because laparoscopic bile duct injuries present in a more occult manner than biliary injuries associated with open cholecystectomy, the importance of the clinical constellation of symptoms can be missed. Several diagnostic errors can occur:

(1) Failure to recognize that ileus, abdominal pain, and distention, which may be normal following an open cholecystectomy, is abnormal following a laparoscopic cholecystectomy.

(2) Failure to recognize that abdominal fluid collections or persistent bilious drainage (from a surgical or postsurgical drain) may represent a bile duct injury.

(3) Failure to recognize an injury during the first clinic (or emergency room) visit; or prior to discharge in a patient who requires a longer (>3 days) hospital stay.

(4) Failure to identify the injury during an exploratory laparotomy for bile ascites.

(5) Failure to obtain preoperative cholangiograms prior to an exploratory laparotomy.

When these errors are made, the injury is generally recognized later, often after 3 weeks, which increases the morbidity of the injury.

Treatment of bile duct injuries

While diagnostic delay contributes to the morbidity of bile duct injuries, the most significant morbidity is accrued when attempts at repair or treatment are unsuccessful or when the length of treatment spans several years.[2] The factors that should be considered in determining the success of a treatment include the initial and long-term success rates, the length of treatment (i.e. the time it takes for the treatment to be completed), and the morbidity and mortality of treatment.

Surgical repair

Most of these injuries and strictures are best repaired surgically. There are three factors that influence the surgical success rate: preoperative diagnostic evaluation, notably cholangiography, the surgical technique, and the experience of the surgeon.

Preoperative cholangiography

Knowledge of the extent and presence of a biliary injury is only possible with complete cholangiography. Patients with a suspected bile duct injury need to have their complete biliary tree imaged using ERCP and PTC if needed before any surgical procedure. In analyzing a large number of patients with bile duct injuries, we noted that patients frequently underwent exploratory operations, or operations to repair an injury, either without preoperative cholangiography (when fluid collections were noted on CT scan or ultrasound), or with incomplete cholangiography.[2] An example of incomplete cholangiography is shown in Fig. 19.4, where an ERCP demonstrates

transection and clipping of the CBD, but does not delineate the proximal bile ducts. Without obtaining a PTC, the surgeon has no knowledge of the extent of the bile duct injury. Since the magnitude of these injuries can be quite variable, from resection of a portion of the hepatic duct, to complete resection of the extrahepatic bile ducts, it would be difficult to impossible for the surgeon to sort this out in the operating room. Further, unless the surgeon knows that there *is* a bile duct injury, the tendency is to conclude that any ductal structure draining bile is the cystic duct stump, and oversew it. We noted that this occurred in about 30% of patients explored without a preoperative cholangiogram or in whom a cholangiogram was obtained during an exploratory laparotomy.[2]

Obtaining a preoperative cholangiogram greatly influenced the outcome of operations performed in response to a bile duct injury. When cholangiograms were not obtained preoperatively (or cholangiograms were obtained intraoperatively), operations to repair duct injuries were successful in only 4% of patients, 67% of patients had an unsuccessful attempt at repair, and the injury was missed in 29% of patients. When patients had an incomplete cholangiogram (imaging of the distal but not proximal biliary tree), attempts to repair the injury were successful in only 31% of patients, and failed in 69% of patients. But, operative repairs were successful in 84% of patients in whom cholangiographic data was complete preoperatively. These data are shown in Fig. 19.5.

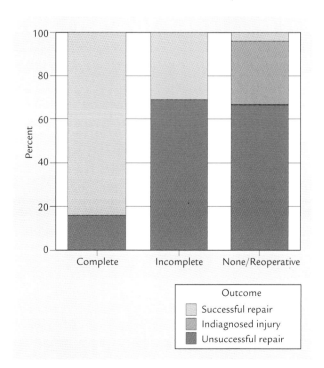

Figure 19.5 Preoperative cholangiography and success of surgical repair.

Surgical technique

The choice and technique of repair correlates with the success rate. When the common duct (or common hepatic duct) has been divided and there is sufficient length to perform an end-to-end anastomosis without tension, this is considered to be an option by many. We have noted, however, that end-to-end anastomoses have a high failure rate. In a large series of patients with laparoscopic bile duct injuries, we noted that all primary end-to-end repairs of class III injuries were unsuccessful when the duct had been divided.[2] Two other reports[3,4] noted similarly poor results (22% success rate) from this type of repair when the injury was repaired at the initial open cholecystectomy. Further, when this approach was used in reparative operations, even by surgeons who specialize in biliary surgery, it similarly had a lower long-term success rate than Roux-en-Y hepaticojejunostomy.[5–8]

The reasons for the high failure rate of end-to-end biliary anastomoses relate to ischemia and tension. The blood supply of the common duct is axial running at 3:00 and 9:00 on the duct. These vessels are small and easily damaged during extensive mobilization of the duct (as would occur during a cholecystectomy if the common duct was mistaken for the cystic duct). In addition, the majority of the blood supply (60%) comes from below, while only 38% comes from above, further contributing to ischemia in the proximal portion of the duct. Further, these ducts are invariably divided with electrocautery and a portion of the duct resected. This leaves damaged tissue, that needs to be debrided, resulting in too great a distance to allow for an end-to-end anastomosis to be performed without tension.

Roux-en-Y hepaticojejunostomy has the best success rate for the repair of a transection or resection injury of the common duct or common hepatic duct. Experienced surgeons report a success rate of 80–99%, and, in series that include less experienced surgeons, the success rate is 60–70%.[2,5–22]

Certain technical factors are important in achieving this high degree of success. The essential elements of a successful hepaticojejunostomy are listed in Table 19.5. We analyzed a large number of bile duct injury repairs, including patients repaired by our group and by surgeons in the community. We noted that when these principles were not employed, there was a high failure rate.[2] These data are shown in Fig. 19.6, where the percentage of successful and unsuccessful repairs utilizing these principles is shown. As can be seen, more than 60% of successful repairs employed preoperative drainage of bilious ascites, debridement of damaged or scarred bile duct, a single-layer

---

Table 19.5 Tenets of a successful surgical repair

- Preoperative eradication of intra-abdominal infection and inflammation
- Viable ductal tissue (excise damaged ductal tissue)
- Single-layer mucosa-to-mucosa anastomosis
- Fine, monofilament, absorbable suture
- Alleviate tension on the anastomoses (tack-up Roux limb)
- Stenting is not necessary (except very small ducts)

---

anastomosis with absorbable suture, and support of the Roux limb. In contrast, only 16% of unsuccessful repairs controlled intra-abdominal infection, 9% debrided scarred and/or damaged ducts, and only 40% used a single-layer anastomosis using absorbable suture with support of the Roux limb.

The question of whether to stent is disputed. Many surgical groups feel strongly that stenting is necessary, we have not found that placement of stents makes a difference in the success of most biliary repairs, and others have reported similar findings. Stenting is useful, however, when very small ducts are repaired (class IV injuries or class III injuries

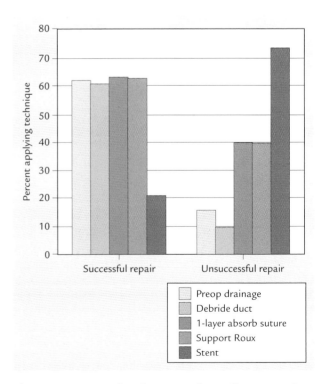

Figure 19.6 Surgical technique and its influence on the success of the repair.

where the resection has been carried high into the porta).

Surgical experience

The third factor that determines the success of a repair is the experience of the surgeon performing the repair. We have found this to be the most important factor in determining whether a patient has a successful repair. In the group of patients we analyzed, we noted that when the injury was repaired by the initial laparoscopic surgeon (or their partner), only 17% of primary repair attempts and no secondary repair attempts were successful. In contrast, 94% of repairs performed by a specialist in biliary surgery were successful.[2] This included primary repairs and secondary repairs following a previously failed repair by the initial laparoscopic surgeon.

Conduct of the operation

Injury detected intraoperatively

If a bile duct injury is detected intraoperatively, there are several issues to consider before proceeding with an operative repair. If the injury is a class I injury, detected with an intraoperative cholangiogram, the repair is usually straightforward. A laparotomy should be performed and the small defect in the common duct repaired with fine (5/0 or 6/0) monofilament absorbable sutures (e.g. Maxon). A CBDE is not needed and there is no need to place a T-tube, this only increases the size of the choledochotomy, and could further injure the duct if it is a normal size (<5 mm).

A class III injury occurs if a class I injury is not recognized before transection of the common duct. If such an injury has occurred, the magnitude of the injury and experience of the surgeon dictate the approach. If the common (or hepatic) duct has been transected or a portion resected, a Roux-en-Y hepaticojejunostomy (or choledochojejunostomy) should be performed if the surgeon feels confident performing the procedure. This should be done rather than attempting an end-to-end anastomosis, because this repair has a higher failure rate than Roux-en-Y hepaticojejunostomy, even in the best circumstances. The Roux-en-Y hepaticojejunostomy should be done with a single-layer, fine monofilament, absorbable suture, and the Roux limb should be supported to alleviate tension on the anastomosis. If the surgeon does not feel comfortable performing the repair, a small tube or tubes (like a feeding tube) can be placed into the injured duct(s) if they are clearly visible, the hepatic bed drained, and the patient referred to a specialist in biliary surgery. If the ducts are not readily identifiable, the hepatic bed should just be drained. A class II injury noted intraoperatively should be dealt with in a similar fashion. No attempt should be made to close the common duct over a T-tube when there is a partial (generally lateral) loss of duct, this will only result in a stricture when the T-tube is removed. The duct should be divided, the distal duct oversewn, and the proximal portion implanted into a Roux limb.

If the class III injury is high (near, at, or above the hepatic duct bifurcation), or if a class IV injury has occurred, these are more difficult injuries to repair. Not only are these ducts small normally, but these repairs often require dissection high into the porta. Unless the surgeon has extensive experience with such a repair, this patient should be referred to a surgeon who specializes in biliary surgery. A small tube or tubes (like a feeding tube) should be placed into the injured duct(s) if they are clearly visible, the hepatic bed drained, and the patient referred to a specialist in biliary surgery. The repair of these types of injuries will be described below.

Elective surgical repair of a bile duct injury

Several factors are important in achieving a successful repair in an elective situation. As previously noted, the intra-abdominal infection and inflammation need to be controlled by percutaneous drainage of any bile ascites, and the injury delineated using ERCP and PTC if needed. For high injuries of the bile ducts and class IV injuries, a PTC catheter placed into the damaged ducts can aid in identification of the ducts. The dissection starts at the liver and proceeds interiorly, taking down all adhesions to the undersurface of the liver and working down to the bile ducts. Once the bile duct has been identified, it should be circled with a vessel loop and the extent of the injury delineated. If the common duct is intact, but strictured, the stricture should be excised, the distal duct oversewn and a Roux-en-Y hepaticojejunostomy performed using the principles outlined above. If the duct has been transected, the proximal duct should be debrided back to healthy tissue, preserving as much duct length as possible, but being sure to get back to healthy, non-scarred tissue for the anastomosis. This, similarly, is repaired with a Roux-en-Y hepaticojejunostomy.

If the injury extends to the bifurcation of the right and left ducts, additional length for the anastomosis can be obtained by exposing the left hepatic duct which has a horizontal course at the base of the quadrate lobe (segment IV). Exposing this allows for a side-to-side anastomosis between the Roux limb and an incision extended into the left hepatic duct. This technique was described by Hepp and Couinaud and has been popularized by Blumgart. If the injury extends above the bifurcation of the right and left hepatic ducts, these ducts need to be re-implanted separately into the Roux limb. For class IV injuries, the right hepatic ducts (or a sectorial duct) are implanted into a Roux limb. No attempt should be made to suture the right hepatic duct to the common hepatic duct, since this would only injure this system as well.

Dilatation and stenting

Another method employed in the treatment of bile duct injuries is balloon dilatation and stenting.[9,23-34] The balloon dilatation can be performed either via an endoscopic approach for primary strictures in which the common duct has not been transected, or via a percutaneous transhepatic route for higher strictures or recurrent strictures following a hepaticojejunostomy. In these techniques, the stricture is traversed with a guidewire and a balloon catheter (angioplasty-type) threaded over this. The stricture is dilated using 4–10 mm balloons and dilatation is carried out until there is no 'waist deformity'. Following this, a stent is placed either transhepatically or endoscopically (depending on the access). Patients are stented for an average of one year (range 0.4–1.5 years). During the treatment period, the patients return for stent changes every 3–4 months. Most patients require numerous dilatation sessions (range 1–10). The treatment can be performed under conscious sedation, but a significant number of

patients find this too painful and require general anesthesia. Patients are hospitalized following the procedure and most require additional hospitalization for the treatment of cholangitis during the treatment period. The total length of hospitalization during treatment averaged 24 days (range 10–38) in the dilatation series reported in the literature. The early success rate at 6 months to 4 years averages 74%. There is considerable variation in success rates, however, with reports ranging from 27% to 95%.[2,9,23-34]

There have also been a small number of reports using metal stents for the treatment of benign strictures. These results have not been as good as balloon dilatation, with early results of 74%, but poor results of 42% at 2 years. In addition, when the treatment fails, the metal stent makes surgical reconstruction of the bile duct treacherous because the metal stent can become incorporated into the ductal tissue, requiring resection of the bile duct incorporated in the stented area. Given the poor results with metal stents and their interference with subsequent surgical reconstruction, these stents should not be used to treat benign strictures.[35-37]

Long-term success rate

Surgical repair versus dilatation and stenting (Fig. 19.7 and Table 19.6)

There have been numerous published series documenting the success rate of treatment of biliary strictures by surgical correction or balloon dilatation and stenting. These series,[2,5-34] listed in the references, are demonstrated graphically (Fig. 19.7) where the long-term success rate with

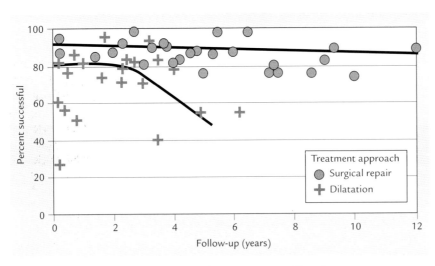

Figure 19.7 Long-term success rate of surgery versus dilatation.

Table 19.6 **Comparison of surgical repair with balloon dilatation and stenting**		
	Surgical repair average (range)	**Balloon dilatation** average (range)
Early success rate (0–4 years) (%)	89 (81–98)	74 (27–95)
Long-term success rate (>4 years) (%)	85 (74–99)	55
Length of treatment (days)	14 (7–27)	365 (146–550)
Hospitalization (days)	14 (7–27)	24 (10–38)
Morbidity (%)	19 (4–39)	28 (5–72)
Mortality (%)	1.6 (0–9)	1.3 (0–22)

surgery (red circles) and balloon dilatation (blue crosses) is shown. Comparison of the two techniques is summarized in Table 19.6. As can be seen, in the first 4 years, the success rates are similar, although surgery is on the average more successful (88%) than balloon dilatation (74%). But, at 5 years, the success rate with balloon dilatation drops to 55% while the surgical success rate continues to be 80–90% in published series followed up to 12.5 years. This superior long-term surgical success rate is important because patients with biliary strictures are typically young with a long life expectancy.

One area, however, where balloon dilatation has proved to be useful is the high recurrent stricture that has already been repaired by an experienced biliary surgeon. In this situation, it is reasonable to attempt balloon dilatation before proceeding with a second reconstruction. This approach can eliminate the need for a second operation in many instances.[9,13] In most dilatation series, however, many patients are treated with dilatation who are good candidates for surgical reconstruction. In general, this approach does not seem warranted.

Length of treatment, morbidity and mortality

One factor often not quantitated in evaluating the success of treatment is how long the treatment takes and the condition of the patient during the treatment phase. Clearly a treatment program that spans many months to years carries a higher morbidity if the patient experiences recurrent episodes of cholangitis during that time. Additionally, during an ongoing treatment program many patients may not be able to work or perform their usual duties, which is also a factor in overall morbidity. As noted above, treatment with balloon dilatation on average takes about 1 year. The morbidity of a long illness is not always appreciated when analyzing these series. We recently studied 90 patients with bile duct injuries resulting from laparoscopic cholecystectomy.[2] In this group there were 26 patients treated with balloon dilatation. Patients treated with balloon dilatation had the longest length of illness. This is shown in Fig. 19.8, where it can be seen that patients whose bile duct injuries were initially repaired by a specialist in biliary surgery had the

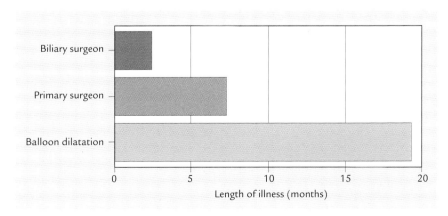

Figure 19.8 Length of illness and the influence of the treating physician.

shortest length of illness (2.5 months); patients whose injuries were repaired by the surgeon performing the cholecystectomy (primary surgeon) had an illness length of 7.3 months; and those treated with balloon dilatation had the longest illness length (19 months). Further, these patients were ill during treatment with balloon dilatation. They suffered from recurrent cholangitis, fatigue, reflux, and depression and most were not able to work at their usual jobs. The contribution each treatment made to the length of illness is shown in Fig. 19.9. It compares: patients who had one successful surgical repair, patients who required two repairs, patients who had an unsuccessful repair and successful balloon dilatation, and patients who had an unsuccessful surgical repair (by the primary surgeon), then unsuccessful balloon dilatation, followed by a successful surgical repair by a specialist in biliary surgery. The most striking finding here is that patients treated with two surgical repairs did not have a prolonged illness following their second repair (their average hospitalization was 11 days), even when it followed a prolonged treatment that included balloon dilatation. Further, patients treated with two surgical repairs had a shorter length of illness than those who underwent balloon dilatation following a failed surgical repair. The overall success of balloon dilatation in our series, 27%, was also lower than other reports. Additionally, reports of cost comparisons in the literature show the two regimens to be equal.[9]

Patients with biliary injuries and strictures who were immediately referred to a specialist in biliary surgery had the best success rate and the shortest length of illness. Those treated by their primary surgeon who required a subsequent repair (83% in our study) and who were then referred to a biliary surgeon had a longer length of illness, but those with the longest illness length were patients treated with balloon dilatation, especially if it followed a failed repair by their primary surgeon.[2]

The reported ranges of morbidity and mortality of surgical repair and balloon dilatation in the literature are surprisingly not all that different.[2,5–34] Surgery: morbidity, 4–29%; mortality, 0–9%; dilatation: morbidity, 5–72%; mortality, 0–22%. But, the real morbidity of an illness relates not just to the complications of treatment, but to the length of time the patient is ill and the number of procedures it takes to achieve a good, long-term result. As noted above, there are many factors that contribute to this including recognition of the problem, the preoperative evaluation, the treatment approach, and the surgeon (or physician) performing the treatment.

Biliary stricture secondary to chronic pancreatitis

Another cause of biliary stricture is chronic pancreatitis. These strictures comprise about 10% of biliary strictures and result from chronic fibrosis of the pancreas resulting in a stricture of the intrapancreatic portion of the common bile duct. The stricture results in cholestasis which is initially manifested by an elevated alkaline phosphatase and later hyperbilirubinemia, which may fluctuate. The clinical presentation of these patients can be quite variable from asymptomatic elevated alkaline phosphatase, intermittent jaundice, persistent jaundice with or without abdominal pain, to cholangitis and even liver abscess. With prolonged cholestasis these patients may develop secondary biliary cirrhosis. Most of these patients also have other complications of chronic pancreatitis including chronic abdominal pain, pancreatic pseudocyst formation, pancreatic insufficiency, and diabetes.

These patients should be evaluated with an abdominal CT scan to look at the pancreas as well as ERCP, which generally demonstrates a long tapered stricture of the intrapancreatic duct. The stricture can

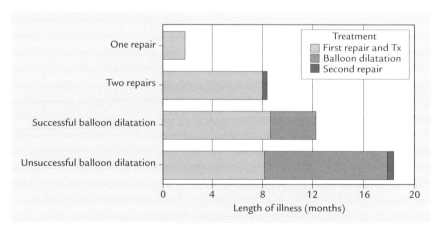

Figure 19.9 Contribution of treatments to length of illness.

also have an hour-glass configuration with stenosis at the point the common bile duct enters the pancreas. CT scan most often shows pancreatic findings consistent with chronic pancreatitis which include calcification of the pancreas, pancreatic stones, a dilated pancreatic duct, fibrosis of the pancreas, and pancreatic pseudocyst. The dilated pancreatic duct can also be seen on the ERCP, often with a chain of lakes appearance. The finding of a pseudocyst in the head of the pancreas associated with a biliary stricture does not indicate that the cyst is the cause of the stricture. Simply draining the cyst will usually not eliminate the stricture, the stricture needs to be treated.

The key is to distinguish a biliary stricture associated with chronic pancreatitis from a pancreatic malignancy. Clinically, most patients with pancreatic carcinoma present with painless jaundice and do not have a long history of pancreatitis and chronic abdominal pain, which is the typical pattern for patients with chronic pancreatitis. The patient with malignancy has progressive elevation of bilirubin, while the patient with a benign stricture may have intermittent hyperbilirubinemia. Also, the bilirubin level tends to be higher in the patient with malignancy. On imaging studies, patients with a pancreatic cancer will generally have a mass in the head of the pancreas, while patients with chronic pancreatitis will generally show diffuse pancreatic enlargement with the signs of chronic pancreatitis noted above. On ERCP, the benign biliary strictures have a long smooth tapering appearance while those associated with malignancy typically show a more abrupt cut-off and are often more irregular.

Surgical treatment of these strictures is indicated if the stricture produces cholestasis, especially in the setting of jaundice, cholangitis, abdominal pain, choledocholithiasis, or hepatic fibrosis.[7,38-47] Many recommend surgical correction when cholestasis is manifested simply by an elevated alkaline phosphatase because of the risk of developing secondary biliary cirrhosis,[38,39,41,44,46,47] and others recommend serial liver biopsies.[48] One of the best studies that examined the incidence of secondary biliary cirrhosis in patients with biliary strictures due to chronic pancreatitis is that of Afrodakis and Kaplowitz,[38] who noted a 29% incidence. Others[43,44,49] have noted a lower incidence of this complication. Additionally, any biliary stricture present should be corrected concurrently during surgical treatment of other complications of chronic pancreatitis.

Because these strictures occur in the distal common bile duct they are easily managed with either a Roux-en-Y choledochojejunostomy or choledochoduodenostomy with excellent results. We prefer to use an end-to-side choledochoduodenostomy for treatment of these lesions. Use of an end-to-side rather than a side-to-side anastomosis prevents possible problems with a sump syndrome, and is an easy procedure. The common duct is transected above the duodenum (after a Kocher maneuver has been performed), the distal end sutured with absorbable suture, and the proximal end implanted into the duodenum using a single layer of fine monofilament absorbable sutures. The gallbladder should always be removed as well to prevent future cholelithiasis.

Summary

In conclusion, the crucial steps in the management of bile ducts injuries and stricture are:

(1) Suspect an injury when the patient's postoperative course is atypical following a laparoscopic or open cholecystectomy, including the presence of abdominal pain, distention, ileus, jaundice, fluid in the abdomen, a persistent bile leak, or a longer than normal hospitalization postoperatively (3 or more days).
(2) Screen with imaging studies (CT, US).
(3) If a fluid collection or bile leak is found, establish drainage to gain control of abdominal infection and *assume that a bile duct injury is present until proven otherwise.*
(4) Define the anatomy of the injury with an ERCP and a PTC if the entire biliary tree is not imaged on the ERCP.
(5) Decide on a course of management.

In considering a plan of management remember that there is no need to rush to surgery, it is important to stabilize the patient, eliminate intra-abdominal infection, delineate the injury, and maximize the possibility for a successful repair. Further, surgeons who specialize in the repair of bile duct injuries have a higher success rate than those with less experience. Finally, non-surgical management of biliary strictures (e.g. balloon dilatation and stenting) may have a higher failure rate than usually reported, does not have a high long-term success rate (compared to surgery), and substantially increases the duration of disability.

Key points

- Suspect bile duct injuries if postoperative course is atypical after cholecystectomy.
- Image: US/CT, and drain fluid collection.
- Define anatomy: ERCP/PTC.
- Refer to specialist center for definiting management.

Suspicion of bile duct injury at cholecystectomy

- Perform cholangiography.
- Convert to laparotomy.
- Small defect in common duct: primary repair.
- Class III: Roux-en-Y hepaticojejunostomy and refer.
- Class IV: immediate referral to tertiary center.
- Advise patient of injury and arrange long-term follow-up.

Suspicion of bile duct injury after cholecystectomy

- Failure to progress in the postoperative period: abdominal pain distention/ileus/nausea fever/leukocytosis.
- Persistent biliary drainage.
- Jaundice.
- Immediately suspect bile duct injury: LFTs US/CT: exclude bile ascites—drain ERCP and/or PTC.
- Refer to tertiary center.

REFERENCES

1. Deziel DJ, Millikan KW, Economou SG, Doolas A, Ko ST, Airan MC. Complications of laparoscopic cholecystectomy: a national survey of 4,292 hospitals and an analysis of 77,704 cases. Am J Surg 1993; 165: 9–14

2. Stewart L, Way LW. Bile duct injuries during laparoscopic cholecystectomy. Factors that influence the results of treatment. Arch Surg 1995; 130: 1123–8; discussion 1129

3. Andren-Sandberg A, Johansson S, Bengmark S. Accidental lesions of the common bile duct at cholecystectomy II. Results of treatment. Ann Surg 1985; 201: 452–5

4. Csendes A, Diaz JC, Burdiles P, Maluenda F. Late results of immediate primary end to and repair in accidental section of the common bile duct. Surg Gynecol Obstet 1989; 168: 125–30

5. Pellegrini CA, Thomas MJ, Way LW. Recurrent biliary stricture. Patterns of recurrence and outcome of surgical therapy. Am J Surg 1984; 147: 175–80

6. Genest JF, Nanos E, Grundfest-Broniatowski S et al. Benign biliary strictures: an analytic review (1970 to 1984). Surgery 1986; 99: 409–13

7. Lillemoe KD, Pitt HA, Cameron JL. Current management of benign bile duct strictures. Advance Surg 1992; 25: 119–74

8. Warren KW, Mountain JC, Midell AJ. Management of strictures of the biliary tract. Surg Clin N Am 1971; 51: 711–31

9. Pitt HA, Kaufman SL, Coleman J et al. Benign postoperative biliary strictures. Operate or dilate? Ann Surg 1989; 210: 417–25; discussion 426–7

10. Frattaroli FM, Reggio D, Guadalaxara A, Illomei G, Pappalardo G. Benign biliary strictures: a review of 21 years of experience. J Am Coll Surg 1996; 183: 506–13

11. Kozicki I, Bielecki K, Kawalski A et al. Repeated rconstruction for recurrent benign bile stricture. Br J Surg 1994; 81: 677–9

12. Raute M, Podlech P, Jaschke W, Manegold BC, Trede M, Chir B. Management of bile duct injuries and strictures following cholecystectomy. World J Surg 1993; 17: 553–62

13. Millis JM, Tompkins RK, Zinner MJ, Longmire WP Jr, Roslyn JJ. Management of bile duct strictures. An evolving strategy. Arch Surg 1992; 127: 1077–82; discussion 1082–4

14. Csendes A, Diaz C, Burdiles P et al. Indications and results of hepaticojejunostomy in benign strictures of the biliary tract. Hepatogastroenterology 1992; 39: 333–6

15. Ross CB, H'Doubler WZ, Sharp KW et al. Recent experience with benign biliary strictures. Am Surg 1989; 55: 64–70

16. Innes JT, Ferrara JJ, Carey LC. Biliary reconstruction without transanastomotic stent. Am Surg 1988; 54: 27–30

17. Way LW, Bernhoft RA, Thomas MJ. Biliary stricture. Surg Clin N Am 1981; 61: 963–72

18. Bergman JJ, van den Brink GR, Rauws EA et al. Treatment of bile duct lesions after laparoscopic cholecystectomy. Gut 1996; 38: 141–7

19. Nealon WH, Urrutia F. Long-term follow-up after bilioenteric anastomosis for benign bile duct strictures. Ann Surg 1996; 223: 639–45; discussion 645–8

20. Soper NJ, Flye MW, Brunt LM et al. Diagnoses and management of biliary complications of laparoscopic cholecystectomy. Am J Surg 1993; 165: 663–9

21. Branum G, Schmitt C, Bailie J et al. Management of major biliary complications after laparoscopic cholecystectomy. Ann Surg 1993; 217: 532–41

22. Trerotola SO, Savader SJ, Lund GB et al. Biliary tract complications following laparoscopic cholecystectomy: imaging and intervention. Radiology 1992; 184: 195–200

23. Vitale GC, George M, McIntyre K, Larson GM, Wieman TJ. Endoscopic management of benign and malignant biliary strictures. Am J Surg 1996; 171: 553–7

24. Kozarek RA, Ball TJ, Traverso LW. Endoscopic treatment of biliary injury in the era of laparoscopic cholecystectomy. Gastrointest Endosc 1994; 40: 10–6

25. Davids PH, Tanka AK, Rauws EA et al. Benign biliary strictures. Surgery or endoscopy? Ann Surg 1993; 217: 237–43

26. Vitale GC, Stephens G, Wieman TJ, Larson GM. Use of endoscopic retrograde cholangiopancreatography in the management of biliary complications after laparoscopic cholecystectomy [published erratum appears in Surgery 1994; 115: 263]. Surgery 1993; 114: 806–12; discussion 812–4

27. Davids PH, Rauws EA, Coene PP et al. Endoscopic stenting for post-operative biliary strictures. Gastrointest Endosc 1992; 38: 12–8

28. Citron SJ, Martin LG. Benign biliary strictures: treatment with percutaneous cholangioplasty. Radiology 1991; 178: 339–41

29. Geenen DJ, Geenen JE, Hogan WJ et al. Endoscopic therapy for benign bile duct strictures. Gastrointest Endosc 1989; 35: 367–71

30. Berkelhammer C, Kortan P, Haber GB. Endoscopic biliary prostheses as treatment for benign postoperative bile duct strictures. Gastrointest Endosc 1989; 35: 95–101

31. Moore AV Jr, Illescas FF, Mills SR et al. Percutaneous dilation of benign biliary strictures. Radiology 1987; 163: 625–8

32. Williams HJ Jr, Bender CE, May GR. Benign postoperative biliary strictures: dilation with fluoroscopic guidance. Radiology 1987; 163): 629–34

33. Mueller PR, vanSonnenberg E, Ferrucci JT Jr et al. Biliary stricture dilatation: multicenter review of clinical management in 73 patients. Radiology 1986; 160: 17–22

34. Vogel SB, Howard RJ, Caridi J et al. Evaluation of percutaneous transhepatic balloon dilatation of benign biliary strictures in high-risk patients. Am J Surg 1985; 149: 73–9

35. Bonnel DH, Liguory CL, Lefebvre JF, Cornud FE. Placement of metallic stents for treatment of postoperative biliary strictures: long term outcome in 25 patients. Am J Roentgenol 1997; 169: 1517–22

36. Hausegger KA, Kugler C, Uggowitzer M et al. Benign biliary obstruction: is treatment with the Wallstent advisable? Radiology 1996; 200: 437–41

37. Tesdal IK, Adamus R, Poeckler C et al. Therapy for biliary stenoses and occlusions with use of three different metallic stents: single-center experience. J Vasc Interven Radiol 1997; 8: 869–79

38. Afroudakis A, Kaplowitz N. Liver histopathology in chronic common biole duct stenosis to chronic alcoholic pancreatitis. Hepatology 1981; 1: 65–72

39. Wilson C, Auld CD, Schlinkert R et al. Hepatobiliary complications in chronic pancreatitis. Gut 1989; 30: 520–7

40. Sarles H, Sahel J. Cholestasis and lesions of the biliary tract in chronic pancreatitis. Gut 1978; 19: 851–7

41. Warshaw AL, Schapiro RH, Ferrucci JT et al. Persistant obstructive jaundice, cholangitis, and biliary cirrhosis due to common duct stenosis in chronic pancreatitis. Gastroenterology 1976; 70: 562–7

42. Petrozza JA, Dutta SK, Latham PS et al. Prevalence and natural history of distal common bile duct stenosis in chronic alcohol-induced pancreatitis. Ann Surg 1989; 210: 608–13

43. Stahl TJ, O'Connor AM, Ansel HJ et al. Partial biliary obstruction caused by chronic pancreatitis. An appraisal of indications for surgical biliary drainage. Ann Surg 1988; 201: 26–32.

44. Araha GV, Prinz RA, Preeark RJ et al. The spectrum of biliary tract obstruction from chronic pancreatitis. Arch Surg 1984; 119: 595–600

45. Yadegar J, Williams RA, Passaro E et al. Common duct stricture from chronic pancreatitis. Arch Surg 1980; 115: 582–6

46. Stabile BE, Wilson SE, Passaro E. Stricture of the common bile duct from chronic pancreatitis. Surg Gynecol Obstet 1987; 165: 121–6

47. Buehler H, Muench R, Schmid M et al. Cholestasis in alcoholic chronic pancreatitis: diagnostic value of transaminase ratio for differentiation between extra- and intrahepatic cholestasis. Scand J Gastroenterol 1985; 20: 851–6

48. Lesur G, Phillippe L, Jean-Francois F et al. Factors predictive of liver histopathological appearance in chronic alcoholic pancreatitis with common bile duct stenosis and increased serum alkaline phosphatase. Hepatology 1993; 18: 1078–81

49. Kalvaria I, Bornman PC, Marks IN et al. The spectrum and natural history of common bile duct stenosis in chronic alcohol-induced pancreatitis. Ann Surg 1989; 210: 608–13

20 Treatment of laparoscopically discovered gallbladder cancer

Yuman Fong and David L Bartlett

Introduction

A great deal of pessimism has traditionally been associated with the treatment of gallbladder cancer. There are many reasons for the general nihilism associated with this disease entity since its first description in 1778.[1] Foremost is the aggressive nature for dissemination of this cancer. Gallbladder cancer spreads early by direct invasion into the liver, by lymphatic metastasis to regional nodes, by peritoneal dissemination to produce carcinomatosis, and by hematogenous means to produce discontiguous liver metastasis and other distant metastases. This cancer, therefore, often presents late when surgical excision is either no longer possible or technically difficult, and alternative therapies are generally ineffective. Therefore, it is not surprising that Blalock recommended in 1924 that surgery be avoided for gallbladder cancer if the diagnosis could be made preoperatively.[2] In fact, until recently, the 5-year survival in most large series was less than 5%, and the median survival was less than 6 months.[3,4] As liver resection has become increasingly safe, significant experience has demonstrated radical surgery to be a sensible option in treatment of this disease and the only potentially curative option.[5,6] Surgical excision is the treatment option of choice for those patients whose gallbladder cancers are confined to the local region of the liver and porta hepatis.

Since the beginning of the last decade, however, gallbladder cancer has taken on a new presentation. With the advent and popularization of laparoscopic cholecystectomy, increasing numbers of cases of gallbladder cancer are being discovered laparoscopically. Currently, approximately 180 000 laparoscopic cholecystectomies are performed in the United States every year for presumed gallstone disease. Since gallbladder cancer is encountered once in every 100 cases of cholecystectomy for gallstones,[6] a significant number of patients will present in this clinical setting. The current chapter will review data addressing the utility of subsequent radical resection for laparoscopically discovered gallbladder cancer. We will begin with a brief review of gallbladder cancer in general, focusing on the natural history and results of surgical treatment. A summary of the data on presentation and results of treatment of laparoscopically discovered disease will be discussed, including the differences of such a clinical scenario from disease discovered by open operation.

Epidemiology

In the United States gallbladder cancer is the most common biliary tract malignancy and the fifth most common gastrointestinal malignancy, with an incidence of 1.2 cases per 100 000 population per year.[7] This cancer is responsible for approximately 2800 deaths per year. The most obvious associated condition for gallbladder cancer is gallstone disease. Between 75 and 98% of all patients with carcinoma of the gallbladder have cholelithiasis.[8] Most importantly, gallbladder cancer will be found once in every 100 cases of presumed gallstone disease.

The natural history of gallbladder cancer has been defined through many retrospective reviews and large surveillance programs. The overall 5-year survival is consistently less than 5%, with a median survival of 5 to 8 months. Piehler et al.[4] reviewed 5836 cases in the world's literature from 1960 to

1978. They reported an overall 5-year survival of 4.1% and a 1-year survival of 11.8%. Only about 25% were resectable for cure, and of those resected for cure, 16.5% survived 5 years.

Perpetuo et al.[3] reviewed the M.D. Anderson experience with gallbladder cancer over 36 years and reported a 5-year survival rate of less than 5% and median survival of 5.2 months. Cubertafond et al.[9] reported the results of a French Surgical Association Survey of 724 carcinomas of the gallbladder. They reported a median survival of 3 months, a 5-year survival rate of 5%, and a 1-year survival rate of 14%. They observed no differences among the different surgical procedures adopted, and concluded that no progress had been made in the treatment of gallbladder cancer. A survey of gallbladder cancer in Wessex, United Kingdom, revealed only four patients out of 95 surviving a duration ranging from 8 to 72 months from the time of diagnosis.[10] A review of gallbladder cancer from Australia revealed a 12% 5-year survival rate, with all survivors having stage I or II disease. The median survival for patients with stage III or IV disease was only 46 days.[11] SEER data from the United States demonstrate similarly unsatisfying results, with only marginal improvement over earlier studies.[7] Overall 5-year survival was reported at 12.3% in 2330 patients.

A multi-institutional review from Japan, on the other hand, reported a 50.7% 5-year survival for 984 patients undergoing radical resection versus 6.2% for 702 patients undergoing more conservative management.[12] These results suggest that it may be possible for surgery to have a role in changing the natural history of this tumor. It is again important to emphasize that there are no good prospective data on the treatment of gallbladder cancer, and no randomized trials comparing extended resection to conservative management. Therefore, controversy regarding management will continue.

Pathology

Carcinomas are difficult to differentiate grossly from chronic cholecystitis at early stages, and are often found incidentally on pathologic section. Even at late stages when tumor can obstruct the common bile duct and produce jaundice, gallbladder cancer is often mistaken for benign disease since associated gallstones and Mirizzi's syndrome are common.[13] A long obstruction of the mid-common bile duct has to be considered gallbladder cancer until proven otherwise. Tumors that arise in the neck and Hartmann's pouch may also infiltrate the common hepatic ducts, making it clinically and radiographically indistinguishable from hilar bile duct tumors.

Approximately 60% of tumors originate in the fundus of the gallbladder, 30% in the body, and 10% in the neck.[14] These tumors most commonly grow in a diffusely infiltrative form,[15] with a tendency to involve the entire gallbladder, and to spread in a subserosal plane which is the same as the surgical plane used for routine cholecystectomy. If such a tumor is unrecognized at the time of surgery, cholecystectomy will incompletely excise disease and lead to dissemination of tumor. Although the nodular type can show early invasion through the gallbladder wall into the liver or neighboring structures, it may be easier to control surgically than the infiltrative form because the margins are better defined. The papillary growth pattern has the best prognosis, because even large tumors have only minimal invasion of the gallbladder wall.[7]

The most common histologic cell type of gallbladder cancers is adenocarcinomas. Other rare subtypes of gallbladder cancer include oat cell carcinomas,[16] adenosquamous tumors,[17] sarcomas, carcinosarcoma, carcinoid, lymphoma, and melanoma.

Patterns of spread

Gallbladder cancer commonly disseminates by four modes of spread:

(1) Direct extension and invasion of adjacent organs,
(2) Lymphatic spread,
(3) Shedding and peritoneal dissemination, and
(4) Hematogenous spread to distant sites.

The gallbladder lies on segments IVb and V of the liver and these segments are involved early in tumors of the fundus and body. Direct extension into vital structures in the proximity of the gallbladder, including the portal vein, hepatic artery, and bile duct, commonly occurs and is a major cause of symptoms. Lymphatic spread of the gallbladder is also common, and most often involves cystic and pericholedochal nodes. Tumor may then pass to nodes posterior to the pancreas, portal vein, and common hepatic artery. Advanced disease may reach the interaortocaval, celiac, and superior mesenteric artery lymph nodes. Gallbladder cancer also has a remarkable propensity to seed and grow in the peritoneal cavity, as well as along needle biopsy sites and in laparoscopic port sites. Hematogenous spread is less common but will present most often as discontiguous liver metastases, and more rarely as lung or brain metastases. At postmortem examination, Perpetuo et al.[3] reported that 91% of patients had liver metastasis and 82% had intra-abdominal lymph node involvement. 60% had

Table 20.1 **Summary of most commonly used staging systems**

Stage	TNM	Modified Nevin	Japanese	Proposed new staging
I	Mucosal or muscular invasion (T1N0M0)	In situ carcinoma	Confined to gallbladder capsule	Mucosal or muscular invasion
II	Transmural invasion (T2N0M0)	Mucosal or muscular invasion	N1 lymph nodes; minimal liver or bile duct invasion	Transmural invasion
III	Liver invasion <2 cm; lymph node mets (T3N1M0)	Transmural direct liver invasion	N2 lymph nodes; marked liver or bile duct invasion	(A) Liver invasion <2 cm (T3N0M0) (B) Liver invasion >2 cm; (T4N0M0)
IV	(1) Liver invasion >2 cm (T4N0M0, TxN1M0) (2) Distant metastases (TxN2M0, TxNxM1)	Lymph node metastasis	Distant metastases	[—]
V	[—]	Distant metastases	[—]	Distant metastases N1 disease (TxN1M0)

peritoneal spread, 32% had lung metastases, and 5% had brain metastases.

Staging

The multitude of staging systems (Table 20.1) used for this disease has made it difficult to compare treatment results. Nevin et al.[18] originally classified patients into five stages based primarily on the thickness of invasion, and combined patients with direct liver extension or distant metastases into stage V. Donahue et al.[19] modified the Nevin system to include tumors with contiguous liver invasion as stage III and non-contiguous liver involvement as stage V. Stage IV continued to include lymph node metastasis. The Japanese Biliary Surgical Society staging system separates tumors into four stages according to the degree of lymph node metastasis, serosal invasion, peritoneal dissemination, hepatic invasion, and bile duct infiltration. The main weakness of this staging system is that lymph node metastases are considered in the same stage as microinvasion of the liver.

We believe that the TNM staging system with minor modifications should be routinely used for uniform comparison of results. Tumors without perimuscular invasion are considered stage I. Tumors with invasion into the perimuscular connective tissue are considered stage II, and liver invasion less than 2 cm is stage III. In addition, nodal metastases to the hepatoduodenal ligament are included in stage III. Stage IV includes patients with liver invasion of greater than 2 cm or patients with N2 nodal metastases or distant metastases. In a recent review of the gallbladder cancer experience at the Memorial Sloan–Kettering Cancer Center it was clear that patients with fundal carcinomas with liver invasion greater than 2 cm had a better prognosis compared to those with nodal metastasis.[6] It is our impression, therefore, that stage III should be divided into IIIA and IIIB. Stage IIIA would include tumors with liver invasion less than 2 cm and no nodal metastasis (T3N0), and stage IIIB would include any N1 nodal metastasis and liver invasion greater than 2 cm (T4N0, any TN1). Stage IV would include only N2 nodal or distant metastases, where there is no reasonable chance for cure.

Clinical presentation

The clinical presentation of gallbladder cancer is identical to the more prevalent biliary colic and/or chronic cholecystitis, making it often difficult to suspect the diagnosis preoperatively. Findings on blood tests also do not easily distinguish gallbladder cancer from benign gallstone disease. Increased alkaline phosphatase and/or bilirubin levels are found in cases of advanced tumors, but may also be found for patients with gallstones. A CEA greater than 4 ng/ml is 93% specific for the diagnosis of gallbladder cancer, but is only 50% sensitive.[20] A serum Ca 19–9 level[21] greater than 20 units/ml has 79.4% sensitivity and 79.2% specificity, but neither test is routine in patients suspected of having benign disease. Vigilance for cancer in examination of

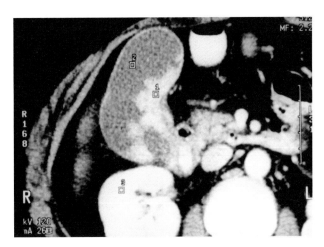

Figure 20.1 CT scan demonstrating a papillary carcinoma of the gallbladder. This patient was subjected to a laparoscopic cholecystectomy in spite of this scan and required a subsequent reoperation for a potentially curative radical resection.

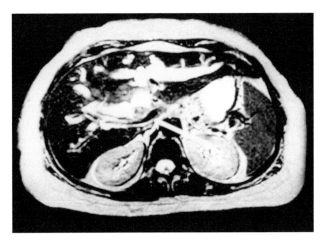

Figure 20.2 Magnetic resonance cholangiopancreatography demonstrating extent of gallbladder cancer. Extension of tumor within and obstructing the common bile duct is shown with isolation of the left and right hepatic duct. The portal vein (white arrow) is patent and not involved by tumor.

preoperative sonograms or CT scans is essential. Any mass associated with the gallbladder (Fig. 20.1), or presence of a porcelain gallbladder should raise concern of gallbladder cancer.

In a report of 42 laparoscopically discovered gallbladder cancers, in only two of the cases did the laparoscopic surgeon suspect a cancer prior to the surgical procedure.[22] The laparoscopic procedure consisted of 19 cases of laparoscopic cholecystectomy, one laparoscopic cholecystectomy with intraoperative cholangiogram, and six laparoscopic biopsies only. There were 16 cases that were converted to open procedures, including 12 open cholecystectomies, three open cholecystectomies with common bile duct exploration, and one cholecystectomy with hepaticojejunostomy. Even at the conclusion of the laparoscopic procedure, in only 20 of the 42 cases was there any suspicion of cancer. This underscores the difficulties in diagnosis of gallbladder cancer and the ease with which this aggressive malignancy is confused with benign stone disease.

Radiologic work-up

Most patients with laparoscopically-discovered gallbladder cancer will have had an ultrasound performed for suspected gallstones. Review of this ultrasound may provide information concerning liver involvement by tumor, biliary extension of tumor, and vascular involvement. Most often though, another cross-sectional imaging test is indicated for assessment of these sites of potential

disease, as well as to assess for presence of nodal disease and signs of carcinomatosis. The combination of CT scanning and ultrasonography[23] is the most common combination for initial assessment, although MRI scanning can be substituted for CT.[24]

If initial assessment indicates laboratory or radiologic evidence of biliary obstruction, assessment of extent of biliary involvement by other imaging techniques may be necessary. Gallbladder cancer can cause obstructive jaundice by direct invasion of the common hepatic duct, or by compression and involvement of the common hepatic duct by pericholedochal lymph nodes. A high correlation between Mirizzi's syndrome and gallbladder cancer exists.[13] Endoscopic or percutaneous cholangiograms are the traditional methods for such assessment. For small tumors the pattern of obstruction seen on PTC or ERCP may assist in differentiating gallbladder cancer from other tumors and from benign disease.[25] More recently, the technique of MR cholangiopancreatography (MRCP) (Fig. 20.2) has improved to become a suitable, non-invasive substitute for direct cholangiography.[26]

Suspicion for main portal venous involvement by tumor, or hepatic arterial involvement by tumor usually prompts angiography to definitively demonstrate unresectability. Improvements in Doppler ultrasound and in MR angiography provide noninvasive substitutes for such assessment. We will often assess a patient presenting with known gallbladder cancer with a single MR scan. Detailed information on liver involvement, biliary extension, vascular proximity and involvement, and nodal

Table 20.2 Findings related to T stage of disease

Stage	Total	Peritoneal metastases (%)	Nodal metastases (%)
T2	9	12	50
T3	16	43	50
T4	16	68	66

T2, submucosal invasion; T3, full thickness invasion through gallbladder wall with <2 cm extension into liver; T4, more than 2 cm extension into liver. From Fong et al.[22]

disease can be gleaned from a single non-invasive test. With the quality of current cross-sectional imaging, it is rare that direct cholangiography or angiography is necessary.

Surgical management

A wide range of operations have been advocated for gallbladder cancer, ranging from simple cholecystectomy alone to combined extended hepatectomy, common bile duct resection, and pancreaticoduodenectomy.[27] There is as yet no consensus as to the extent of surgery.[28] A survey of prominent gastrointestinal surgeons in the United States indicated that 49% recommended lymph node dissection and 64% recommended some form of liver resection for stage T2–4 disease. The nihilistic attitude toward this disease is reflected by the recommendation of 21% of surgeons answering this survey to perform only a simple cholecystectomy for node-positive disease.[28]

Data would indicate that a potentially curative approach for gallbladder cancer, except for disease at the earliest stages, would require a liver resection and a lymphadenectomy. It is clear from pathologic data that T2, T3, or T4 tumors were all associated with greater than a 50% chance of metastases to the regional lymph nodes (Table 20.2). As liver resections have become increasingly safe, increasing numbers of surgical centers are performing radical resections for this disease, and data are consequently accumulating that are justifying such an aggressive approach. We will review the data supporting radical resection for gallbladder cancer at various stages of disease. Then a discussion of the justification of such treatment in patients with laparoscopically discovered gallbladder cancer will be presented.

The most practical way of thinking about laparoscopically-discovered gallbladder cancer is to base therapy on clinical T stage of disease. Not only is there a close correlation of T stage with prognosis, but patients presenting in this setting will usually have had the gallbladder excised and the extent of local disease defined pathologically. Knowing the likelihood of further local, nodal, peritoneal disease will allow for rational therapeutic choices.

Tumors confined to the muscular coat (T1 tumors)

There are abundant data to indicate that early gallbladder cancer that has not penetrated through the muscular layer of the gallbladder is adequately treated by simple cholecystectomy. Tsukada et al.[29] demonstrated that in 15 cases with T1 lesions, there were no cases with lymph node metastasis. Table 20.3 summarizes results of resection for stage I disease. After simple cholecystectomy alone, the 5-year survival was 78–100%.[30,31] In a report of 56 patients treated with simple cholecystectomy alone, only two patients recurred and went on to die of their disease. Both of these had submucosal spread of the tumor to involve the cystic duct margin.[32]

When patients present after laparoscopic cholecystectomy with a pathologic diagnosis of T1 gallbladder cancer, the most important maneuver is a careful review of the pathology. Care must be taken to verify no areas of deeper invasion, and to verify negative margins including the cystic duct stump. If the gallbladder margin is involved by tumor, a liver resection is required. If the cystic duct stump is involved, an excision of the common bile duct including the junction with the cystic duct is indicated. No nodal dissection is necessary.

Tumor invading into the subserosal layer (stage II)

Although T2 tumors by definition have not transgressed the serosal plane, the recommended management for stage II disease is an extended or radical cholecystectomy to include a liver resection and regional lymph node dissection, as described above. The reasons for such a recommendation are related to the pattern of spread of disease. In the most common infiltrative form of gallbladder cancer,[15] the gallbladder cancer often spreads in a subserosal plane, which is the same as the surgical plane used for routine cholecystectomy. This results in a high likelihood of positive margins after simple cholecystectomy. In the review by Yamaguchi and Tsuneyoshi,[30] patients had tumor extending into the subserosal layer and 11 of these had positive microscopic margins after simple cholecystectomy. Furthermore, the likelihood of metastatic disease to

Table 20.3 **Actuarial survival results reported in retrospective reviews after resection of stage I gallbladder cancers**

Author	Year	N	Procedure	3-year survival (%)	5-year survival (%)
Ouchi et al.[61]	1987	14	Not specified	78	71.4
Yamaguchi and Enjoji[17]	1988	11	Not specified	100	Not reported
Donohue et al.[19]	1990	6	Simple cholecystectomy: 83%	100	100
Gall et al.[35]	1991	7	Simple cholecystectomy	86	86
Ogura et al.[a12]	1991	366	Not specified	87	78
Shirai et al.[62]	1992	39	Simple cholecystectomy	100	100
Yamaguchi and Tsuneyashi[30]	1992	6	Simple cholecystectomy	100	100
Shirai et al.[32]	1992	56	Simple cholecystectomy	100	100
		38	Extended cholecystectomy	100	100
Matsumoto et al.[5]	1992	4	Extended cholecystectomy	100	100
Oertli et al.[55]	1993	6	Simple cholecystectomy	100	100
de Aretxabala et al.[63]	1992	32	Simple cholecystectomy: 69%	94	94

[a] Multi-institutional survey.

regional lymph nodes exceeds 50%.[6,22,29] Indeed, it is perhaps this group of T2 lesions which will have the best chance of benefiting from definitive extended re-resection,[33] with 5-year survival of patients subjected to simple cholecystectomy being 20–57% and survival of patients subjected to radical resection being 80–100% (Table 20.4).

For patients presenting with T2 gallbladder cancer discovered at laparoscopic cholecystectomy, a re-exploration with the intent to perform a liver resection, and regional nodal dissection is recommended. During this re-exploration, inflammation from the previous operation will make it difficult to determine the exact extent of disease. The patients must be informed that final pathology may not demonstrate residual tumor.

Advanced tumors (stage III and IV)

Patients with T3 or T4 gallbladder cancer will present after laparoscopic cholecystectomy not only with an obvious pathologically positive margin for tumor, but also with a hepatic mass on cross-sectional imaging. Debate raged in the past regarding justification of radical surgery for such advanced disease. As radical resections have become increasingly safe, the literature is abundant with reports of long-term survivors after aggressive surgical management; Table 20.5 reviews these studies. Onoyama et al[34] reported a 63.6% 5-year survival for Japanese Biliary Surgical Society stage II and 44.4% 5-year survival for stage III disease after extended cholecystectomy (these stages combined represent AJCC

stage III). They reported an 8.3% 5-year survival for stage IV disease. In addition, they noted a 5-year survival rate of 60% for patients having metastatic disease to N1 nodes. Shirai et al.[32] reported a 45% 5-year survival for patients with node-positive tumors, documenting nine patients surviving over 5 years after radical resection. Gall et al.[35] reported that four of eight patients undergoing curative resection for AJCC stage III and IV gallbladder carcinoma at the initial operation were alive after 81, 50, 13, and 8 months. Our data from the Memorial Sloan–Kettering Cancer Center revealed a 67% actuarial 5-year survival for patients with completely resected stage III and 33% 5-year survival for patients with completely resected stage IV tumors.[6] These results represent marked alteration of the natural history of this tumor.

These data would indicate that radical surgery for advanced gallbladder cancer may be potentially curative. Patients presenting with T3 and T4 disease after laparoscopic cholecystectomy should have imaging performed to rule out signs of unresectable disease, including discontiguous liver metastases or signs of carcinomatosis. Barring any contraindications to surgery, patients should be re-explored for radical resection of tumor, which usually requires a major liver resection and regional lymphadenectomy.

Re-resection after laparoscopic cholecystectomy

Data available for re-resection for gallbladder cancer treated initially with open simple cholecystectomy

Table 20.4 Actuarial survival results reported in retrospective reviews after resection of stage II gallbladder cancers

Author	Year	N	Procedure	3-year survival (%)	5-year survival (%)
Yamaguchi and Enjoji[17]	1988	73	Not specified	40.1	Not reported
Donohue et al.[19]	1990	12	67% Extended chole	58	22
Ogura et al.[12]	1991	499	Not specified	53	37
Gall et al.[35]	1991	7	86% Simple chole	86	86
Shirai et al.[62]	1992	35	Simple chole	57	40.5
		10	Extended chole	90	90
Yamaguchi and Tsuneyashi[30]	1992	25	Simple chole	36	36
Matsumoto et al.[5]	1992	9	Extended chole	100	100
Oertli et al.[55]	1993	17	Simple chole	29	24
Cubertafond et al.[a9]	1994	52	88% Simple chole	20	Not reported
Bartlett et al.[6]	1996	8	Extended chole	100	88
Paquet[33]	1998	5	Extended chole	100	80

[a] Multi-institutional survey.
Chole, cholecystectomy.

Table 20.5 Actuarial survival results reported in retrospective reviews after resection of stage III and IV gallbladder cancers

Author	Year	N	Stage	3-year survival (%)	5-year survival (%)	Comments
Matsumoto et al.[5]	1992	8	III	38	—	Majority with common bile duct resection
Chijiiwa and Tanaka[38]	1994	12	III	80	—	Extended resections only
Onoyama et al.[34]	1995	12	III	44	44	Extended resections only
Bartlett et al.[6]	1996	8	III	63	63	Extended resections only
Ouchi et al.[61]	1987	12	III/IV	17	—	Extended resections only
Nakamura et al.[65]	1989	13	III/IV	16	16	Includes 5 HPD, 10 extended hepatectomy
Donohue et al.[19]	1990	17	III/IV	50	29	Extended resections only
Gall et al.[35]	1991	8	III/IV	50	—	Includes only curative resection at initial surgery
Shirai et al.[62]	1992	20	III/IV	—	45	All patients have lymph node metastases
Ogura et al.[12]	1991	453	IV	18	8	Multi-institutional series with 25% simple cholecystectomy
Todoroki et al.[51]	1991	27	IV	7	—	All patients had IORT
Nimura et al.[27]	1991	14	IV	10	—	All patients underwent HPD
Matsumoto et al.[5]	1992	27	IV	25	—	Includes 3 HPD, 6 extended hepatectomy, 11 cbd resection
Chijiiwa and Tanaka[64]	1994	11	IV	11	—	Extended resections only
Onoyama et al.[34]	1995	14	IV	8	8	Japanese staging
Bartlett et al.[6]	1996	7	IV	25	25	Long-term survivors with no lymph node metastases

HPD, hepatopancreatoduodenectomy; IORT, intraoperative radiation therapy.

suggest that, for tumors with a depth of penetration greater or equal to T2, a radical re-resection is warranted.[36] The prognosis for patients subjected to two operations for gallbladder cancer is thought to be less favorable than for patients treated with a single procedure. Gall et al.[35] reported a median survival of 42 months for patients undergoing a curative resection at the first operation versus 12.5 months for those undergoing a curative resection at a second operation. It is clear from their results that the best outcome is seen in patients subjected to appropriate initial management.

Laparoscopic cholecystectomy has given birth to an entirely new clinical entity since 1989, namely that of a laparoscopically-discovered gallbladder cancer. To date, few data have addressed the need and utility of radical re-resection after gallbladder cancer is discovered. We reported a series of 42 gallbladder cancers discovered at laparoscopy.[22] One patient with T1 gallbladder cancer was advised that his laparoscopic cholecystectomy was a definitive procedure, and no additional therapy was undertaken. All other patients underwent abdominal and pelvic CT scanning, chest radiography, and either a Doppler ultrasound or an MRI for evaluation of portal venous tumor involvement as well as evaluation of portal lymphadenopathy. Of the 41 patients with T2, T3, or T4 disease, five were not offered further surgery due to unresectable disease discovered by imaging. The remaining 36 patients were subjected to surgical exploration, with 17 additional patients found to be unresectable. The median

follow-up of the resected patients was 16 months. At the time of writing, only three of these 19 patients subjected to re-resection have died, and the median survival has not been reached (Fig. 20.3). The survival of these re-resected patients is remarkably different from those found unresectable. The median survival of those not resected was 4 months. The difference in survival of the resected and non-resected patients is statistically significant to the $P < 0.0001$ level. These data would indicate that such re-exploration and resection are justified and useful.

Liver resection

Except for the patient with T1 tumors who has a positive cystic duct margin, all other patients undergoing re-exploration for re-resection should have some form of liver resection (radical cholecystectomy). This is because of the possibility of residual disease in the gallbladder bed. Even patients with T2 tumors have a likelihood of residual gallbladder bed disease because the most common plane for simple cholecystectomy is subserosal. Recommendations for liver resection for gallbladder cancer have ranged from a limited wedge excision of 2 cm of liver around the gallbladder bed to routine extended right hepatic lobectomy. We prefer an anatomic segment IVb and V resection when possible, because this anatomic operation allows the greatest chance of tumor clearance while minimizing the amount of functional liver removed.

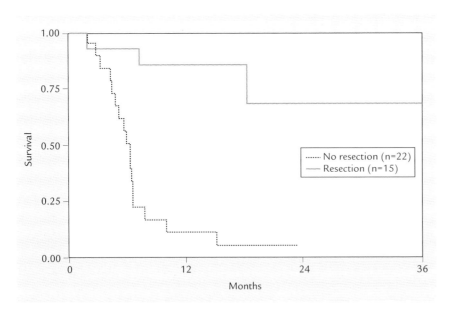

Figure 20.3 Comparison of survival of patients discovered by laparoscopy to have gallbladder cancer related to further surgical treatment. Patients found to be untreatable by further surgery (dashed line) are compared to those subjected to further resection of tumor (solid line) ($P < 0.0001$).

In cases of previous cholecystectomy, such a limited resection may not be possible. Scars from the previous surgery may be difficult to distinguish from tumor and a more radical resection may be necessary to ensure complete eradication of disease. It must be emphasized that complete excision of any suspicious areas must be performed since any residual tumor will result in recurrence. A recurrence of tumor is usually rapidly fatal. Often, therefore, a right lobectomy or trisegmentectomy will be necessary.

Lymph node dissection

Studies of lymphatic spread of gallbladder cancer have been published and reviewed.[37] Recommendations for lymph node dissection for gallbladder cancer have ranged from excision of the cystic duct node alone to en bloc portal lymphadenopathy with pancreaticoduodenectomy.[5] Justification for more radical procedures comes from the propensity for early spread to superior anterior and posterior pancreaticoduodenal nodes. Combined liver and pancreatic resections have high operative mortalities of near 20%, and are not justified by long-term results.

The concept of portal lymphadenectomy for tumor penetrating the gallbladder beyond T2 is supported by our findings of positive nodes in over 50% of patients with T2, T3, or T4 gallbladder cancer.[22] We also believe that an adequate portal lymphadenectomy requires resection of the common bile duct. Particularly in patients who had just had a cholecystectomy, the portal lymph nodes are often intimately associated with the bile duct. Resection of the common bile duct greatly facilitates nodal clearance. In general, a full Kocher maneuver should be performed and lymphatic tissue should be dissected behind the duodenum and pancreas and swept superiorly. Any interaortocaval nodes or superior mesenteric nodes should be included in the specimen if possible. The common bile duct should be transected as it courses posterior to the duodenum into the pancreas. The portal vein and hepatic artery should be skeletonized and all tissue swept superiorly along with the transected duct. At the confluence of the right and left hepatic ducts, the common bile duct should be divided again (assuming the cystic duct does not enter the right hepatic duct). A Roux-en-Y hepaticojejunostomy should be performed to re-establish biliary–enteric continuity.

Laparoscopic port sites

A number of studies have demonstrated the propensity of tumor to recur in the laparoscopic port sites

Table 20.6 Recurrence of tumor in laparoscopic port sites

Author	N	Port
Drouard et al.[38]	1	Umbilical
Clair et al.[39]	1	Umbilical
Landen[40]	1	Umbilical
Fligelstone et al.[41]	1	Umbilical
Fong et al.[42]	2	Umbilical
Nduka et al.[44]	1	Epigastric
Nally and Preshaw[44]	1	Umbilical
Kim and Roy[45]	1	Umbilical

(Table 20.6).[38–45] This tumor has a great potential for seeding and dissemination. Indeed, our preliminary report of the first ten patients we encountered with laparoscopically-discovered gallbladder cancer included two patients in whom the tumor recurrence was found in the port site.[42] The incidence of peritoneal metastases is higher than reported in the prelaparoscopic age.[5] It has become our standard practice to excise laparoscopic port sites at the re-exploration. During re-exploration, therefore, care must be taken to perform a full abdominal inspection to rule out peritoneal disease. Whether such excision of port sites is useful requires further investigation, since port recurrence may be just a marker for diffuse peritoneal dissemination of disease.

Complications

The operations described above are extensive procedures with substantial risks, particularly since the majority of patients undergoing treatment for gallbladder cancer are in their seventh or eighth decade of life and may be at increased risk as a consequence of concomitant medical problems. In a multi-institutional review of 1686 gallbladder cancer resections from Japan, a comparison of morbidity by procedure was made.[12] A morbidity of 12.8% was reported for cholecystectomy, 21.9% for extended cholecystectomy, and 48.3% for hepatic lobectomy. The mortality rates were 2.9%, 2.3%, and 17.9%, respectively. There were 150 hepatopancreatoduodenectomies for gallbladder cancer, with a 54% morbidity rate, and a 15.3% mortality rate. The morbidity and mortality rates of major liver resections have decreased in later reports, even in the aged population.[46] In our report of re-resection for laparoscopically-discovered gallbladder cancer, all resected patients were subjected to some form of liver resection and the operative mortality was 5%.[22]

The most common complications are bile collections, liver failure, intra-abdominal abscess, and respiratory failure. The risk of resection for each patient and for each type of resection needs to be weighed against their chance of benefiting from the procedure based on their stage of disease.

Adjuvant therapy

Because of the rarity of this disease in general, as well as the rarity of completely resected gallbladder cancers, there are no prospective, randomized studies examining the utility of adjuvant therapy for gallbladder cancer. All data available are derived from retrospective series. Data do not support the routine use of chemotherapy.[47–49]

Data regarding radiation therapy are more substantial, but still far from conclusive.[50] Todoroki et al.[51] examined intraoperative radiation therapy after complete resection for stage IV gallbladder cancer. They reported a 10.1% 3-year survival for patients receiving intraoperative radiation therapy versus 0% for surgery alone. Bosset et al.[52] examined postoperative external beam irradiation after complete resection in seven patients. They concluded that it was a safe treatment, and five of the seven patients were still alive at a median follow-up of 11 months. Hanna and Rider[53] reported radiation therapy in 51 patients and reported survival to be significantly longer in patients receiving postoperative radiotherapy compared with those who had surgery alone. In a retrospective review from Finland, the median survival of patients receiving postoperative radiation was 63 months compared with 29 months for patients receiving surgery alone.[54] Currently, in patients with node-positive disease, we are recommending radiation therapy. Chemotherapy is only used as a potential radiation sensitizing agent.

Palliative management

Palliative therapy should be considered in the context that the median survival for patients presenting with unresectable gallbladder cancer is 2 to 4 months.[55,56] The goal of palliation should be relief of pain, jaundice, and bowel obstruction and prolongation of life. These should be done as simply as possible given the aggressive nature of this disease. Biliary bypass for obstruction can be difficult because of advanced disease in the porta hepatis. A segment III bypass is usually necessary if surgical bypass is chosen to relieve jaundice.[57,58]

Such bypasses have a 12% 30-day mortality rate, however.[58] In the event of a preoperative diagnosis of advanced, unresectable gallbladder cancer in the jaundiced patient, therefore, a non-invasive radiologic approach to biliary drainage is justified.

Systemic chemotherapy[59] and radiation therapy[60] have little effect on this tumor. Patients with unresectable disease and good functional status who desire therapy should be directed to investigational studies to determine whether any novel therapies may be useful.

Summary

Gallbladder cancer is an aggressive disease with a dismal prognosis. It should not, however, be approached with a fatalistic attitude because appropriate work-up and extended resection can result in a cure. Gallbladder cancer will be encountered once every 100 times a gallbladder is removed for presumed benign gallstone disease. For patients discovered during pathologic analysis to have a T1 cancer, no further therapy is indicated as long as all margins are negative including the cystic duct margin.[61,62] However, T2, T3, or T4 tumors deserve consideration for re-exploration.[63–69] Selection for re-resection relies on evaluation of general medical fitness and rigorous radiologic work-up to rule out disseminated disease. Evidence of N2 disease on preoperative work-up precludes a curative resection as no long-term survivors have been reported with gross N2 disease. These patients should be treated only as symptoms develop, with no reoperation for curative resection. Those re-explored for resection should undergo a standard extended cholecystectomy including an extensive nodal dissection to include the superior pancreaticoduodenal nodes and a skeletonization of the vessels in the porta hepatis. If the nodal dissection is compromised by the presence of the common bile duct, then this should be resected. In addition, a segment IVb and V resection of the liver or extended resection of the liver should be included, as dictated by the location of the tumor and surrounding inflammation and scar tissue.

Key points

- Gallbladder cancer will be found in 1 per 100 cholecystectomy specimens. (Incidence 1.2 cases per 100 000 population per year).
- 75–98% association with cholelithiasis.

- A long obstruction of the mid-common bile duct is gallbladder cancer until proven otherwise.
- Radiologic investigation of gallbladder cancer:
  US
  MRCP
  CT
  ERCP/PTC if jaundiced
  Angiography.

- Surgical management:
  Stage 1 (T1N0M0): cholecystectomy alone
  Stage II (T2N0M0)
  Stage III (T3N0M0) } Radical cholecystestomy
  ± liver invasion <2 cm
  Stage IV (T4N0M0) ± liver invasion >2 cm
  No dissemination: extended hepatectomy
  Widespread dissemination: no surgical option

REFERENCES

1. Kato S, Nakagawa T, Kobayashi H, Arai E, Isetani K. Septum formation of the common hepatic duct associated with an anomalous junction of the pancreaticobiliary ductal system gallbladder cancer: report of a case. Surg Today 1994; 24: 534–7
2. Blalock AA. A statistical study 888 cases of biliary tract disease. Johns Hopkins Hosp Bull 1924; 5: 391–409
3. Perpetuo MD, Valdivieso M, Heilbrun LK, Nelson RS, Connor T, Bodey GP. Natural history study of gallbladder cancer: a review of 36 years experience at M.D. Anderson Hospital and Tumor Institute. Cancer 1978; 42: 330–5
4. Piehler JM, Crichlow RW. Primary carcinoma of the gallbladder. Surg Gynecol Obstet 1978; 147: 929–42
5. Matsumoto Y, Fujii H, Aoyama H, Yamamoto M, Sugahara K, Suda K. Surgical treatment of primary carcinoma of the gallbladder based on the histologic analysis of 48 surgical specimens. Am J Surg 1992; 163: 239–45
6. Bartlett DL, Fong Y, Fortner JG, Brennan MF, Blumgart LH. Long-term results after resection for gallbladder cancer. Ann Surg 1996; 224 (5): 639–46
7. Carriaga MT, Henson DE. Liver, gallbladder, extrahepatic bile ducts, and pancreas. Cancer 1995; 75(Suppl 1): 171–90
8. Wanebo HJ, Vezeridis MP. Treatment of gallbladder cancer. Cancer Treat Res 1994; 69: 97–109
9. Cubertafond P, Gainant A, Cucchiaro G. Surgical treatment of 724 carcinomas of the gallbladder. Results of the French Surgical Association Survey. Ann Surg 1994; 219: 275–80
10. Carty NJ, Johnson CD. Carcinoma of the gallbladder: a survey of cases in Wessex 1982–1989. J R Coll Surg Edin 1991; 36: 238–41
11. Wilkinson DS. Carcinoma of the gallbladder: an experience and review of the literature. NZ J Surg 1995; 65: 724–7
12. Ogura Y, Mizumoto R, Isaji S, Kusuda T, Matsuda S, Tabata M. Radical operations for carcinoma of the gallbladder: present status in Japan. World J Surg 1991; 15: 337–43
13. Redaelli CA, Buchler MW, Schilling MK et al. High coincidence of Mirizzi syndrome and gallbladder carcinoma. Surgery 1997; 121: 58–63
14. Albores-Saavedra J, Nadji M, Henson DE. Intestinal-type adenocarcinoma of the gallbladder. A clinicopathologic study of seven cases. Am J Surg Pathol 1986; 10: 19–25
15. Sumiyoshi K, Nagai E, Chijiiwa K, Nakayama F. Pathology of carcinoma of the gallbladder. World J Surg 1991; 15: 315–21
16. Henson DE, Albores-Saavedra J, Corle D. Carcinoma of the gallbladder. Histologic types, stage of disease, grade, and survival rates. Cancer 1992; 70: 1493–7
17. Yamaguchi K, Enjoji M. Carcinoma of the gallbladder – a clinicopathology of 103 patients and a newly proposed staging. Cancer 1988; 62: 1425–32
18. Nevin JE, Moran TJ, Kay S, King R. Carcinoma of the gallbladder: staging, treatment, and prognosis. Cancer 1976; 37: 141–8
19. Donohue JH, Nagorney DM, Grant CS, Tsushima K, Ilstrup DM, Adson MA. Carcinoma of the gallbladder. Does radical resection improve outcome? Arch Surg 1990; 125: 237–41
20. Strom BL, Maislin G, West SL et al. Serum CEA and CA 19–9: potential future diagnostic or screening tests for gallbladder cancer? Int J Cancer 1990; 45: 821–4
21. Ritts RE, Nagomey DM, Jacobson DJ, Talbot RW, Zurawski VR Jr. Comparison of preoperative serum CA19–9 levels with results of diagnostic imaging modalities in patients undergoing laparotomy for suspected pancreatic or gallbladder disease. Pancreas 1999; 9: 707–16
22. Fong Y, Heffeman N, Blumgart LH. Gallbladder carcinoma discovered during laparoscopic cholecystectomy: aggressive reresection is beneficial. Cancer 1998; 83: 423–7
23. Chijiiwa K, Sumiyoshi K, Nakayama F. Impact of recent advances in hepatobiliary imaging techniques on the preoperative diagnosis of carcinoma of the gallbladder. World J Surg 1991; 15: 322–7
24. Wilbur AC, Gyi B, Renigers SA. High-field MRI of primary gallbladder carcinoma. Gastrointest Radiol 1988; 13: 142–4
25. Collier NA, Carr D, Hemingway A, Blumgart LH. Preoperative diagnosis and its effect on the treatment of carcinoma of the gallbladder. Surg Gynecol Obstet 1984; 159: 465–70

26. Schwartz LH, Coakley FV, Sun Y, Blumgart LH, Fong Y, Panicek DM. Neoplastic pancreaticobiliary duct obstruction: evaluation with breath-hold MR cholangiopancreatography. AJR 1998; 170 (6): 1491–5

27. Nimura Y, Hayakawa N, Kamiya J et al. Hepatopancreatoduodenectomy for advanced carcinoma of the biliary tract. Hepatogastroenterology 1991; 38: 170–5

28. Gagner M, Rossi RL. Radical operations for carcinoma of the gallbladder: present status in North America. World J Surg 1991; 15: 344–7

29. Tsukada K, Kurosaki I, Uchida K et al. Lymph node spread from carcinoma of the gallbladder. Cancer 1997; 80: 661–7

30. Yamaguchi K, Tsuneyoshi M. Subclinical gallbladder carcinoma. Am J Surg 1992; 63: 382–6

31. Shirai Y, Yoshida K, Tsukada K, Muto T. Inapparent carcinoma of the gallbladder. An appraisal of a radical second operation after simple cholecystectomy. Ann Surg 1992; 215: 326–31

32. Shirai Y, Yoshida K, Tsukada K, Muto T, Watanabe H. Radical surgery for gallbladder carcinoma. Long-term results. Ann Surg 1992; 216: 565–8

33. Paquet KJ. Appraisal of surgical resection of gallbladder carcinoma with special reference to hepatic resection. J HBP Surg 1998; 5: 200–6.

34. Onoyama H, Yamamoto M, Tseng A, Ajiki T, Saitoh Y. Extended cholecystectomy for carcinoma of the gallbladder. World J Surg 1995; 19: 758–63

35. Gall FP, Kockerling F, Scheele J, Schneider C, Hohenberger W. Radical operations for carcinoma of the gallbladder: present status in Germany. World J Surg 1991; 15: 28–36

36. Shirai Y, Yoshida K, Tsukada K, Muto T. Inapparent carcinoma of the gallbladder – an appraisal of a radical second operation after simple cholecystectomy. Cancer 1988; 62: 1422–32

37. Boerma EJ. Towards an oncological resection of gall bladder cancer. Eur J Surg Oncol 1994; 20: 537–44

38. Drouard F, Delamarre J, Capron J. Cutaneous seeding of gallbladder cancer after laparoscopic cholecystectomy. N Engl J Med 1991; 325: 1316

39. Clair DG, Lautz DB, Brooks DC. Rapid development of umbilical metastases after laparoscopic cholecystectomy for unsuspected gallbladder carcinoma. Surgery 1993; 113: 355–8

40. Landen SM. Laparoscopc surgery and tumor seeding. Surgery 1993; 114: 131–2

41. Fligelstone L, Rhodes M, Flook D, Puntis M, Crosby D. Tumour inoculation during laparoscopy. Lancet 1993; 342: 368–9

42. Fong Y, Brennan MF, Turnbull A, Coit DG, Blumgart LH. Gallbladder cancer discovered during laparoscopic surgey – potential for iatrogenic dissemination. Arch Surg 1993; 128: 1054–6

43. Nduka CC, Monson JRT, Menzies-Gow N, Darzi A. Abdominal wall metastases following laparoscopy. Br J Surg 1994; 81: 648–52

44. Nally C, Preshaw RM. Tumour implantation at umbilicus after laparoscopic cholecystectomy for unsuspected gallbladder carcinoma. Can J Surg 1994; 37: 243–4

45. Kim HJ, Roy T. Unexpected gallbladder cancer with cutaneous seeding after laparoscopic cholecystectomy. South Med J 1994; 87: 817–20

46. Fong Y, Blumgart LH, Fortner JG, Brennan MF. Pancreatic or liver resection for malignancy is safe and effective for the elderly. Ann Surg 1995; 222: 426–37

47. Chao TC, Jan YY, Chen MF. Primary carcinoma of the gallbladder associated with anomalous pancreaticobiliary duct junction. J Clin Gastroenterol 1995; 21: 306–8

48. Oswalt CE, Cruz AB Jr. Effectiveness of chemotherapy in addition to surgery in treating carcinoma of he gallbladder. Rev Surg 1977; 34: 436–8

49. Morrow CE, Sutherland DE, Florack G, Eisenberg MM, Grage TB. Primary gallbladder carcinoma: significance of subserosal lesions and results of aggressive surgical treatment and adjuvant chemotherapy. Surgery 1983; 94: 709–14

50. Todoroki T. Radiation therapy for primary gallbladder cancer. Hepatogastroenerology 1997; 44: 1229–39

51. Todoroki T, Iwasaki Y, Orii K et al. Resection combined with intraoperative radiation therapy (IORT) for stage IV (TNM) gallbladder carcinoma. World J Surg 1991; 15: 357–66

52. Bosset JF, Mantion G, Gillet M et al. Primary carcinoma of the gallbladder. Adjuvant postoperative external irradiation. Cancer 1989; 64: 1843–7

53. Hanna SS, Rider WD. Carcinoma of the gallbladder or extrahepatic bile ducts: the role of radiotherapy. Can Med Assoc 1978; 118: 59–61

54. Vaittinen E. Carcinoma of the gall-bladder. A study of 390 cases diagnosed in Finland 1953–1967. Ann Chirurg Gynaecol Fenn Suppl 1970; 168: 1–81

55. Oertli D, Herzog U, Tondelli P. Primary carcinoma of the gallbladder: operative experience during a 16 year period. Eur J Surg 1993; 159: 415–20

56. Wanebo HJ, Castle WN Fechner RE. Is carcinoma of the gallbladder a curable lesion? Ann Surg 1982; 196: 624–31

57. Bismuth H, Corlett MB. Intrahepatic cholangioenteric anastomosis in carcinoma of the hilus of the liver. Surg Gynecol Obstet 1975; 140: 170–6

58. Kapoor VK, Pradeep R, Haribhakti SP, Sikora SS, Kaushik SP. Early carcinoma of the gallbladder: an elusive disease. J Surg Oncol 1996; 62: 284–7

59. Taal BG, Audisio RA, Bleiberg H et al. Phase II trial of mitomycin C (MMC) in advanced gallbladder and biliary tree carcinoma. An EORTC gastrointestinal tract cancer cooperative group study. Ann Oncol 1993; 607–9

60. Houry S, Schlienger M, Huguier M, Lacaine F, Penne F, Laugier A. Gallbladder carcinoma: role of radiation therapy. Br J Surg 1989; 76: 448–50

61. Ouchi K, Owada Y, Matsuno S, Sato T. Prognostic factors in the surgical treatment of gallbladder carcinoma. Surgery 1987; 101: 731–7

62. Shirai Y, Yoshida K, Tsukada K, Muto T, Watanabe H. Early carcinoma of the gallbladder. Eur J Surg 1992; 158: 545–8

63. de Aretxabala X, Roa I, Burgos L et al. Gallbladder cancer in Chile. A report on 54 potentially resectable tumors. Cancer 1992; 69: 60–5

64. Chijiiwa K, Tanaka M. Carcinoma of the gallbladder: an appraisal of surgical resection. Surgery 1994; 115: 751–6

65. Nakamura S, Sakaguchi S, Suzuki S, Muro H. Aggressive surgery for carcinoma of the gallbladder. Surgery 1989; 106: 467–73

66. Fong YM. Gallbladder cancer: recent advances and current guidelines for surgical therapy. Adv Surg 2001; 35: 1–20

67. Whalen GF, Bird I, Tanski W, Russell JC, Clive J. Laparoscopic cholecystectomy does not demonstrably decrease survival of patients with serendipitously treated gallbladder cancer. J Am Coll Surg 2001; 192 (2): 189–95

68. Fong Y, Jarnagin W, Blumgart LH. Gallbladder cancer: comparison of patients presenting initially for definitive operation with those presenting after prior noncurative intervention. Ann Surg 2000; 232 (4): 557–69

69. Todoroki T, Takahashi H, Koike N et al. Outcomes of aggressive treatment of stage IV gallbladder cancer and predictors of survival. Hepatogastroenterology 1999; 46 (28): 2114–21

21 Minimal access pancreatic surgery

Michael PN Lewis and Michael Rhodes

The advances in minimal access techniques have been difficult to apply to the pancreas primarily due to its position deep within the abdomen, making accessibility a key issue. Nevertheless, many pancreatic surgical techniques can and have been performed using laparoscopic or endoscopic approaches. While more conventional approaches are still used for the majority of pancreatic operations there has been some success with the introduction of minimally invasive techniques in the diagnosis and treatment of pancreatic disease. Most notable success has been in the use of laparoscopy for the staging of pancreatic tumours, for treatment of pancreatic pseudocysts and the use of endoscopic techniques in diagnosis and therapy. Pancreatic surgery is certainly an area where there is further scope for the development of minimally invasive techniques, while current conventional access results in a large degree of surgical trauma and its attendant high morbidity and mortality.

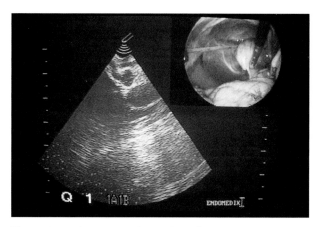

Figure 21.1 Laparoscopic staging of pancreatic malignancy: 5 and 10 mm ultrasound probes may be of use in the preoperative staging of pancreatic malignancy. Here a routine preoperative staging is being undertaken and the probe is seen resting on the right lobe of the liver.

Diagnostic laparoscopy and staging

The use of laparoscopy as a diagnostic tool in pancreatic disease is gaining wider acceptance. The most valuable application would appear to be the use of laparoscopy and laparoscopic ultrasound in the staging of pancreatic malignancies. Laparoscopy in the staging of pancreatic cancer has been advocated since 1978,[1] and the advent of laparoscopic ultrasonography (Fig. 21.1) has improved the yield.[2,3] This is primarily by the detection of small 'occult' intraperitoneal metastases that cannot be visualized by current radiological techniques. Laparoscopic ultrasound allows full assessment of pancreatic tumour invasion, local and regional lymph node status and hepatic metastases.

Pancreatic cancer has a very poor prognosis and potentially curative resection carries, at best, a 5-year survival of 5%. As a sizeable proportion of patients with pancreatic cancer are found to be inoperable at laparotomy (Figs 21.2 and 21.3), surgeons have looked at ways of decreasing the rate of unnecessary laparotomies in these patients and improving patient selection.[4,5] By identifying patients more likely to benefit from surgery the clinician can hope to improve the survival statistics for pancreatic resection. Various modes of radiological investigations have increased the staging yield, but all are unable to exclude minute peritoneal or hepatic metastases.

Coley et al.[6] found that spiral CT, the most utilized radiological investigation, has a positive predictive value of irresectability of 92% and macroscopic clearance prediction of 87%. These figures suggest

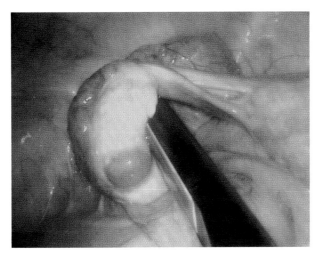

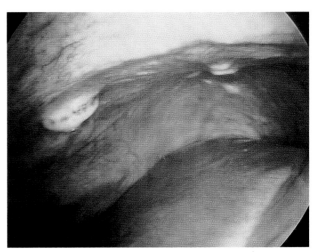

Figure 21.2 Laparoscopic staging of pancreatic malignancy: while high resolution CT scanning and MRI can detect many metastases from pancreatic carcinoma, laparoscopy adds specificity and sensitivity to the preoperative staging of pancreatic malignancy. Here a 1 cm lesion attached to the right ovary was biopsied and found to be metastatic pancreatic adenocarcinoma.

Figure 21.3 Laparoscopic staging of pancreatic malignancy: laparoscopy is particularly helpful in detecting small peritoneal deposits, often found in pancreatic malignancy and almost impossible to detect on CT. Here a patient with a 2 cm lesion in the head of the pancreas, which appeared resectable on CT, is found to have several small peritoneal deposits.

that further investigations may be unnecessary and that spiral CT alone should give enough information for the surgeon to decide on a path of resection or palliation.[7] However, laparoscopic ultrasound can improve on the staging of spiral CT. In particular, the presence of occult metastases can be readily visualized and can change the decision regarding resectability of tumours in 25–73% of patients.[3,8] Furthermore, laparoscopic ultrasound is better than CT at the detection of vascular invasion.[9]

We have used laparoscopy and laparoscopic ultrasound to assess 88 consecutive patients with upper gastrointestinal malignancy over a 3-year period, of whom 32 had pancreatic adenocarcinoma. These 32 patients were a select group deemed potentially resectable and were from a total of 173 patients referred to our unit with pancreatic carcinoma during the 3-year study period. All underwent elective laparoscopy under general anaesthesia as previously described.[10]

Laparoscopy was performed using a Hasson technique with one or two 10 mm ports in the right and left flank if needed for the laparoscopic ultrasound probe. A 7.5 MHz linear array ultrasound probe with non-flexible head (Aloka, Keymed, Southend, UK) was used to assess intrahepatic metastases, and to evaluate the involvement of the portal and superior mesenteric vein in pancreatic cancer. It was also used to assess coeliac and superior mesenteric arteries and to examine lymph nodes around the coeliac axis. Under direct laparoscopic vision, biopsies were taken from metastatic

lesions. In patients with obstructive jaundice and the presence of obvious metastatic disease, a biliary bypass was performed laparoscopically during the same session.[11]

Criteria for unresectability of a primary tumour included definite peritoneal or liver metastases, obstruction or invasion of the superior mesenteric vein (SMV) or superior mesenteric–portal vein confluence (SMPVC) and/or tumour encasement of the coeliac or superior mesenteric artery (SMA). Bilobar or extrahepatic metastatic involvement excluded patients assessed for possible hepatectomy. Patients assessed as suitable for curative surgery were scheduled for laparotomy 2 weeks later. This allowed time to examine biopsies carefully, to inform and prepare the patient thoroughly and to organize theatre accordingly.

In our experience, laparoscopy and laparoscopic ultrasound provide a specificity of 76% when assessing the resectability of pancreatic adenocarcinoma. This is similar to the findings of John et al.[3] who demonstrated that laparoscopy alone provides specificity for resectability of 50%, which is increased to 88% with the addition of laparoscopic ultrasound. Warshaw et al.[4] found that laparoscopy alone detected unsuspected small but visible abdominal metastases in nearly half the patients who came to laparotomy with pancreatic cancer and most workers in the area suggest that laparoscopy should be performed in all patients in whom a laparotomy for pancreatic carcinoma is contemplated.[4,12–14] Several authors have found that the combination of diagnostic laparoscopy with laparoscopic ultrasound in the staging of pancreatic cancer further increased the percentage of patients found to have metastatic disease.[3,15] The use of staging laparoscopy with laparoscopic ultrasonography has also been shown to increase the resectability rate in patients with liver tumours.[16] Other authors have shown that information derived exclusively from the ultrasound component of the laparoscopic examination directly affected patient management.[17]

While there is no doubt that laparoscopic staging of pancreatic tumours is accepted practice in many centres and that just over half of our patients have avoided an unnecessary laparotomy, it is perhaps most helpful to concentrate on those in whom laparoscopy failed to detect disseminated disease. Laparoscopy failed to detect irresectable tumour in three key areas: around the portal vein, posteriorly on the bare area of the liver and in lymph nodes around the mesocolon or porta hepatis. Portal vein involvement by pancreatic tumour is very difficult to assess prior to a formal dissection and our policy is always to offer surgery if laparoscopy and laparoscopic ultrasound suggested any hope of removing a pancreatic tumour from the portal vein. It is perhaps not surprising that a Whipple's resection had to be abandoned in three cases due to larger than expected pancreatic tumours that were either adherent to or actually involving the portal/superior mesenteric veins. In one case, a tumour within the uncinate process of the pancreas had actually invaded the superior mesenteric vein beneath the transverse mesocolon, an area which we had failed to examine adequately at laparoscopy. This problem may be overcome by reflecting the transverse colon and mesocolon cranially, a manoeuvre which we now routinely employ when staging carcinoma of the pancreas.

Bilateral liver metastases are usually picked up by laparoscopy and laparoscopic ultrasound, but in two of our patients, small metastases (<1 cm diameter) were missed in the posterior part of segment VIII of the liver (the bare area). Our suspicion is that this may be due to the use of a rigid ultrasound probe, with which it may be difficult to examine the posterior part of the liver. A flexible tip probe may be more useful in this context, but we have no experience with such an instrument.

Three further patients had unexpected lymph node metastases, one along the lesser omentum, one at the hilum of the liver and the third at the base of the mesocolon. Once again, these missed lymph nodes, which all contained tumour on frozen section during the laparotomy, might have been identified by more detailed examination of the areas in question at laparoscopy. The addition of a flexible tipped ultrasound probe, together with the lessons learned during our 3-year study, would suggest that it should be possible to determine the resectability of pancreatic and hepatic tumours with a specificity approaching 90% using this technique. However, there are still problems in assessing the state of the portal vein in pancreatic carcinoma and our policy remains one of a trial dissection, if there appears to be the possibility of a successful resection.

The results of our study are similar to previous authors who have studied the use of laparoscopy and laparoscopic ultrasound to stage intra-abdominal malignancy.

Laparoscopic staging will not supplant preoperative imaging tests such as ultrasound or CT scanning, but it will provide additional information in patients with upper gastrointestinal malignancy. Laparoscopic staging may decrease overall morbidity, operating costs and hospitalization in those patients who avoid an unnecessary laparotomy and additional palliative procedures can be performed at the same time as staging. On the basis of our 3-year prospective study we conclude that laparoscopy and laparoscopic ultrasound are valuable tools in the management of upper gastrointestinal malignancies.

Laparoscopic palliative bypass

Laparoscopic biliary or duodenal bypass of pancreatic tumours has been gaining wider acceptance with the rise in laparoscopic staging.[11,18–21] For biliary bypass the standard procedure should still be endoscopic retrograde cholangiopancreatography and stent placement. This carries a smaller morbidity and mortality than operative bypass and is usually fairly quick and simple to perform.[22–24] It does have a higher incidence of late failure necessitating change of stent (usually due to encrustation of the stent), but it is still the procedure of choice for biliary obstruction due to pancreatic tumours. The incidence of stent blockage is decreasing with the advent of better designed stents. However, in patients in whom endoscopic stenting is not technically possible or in whom patient preference is for operative bypass, then laparoscopic bypass should be considered. A minimally invasive approach to surgical bypass is very pertinent to these patients in whom the median survival from diagnosis is only 150 days. Thus any improvement in postoperative recovery time is of major benefit to the patient in whom quality of life is paramount.

Laparoscopic bypass by means of cholecystojejunostomy was first described in 1992[20,25] and similarly laparoscopic gastrojejunostomy for duodenal obstruction in the same year.[26] While the use of prophylactic gastrojejunostomy is advocated in open surgery for biliary bypass of pancreatic tumours (in which patient group 25% will go on to develop duodenal obstruction) its associated morbidity makes it harder to justify as a prophylactic procedure when it can be done if required by a minimally invasive route. For this reason we do not routinely perform a gastrojejunostomy at the time of laparoscopic biliary bypass. However, most patients undergoing laparoscopic biliary bypass are done due to failure of endoscopic stenting. The main cause of failure of endoscopic stenting is inability to pass the duodenoscope beyond a large tumour invading the duodenum. It is not unusual, therefore, to have impending duodenal obstruction at the time of surgery, making gastrojejunostomy advantageous.

Technique

The patient is placed supine and a standard umbilical 10 mm port site is used for the laparoscope. Additionally, a 12 mm port is placed in the right flank for an endoscopic linear stapler, and two further 5 mm ports in either flank for graspers and suture holders.

It is mandatory to perform a cholangiogram through the gallbladder if the surgeon plans to perform a cholecystojejunostomy. This is because it is often very difficult to assess cystic duct patency and proximity to the tumour from below by means of an ERCP. Contrast is by definition injected under very low pressure at ERCP, because of the presence of a biliary stricture, through which it had not been possible to pass a stent (otherwise the patient would not need to be considered for laparoscopic biliary bypass). By infusing 50 ml of contrast into the gallbladder after first removing an equivalent amount of bile under continuous flouroscopic screening (Figs 21.4 and 21.5), it is usually possible to delineate the junction between the cystic and hepatic ducts. As long as there is 1 cm clearance between the junction and the pancreatic tumour, then laparoscopic bypass is likely to succeed. If, however, tumour is involved or near the cystic duct the biliary system should be decompressed above at the common hepatic duct with a choledochojejunostomy. One trick with a cholangiogram undertaken through the gallbladder is to be patient, as there are often small plugs of mucus obstructing the cystic duct (even in the presence of a grossly distended gallbladder) and it may require quite a head of pressure from the contrast medium to dislodge these. In order to obtain this, it is best to use the Reddick/Olsen cholangiogram forceps (Stortz, Germany) in order to close the hole in the

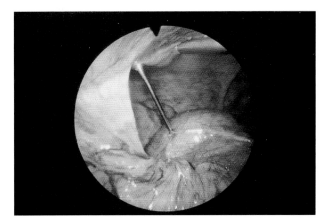

Figure 21.4 Laparoscopic cholecystojejunostomy: initial decompression of the gallbladder is best effected with a Verres needle placed through the abdominal wall and into the gallbladder under direct vision. After aspiration of 50–100 ml of bile, a cholangiogram (Fig. 21.5) may be performed to ensure a patent cystic duct prior to using the gallbladder for biliary bypass.

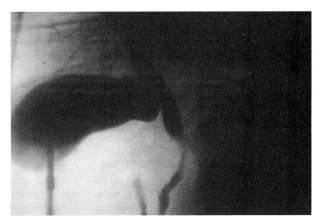

Figure 21.5 Laparoscopic cholecystojejunostomy: cholangiography is essential prior to electing for a cholecystojejunostomy in patients with pancreatic cancer. It allows demonstration of the bile duct stricture from above and unless there is at least 1 cm of bile duct above the stricture before the cystic duct entry, the gallbladder is unlikely to provide effective biliary bypass in the longer term. Often, the cystic duct contains small mucous plugs and contrast may need to be infused into the gallbladder under a fair amount of pressure. It is helpful if C-arm screening is used to obtain dynamic images as contrast is infused.

gallbladder snugly around the cholangiogram catheter (Fig. 21.2). It is interesting to note that in our own experience,[11] distension of the gallbladder is not a good indication of either a patent cystic duct or anatomy which would favour the use of the gallbladder as a conduit for bile. It may be that the lack of a cholangiogram, prior to cholecystojejunostomy in the era of open surgery, is what led to its

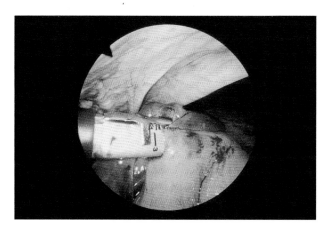

Figure 21.6 Laparoscopic cholecystojejunostomy: the simplest way to approximate the jejunum and gallbladder is using a linear cutting stapler. Here the jejunum and gallbladder are shown with the stapler in place.

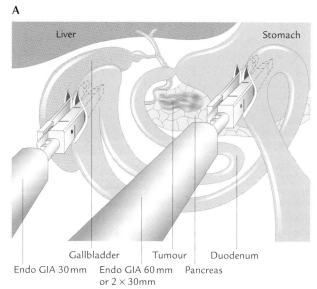

A

Liver   Stomach

Gallbladder   Tumour   Duodenum
Endo GIA 30 mm   Endo GIA 60 mm Pancreas
                  or 2 × 30mm

B

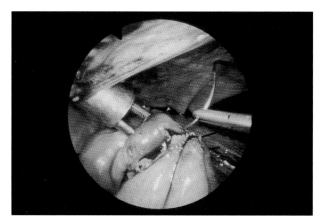

Figure 21.7 After firing the stapler, the remaining hole may be closed with a suture of the surgeon's choice—here 2/0 silk is being used.

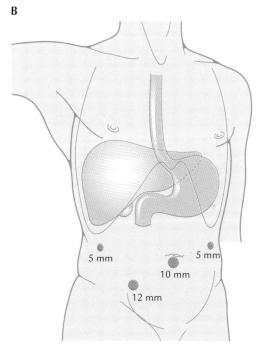

5 mm   5 mm
          10 mm
     12 mm

Figure 21.8 Diagramatic representation of laparoscopic cholecystojejunostomy and gastroenterostomy and schematic illustration of port placement for this operation.

10% failure rate and subsequent disrepute as a means of biliary bypass in pancreatic cancer.

If a single biliary anastomosis is performed, a loop of proximal jejunum should be brought up to the gallbladder such that it is as close to the duodeno–jejunal flexure as possible without creating tension on the loop. If a double anastomosis is performed then the gastrojejunostomy should be performed first again, using a loop of jejunum as proximal to the duodeno–jejunal flexure as possible without tension and more distal jejunum used for the biliary anastomosis (Fig. 21.6).

Cholecystojejunostomy or choledochojejunostomy can be performed using a simple suture technique or with a stapled and sutured technique (Figs 21.7 and 21.8). The jejunal loop should be held in approximation to the gallbladder fundus. The jejunum should be incised for approximately 2 cm

longitudinally on its antimesenteric border using diathermy and a similar 2 cm incision made in the fundus of the gallbladder or longitudinally along the common hepatic duct. The gallbladder or hepatic duct should be aspirated of bile as much as possible to avoid unnecessary contamination of the peritoneum. Simple suture technique involves suturing the anastomosis with a continuous seromuscular posterior layer using 2/0 vicryl or monocryl, followed by a continuous anterior layer, again with a seromuscular stitch. The stapled and sutured technique involves the use of an endoscopic linear stapler cutter for the main part of the anastomosis, with a sutured closure of the remaining enterotomy. The stapler is passed down the 12 mm port and opened. While the fundus of the gallbladder and the jejunal loop are held in apposition the two limbs of the stapler are passed into 1 cm linear incisions in the gallbladder and jejunum and the stapler closed. At this point, prior to firing of the staple gun the surgeon should ascertain that the stapler is in the correct position with the antimesenteric border of the jejunum held with the gallbladder wall. The stapler is fired and the remaining enterotomy closed with a continuous seromuscular 2/0 vicryl stitch. If a larger anastomosis is required the stapler can be reloaded following the first firing and again fired to lengthen the anastomosis. For a stapled sutured choledochojejunostomy it is usually best to fire the stapler through a left sided port to gain correct alignment along the longitudinal axis of the common hepatic duct. Following firing of the stapler the remaining defect is closed using a continuous seromuscular 2/0 vicryl suture. Postoperatively, patients are encouraged to mobilize and drink freely on the morning following surgery.

Gastrojejunostomy is usually performed at the same time as cholecystojejunostomy (Fig. 21.9). The same patient position and port placements are used. The proximal jejunum is brought antecolic and positioned along the gastric antrum in an isoperistaltic orientation. A longitudinal cut is made using diathermy for 2 cm along the antimesenteric border of the jejunum and opposing stomach and a

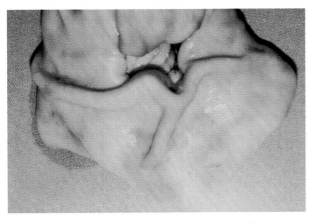

Figure 21.9 Laparoscopic gastroenterostomy (illustration courtesy of Professor Les Nathanson, Brisbane). Experimental work in dogs has shown that stapled gastroenterostomies often stenose significantly after 12 weeks. If only a single firing of the 30 mm linear stapler cutter is used, gastric outlet obstruction is a common problem and it is therefore advisable to use two firings of this stapling gun to ensure an adequate lumen. This illustration shows a 3 cm anastomosis after 12 weeks and it has closed almost completely.

continuous full thickness posterior layer is sutured using 2/0 vicryl or monocryl, followed by a continuous anterior layer, again with a full thickness stitch. Alternatively, a similar stapled sutured technique can be used with a 10 mm linear stapler cutter being passed through a 12 mm port in the right flank. The jaws of the stapler are passed down into the stomach and jejunum and closed. The stapler is then fired after the alignment of the stapler cutter has first been checked. The remaining enterotomy is closed using a continuous full thickness suture with 2/0 vicryl. Postoperatively the patient is encouraged to mobilize as soon as possible and to drink freely from 24 hours. We do not routinely drain the abdomen in such cases.

Although most patients with pancreatic cancer are successfully palliated by endoscopic insertion of a biliary stent there will remain a small proportion in whom laparoscopic bypass is a valid and minimally invasive alternative. Laparoscopic gastrojejunostomy can also be performed for those patients with added duodenal obstruction.

Endoscopic techniques in pancreatic disease

Pancreatography

Endoscopic retrograde pancreatography is now an established and important diagnostic tool for diseases of the pancreas. Further endoscopic developments have made possible diagnostic procedures such as endoscopic ultrasonography, pancreatic sphincter manometry[27,28] and measurement of pancreatic blood flow.[29]

Endoscopic therapy for diseases of the pancreas can be divided into those for acute pancreatitis and those for chronic pancreatitis. In acute biliary pancreatitis endoscopic sphincterotomy (ES) is a controversial topic. Two large randomized trials of ERCP and ES within the first 72 hours of admission with biliary pancreatitis found a lower morbidity and mortality for ES only in severe pancreatitis.[32,31]

Current opinion would suggest that endoscopic sphincterotomy is reserved for the treatment of severe biliary pancreatitis and for those patients in whom the disease does not settle within 4 to 5 days or in whom symptoms of cholangitis are present.

Endoscopic therapies for chronic pancreatitis include endoscopic pancreatic sphincterotomy, insertion of ductal stents, stone lithotripsy and the endoscopic drainage of pseudocysts. Patients with chronic pancreatitis have abdominal pain of varying intensity. The most widely held view amongst endoscopists is that the pain is related to high intraductal pressures.[32–38] The therapeutic hope is that relief of increased ductal pressure by sphincterotomy or the insertion of a pancreatic duct stent will relieve pain by relieving the ductal pressure. Surgical decompression of the pancreatic duct in patients with chronic pancreatitis results in improvement of pain.[39] It is not surprising that endoscopic decompression has been studied. Results from endoscopic stenting of the pancreatic duct shows that it carries a relatively low morbidity rate of between 5 and 18% and a mortality rate of 0–3%. Improvement of pain is seen in 50–94% of patients.[40–45] The major drawback behind endoscopic stenting of the pancreatic duct is the poor long-term outcome. Most stents will block or displace over time. Furthermore the stents can induce inflammatory changes similar to those of chronic pancreatitis and block side branches along the section of the duct through which the stent passes. Pancreatic stents rarely work for longer than 3 months and should be removed after this time to avoid undue stent-associated inflammation. If there has been no improvement in pain then the stent should be removed after one month.[40] Further improvements in the technical aspect of pancreatic stents may improve the potential for their use and certainly more studies are required to ascertain their optimal use. At present pancreatic stenting is certainly worth considering in patients with severe pain from chronic pancreatitis who are too infirm for surgery or in patients with small pancreatic ductal strictures.

Pancreatic pseudocysts

The treatment of pancreatic pseudocysts has undergone a small revolution in the last ten years.[46] The advent of percutaneous and endoscopic stenting and laparoscopic surgery for pancreatic pseudocysts has provided the clinician with a greatly improved stock of therapeutic procedures for this condition.[46,47]

A true pancreatic pseudocyst is a pancreatic fluid collection whose capsule is composed of inflammatory fibrous tissue. The fluid within is rich in amylase and derived from acute inflammatory exudate following pancreatitis or from a pancreatico-cystic tract that may still be patent at the time of diagnosis. There are three common causes that lead to different types of pseudocyst: acute pancreatitis, chronic pancreatitis (CP) and trauma. However, the distinction between the first two becomes blurred in cases of acute alcoholic pancreatitis in which the pancreatic duct may have been diseased prior to the acute attack.

Following acute pancreatitis it is common for a proportion of cysts and acute fluid collections to regress if left alone.[48–50] While some pseudocysts regress if left to their own devices, this cannot be anticipated on an individual basis. The chances of spontaneous regression appear to diminish the longer the cyst is present and the longer the pseudocyst is present, the greater the risk of complications arising from it. There thus comes a time when it is expedient to treat the pseudocyst and this is generally thought to be between 6 and 12 weeks from diagnosis.[51–56] Pseudocysts of chronic pancreatitis should be treated on initial presentation as they rarely regress spontaneously.[51,57,58]

When the pseudocyst is emptied and allowed to drain freely the cavity should obliterate with time. This principle underlines successful treatment which can be performed by either internal or external drainage or resection. Adequate therapy should have a lower morbidity and mortality rate than leaving the cyst alone and, although good results can be achieved by external drainage of the pseudocyst or resection,[59,60] optimal treatment is best achieved by internal drainage into a viscus either surgically[61] or by other techniques. Internal endoscopic or laparoscopic drainage procedures utilize either stomach, duodenum or jejunum for anastomosis to the wall of the pseudocyst for internal drainage.

Endoscopic internal drainage

There has been a dramatic upsurge in endoscopic techniques for internal drainage of pancreatic pseudocysts.[62,63]

There are three prerequisites for endoscopic drainage. First the cyst should cause a visible bulge into the lumen of the stomach or duodenum, second there should be no vascularities within the area and third the cyst should be less than 1 cm from the lumen. The most common method employed uses the insertion of a guidewire from the duodenum or stomach into the cyst and subsequent passage of a plastic stent over the guidewire. The stent may be either a pigtail or a straight plastic stent, although there is an increased risk with the latter of the danger of displacement of the stent into the cyst cavity. Endoscopic ultrasound should be utilized first to check for large vessels at the site of potential puncture. Endoscopic retrograde pancreatography gives valuable information with regard to ductal communication with the pseudocyst[64] and for smaller cysts within the pancreatic parenchyma and with a ductal connection, trans-sphincteric stenting and drainage will allow drainage and maintain ductal calibre.[65]

Complication rates and success rates with these techniques were initially fairly high, although they are improving and most recent studies suggest rates comparable to surgery.[65–68] Success rates are around 95% with complication rates of between 5 and 19% and recurrence rates of 12 to 23%. It is difficult to compare endoscopic and surgical therapy as they are usually used on different populations of patients. An adequate prospective randomized trial would be inhibited by the exclusion criteria of endoscopic treatment. At present it is reasonable to propose endoscopic therapy in patients with the three prerequisites outlined above if there is access to a centre with the necessary expertise and equipment.

Laparoscopic pseudocystogastrostomy

Laparoscopic internal drainage procedures for pancreatic pseudocysts are a fairly recent addition to the treatment of this condition.[69,70]

With any surgical procedure on a pancreatic pseudocyst it is important to aspirate the pseudocyst fluid completely and examine the entire wall carefully to exclude an associated neoplasia. A biopsy of the wall should also be taken. The cyst wall should be thick enough and resistant enough to contain and hold the stitches. A study in dogs has suggested that it takes 6 weeks from the episode of pancreatitis for the cyst wall to mature enough for adequate anastomosis and this is another reason to wait before surgery.[54] Meticulous haemostasis, observation and care during surgery will ameliorate postoperative haemorrhage. The pseudocyst wall is usually in contact with large arteries, which have a habit of bleeding. The major cause of postoperative mortality is haemorrhage, either from the cyst wall or the anastomosis, especially in larger pseudocysts,[71] and it is not uncommon for the cystic fluid or acidic gastric contents to erode vessels around the anastomosis or within the wall in the postoperative period.

Technique

The patient should be placed supine. An umbilical port site should be placed for the laparoscope and two to three further ports added for instrumentation. We use a technique whereby the pseudocyst is first identified through the stomach with laparoscopic ultrasound. The anterior stomach wall is then incised longitudinally using diathermy and the stomach opened. The bulge of the pseudocyst through the posterior stomach wall should then be apparent. Aspiration of the pseudocyst at this point should be performed to identify the correct placement and so avoid major vascular injury. The posterior gastric wall and the conjoined fibrotic wall of the pseudocyst are then incised using diathermy and

an endoscopic stapler used to staple across the walls and thus create a large stoma between cyst and stomach. The cyst wall should be biopsied at this point and careful attention should be given to haemostasis in order to avoid the common postoperative complication of haemorrhage. The anterior gastric wall is next sutured with 2/0 vicryl and surgery concluded.

Percutaneous cystogastrostomy

Percutaneous cystogastrostomy is a technique originally described in 1985,[72] which requires a deal of expertise, but very good results have so far been published.[73] Under general anaesthesia a pigtail stent, guided by ultrasound scanning, is passed through both anterior and posterior walls of the stomach and into the cyst. An endoscopic grasper then holds the catheter while the trocar is withdrawn so that the proximal end of the stent curls up within the gastric lumen. This technique would appear to have a low morbidity and cyst recurrence rate.

Laparoscopic pancreatic resection

Theoretically, there is a great advantage to laparoscopic techniques for pancreatic resection. The amount of surgical trauma involved using conventional techniques is considerable and therefore associated with much attendant co-morbidity. Minimal access techniques for pancreatic resection have therefore been applied with varying degrees of success.

Pancreaticoduodenectomy

The most common surgical procedure on the pancreas still presents a number of problems for laparoscopic surgeons. Pancreaticoduodenectomy requires skilful and meticulous dissection, haemostasis and anastomoses, all of which are exceedingly difficult to perform with the limited hand co-ordination and feedback currently inherent in laparoscopic surgery. Nevertheless, pancreaticoduodenectomy has been performed in patients using laparoscopic techniques.[74] In the porcine model this procedure was time-consuming (5 to 7.5 hours) and associated with a failure rate of 50%, an anastomotic leak rate of up to 66% and widespread jejunal ecchymoses from extensive manipulation.[75] Laparoscopic dissection followed by minilaparotomy pancreaticoduodenectomy has been performed successfully in a patient with pancreatic cancer,[76]

A

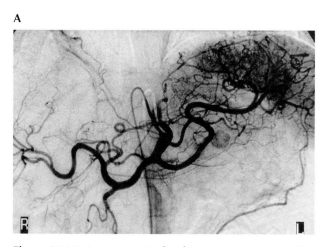

B

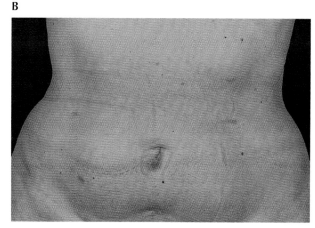

Figure 21.10 Laparoscopic distal pancreatectomy: a 69-year-old woman presented with repeated faints and investigation suggesting an insulinoma. Angiography (A) revealed a small tumour blush in the tail of the pancreas and she underwent laparoscopic distal pancreatectomy. (B) The operation was effected through four ports. The pancreas was divided using a linear stapler cutter and the whole procedure took under 2 hours. Postoperative hospital stay was 3 days and the patient returned to work within 2 weeks. There had been no recurrence of her symptoms during the next 3 years' follow-up and histology of the resected specimen confirmed a small insulinoma.

although further results are still awaited. While very few centres are performing laparoscopic pancreaticoduodenectomy in patients this is still a risky and unproven technique and should not be recommended at the present time. Improvements in laparoscopic equipment and techniques may bring the operation into the mainstream in the future.

Distal pancreatectomy

In contrast to pancreaticoduodenectomy, distal pancreatectomy is a feasible and relatively widely accepted procedure (Fig. 21.10). It was first performed by Sussman et al.[77] in 1996 for a patient with an insulinoma in the tail of the pancreas, and by Cuschieri et al.[78] for a patient with chronic pancreatitis. Subsequently there have been several reports of laparoscopic distal pancreatectomy. Cuschieri has performed a 70% pancreatectomy with splenectomy for five patients with intractable pain from chronic pancreatitis. The mean operating time was 4.5 hours with minimal morbidity and a mean hospital stay of 6 days. The procedure would therefore appear to be safe and to be associated with faster recovery than conventional techniques. Current indications for distal pancreatectomy include chronic pancreatitis affecting mainly the body and tail, isolated benign neuroendocrine or malignant tumours of the distal pancreas and small pancreatic pseudocysts and abscesses of the tail of the pancreas. However, caution should be observed with all cases of malignant tumours resected through laparoscopy. At the present time curative resection has not been proven to be adequate by laparoscopic techniques.

Technique

Although the operation can be performed by a retroperitoneal technique, we shall concentrate on the more standard laparoscopic approach. The patient is positioned supine and exposure can be facilitated by raising the left upper quadrant with a small sandbag. The technique of laparoscopic distal pancreatectomy involves standard insufflation of the peritoneum. To approach the pancreas the lesser sac should be opened through the infragastric route by careful dissection of the omentum off the left side of the transverse colon. The omentum can then be partially lifted up and to the right to expose the left hand side of the lesser sac and the tail of the pancreas. The pancreas should then be examined by ultrasonography and the precise resection margins identified. Care should be taken to identify the splenic vessels and these should be avoided if the spleen is not to be resected at the same time. Dissection of the inferior edge of the pancreas at the resection margin should now be undertaken. The pancreas can be transected using an endoscopic stapling device. This often requires more than one firing of the stapler, especially if the pancreas is calcified and diseased from chronic pancreatitis. The size of staple is important; the pancreas is a vascular gland and staples should be strong enough to prevent bleeding from the transected edge and to prevent pancreatic duct leakage. The tail should now be dissected free from loose attachments of the retroperitoneum, lienorenal ligament and the splenic vessels. The resected specimen should be placed in an endoscopic retrieval bag and removed through the largest port. This may need to be enlarged in order to deliver the specimen. Unlike the spleen it is important to remove the pancreas whole in order for adequate histological assessment of the resection margins, although this does not apply if pancreatectomy is performed for chronic pancreatitis. The lesser sac should be drained following surgery to control any small pancreatic leaks.

Key points

- Roles of laparoscopy in pancreatic surgery:
  Staging pancreatic tumours

  Treatment of pancreatic pseudocysts
  Palliative surgical biliary bypass and gastroenterostomy.
- Laparoscopic staging of pancreatic tumours:
  Visual detection of small metastases (peritoneum and liver)
  Intraoperative ultrasound
  Peritoneal cytology.
- Laparoscopic palliative bypass surgery for pancreatic carcinoma:
  Always obtain transcystic cholangiography to assess patency of cystic duct.

REFERENCES

1. Cuschieri A, Hall A, Clarke J. Value of laparoscopy in the diagnosis and management of pancreatic carcinoma. Gut 1978; 19: 672–7

2. Jakimowicz J. Technical and clinical aspects of intraoperative ultrasound applicable to laparoscopic ultrasound. Endosc Surg Allied Technol 1994; 2: 119–26

3. John T, Greig J, Carter D, Garden O. Carcinoma of the pancreatic head and periampullary region. Tumour staging with laparoscopy and laparoscopic ultrasonography. Ann Surg 1995; 221: 156–64

4. Warshaw AL, Tepper JE, Shipley WU. Laparoscopy in the staging and planning of therapy for pancreatic cancer. Am J Surg 1986; 151: 76–80

5. Warshaw AL, Gu ZY, Wittenberg J, Waltman AC. Preoperative staging and assessment of resectability of pancreatic cancer. Arch Surg 1990; 125: 230–3

6. Coley S, Strickland N, Walker J, Williamson R. Spiral CT and the preoperative assessment of pancreatic adenocarcinoma. Clin Radiol 1997; 52: 24–30

7. Gloor B, Todd K, Reber H. Diagnostic workup of patients with suspected pancreatic carcinoma: the University of California–Los Angeles approach. Cancer 1997; 79: 1780–6

8. Schrenk P, Wayand W. Value of diagnostic laparoscopy in abdominal malignancies. Int Surg 1995; 80: 353–5

9. Hann L, Conlon K, Dougherty E, Hilton S, Bach A, Brennan M. Laparoscopic sonography of peripancreatic tumors: preliminary experience. AJR 1997; 169: 1257–62

10. Cuschieri A. Laparoscopic surgery of the pancreas. J R Coll Surg Edin 1994; 39: 178–84

11. Rhodes M, Nathanson L, Fielding G. Laparoscopic biliary and gastric bypass: a useful adjunct in the treatment of carcinoma of the pancreas. Gut 1995; 36: 778–80

12. Cuschieri A. Value of laparoscopy in hepatobiliary disease. Ann R Coll Surg Engl 1975; 57: 33–8

13. Cuschieri A. Laparoscopy for pancreatic cancer: does it benefit the patient? Eur J Surg Oncol 1988; 14: 41–4

14. Murugiah M, Paterson-Brown S, Windsor JA, Miles WF, Garden OJ. Early experience of laparoscopic ultrasonography in the management of pancreatic carcinoma. Surg Endosc 1993; 7: 177–81

15. Bemelman WA, de Wit LT, van Delden OM et al. Diagnostic laparoscopy combined with laparoscopic ultrasonography in staging of cancer of the pancreatic head region [see comments]. Br J Surg 1995; 82: 820–4

16. John TG, Greig DJ, Crosbie JL, Miles WFA, Garden OJ. Superior staging of liver tumours with laparoscopy and laparoscopic ultrasound. Ann Surg 1994; 220: 711–9

17. Rifkin MD, Rosato FE, Branch M, Foster J, Yang SL, Barbot DJ, Marks GJ. Intra-operative ultrasound of the liver. An important adjunctive tool for decision making in the operating room. Ann Surg 1987; 205: 466–72

18. Nathanson L. Laparoscopy and pancreatic cancer: biopsy, staging and bypass. Ballieres Clin Gastroenterol 1993; 7: 941–60

19. Nathanson L, Shimi S, Cuschieri A. Sutured laparoscopic cholecystojejunostomy evolved in an animal model. J R Coll Surg Edin 1992; 37: 215–20

20. Shimi S, Banting S, Cuschieri A. Laparoscopy in the management of pancreatic cancer: endoscopic cholecystojejunostomy for advanced disease. Br J Surg 1992; 79: 317–9

21. Hawsali A. Laparoscopic cholecysto-jejunostomy for obstructing pancreatic cancer. J Laparoendosc 1992; 2: 351–5

22. Dowsett J, Russell R, Hatfield A et al. Malignant obstructive jaundice: what is the best management? A randomised trial of surgery versus endoscopic stenting. 1988; 29: A1493

23. Andersen J, Sarensen S, Fruse A, Rokkjaer M, Mateen P. Randomised trial of endoscopic endoprothesis versus operative bypass in malignant obstructive jaundice. Gut 1989; 30: 1132–5

24. Shepherd H, Royle G, Ross A, Diba A, Arthur M, Colin-Jones D. Endoscopic biliary prosthesis in the palliation of malignant obstruction of the distal common bile duct: a randomisd trial. Br J Surg 1988; 75: 1166–8

25. Fletcher D, Jones R. Laparoscopic cholecystojejunostomy as palliation for obstructive jaundice in inoperable carcinoma of the pancreas. Surg Endosc 1992; 6: 147–9

26. Wilson R, Varma J. Laparoscopic gastroenterostomy for malignant duodenal obstruction. Br J Surg 1992; 79: 1348

27. Raddawi H, Geenen J, Hogan W, Dodds W, Venu R, Johnson G. Pressure measurements from biliary and pancreatic segments of sphincter of Oddi – comparison between patients with functional abdominal pain, biliary or pancreatic disease. Dig Dis Sci 1991; 36: 71–4

28. Lans J, Parikh N, Geenen J. Applications of sphincter of Oddi manometry in routine clinical investigations. Endoscopy 1991; 23: 139–43

29. Lewis M, Lo S, Reber P et al. Endoscopic measurement of pancreatic blood flow: alterations In patients with chronic pancreatitis. Gastroenterology 1996; 110: A411

30. Fan S, Lai E, Mok F. Early treatment of acute biliary pancreatitis by endoscopic papillotomy. N Engl J Med 1993; 328: 228–32

31. Neoptolemos J, Carr-Locke D, London N. Controlled trial of urgent endoscopic retrograde cholangiopancreatography and endoscopic sphincterotomy versus conservative treatment for pancreatitis due to gallstones. Lancet 1988; 2: 979–83

32. Widdison AL, Alvarez C, Karanjia ND, Reber HA. Experimental evidence of beneficial effects of ductal decompression in chronic pancreatitis. Endoscopy 1991; 23: 151–4

33. Karanjia N, Widdison A, Leung F, Alvarez C, Lutrin F, Reber H. Compartment syndrome in experimental chronic obstructive pancreatitis: effect of decompressing the main pancreatic duct. Br J Surg 1994; 81: 259–64

34. Sarles H, Bernard JP, Johnson C. Pathogenesis and epidemiology of chronic pancreatitis. Ann Rev Med 1989; 40: 453–68

35. Jalleh R, Aslam M, Williamson R. Pancreatic tissue and ductal pressures in chronic pancreatitis. Br J Surgery 1991; 78: 1235–7

36. Ebbehoj N, Borly L, Madsen P, Svendsen L. Pancreatic tissue pressure and pain in chronic pancreatitis. Pancreas 1986; 1: 556–8

37. Madsen P, Winkler K. The intraductal pancreatic pressure in chronic obstructive pancreatitis. Scand J Gastroenterol 1982; 19: 553–4

38. Bradley E. Pancreatic duct pressure in chronic pancreatitis. Am J Surg 1982; 144: 313–6

39. Alvarez C, Widdison AL, Reber HA. New perspectives in the surgical management of chronic pancreatitis. Pancreas 1991; 6 (Suppl 1): S76–81

40. Huibregste K, Smits M. Endoscopic management of diseases of the pancreas. Am J Gastroenterol 1994; 89: S66–S77

41. Cremer M, Deviere J, Delhaye M. Stenting in severe chronic pancreatitis: results of medium term follow-up in seventy-six patients. Endoscopy 1991; 23: 171–6

42. Grimm H, Meyer W, Nam V. New modalities for treating chronic pancreatitis. Endoscopy 1989; 21: 70–4

43. Fuji T, Amano H, Ohmura E. Endoscopic pancreatic sphincterotomy: technique and evaluation. Endoscopy 1989; 21: 27–30

44. Kozarek R, Patterson D, Ball T. Endoscopic placement of pancreatic stents and drains in the management of pancreatitis. Ann Surg 1988; 209: 261–6

45. McCarthy J, Geenen J, Hogan W. Preliminary experience with endoscopic stent placement in benign pancreatic diseases. Gastrointest Endosc 1988; 34: 16–8

46. Adams DB, Anderson MC. Changing concepts in the surgical management of pancreatic pseudocysts. Am Surg 1992; 58: 173–80

47. Grace PA, Williamson RC. Modern management of pancreatic pseudocysts. Br J Surg 1993; 80: 573–81

48. Czaja AJ, Fisher M, Marin GA. Spontaneous resolution of pancreatic masses (pseudocysts?) – development and disappearance after acute alcoholic pancreatitis. Arch Intern Med 1975; 135: 558–62

49. Beebe DS, Bubrick MP, Onstad GR, Hitchcock CR. Management of pancreatic pseudocysts. Surg Gynecol Obstet 1984; 159: 562–4

50. Yeo C, Bastides J, Lynch-Nyhan A, Fishman E, Zinner M, Cameron J. The natural history of pancreatic pseudocysts documented by computed tomography. Surg Gynecol Obstet 1990; 170: 411–7

51. Warshaw AL, Rattner DW. Timing of surgical drainage for pancreatic pseudocyst. Clinical and chemical criteria. Ann Surg 1985; 202: 720–4

52. Anderson MC, Adams DB. Pancreatic pseudocysts. When to drain, when to wait. Postgrad Med 1991; 89: 199–200

53. Frey CF. Pancreatic pseudocyst—operative strategy. Ann Surg 1978; 188: 652–62

54. Warren W, March W, Mullen W. Experimental production of pseudocysts of the pancreas with preliminary observations on internal drainage. Surg Gynecol Obstet 1957; 105: 385–92

55. Mullins R, Malagoni M, Bergamini T, Casey J, Richardson J. Controversies in the management of pancreatic pseudocysts. Am J Surg 1988; 155: 165–72

56. Desa L, Williamson R. On-table pancreatography: importance in planning operative strategy. Br J Surg 1990; 77: 1145–50

57. Crass R, Way L. Acute and chronic pancreatic pseudocysts are different. Am J Surg 1981; 142: 660–3

58. Williams KJ, Fabian TC. Pancreatic pseudocyst: recommendations for operative and nonoperative management. Am Surg 1992; 58: 199–205

59. Andersson R, Janzon M, Sundberg I, Bengmark S. Management of pancreatic pseudocysts. Br J Surg 1989; 76: 550–2

60. Adams DB, Anderson MC. Percutaneous catheter drainage compared with internal drainage in the management of pancreatic pseudocyst. Ann Surg 1992; 215: 571–6

61. Moran B, Rew DA, Johnson CD. Pancreatic pseudocyst should be treated by surgical drainage. Ann R Coll Surg Engl 1994; 76: 54–8

62. Dohmoto M, Rupp KD. Endoscopic drainage of pancreatic pseudocysts. Surg Endosc 1992; 6: 118–24

63. Froeschle G, Meyer-Pannwitt U, Brueckner M, Henne-Bruns D. A comparison between surgical, endoscopic and percutaneous management of pancreatic pseudocysts – long term results. Acta Chir Belg 1993; 93: 102–6

64. Weltz C, Pappas TN. Pancreatography and the surgical management of pseudocysts. Gastrointest Endosc Clin N Am 1995; 5: 269–79

65. Barthet M, Sahel J, Bodiou-Bertei C, Bernard J-P. Endoscopic transpapillary drainage of pancreatic pseudocysts. 1995; 3: 208–13

66. Binmoeller K, Seifert H, Walter A, Soehendra N. Transpapillary and transmural drainage of pancreatic pseudocysts. Gastrointest Endosc 1995; 42: 219–24

67. Cremer M, Deviere J, Engelholm L. Endoscopic management of cysts and pseudocysts in chronic pancreatitis: long-term follow-up after 7 years of experience. Gastrointest Endosc 1989; 35: 1–9

68. Lawson JM, Baillie J. Endoscopic therapy for pancreatic pseudocysts. Gastrointest Endosc Clin N Am 1995; 5: 181–93

69. Frantzides C, Ludwig K, Redlich P. Laparoscopic management of a pancreatic pseudocyst. J Laparoendosc Surg 1995; 4: 55–9

70. Trias M, Targarona E, Balague C, Cifuentes A, Taura P. Intraluminal stapled laparoscopic cystogastrostomy for treatment of pancreatic pseudocyst. Br J Surg 1995; 82: 403

71. Johnson LB, Rattner DW, Warshaw AL. The effect of size of giant pancreatic pseudocysts on the outcome of internal drainage procedures. Surg Gynecol Obstet 1991; 173: 171–4

72. Hancke S, Henriksen F. Percutaneous pancreatic cystogastrostomy guided by ultrasound scanning and gastroscopy. Br J Surg 1985; 72: 916–7

73. Henriksen FW, Hancke S. Percutaneous cystogastrostomy for chronic pancreatic pseudocyst. Br J Surg 1994; 81: 1525–8

74. Gagner M, Pomp A. Laparoscopic pylorus-preserving pancreaticoduodenectomy. Surg Endosc 1994; 8: 407–10

75. Jones D, Wu J, Soper N. Laparoscopic pancreaticoduodenectomy in the porcine model. Surg Endosc 1997; 11: 326–30

76. Uyama I, Ogiwara H, Iada S, Takahara T, Furuta T, Kikuchi K. Laparoscopic minilaparotomy pancreaticoduodenectomy with lymphadenectomy using an abdominal wall lift method. Surg Laparosc Endosc 1996; 6: 405–10

77. Sussman L, Christie R, Whittle D. Laparoscopic excision of distal pancreas including insulinoma. Aust NZ J Surg 1996; 66: 414–6

78. Cuschieri A, Jakimowicz J, van-Spreeuwel J. Laparoscopic distal 70% pancreatectomy and splenectomy for chronic pancreatitis. Ann Surg 1996; 223: 280–5

22 Carcinoma of the head of the pancreas involving the portal vein

Lawrence E Harrison, Kevin C Conlon and Murray F Brennan

Introduction

Even though surgical resection remains the only potentially curative treatment for adenocarcinoma of the pancreas, only 10–20% of patients are candidates for pancreatic resection.[1,2] This low resectability rate reflects the advanced stage of disease at the time of diagnosis, with almost 50% of patients having distant spread of tumor and approximately one-third manifesting locally advanced disease. Most agree that distant metastases constitute an absolute contraindication for pancreatic resection. Locally advanced disease, which includes regional adenopathy and/or major vascular involvement, may also preclude curative resection. For many, the inability to dissect the pancreas from the portal vein (PV) or superior mesenteric vein (SMV) has historically been a contraindication for resection of patients with adenocarcinoma of the pancreas. Not infrequently, isolated local invasion of the PV or SMV may be the only obstacle to resection.

In an attempt to improve resectability and cure rates, excision of the pancreatic tumor in combination with resection of the major peripancreatic vascular structures and regional lymphadenectomy has been pursued. Although first reported in the early 1950s,[3,4] the technique of major vascular resection was initially popularized by Fortner in the 1970s.[5] Fortner described an operation in which the pancreatic resection included an en bloc regional lymph node dissection, peripancreatic soft tissue resection and resection of the portal vein (type I regional pancreatectomy). A type II operation was the same operation as a type I, but with resection and reconstruction of a segment of a major artery in the regional dissection.[6] While these extended resections led to an improved resectability rate, high morbidity and mortality rates and failure to convincingly improve long-term survival dissuaded most surgeons from pursuing the 'regional' pancreatectomy.[7,8]

Since Fortner's original report, pancreatic resection with vascular reconstruction has undergone considerable evolution and refinement with an acceptable morbidity and mortality. While arterial resection still carries a high morbidity and mortality,[9,10] extended pancreatic resections with venous reconstruction are feasible and may render patients free of gross tumor. However, the central issues concerning portal vein resection for pancreatic adenocarcinoma are: whether these resections can be performed safely and to what extent vascular involvement affects overall survival for patients undergoing pancreatic resection. This chapter summarizes data regarding major vascular resection (with emphasis on portal vein resection (PVR)) for adenocarcinoma of the head of the pancreas as it pertains to technique and outcome measures.

Preoperative clinical evaluation and diagnostic imaging

In terms of major vascular involvement, signs and symptoms of portal hypertension suggestive of PV occlusion are important to elicit, since this often translates into unresectable locally advanced disease. After a complete history and physical examination, the next most important diagnostic tool for the general diagnosis and staging of pancreatic cancer is a high quality CT scan. Standard protocol should include a helical CT scan, including oral and intravenous contrast with 3 mm sections through the pancreas.

After ruling out distant disease, evaluation of the mesenteric vasculature is the next step prior to exploration. For patients with locally advanced tumors by CT scan, portal vein invasion is a common finding on preoperative imaging. Tumors large enough or inopportunely placed to involve the PV often involve the superior mesenteric artery (SMA). However, isolated PV involvement is not infrequently seen. Therefore, in the absence of distant metastatic disease and obvious arterial involvement, patients with suspected isolated portal vein involvement should still be considered candidates for resection.

Historically, surgeons have relied on angiography to determine vascular involvement by tumor. During the venous phase of a mesenteric angiogram, the PV can be visualized and tumor invasion is suggested by narrowing of the vessel. Nakao and colleagues, using a grading system from A through D, correlated angiographic evidence of PV tumor invasion with histologic invasion and outcome. They demonstrated that no histologic invasion was noted in type A (normal) portagrams. As the narrowing progressed from unilateral (type B) to bilateral (type C) to marked stenosis or obstruction (type D), the percentage and degree of histologic invasion by tumor increased, which correlated with outcome.[11] Similar grading systems have also been used to predict resectability and outcome after PVR. Using angiography in a series of patients undergoing PVR, Ishikawa et al.[12] developed a grading system to classify tumor invasion of the PV/SMV based on the mesenteric angiogram. By retrospective analysis, they suggested that patients whose angiogram showed less than semicircular encroachment or invasion <1.2 cm in length benefited from PVR.

Most surgeons have abandoned the use of mesenteric angiography for preoperative evaluation of patients with peripancreatic masses since a high quality CT scan evaluates tumor invasion of the PV and SMA as well as, if not better than, angiography. A contrast enhanced helical CT scan of the abdomen with thin cuts through the pancreas allows very accurate evaluation of the SMV–PV complex, as well as arterial involvement by the tumor (Fig. 22.1). In addition to imaging of the pancreas with one breath hold, which suppresses motion artifact, it also allows quick arterial enhancement and a second pass provides a portal phase, as well. In most centers, the CT scan has supplanted the use of angiography to determine vascular involvement of peripancreatic tumors. At the present time, a quality CT scan should be considered the standard of care for evaluation of tumor involvement of the PV/SMV.

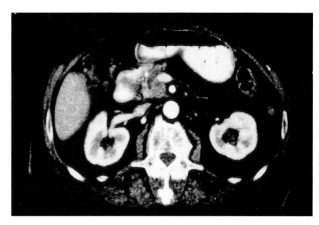

Figure 22.1 CT imaging demonstrates a pancreatic head mass involving the superior mesenteric vein with a clear fat plane surrounding the superior mesenteric artery.

Ultrasonography also plays a role in imaging the PV and may have clinical application. Transabdominal or endoscopic ultrasound may detect PV invasion and thrombosis. More recently, laparoscopic ultrasound has been used to stage patients with peripancreatic masses and has been found to be a useful method to detect tumor involvement of the PV[13,14] (Fig. 22.2 A, B). A novel method of PV evaluation employs intraportal endovascular ultrasonography (IPEUS) placed either by a percutaneous transhepatic route or intraoperatively by cannulation of a branch of the SMV. In a 1995 study, findings of IPEUS were confirmed by pathologic examination of resected PV specimens and results were compared to angiography and CT scan. The authors reported that the sensitivity and specificity of IPEUS was 100% and 93.3%, respectively, for predicting histologic invasion of the PV, which was superior to both angiography and CT scanning.[15] This technique, although interesting and technically challenging, would seem unlikely to gain acceptance as a routine test.

Magnetic resonance imaging (MRI) may ultimately be the procedure of choice for the evaluation of pancreatic cancer. In particular, some studies suggest that MRI provides accurate evaluation of tumor invasion of the PV/SMV. In a study of 20 patients with peripancreatic tumors, McFarland and colleagues demonstrated that MR angiography provided a positive predictive value of 100% when compared to intraoperative findings of PV invasion.[16] Trede and colleagues[17] prospectively staged 47 consecutive patients with presumed peripancreatic malignanices with preoperative MRI, CT, ultrasound and angiography and confirmed their radiological findings with surgical exploration. In terms of vascular invasion, MRI was found to be the most sensitive, specific and accurate staging method (Table 22.1). In addition to vascular evaluation, MRI

A

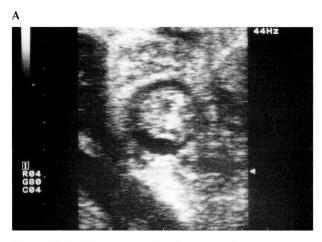

B

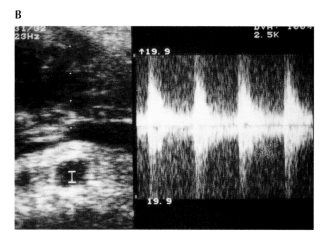

Figure 22.2 (A) Laparoscopic ultrasound demonstrating tumor thrombus within the portal vein. (B) Laparoscopic ultrasound with SMA Doppler: pancreatic mass encircling the splenic vein–portal vein confluence.

Table 22.1 Preoperative imaging: evaluation of vascular involvement

	Sensitivity (%)	Specificity (%)	Accuracy (%)
MRI	81	96	89
Ultrasound	81	84	83
CT	74	85	80
Angiography	43	100	69

was highly accurate in predicting liver metastasis, lymph node involvement and extrapancreatic tumor extension. While promising, this imaging modality will require additional evaluation before clinicians use it in lieu of a CT scan.

By whatever imaging modality, evaluation of the PV, SMV and mesenteric arterial vessels is necessary prior to exploration. While our philosophy is that isolated PV involvement is not a contraindication to resection, we are reluctant to resect patients with evidence of PV thrombosis, either by clinical signs or radiographic evidence of PV clot or associated varices. Unfortunately, significant PV involvement is usually associated with SMA or celiac artery involvement and such involvement should be considered an absolute contraindication to resection.

Intraoperative evaluation

Once the patient has been determined to be a surgical candidate and appears resectable by radiographic

criteria, the next step in evaluation is staging laparoscopy. The use of laparoscopy has significantly reduced the percentage of patients undergoing an open exploration without resection. Prior to laparoscopy at Memorial Sloan–Kettering Cancer Center (MSKCC), only 35% of surgically explored patients with peripancreatic tumors underwent curative resection. Since the introduction of laparoscopic staging, our resectability rate at laparotomy has increased to over 75% and with laparoscopic ultrasound, 90%. Importantly, those patients deemed unresectable by laparoscopy have a minimally morbid procedure with a median length of hospital stay of 1 day, which is significantly less than an open exploration without resection (median 7 days). In addition to patient comfort, laparoscopy offers considerable cost savings. Laparoscopy is an essential step in staging peripancreatic tumors and in our opinion, should be considered standard of care[18] (see Chapter 21).

Laparoscopy can be performed immediately prior to the definitive resection or as a separate outpatient procedure. After general anesthesia, a port is placed using an open technique in the periumbilical position and the abdomen is insufflated. In addition to the periumbilical camera port, right and left upper quadrant ports are placed. Additional ports can be used, according to need. After a 30° angled telescope is introduced in the peritoneal cavity, the patient undergoes a methodical evaluation. First, with the patient in a neutral position, the primary tumor is assessed, noting local extent and fixation to other organs, such as colon, spleen or stomach. The peritoneal surfaces are inspected for metastatic deposits and the transverse mesocolon is examined from below to ensure no transperitoneal invasion. The presence of varices is also noted, reflecting portal, splenic or superior mesenteric venous obstruction. The right and left lobes of the liver are then inspected. In addition, the liver parenchyma is palpated to identify deep lesions. Laparoscopic ultrasound probes may assist in identifying deep parenchymal lesions. Next, by accessing the right upper quadrant port, the laparoscope may enter the foramen of Winslow and periportal lymph nodes may be biopsied, if required. Next, the omentum is identified and retracted toward the left upper quadrant. This allows inspection of the mesocolon and ligament of Trietz. Finally, the gastrohepatic omentum is incised, exposing the caudate lobe of the liver, vena cava and celiac axis. Celiac, portal or perigastric lymph nodes may be excised or sampled with a biopsy forceps.

Technique of portal vein resection

For patients with otherwise resectable lesions, a standard pancreatic resection is performed. In most cases, intraoperative assessment will reveal adherence of the tumor to the PV or SMV, often on the lateral aspect of the vein after the gland has been divided. At this point, the dissection is nearly complete and the final step prior to removal of the specimen is the segmental resection of the PV.

The first step for PVR is proximal and distal control of the PV. Clamp placement and approach to the splenic vein will depend on tumor location. For SMV lesions, the splenic vein is spared by placing the proximal clamp at or just distal to the splenic–portal vein confluence (Fig. 22.3). For low PV lesions, the splenic vein can be maintained by placing the proximal clamp at an angle, as shown in Fig. 22.4. For mid or high PV involvement, ligation and division of the splenic vein facilitates primary reconstruction by improving mobility of the proximal and distal segments of the vein (Fig. 22.5). While splenic vein ligation is usually tolerated without sequela, there have been reports of upper gastrointestinal hemorrhage as a result of portal hypertension after splenic vein ligation and some recommend splenic vein preservation whenever possible.[19]

After transection of the portal vein segment and removal of the specimen, a primary anastomosis with monofilament suture is almost always possible with elevation of the small bowel mesentery with the patient in the Trendelenberg position. If the splenic vein is preserved for a mid or high PV involvement, mobility of the PV is severely limited and an interposition graft is usually required (especially if the segmental resection is greater than 2 cm). If a conduit is required, autologous (internal jugular, left renal or saphenous vein) tissue is

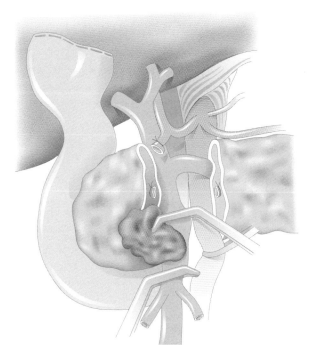

Figure 22.3 Technique of portal vein resection. Tumor involving the SMV: proximal and distal control of the portal vein can be accomplished without sacrificing the splenic vein.[31]

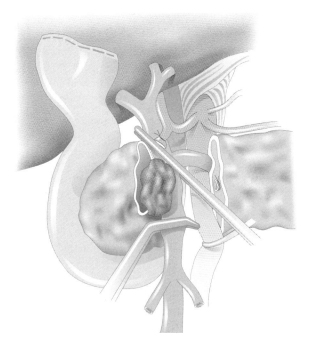

Figure 22.4 Technique of portal vein resection. Tumor involving the distal portal vein: by placing the proximal vascular clamp at an angle, the splenic vein can be maintained.[31]

preferred to synthetic material because of higher patency rates.[20] If the left renal vein is to be used as a conduit, an extended Kocherization is performed to expose the vena cava and left renal vein. It is important to note that at least 3–4 cm of the renal

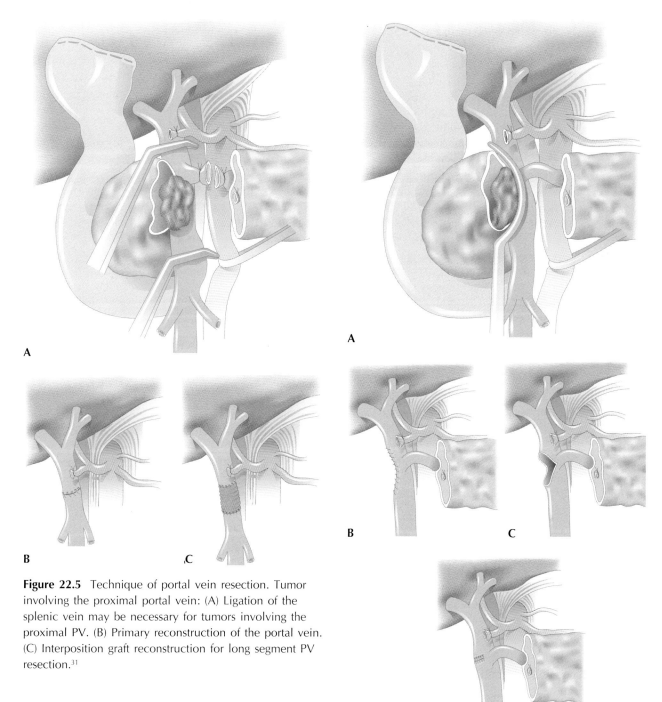

Figure 22.5 Technique of portal vein resection. Tumor involving the proximal portal vein: (A) Ligation of the splenic vein may be necessary for tumors involving the proximal PV. (B) Primary reconstruction of the portal vein. (C) Interposition graft reconstruction for long segment PV resection.[31]

Figure 22.6 Technique of portal vein resection: (A) For minimal tumor invasion of the lateral wall, a side-biting vascular clamp is used to perform a lateral venorraphy. Care must be used not to narrow the portal vein. (B) Primary reconstruction of the portal vein (C) V-plasty repair for minimal lateral wall invasion. (D) Primary repair after V-plasty.[31]

vein can be harvested without compromising kidney function, as long as the gonadal vein is preserved. If vascular reconstruction is prolonged, the SMA may be temporarily occluded to prevent vascular congestion of the bowel.

A lateral venorraphy for adequate tumor clearance may also be used. This is usually accomplished by placing a vascular clamp on the lateral aspect of the portal vein after the pancreas is divided (Fig. 22.6). With lateral venography, a word of caution must be given regarding narrowing the PV. If too much of the lateral wall is resected, PV congestion and thrombosis will occur. Revision after a lateral venorraphy for narrowing often requires a long segmental resection. This will result in a much longer segment of

resected vein than would originally be required if a segmental resection was attempted primarily. This increases PV clamp and operative time and almost always requires an interposition graft.

Should isolated portal vein involvement preclude pancreatic resection?

The rationale for performing pancreatectomy with PVR is based on the fact that patients with adenocarcinoma of the pancreas who undergo pancreatic resection have a significantly longer survival than those patients who undergo palliative bypass or no operation[1] (Fig. 22.7). In addition, some groups have proposed that locally advanced disease should not be a contraindication to resection, as resection provides the best palliation.[21] Therefore, if patients have an improved survival and better palliation after pancreatic resection, and PVR allows an increase in resectability, then patients should benefit from pancreatic resection with PVR.

However, prior to recommending PVR for isolated PV involvement, issues of safety and survival need to be addressed. For PVR to be of benefit, survival after pancreatic resection with PVR should approach that of those resections without PVR and should surpass that of either palliative bypass or non-operative supportive care. In addition, it should be possible to perform PVR without significantly increasing the postoperative mortality and morbidity of a standard pancreatic resection. The recent literature addressing these two issues is summarized below.

Safety of portal vein resection

Most surgeons do not perform vascular resections for tumor invasion because of earlier reports of high morbidity and mortality without obvious benefit to the patient.[7] However, prior to deeming all patients unresectable because of vascular involvement, it is important to distinguish PVR for isolated PV involvement from resections involving arterial reconstructions. The high morbidity and mortality rates originally reported by Fortner were associated with major arterial reconstructions (type II resection). While select groups continue to perform arterial resections for tumor invasion, high rates of postoperative deaths and complications are still reported.[9,10] For Fortner's type I resection (PV only), acceptable mortality rates are reached and recent data support the contention that isolated PVR in the absence of arterial resection is well tolerated.

Of 390 patients who underwent resection for histologically confirmed adenocarcinoma of the pancreas between October 1983 and December 1996 at MSKCC, 64 (16%) were identified as having isolated clinical involvement of the portal vein and underwent pancreatic resection with PVR. Measures of clinical outcome of the PVR group were compared to a similar group of patients undergoing pancreatic resection with curative intent without portal vein resection over this same time period. Operative procedures included pancreaticoduodenectomy (N = 48), total pancreatectomy (N = 8) or distal subtotal pancreatectomy (N = 8).

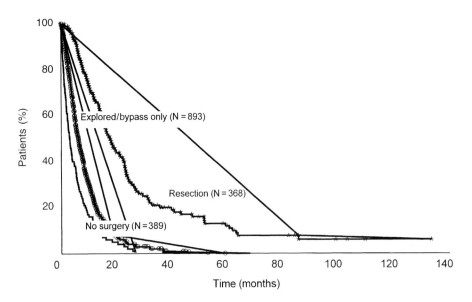

Figure 22.7 Survival of patients with adenocarcinoma of the pancreas at MSKCC. Patients able to undergo resection have a significantly longer survival compared to those undergoing bypass or no surgery.

Table 22.2 Memorial Sloan–Kettering Cancer Center experience with portal vein resection (PVR) for pancreatic adenocarcinoma

	PVR (N = 64)	No PVR (N = 326)
Operative factors		
EBL (ml)	1800 (350–8500)[a]	1200 (130–7600)
Transfusion (units PRBC)	3 (0–13)[a]	1 (0–13)
Operative time (hours)	7.0 (2.8–14.5)[a]	5.8 (2–11.3)
Tumor characteristics		
Tumor size (cm)	4.0 (1.1–12)[a]	3.5 (0.5–16)
No. of margin positive (%)	17 (27)	77 (24)
No. of lymph node positive (%)	34 (53)	178 (55)
Differentiation (%)		
Good	20	18
Moderate	47	53
Poor	33	29
Outcome		
LOS (days)	20 (8–125)[a]	14 (5–88)
Reoperative rate	10 (16%)	41 (13%)
Operative mortality	3 (5%)	10 (3%)

LOS: length of hospital stay; EBL: estimated blood loss.
[a] $P < 0.01$

Of the 64 patients who underwent PVR, 44 had a primary end-to-end anastomosis and 20 patients underwent lateral venorraphy of the portal vein. Total anesthesia time was significantly longer for those patients undergoing PVR (7.0 hours (range 2.8–14.5 hours)) compared with those not requiring PVR (5.8 hours (range 2–11.3 hours), $P < 0.01$). Estimated intraoperative blood/fluid loss and transfusion requirements were also significantly increased in the PVR group (1800 ml (range 350–8500 ml); 3 units (range 0–13)) compared to those patients undergoing pancreatic resection without vascular excision (1200 ml (range 130–7600 ml); 1 unit (range 0–13)), ($P < 0.01$) (Table 22.2).

Of the 64 patients undergoing PVR, 10 (16%) required surgical re-exploration. Only one patient undergoing PVR required reoperation for PV thrombosis and, during our more recent experience with PVR, we have not documented any evidence of delayed PV thrombosis, including clinical ascites or bleeding varices. Importantly, portal vein resection did not alter the cause for re-exploration (Table 22.3). The median length of hospital stay was significantly longer for those patients undergoing PVR (20 days (range 8–125)) compared to those patients not requiring PVR (14 days (range 5–88)). There were three postoperative deaths in the PVR group,

Table 22.3 Memorial Sloan–Kettering Cancer Center experience with PVR: reoperation for pancreatic resection

Reason for reoperation	No PVR	PVR
Bleeding	19	4
Abscess	16	3
Wound	2	1
Portal vein obstruction	0	1
Other	4	1
Total	41 (13%)	10 (16%)

yielding an in-hospital mortality rate of 5%. However, this was not significantly different from the operative mortality rate seen in those patients not undergoing PVR (ten patients (3%)).

These data are similar to other reports evaluating the safety of portal vein resection. Allema et al.[22] evaluated 20 patients with pancreatic adenocarcinoma requiring portal vein resection for suspicion of macroscopic tumor involvement. They reported that minor and major morbidity were similar between those patients undergoing PVR and those undergoing pancreatic resection without portal venous reconstruction. The was no difference in the postoperative mortality in the PVR group (3/20) compared to the non-PVR group (11/156). Importantly, two of the three postoperative deaths after PVR were in patients undergoing total pancreatectomy. The experience at M.D. Anderson with PVR also demonstrates that resection of the PV can be performed safely. Fuhrman and colleagues[23] noted that PVR added approximately an hour and a half to the operative procedure. They also reported an increase in blood loss and transfusion requirement for PVR. On the other hand, the median hospital stay after PVR (16 days) was not different from those patients undergoing standard pancreaticoduodenectomy (17 days). The postoperative complication rates were equivalent (28% for standard pancreatectomy versus 30% for PVR) and a low operative mortality after PVR (4%) was also achieved.

Pichlmayr's group reported a series of 75 patients undergoing extended resection for pancreatic adenocarcinoma.[10] Of these, 19 underwent isolated PVR with a 5.3% 30-day mortality rate and a relaparotomy rate of 21.1%. Importantly, when PVR was associated with resection of other organs (including arterial resections), the mortality dramatically increased to over 20%. These results are similar to Fortner's results with the type II regional pancreatectomies. Takahashi and colleagues reported a similar (10%) operative mortality for pancreatic resection involving PVR (N = 63) and for those patients not requiring PVR (N = 70). However, for patients undergoing both PVR and arterial resection, the operative mortality rose to nearly 44% (N = 16).[9]

In summary, for those centers performing a significant number of pancreatic resections annually, the postoperative mortality rate after standard resection ranges from 1 to 5%.[24] Similar postoperative mortality rates have been achieved after PVR. The technical safety of PVR is well documented, and in the absence of arterial resection, PVR is well tolerated. Therefore, PVR for isolated involvement of the PV should not be a contraindication to resection based on a prohibitive morbidity or mortality.

Survival after portal vein resection for pancreatic adenocarcinoma

While Fortner introduced the concept that PVR is technically feasible and recent large series confirm the safety of the procedure, the question of whether portal vein resection for clinically apparent portal vein involvement impacts on survival needs to be evaluated. While some groups have reported that extended pancreatic resections improve overall survival for patients with pancreatic carcinoma,[25,26] these results have not been consistently reproduced. While it is doubtful that PVR by itself improves survival, equivalent survival to resected patients not requiring PVR suggests that isolated portal vein involvement should not be a deterrent to resection.

Comparing known prognostic factors for adenocarcinoma of the pancreas,[27–29] the percentage of patients in the MSKCC series with positive lymph nodes, tumor differentiation and microscopically positive margins was similar for those patients undergoing PVR compared to a standard pancreatectomy. A similar distribution of prognostic determinants between no PVR and PVR has been noted by others.[22,23] Allema and colleagues noted no difference in the percentage of patients with lymph node metastases or tumor differentiation between those patients requiring PVR and those who did not.[22] The M.D. Anderson series also noted no difference in margin status or node positivity. However, perineural invasion was significantly higher in the PVR group.[23] The only negative prognostic factor associated with PVR in our series was a larger tumor size, which has also been reported by Fortner.[30] Median tumor size was significantly larger in those patients undergoing PVR (4 cm (range 1.1–12)) compared to the control group (3.5 cm (range 0.5–16), $P < 0.01$). In addition, 34% of patients undergoing standard pancreatic resection had tumors less than or equal to 2.5 cm, compared to only 17% of patients requiring PVR. While some have noted this size discrepancy after pancreatectomy with PVR,[22] others have reported similar tumor sizes.[23]

Although tumor size is a negative prognostic factor for adenocarcinoma of the pancreas,[27,28,30] the overall survival of patients undergoing pancreatic resection with PVR appears to be similar to those patients undergoing a standard pancreatectomy. Importantly, both procedures have a superior outcome compared to palliative bypass or non-operative treatment.[27] Of the 64 patients undergoing PVR at MSKCC, overall median survival was 13 months (range < 1–109 months), which was not statistically different from those patients undergoing pancreatic resection without PVR (17 months (range < 1–132)). No difference in survival was detected when the patients were stratified according to operative procedure (Fig. 22.8 A–D).[31] Takahashi et al.[9] reporting on 63 patients requiring PVR for pancreatic adenocarcinoma, observed that those patients with negative margins after resection had a 5-year survival of 14%. They also demonstrated no difference in survival

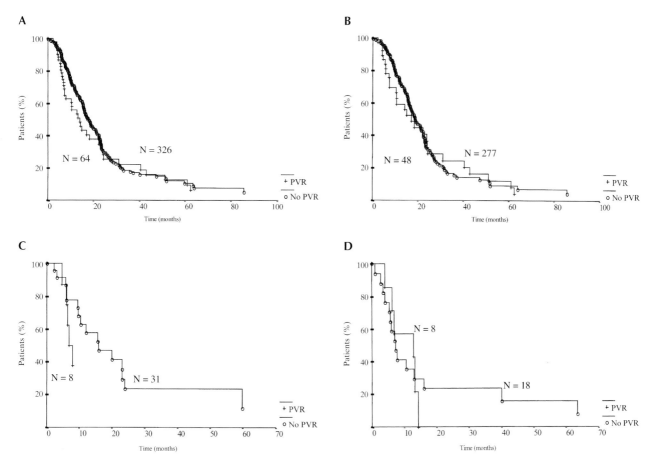

Figure 22.8 MSKCC experience with PVR: survival PVR versus no PVR (A) overall survival, (B) pancreaticoduodenectomy, (C) distal subtotal pancreatectomy and (D) total pancreatectomy: there was no significant difference in survival of any group.

Table 22.4 Portal vein resection for suspected clinical involvement: summary of the literature

Author	Country	N	Operative mortality	LOS (days)	Node positivity	Positive margins	Histologic invasion of PV/SMV (%)	Survival
Harrison et al.[31]	USA	58	3 (5%)	15	30 (52%)	15 (27%)	NR	13 months
Fuhrman et al.[23]	USA	23	1 (4%)	17	9 (39%)	4 (17%)	NR	NR
Allema et al.[22]	Netherlands	20	3 (15%)	NR	14 (70%)	17 (85%)	50	7 months
Roder et al.[32]	Germany	22	0 (0%)	28	17 (77.3%)	15 (68%)	61.3	8 months
Klempnauer et al.[10]	Germany	19	1 (5.3%)	29.9	NR	NR	NR	16.8%
Launois et al.[33]	France	9	0 (0%)	30.5	NR	NR	NR	6.1 months
Tashiro et al.[34]	Japan	17	1 (5.9%)	NR	9 (53%)	NR	25.9	NR
Ishikawa et al.[12]	Japan	30	1 (3.3%)	NR	28 (93%)	NR	85.7	18%
Takahashi and Tsuzuki[9]	Japan	63	6 (9.5%)	NR	NR	24 (38%)	61	14%

NR: not recorded.

between those patients undergoing pancreatic resection with or without PVR. Ishikawa et al. reported a 29% 3-year and an 18% 5-year survival after pancreatectomy with PVR.[12] Similar survival data have been reported by others,[10,26] and are summarized in Table 22.4.

Not all centers report equivalent survival for patients undergoing PVR compared to a standard pancreatic resection. Roder et al.[32] compared 22 patients undergoing pancreaticoduodenectomy with PVR to 89 patients without PVR. Of the patients undergoing PVR, none survived longer than 16 months and the overall survival (median survival = 8 months) was statistically less than for those undergoing standard resection. They reported similar results with distal common bile duct adenocarcinoma. Launois and colleagues, reporting their experience with total pancreatectomy for adenocarcinoma of the pancreas, noted that the mean survival for those patients undergoing PVR (N = 9) was 6.1 months compared to 18 months for standard total pancreatectomy.[33] However, conclusions regarding poor survival after PVR are limited based on the small number of PVRs in this series and evaluation of the subset of patients undergoing total pancreatectomy.

While agreement in the literature is not unanimous, recent data emerging from large series evaluating PVR for isolated tumor invasion suggest that survival is similar to standard pancreatic resection. The reason for this similar overall survival between patients undergoing PVR and those requiring only pancreatic resection is probably multifactorial. One factor that may contribute to similar survival rates is based on the fact that since the overall prognosis for adenocarcinoma of the pancreas is so dismal, it is difficult to detect small differences in survival after any intervention. While patients requiring PVR may in fact do worse, any difference may be overshadowed by the overall poor outcome.

Beyond this pessimistic rationale, another reason for similar survival may be based on the fact that the need for portal vein resection is not a predictor of aggressive tumor biology, but rather a reflection of tumor size and location. In our series and others, tumors were larger in those patients requiring PVR and, by sheer mass effect, such tumors may involve the portal vein. Importantly, these patients are self-selected by virtue of having locally advanced disease without evidence of arterial involvement and distant tumor spread.

A third rationale for the similar survivorship is that the resections reported in all series are performed for clinical suspicion of portal vein involvement. Multivariate analysis evaluating prognostic factors for survival after resection for adenocarcinoma of the pancreas demonstrates that, while portal vein resection itself is not a negative prognostic indicator, portal vein invasion is a factor of poor outcome.[27–29] True vascular invasion is difficult to differentiate from inflammatory adhesions by preoperative imaging and conventional surgical exploration. Up to 50% of tumors thought to have vascular invasion intraoperatively are subsequently found to only have inflammatory adhesions to the portal vein after histologic examination (Table 22.4). Tashiro et al. noted that 35% of the 17 patients undergoing PVR for adenocarcinoma of the pancreas had no true histologic invasion of the PV, although macroscopic invasion of the PV was suspected during surgery.[34] Of the 17 patients resected, 11 patients had involvement of the adventia and media and only two patients had histologic tumor involvement of the intima.

The difference in survival between adhesion only versus true invasion is well documented. In a series of 31 patients undergoing PV/SMV resection for suspected tumor invasion, only 19 (61%) had histologic confirmation of true tumor invasion. Those patients without histologic invasion had a significantly improved survival compared to those with invasion[32] (Fig. 22.9). In addition to the presence and absence of invasion, the degree of invasion correlates with survival. Nakao et al. performed 89 PV and/or SMV resections for clinical suspicion of tumor involvement during exploration.[11] By histologic examination, the degree of carcinoma invasion into the PV or SMV was subsequently classified into one of the following three grades: grade 0, no carcinoma into the wall of the vein; grade I, invasion of tumor into the tunica adventitia or media; grade II, invasion into the tunica intima. The survival rate associated with no histologic invasion (grade 0) was significantly higher than that associated with invasion into the intima (grade II) (Fig. 22.10). The relationship between depth of cancer invasion of the portal vein and survival has been confirmed by others.[9] Most likely, a combination of the above arguments contributes to the similar survival between patients undergoing PVR and those requiring standard pancreatic resection. Regardless of the rationale, the data are compelling that PVR can be performed safely and that patients requiring PVR for isolated clinical involvement by tumor have a similar outcome compared to those without PVR.

Summary

When it comes to the treatment of pancreatic cancer, it has been said that physicians are divided into one of three camps: the nihilists, the realists and the activists.[35] Nihilists champion palliative and even non-operative approaches to a disease with a poor long-term outcome. Activists recommend extended surgical extirpation with extensive lymphadenectomy for all patients. Finally, the realists select from the armamentarium of the previous two, based on tumor extent and biology.

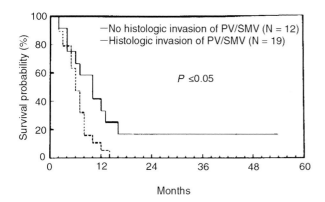

Figure 22.9 Histologic invasion of the PV/SMV: comparison of survival. Patients without pathologic documentation of invasion did statistically better than those with true histologic involvement. (From Roder et al.[32])

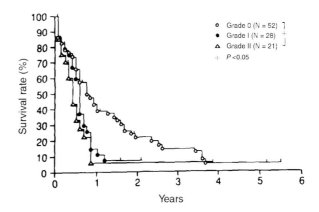

Figure 22.10 Survival according to the degree of histologic invasion of the PV/SMV. Grade 0: no carcinoma into the wall of the vein; grade I: invasion of tumor into the tunica adventitia or media; grade II: invasion into the tunica intima. (From Nakao et al.[11])

While distant metastases remains an absolute contraindication to resection for adenocarcinoma of the pancreas, extended resection for locally advanced disease may be indicated for a select group of patients. Most believe that arterial involvement remains a contraindication for resection based on high operative morbidity and mortality and poor long-term outcome. One the other hand, PVR for isolated PV involvement can be performed safely with a low perioperative mortality rate and overall survival is equal to those patients undergoing standard pancreatectomy. Therefore, suspected isolated portal vein involvement frequently does not preclude operability and, by itself, should not be a contraindication for pancreatic resection.

Key points

- Not infrequently, isolated local invasion of the portal or superior mesenteric vein may be the only obstacle to resection.
- Preoperative evaluation:
  Spiral CT
  Under evaluation
    Intraportal endovascular ultrasonography
    MRI.
- Intraoperative evaluation:
  Staging laparoscopy and ultrasound.
- Arterial involvement is a contraindication to radical resection because of high operative mortality and poor long-term outcome.

REFERENCES

1. Brennan MF, Kinsella TJ, Casper ES. Cancer of the pancreas. In: DeVita VT, Hellman S, Rosenberg SA, eds. Cancer: principles & practice of oncology. Philadelphia: J.B. Lippincott, 1993: 849–82

2. Brennan MF, Moccia RD, Klimstra D. Management of adenocarcinoma of the body and tail of the pancreas. Ann Surg 1996; 223: 506–12

3. Child CG, Gore AL, O'Neill EA. Pancreaticoduodenectomy with resection of the portal vein in the Macaca mulatta monkey and in man. Surg Gynecol Obstet 1952; 94: 31–45

4. Moore G, Sako Y, Thomas L. Radical pancreatectomy with resection and reanastomosis of the superior mesenteric vein. Surgery 1951; 30: 550–3

5. Fortner JG. Regional resection of cancer of the pancreas: a new surgical approach. Surgery 1973; 73: 307–20

6. Fortner JG. Technique of regional subtotal and total pancreatectomy. Am J Surg 1985; 150: 593–600

7. Sindelar W. Clinical experience with regional pancreatectomy for adenocarcinoma of the pancreas. Arch Surg 1989; 124: 127–32

8. Mukaiya M, Hirata K, Satoh T et al. Lack of survival benefit of extended lymph node dissection for ductal adenocarcinoma of the head of the pancreas: retrospective multi-institutional analysis in Japan. World J Surg 1998; 22:2 48–253

9. Takahashi S, Tsuzuki T. Combined resection of the pancreas and portal vein for pancreatic cancer. Br J Surg 1994; 81: 1190–3

10. Klempnauer J, Ridder G, Becklas H, Pichlmayr R. Extended resections of ductal pancreatic cancer – impact on operative risks and prognosis. Oncology 1996; 53: 47–53

11. Nakao A, Harada A, Nonami T, Kaneko T, Inoue S, Takagi H. Clinical significance of portal invasion by pancreatic head carcinoma. Surgery 1995; 117: 50–5

12. Ishikawa O, Ohigashi H, Imaoka S et al. Preoperative indications for extended pancreatectomy for locally advanced pancreas cancer involving the portal vein. Ann Surg 1992; 215: 231–6

13. Minnard A, Conlon KC, Hoos A, Dougherty E, Hann L, Brennan M. Laparoscopic ultrasound enhances standard laparoscopy in the staging of pancreatic cancer. Ann Surg 1998; 228: 182–7

14. John TG, Greig JD, Carter DC, Garden OJ. Carcinoma of the pancreatic head and periampullary region: tumor staging with laparoscopy and laparoscopic ultrasonography. Ann Surg 1995; 221: 156–64

15. Kaneko T, Nakao A, Inoue S et al. Intraportal endovascular ultrasonography in the diagnosis of portal vein invasion by pancreatobiliary carcinoma. Ann Surg 1995; 222: 711–8

16. McFarland EG, Kaufman JA, Saini S et al. Preoperative staging of cancer of the pancreas: value of MR angiography versus conventional angiography in detecting portal venous invasion. AJR 1996; 166: 37–43

17. Trede M, Rumstadt B, Wendl K et al. Ultrafast magnetic resonance imaging improves the staging of pancreatic tumors. Ann Surg 1997; 226: 393–407

18. Conlon KC, Dougherty E, Klimstra DS, Coit DC, Turnbull ADM. The value of minimal access surgery in the staging of patients with potentially resectable peripancreatic malignancy. Ann Surg 1996; 223: 134–40

19. Evans DB, Lee JE, Leach SD, Fuhrman GM, Cusack JC, Rich T. Vascular resection and intraoperative radiation therapy during pancreaticoduodenectomy: rationale and technique. Adv Surg 1996; 29: 235–62

20. Leach SD, Lowry AM, Fuhrman GM, Lee JE, Curley SA, Evans DB. Pancreatic malignancy involving the superior mesenteric–portal vein confluence is not a contraindication to pancreaticoduodenectomy (abstract). Gastroenterology 1995; 108: 1228

21. Lillemoe KD, Cameron JL, Yeo CJ et al. Pancreaticoduodenectomy: does it have a role in the palliation of pancreatic cancer? Ann Surg 1996; 223: 718–28

22. Allema JH, Reinder ME, van Gulik TM et al. Portal vein resection in patients undergoing pancreaticoduodenectomy for carcinoma of the pancreatic head. Br J Surg 1994; 81: 1642–6

23. Fuhrman GM, Leach SD, Staley CA et al. Rationale for en bloc vein resection in the treatment of pancreatic adenocarcinoma adherent to the superior mesenteric–portal vein confluence. Ann Surg 1996; 223: 154–62

24. Lieberman MD, Kilburn H, Lindsey M, Brennan MF. Relation of perioperative deaths to hospital volume among patients undergoing pancreatic resection for malignancy. Ann Surg 1995; 222: 638–45

25. Satake K, Nishiwaki H, Yokomatsu H et al. Surgical curability and prognosis for standard versus extended resection for T1 carcinoma of the pancreas. Surg Gynecol Obstet 1992; 175: 259–65

26. Manabe T, Ohsio G, Baba N. Radical pancreatectomy for ductal cell carcinoma of the head of the pancreas. Cancer 1989; 64: 1132–7

27. Geer RJ, Brennan MF. Prognostic indicators for survival after resection of pancreatic adenocarcinoma. Am J Surg 1993; 165: 68–73

28. Cameron JL, Crist DW, Sitzman JV et al. Factors influencing survival after pancreaticoduodenectomy for pancreatic resection. Am J Surg 1991; 161: 120–4

29. Allema JH, Reinders ME, van Gulik TM et al. Prognostic factors for survival after pancreaticoduodenectomy for patients with carcinoma of the pancreatic head region. Cancer 1994; 75: 2069–76

30. Fortner JG, Klimstra DS, Senie RT, Maclean BJ. Tumor size is the primary prognosticator for pancreatic cancer after regional pancreatectomy. Ann Surg 1996; 223: 147–53

31. Harrison LE, Klimstra D, Brennan MF. Isolated portal vein resection in pancreatic adenocarcinoma. A contraindication for resection? Ann Surg 1996; 224: 342–9

32. Roder JD, Stein HJ, Siewert JR. Carcinoma of the periampullary region: who benefits from portal vein resection? Am J Surg 1996; 171: 170–5

33. Launois B, Franci J, Bardaxoglou E et al. Total pancreatectomy for ductal adenocarcinoma of the pancreas with special reference to resection of the portal vein and multicentric cancer. World J Surg 1993; 17: 122–7

34. Tashiro S, Uchino R, Hiraoka T et al. Surgical indication and significance of portal vein resection in biliary and pancreatic cancer. Surgery 1991; 109: 481–7

35. Trede M. Treatment of pancreatic carcinoma: the surgeon's dilemma. Br J Surg 1987; 74: 79–80

23 Neuroendocrine pancreatic tumors

Steven N Hochwald and Kevin Conlon

Introduction

Pancreatic endocrine tumors are benign or malignant epithelial tumors that show evidence of endocrine cell differentiation. Pancreatic endocrine tumors are uncommon, representing <5% of pancreatic tumors in surgical series.[1,2] Clinically silent endocrine tumors have been detected in 0.3 to 1.6% of unselected autopsies in which only a few sections of the pancreas were examined and in up to 10% of autopsies in which the whole pancreas was systematically investigated both grossly and microscopically. Most tumors from these series are small (less than 1 cm), in elderly patients (mean age of 70 years) and benign (clinically silent microadenomas).

Pancreatic endocrine tumors can be broadly classified as functional or non-functional. Despite changing trends, the majority of clinically relevant pancreatic endocrine tumors are functional.[3] The proportion of non-functioning tumors, in series of islet cell neoplasms, has varied over time, ranging between 15 and 53% of cases.[4-7] While the definition of non-functional has been inconsistent in many reports, increased use of more sophisticated imaging modalities has allowed clinically silent intra-abdominal masses to be identified incidentally and many series report an increased incidence of non-functioning neoplasms.[8,9] Overall, the reported 35–50% incidence of non-functioning endocrine tumors suggest that non-functional tumors are at least as common as insulinomas and more common than all of the remaining pancreatic endocrine tumor types.[2]

Functional endocrine tumors of the pancreas are peptide-secreting neoplasms leading to clinical presentation with a defined syndrome related to the effects of an abnormally elevated plasma peptide level. These peptides may or may not occur naturally in the pancreas, and a given tumor may secrete multiple peptides. It is on the basis of the primary functional peptide hormone secreted that each tumor is named; e.g., gastrinoma, insulinoma.

Non-functioning islet cell tumors are pancreatic neoplasms with endocrine differentiation in the absence of a clinical syndrome of hormone hyperfunction. Despite the presence of hormones in tumor cells at immunohistochemistry, many of these tumors lack evidence of increased serum hormonal levels. Tumors releasing increased amounts of hormone in the blood stream without evidence of a hyperfunctional syndrome are also often reported as non-functioning tumors. Several explanations can be given for why these non-functioning tumors are hormonally silent. One reason is that the principal hormone secreted by the tumor may cause no specific clinical signs, although it is released in excess. In some situations, the tumor makes a functionally inert hormone, which is recognized by an antibody directed against a functional hormone. As the specificity of antibodies improves, such false positives should disappear. A second possibility is that the amount of hormone produced may be too small to cause symptoms. Third, the tumor may secrete a precursor hormone that is functionally inert or the hormonal product of the tumor may not yet be identified.

Pancreatic endocrine tumors may occur at any age, although they are rare in children. The age range in one series of 125 patients was 3 months to 80 years, with a mean of 51 years.[10] There have been no described significant differences in incidence by sex.

No differences in histologic pattern have been found in non-functioning as compared to functioning tumors. During embryogenesis pancreatic islets are known to form mostly through cellular buds originating from intralobular ductules. Although this process normally ends before birth, it may persist or

Table 23.1 Comparison of functional endocrine tumors (adapted from Mozzell et al.[13])

Tumor type	Pancreatic associated primary (%)	Malignancy rate (%)	Metastatic rate (%)	Multicentricity (%)	Size	MEN-1 (%)
Gastrinoma	30	60	50–80	20–40	Medium	18–41
Insulinoma	95–99	5–16	31	10	Small	4–10
Glucagonoma	100	82	>50	2–4	Large	Rarely
VI Poma	100	50	50	20	Small	4
Somatostatinoma	68	>90	75	10	Large	Unknown

reappear in many proliferative diseases of the endocrine pancreas, including pancreatic involvement of type I MEN syndrome or solitary endocrine tumors arising in the adult pancreas.[2] Since islet cells often have hormone co-expression during early fetal development, it is thought that the origin of pancreatic endocrine tumors is from multipotent cells in ductular epithelium, which can differentiate towards the various cell lines found in these tumors.[11,12]

Clinically, functional and non-functional tumors present in diverse manners with varied treatment dilemmas. Presentation in functional tumors is usually due to symptoms from the hypersecretion of a particular hormone, while in non-functional tumors it is usually due to an effect of the tumor mass. We will separately discuss the treatment challenges of these two tumor types, but attempts will be made to identify where therapeutic algorithms may overlap for these tumors.

Functional islet cell tumors

Functional tumors vary with regard to size, location, age distribution, sex distribution, propensity for malignancy, and metastatic potential in accordance with the individual tumor type (Table 23.1).[13] As with most endocrine tumors, the clinical morbidity and mortality associated with the tumor are due to hormone hypersecretion. Most tumors are slow growing and well differentiated.

Insulinoma

Insulinoma is a neoplasm that arises from the pancreatic insulin producing beta cells. Unlike other gastrointestinal endocrine tumors, which are malignant in more than 60% of cases, 90% of insulinomas are benign, solitary growths that occur almost exclusively within the pancreatic parenchyma (Table 23.1). They occur throughout the head, body and tail of the pancreas with equal frequency.[14] Three per cent are in the uncinate and 2–3% are ectopic. Ectopic insulinomas are usually found in the duodenal mucosa, the hilum of the spleen, or in the gastrocolic ligament.[13]

The well-known symptoms associated with hypoglycemia and inappropriate hyperinsulinism occur in a fasting state. The symptoms of headache, blurred vision, incoherence, convulsions, and coma are due to the deleterious effect of hypoglycemia on cerebral function. The symptoms of sweating, weakness, hunger, palpitation and trembling are homeostatic responses to hypoglycemia, involving secretion of catecholamines.[15] The development of these symptoms and the presence of fasting hypoglycemia (glucose ≤40 mg/dl) and hyperinsulinism (>5 U/ml) during a supervised 72-hour in-hospital fast has been the gold standard in establishing the diagnosis.[16] In fact, a 72-hour fast is rarely needed, since one-third of patients develop symptoms within only 12 hours, at least 80% within 24 hours, 90% in 48 hours and 100% in 72 hours.[17] Elevated plasma levels of C peptide and proinsulin are confirmatory.

Once the biochemical diagnosis of insulinoma has been achieved, diagnostic testing should be performed in an effort at tumor localization. The preoperative localization of insulinomas has received a tremendous amount of attention in recent years. However, as of yet, no single technique has been accepted that is accurate, independent of operator expertise, safe, non-invasive and inexpensive. A multitude of localization modalities has been devised with a wide disparity in reported success rates and expenses (Table 23.2).[17]

Imaging for suspected islet cell tumors is important in the preoperative period for planning therapy.

Table 23.2 Sensitivity (%) of localization modalities for insulinoma (adapted from Grant[17])

Center	Transabdominal ultrasonography	CT	Angiography	Portal venous sampling	MR imaging	Intraoperative ultrasonography	Palpation
Ann Arbor[25]		26	44	94	0		
NIH[103]	26	17	35	77	25	92	64
Sweden[104]	11	43	54	63			
France[105]	40	50	44	89			
Italy[106]	15	60	75			100	82
Mayo Clinic[107] (1982–87)	59	36	53			90	90
Mayo Clinic (1980–95)	64	26	47		16	95	90

Metastases must be identified preoperatively so that the operative approach can be determined or unnecessary surgery can be abandoned. Non-invasive imaging studies most frequently utilized include CT and MRI and are considered standard radiological modalities for imaging of suspected insulinomas. Because results with dynamic CT for localization of insulinomas have been poor (Table 23.2), spiral CT has replaced dynamic CT for pancreatic imaging in most centers (Fig. 23.1). In one report, nine of eleven tumors could be located using two-phase spiral CT.[18] However, the sensitivity of spiral CT in tumor localization remains to be determined in larger numbers of patients.[17] Pancreatic endocrine tumors typically have a low signal intensity on T1-weighted MR images. They demonstrate high signal intensity on T2-weighted images. MRI with gadolinium contrast is more sensitive for the detection of vascular tumors than is CT with standard intravenous iodinated contrast agents and may therefore permit detection of insulinomas that cannot be identified on CT.[19,20] MRI is likely to become more important for localization of insulinomas, but its role is not yet established.

Other modalities that have been utilized in the localization of insulinomas include somatostatin receptor scintigraphy and endoscopic ultrasound. The sensitivity of somatostatin receptor scintigraphy for the detection of islet cell tumors should be independent of tumor size and depend only on tumor expression, and cellular and total number of somatostatin receptors. Unfortunately, tumors with low somatostatin receptor density may not be imaged. Only 60–70% of insulinomas have been found to express this receptor[21,22] and, therefore, the sensitivity of somatostatin receptor scintigraphy is approximately 50%.[23]

Endoscopic ultrasound, in experienced hands, may be quite sensitive in localization of insulinomas. In

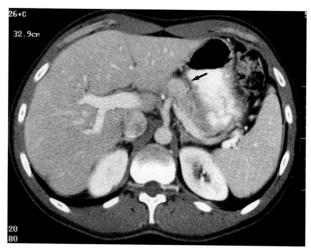

Figure 23.1 Spiral CT of insulinoma in body of pancreas. Arrow indicates tumor which is enhancing with contrast material. The patient underwent an enucleation of this tumor.

one review, seven of ten patients had insulinomas ranging in size from 1.5 to 2.2 cm. Two of three missed tumors were in the head of the pancreas.[24] Despite this, endoscopic ultrasound has several disadvantages. It has difficulty visualizing tumors in the tail of the pancreas. In addition, it is invasive, requiring monitored sedation, and is highly operator dependent.

Invasive localization tests include arteriography and portal venous sampling. Routine arteriography is no longer recommended in the localization of insulinomas, it has been replaced by other modalities due to its invasive and user dependent nature. Portal venous sampling has been considered by some to be the single best test for localizing insulinomas.[25] The technique involves catheter placement through the liver percutaneously and positioned in the portal system. More than 20 blood samples are taken from different veins that drain the pancreas and are tested for insulin to localize the insulinoma. The false positive rate has been shown to be low and sensitivity ranges from 63 to 94% (Table 23.2). However, this technique is user dependent and does not localize the tumor precisely, rather indicating a region of the pancreas that may harbor the tumor. In addition, complications such as hemobilia and hepatic bleeding may occur as a result of this procedure. An invasive technique utilizing selective arteriographic injection of calcium while measuring hepatic venous insulin levels has yielded excellent tumor localization rates.[26] This study is becoming the invasive localizing study of choice, since it may be less user dependent and can be performed more easily than selective portal venous sampling.

Due to the limitations of both invasive and non-invasive imaging in the work-up of suspected insulinomas, some centers recommend non-invasive imaging followed by surgical exploration with the use of intraoperative ultrasound. In selected patients, the Mayo Clinic reports a cure rate of 97.7% using this regimen for benign insulinomas.[17] The use of intraoperative ultrasonography has enhanced the surgeon's ability to localize insulinomas. Additional information provided by intraoperative ultrasonongraphy includes defining the relationship of the tumor to the pancreatic and bile ducts, and adjacent blood vessels.[17]

Our current recommendations in patients who meet biochemical criteria for insulinoma are to perform preoperative non-invasive radiologic imaging consisting of spiral CT scanning or quality MR imaging. If this is negative and the patient has no family history or signs of MEN syndrome, the patient should go to operative exploration. At surgery, intraoperative ultrasound should be utilized, if necessary to localize the tumor.

In general, insulinomas are usually reddish purple or white and easily identified at operation. To confirm findings or to help localize deep parenchymal lesions, intraoperative ultrasonography can be utilized. In this way, the relationship of the pancreatic duct and other vascular structures to the tumor can be demonstrated. Even if one tumor is found, the entire pancreas should be explored. Enucleation is carefully done to avoid injury to the pancreatic duct. The tumor is enucleated by dissecting immediately adjacent to the tumor, bluntly separating the tumor from normal pancreas using fine instruments and a small sucker. The area is left open and is often drained. The use of a drain is not mandatory if there is minimal disruption of pancreatic parenchyma. Distal pancreatectomy may be necessary in larger, deeper tumors, or if the tumor involves the pancreatic duct. For larger lesions of the pancreatic head subtotal pancreatectomy or a pancreaticoduodenectomy may be required.

When an insulinoma has not been identified at the first operation and reoperation is contemplated, referral to a center with considerable experience is mandatory. Since insulinomas are equally distributed throughout the pancreas, success is proportional to the percentage of pancreas removed. Therefore, a blind distal resection would be effective in only 50% of cases and is not recommended. We and others would recommend that the abdomen be closed and the diagnosis be reconfirmed. Extensive preoperative localization should be performed prior to a re-exploration.[17] In one report, with the introduction of intraoperative ultrasound, 15 of 16 reoperated patients have been cured of their disease.[17]

Although infrequent, malignant insulinomas may be found at exploration. The most common sites for metastasis are the liver and adjacent lymph nodes. In the event that metastases are found, there is a relevant role for debulking the tumor, because a survival advantage has been demonstrated for removing as much tumor as possible.[27] In addition, debulking may assist in temporary alleviation of hypoglycemia. Attempts at resection or debulking of hepatic metastases may also be palliative or, rarely, curative.[13]

Gastrinoma

Gastrinomas are the second most common functioning islet cells tumors of the pancreas, occurring one-half as often as insulinomas.[14] These tumors are generally small and occur more frequently (3:2) in males than in females.[28,29] Gastrinomas may occur from childhood into old age, but the majority of cases occur between the fourth and sixth decades of life.[13]

The Zollinger–Ellison syndrome (ZES), originally described in 1955, includes non-insulin-producing tumors of the pancreas, acid hypersecretion and fulminant peptic ulcer disease.[30] The more proper designation for this syndrome today is gastrinoma, as one or more of the initially described components of ZES may not be present. Historically, this disease was recognized following a protracted course of ulcer disease with delays in diagnosis ranging from 3 to 9 years.[14] At present, patients with gastrinoma resemble the typical peptic ulcer patient. The most common presenting symptom of gastrinoma is epigastric pain and most patients will have a solitary ulcer. These ulcers are often <1 cm in diameter and 75% occur in the first portion of the duodenum.

Less commonly, patients with gastrinomas may have recurrent, multiple and atypically located ulcers, for example in the distal duodenum (14%) or jejunum (11%).[31] Perforated ulcer remains a common complication with 7% of patients with gastrinomas presenting with perforation of the jejunum.[32] Interestingly, as many as 20% of patients have no evidence of ulcer disease and present with the secretory effects of the tumor.[33]

Diarrhea occurs in 40% of patients with gastrinoma and is caused by gastric acid hypersecretion that increases intestinal transit time, leading to malabsorption. Control of stomach acid output by either total gastrectomy or medications has been shown to control the diarrhea in nearly all patients.[34] A significant proportion of patients with gastrinoma will experience esophageal abnormalities including dysphagia and esophagitis. Indeed, ulceration, stricture formation and perforation have been reported in this disease.[35] Medical management of esophageal disease requires strict control of acid secretion by the stomach.

Measurement of the fasting serum concentration of gastrin is the best single screening test for gastrinoma, as more than 99% of patients with gastrinomas will have abnormally elevated levels (>100 pg/ml). Ideally, for gastrin levels to be most accurate, all antisecretory medications should be stopped for several days prior to testing. The second critical exam is the determination of basal acid output (BAO). This is defined as a BAO greater than 15 mEq/h in patients without previous surgery to reduce gastric acid secretion, or greater than 5 mEq/h in patients with prior acid-reducing operations.[31] The measurement of gastric acid output helps to exclude other causes for hypergastrinemia such as gastric outlet obstruction, antral G-cell hyperplasia, postvagotomy state, and retained antrum. In patients with achlorhydria, such as those with pernicious anemia and atrophic gastritis, failure of acid-induced feedback inhibition results in elevated serum gastrin levels. Therefore, measurement of serum gastrin levels alone in these patients will be inaccurate 50% of the time in the diagnosis of gastrinoma.[34]

If there is any diagnostic uncertainty or if the serum gastrin level is only moderately elevated, a secretin stimulation test is indicated. This test involves an intravenous bolus of 2 U/kg of secretin and then serum levels of gastrin are determined at 0, 2, 5, 10 and 20 minutes. Patients with gastrinomas have gastrin level elevations of 200 pg/ml or more above the fasting value.[14] A positive secretin test is very useful in the differential diagnosis of gastrinoma from antral G-cell hyperplasia. The latter is also characterized by gastrin hypersecretion and hyperacidity. However, gastrin secretion in antral G-cell hyperplasia does not rise after administration of a secretin bolus.[13] The secretin test has also been used to follow patients following surgical resection of gastrinoma to evaluate for the presence of recurrent or persistent disease. Patients with persistent or recurrent gastrinoma will have an abnormal secretin test before they develop an elevated basal gastrin level or imageable disease.[36]

With the advent of potent gastric antisecretory medications, acid hypersecretion can be effectively controlled in all patients with gastrinoma. Therefore, for control of gastric acid output, total gastrectomy is no longer indicated in the management of these patients.[31] Proton pump inhibitors are the medical treatment of choice when H_2-receptor antagonists have failed because of escape or unwanted side effects. Patients with gastrinoma require greater doses of medication than patients with typical peptic ulcer disease. In one study, the mean total dose of omeprazole to control gastric acid output in 63 patients with gastrinoma was 80 mg per day.[37] Despite this, there is concern whether prolonged high dose omeprazole is safe in humans. Experiments in rodents have shown that prolonged omeprazole use is associated with the development of gastric carcinoid tumors.[38] In fact, the development of diffuse malignant gastric carcinoids has been observed in a few patients with gastrinoma and MEN-1 maintained on omeprazole for prolonged time periods.[37]

Precise localization of all gastrinomas is critical for defining an appropriate therapeutic strategy. Gastrinomas are mainly located in the gastrinoma triangle (Fig. 23.2).[39] Primary gastrinomas can also be observed, but less frequently, in the distal duodenum

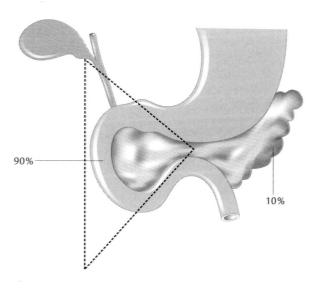

Figure 23.2 Anatomic triangle in which gastrinomas are most often found. (From Mozzell et al.[13])

or jejunum and in other parts of the pancreatic gland. Ectopic gastrinomas are rare but hard to localize preoperatively (ovaries, gallbladder). In sporadic gastrinoma, the primary tumor is often single or associated with peripancreatic metastatic lymph nodes.[33,40] It is thought that primary gastrinomas can be located in lymph nodes because resection of lymph nodes has rarely been associated with long-term cure.[33,40,41] Data indicate that about 30% of gastrinomas are pancreatic and the others are extra-pancreatic, mainly duodenal.[33,41,42] In MEN-1, the endocrine tumors are often multiple and can be located both in the pancreatic gland and the duodenum.[37]

The ability of imaging modalities to localize primary gastrinoma and gastrinoma metastatic to the liver is summarized in Tables 23.3 and 23.4. At the time of diagnosis, approximately 25–40% of patients will have liver metastases, therefore, imaging studies must carefully assess the liver. Although non-invasive modalities for tumor localization have high specificity, their sensitivity is often low. In addition, the sensitivities of ultra-sonography and CT scanning are much lower for duodenal gastrinomas than for pancreatic gastrinomas and depend on tumor size.[43] Approximately 30% of gastrinomas between 1 and 3 cm are seen on CT, while nearly all larger tumors are imaged. CT detects 80% of pancreatic gastrinomas but only 35% of extrapancreatic tumors. Modern MRI technology has demonstrated improved ability to detect liver metastases with an 83% sensitivity and 88% specificity.[44] Despite the widespread use of computed tomography and magnetic resonance imaging, 50% of primary tumors will not be identified on conventional preoperative imaging studies.[37]

Somatostatin receptor scintigraphy (SRS) has been suggested to be the non-invasive imaging study of choice to localize primary and metastatic gastrinomas. Studies have demonstrated that gastrinomas have high densities of somatostatin receptors and that these can be used to image these tumors using radiolabeled somatostatin analogs (Table 23.3).[22,23] In a study of 35 patients, SRS detected 67% of all gastrinomas found at exploration, including 52% of primary gastrinomas found and 80% of lymph nodes containing metastatic gastrinoma. Therefore, SRS missed approximately one-third of all extra-hepatic gastrinomas that were found at exploration. Of note, SRS detected only 30% of duodenal gastrinomas but detected 90% of pancreatic gastrinomas. Similar to several other studies, the investigators found that SRS was significantly more sensitive than conventional imaging studies and, on a lesion-by-lesion basis, was even more sensitive than all conventional imaging studies combined. The addition of all conventional studies to SRS detected only three (4%) additional lesions found at exploration in three patients.[45]

The potential benefit of endoscopic ultrasound for preoperative imaging is that it can visualize small tumors and may help distinguish the primary tumor from lymph node and liver metastases. In a study of 22 patients, EUS had a sensitivity of 50%, 75% and 63% for duodenal, pancreatic and lymph node gastrinoma, respectively.[46] Currently, studies suggest that EUS has a sensitivity of 50% to 75% and a specificity of 95% in the localization of gastrinomas.[24,46]

Techniques such as portal venous sampling of gastrin and angiography with intra-arterial injection of secretin with venous sampling of gastrin have been shown to have good sensitivity for gastrinoma detection (Table 23.4) However, since 80% of gastrinomas are located in a relatively small anatomical area, the gastrinoma triangle, performing a study that indicates a region that may harbor a tumor does not add much information. Secretin angiography may be indicated for selection of patients that may benefit from an aggressive approach (e.g. pancreati-coduodenectomy) for a locally advanced or locally recurrent gastrinoma. A secretin angiogram may be indicated to determine whether all tumor is localized within the planned resection.[37]

Table 23.3 **Sensitivity of non-invasive imaging studies for localization of primary and metastatic gastrinoma (adapted from Norton[57])**		
Imaging study	Extrahepatic primary (%)	Liver (%)
Ultrasound	9	48
CT	31	42
MR	30	71
SRS	58	92

Table 23.4 **Sensitivity of invasive imaging studies for localization of gastrinoma (adapated from Norton[37])**		
Imaging modality	Primary (%)	Liver (%)
Endoscopic ultrasound	50–75	NA
Angiogram	28	62
Portal venous sampling	73	NA
Secretion angiogram	78	41

In our opinion, preoperative evaluation in patients with gastrinoma should include:

(1) Endoscopy to evaluate for the presence of duodenal gastrinoma,
(2) Spiral CT scan to evaluate the pancreas, lymph nodes and liver (consider MR imaging if CT not adequate or further evaluation of liver is needed), and
(3) SRS for global evaluation of tumor extent.

Despite these tests, a significant percentage of patients will not have their tumors detected before surgery. Therefore, a thorough surgical exploration is indicated.

All patients with sporadic gastrinoma should undergo localization studies and be considered for exploratory laparotomy for potential cure. Since gastrinomas are relatively indolent, it has not been shown that resection of the primary tumor extends survival. However, evidence suggests that resection of primary gastrinoma decreases the incidence of liver metastases. Patients with liver metastases from gastrinoma will eventually die of disease. Therefore, it is reasonable to assume that resection of the primary should prolong survival.[37]

When exploring a patient for gastrinoma, a meticulous intraoperative approach is necessary. Gastrinomas that were previously missed have often subsequently been found to be in the duodenal wall. Gastrinomas are located in more proximal portions of the duodenum and the tumor density decreases more distally (Fig. 23.3). Simple palpation through the bowel wall without opening the duodenum will miss small duodenal tumors. Endoscopic transillumination and extensive duodenotomy have been found to improve localization of duodenal primaries.[16] Care to identify the ampulla and the pancreatic duct must be used when attempting to remove medial wall gastrinomas.

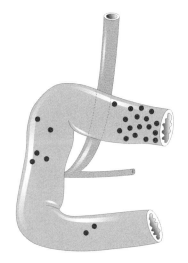

Figure 23.3 Location of 24 duodenal gastrinomas in patients with Zollinger–Ellison syndrome. Seventeen tumors were in the first portion, five were in the second, and two were in the third. (From Thorn et al.[47])

Gastrinomas within the pancreatic head should be enucleated and those in the body or tail of the pancreas should be resected by either subtotal or distal pancreatectomy. Whether tumors are actually in lymph nodes near the pancreatic head or in the pancreas itself is determined by frozen section. If tumor is found only in lymph nodes, other lymph nodes should be identified and removed. A search must then be made for a duodenal wall primary gastrinoma. Duodenal tumors should be resected with a narrow margin of duodenum around the tumor. Distant metastases to the liver should be resected if all tumor can be completely and safely removed.

With increased awareness of duodenal tumors, the operative detection rate is greater than 90% and the immediate cure rate is between 60 and 90% (Table 23.5).[28,48,49] The long-term cure rate is about one-half the immediate cure rate. Patients with resectable

Table 23.5 Results of surgery for localized sporadic and MEN-1 gastrinoma (adapted from Norton[37])

Series	Sporadic or MEN	N	No. with tumor found (%)	No. disease-free (%)
Norton et al.[33]	S	73	56 (77)	37 (50)
Howard et al.[48]	S	11	10 (91)	9 (82)
Thompson et al.[49]	S	5	5 (100)	5 (100)
McArthur et al.[108]	S	22	9 (41)	2 (9)
Melvin et al.[109]	MEN	19	17 (90)	1 (5)
MacFarlane et al.[53]	MEN	10	10 (100)	0 (0)
Jaskowial et al.[110]	S/MEN[a]	17	17 (100)	5 (30)[b]

[a] Reoperation for localized recurrent gastrinoma.
[b] Each of the five patients who were disease-free had sporadic gastrinoma
MEN, Multiple endocrine neoplasia type 1; S, sporadic.

disease have excellent survival (5-year: 70%, 10-year: 50%) but those with unresectable multiple metastases have a 5-year survival rate of only 20–38%.[33,50] Removal of all tumor or surgical debulking prolongs life expectancy in selected patients with metastatic disease.[16] Prospective studies indicate that aggressive resection of metastatic disease in patients who have resectable disease by radiologic criteria had a 5-year survival of 79% compared with 28% in patients with inoperable metastatic disease.[50,51] Patients who have solitary, localized metastatic disease appear to benefit most from this aggressive approach.

The management of gastrinoma in patients with MEN-1 is controversial.[52] Neuroendocrine tumors of the pancreas and duodenum are frequently multiple in this syndrome, making it difficult to determine which tumor is responsible for the clinical features. The role of surgery in these patients is not clear as few are cured and the islet cell tumors are thought to be less malignant than those seen in non-familial forms of the disease. A study has shown that, even when procedures to explore the duodenum and remove duodenal tumors were used, complete remission was uncommon because 86% of tumors had metastasized to lymph nodes and 43% of patients had multiple tumors.[53] Nevertheless, some authors advocate an aggressive approach to these patients including:

(1) Performance of a distal pancreatectomy in every patient to remove tumors in the neck, body or tail,
(2) Duodenotomy in every patient to remove small duodenal wall tumors, and
(3) Peripancreatic lymph node dissection in any MEN-1 patient with a duodenal neuroendocrine tumor or a pancreatic tumor 2 cm in diameter or larger.[54]

Using this approach in 38 patients resulted in 5-, 10- and 15-year survival rates of 98%, 98% and 96%, respectively. There was no operative mortality and no patient subsequently died of MEN-1 related disease. Two-thirds of the patients with gastrinomas remained eugastrinemic.[54] A practical approach may be to perform imaging studies consisting of a CT scan and SRS in patients with MEN-1 and suspected gastrinoma. Those patients with tumors that are large (>2 cm) have a significant probability of metastases to the liver and the tumors are resected according to their malignant potential. Other patients with MEN-1 and gastrinoma may be treated with medication to control gastric secretion.

Glucagonoma

Glucagonomas are usually large tumors (>5 cm) and occur most often in the body and tail of the pancreas and are rarely extrapancreatic (Table 23.1).[13,16] The incidence of glucagonoma is considerably less than insulinoma and gastrinoma and is estimated to be one in 20 million to one in 30 million. The exact incidence is unknown because glucagonomas may be underdiagnosed since they remain asymptomatic until they grow large, and may be misdiagnosed since the symptoms of excess glucagon can be attributed to other causes. The mean age at diagnosis is approximately 55 years. As glucagonoma may be associated with MEN-1 syndrome, patients and their families should be screened for other endocrinopathies.

Patients usually present with symptoms of weight loss, glucose intolerance and migratory necrolytic dermatitis. This rash begins as erythematous macules and papules on the face, abdomen, groin and extremities. Other findings which are less common include stomatitis, glossitis and diarrhea. Glucagonoma is diagnosed by characteristic findings on biopsy of the rash. However, serum levels of glucagon exceeding 1000 pg/ml are diagnostic.[13,16] Although several symptomatic patients with glucagonomas have been found with glucagon concentrations below 1000 pg/ml, most glucagon concentrations of this magnitude have been in asymptomatic patients with small tumors. Glucagon concentrations can be elevated in other disease processes such as hepatic or renal insufficiency and after excessive exercise or severe stress. Elevation can also occur with diabetic ketoacidosis, septicemia and the use of oral contraceptives.

Glucagonomas are less difficult to localize preoperatively than other endocrine tumors of the pancreas because of their size at presentation. The improved technology and widespread use of CT scanning have decreased the importance of angiography and CT scanning is the technique of choice both to localize the primary tumor and to demonstrate metastatic disease.

The management of patients with a glucagonoma is directed towards control of the tumor and its hormonally related symptoms. When the tumor is still localized to the pancreas, surgical resection is the optimal treatment because it can completely reverse all clinical manifestations of the syndrome and result in a lasting cure. Only occasionally are these tumors amenable to enucleation. The high rate of malignancy together with a greater than 50% rate of metastases demands an aggressive resection strategy for glucagonomas.[13] As much tumor as possible should be removed, including nodal metastases and lesions in the liver that can be safely wedged out. Formal hepatic resection is indicated if all gross tumor can be excised. Tumor debulking can provide dramatic and rapid improvement in many glucagonoma symptoms. A marked and prolonged decline in serum glucagon is possible with palliative resection, so the hormonal manifestations of this disorder disappear or are relieved for many years. Repeat debulking of recurrent or metastatic disease may also prolong survival.[55]

Since these tumors are slow growing, the results of resection plus chemotherapy have resulted in 5-year survival rates of 50%.[56] Streptozotocin as a single agent has produced a biochemical response (reduction in serum hormone levels by at least 50%) in 64% of patients treated and a tumor response (regression of tumor size by at least 50%) in 50% of patients.[57] However, most investigators have found a lower response rate than this. Symptoms of glucagonoma may be successfully controlled with the use of somatostatin analog.[58]

VIPoma

VIPoma syndrome characterized by watery diarrhea, hypokalemia and achlorhydria (WDHA) was first described in 1958 by Verner and Morrison.[59] Vasoactive intestinal peptide was first isolated from bovine intestine in 1970 and soon after it was shown that extracts of peptides from tumor and plasma of patients with WDHA produced similar symptoms in dogs.[13,60] The first report of a surgical cure was in 1978 when excision of a VIPoma in a patient with WDHA syndrome completely relieved the symptoms as plasma VIP levels dropped to normal.[13] Since that time, 201 cases have been reported in the literature.[61]

VIPomas are predominantly in the pancreas (90%) and extrapancreatic tumors are very rare, except in children.[14] Pancreatic VIPomas are usually solitary, small in diameter and in the body or tail of the pancreas 75% of the time (Table 23.1).[61] Approximately 50% of pancreatic VIPomas are malignant and one-half of these are metastatic to the liver or regional lymph nodes at diagnosis. Less than 5% of patients with VIPoma of the pancreas have MEN-1.[14] The tumors have a bimodal distribution which is related to histologic type. In a study of 62 patients, 52 had pancreatic VIPomas and 10 had extrapancreatic ganglioneuromas. The extrapancreatic sites (adrenal, mediastinal, retroperitoneal) occur predominantly in the pediatric population and demonstrate a less aggressive course, with only a 10% rate of metastasis.[61]

Diagnosis includes an evaluation of the diarrhea for a secretory nature. This can be confirmed with a trial of fasting for 48–72 hours, which will have no major effect on the diarrhea due to VIPomas. The fecal content of potassium and sodium is determined. The sum of twice the sodium plus the potassium should equal isotonicity in a secretory diarrhea. All infectious causes of diarrhea must be excluded. A fasting plasma VIP level of more than 200 pg/ml is required to establish the diagnosis.[14,62]

Spiral CT scanning should be used to localize VIPomas. With small lesions, other modalities such as SRS or angiography may occasionally be necessary to help identify tumor location.[63]

Surgical excision remains the only effective method of cure. Preoperative restoration of extracellular volume status and correction of electrolyte abnormalities must be accomplished. The fluid and electrolyte imbalance should be reversed slowly because of its chronic nature. Octreotide acetate is useful in promptly inhibiting VIP secretion from the tumor and stopping the diarrhea.[55] A careful surgical exploration including evaluation of the retroperitoneum, both adrenal glands and the pancreas should be performed. Surgical therapy consists of enucleation or pancreaticoduodenectomy for pancreatic head tumors. Body and tail tumors are best managed by distal pancreatectomy. Complete resection of these tumors delivers full symptomatic relief. If all apparent tumor cannot be resected or if there is metastatic disease, surgical debulking remains a useful option. VIP levels are an excellent tumor marker for recurrence. If there is recurrence, repeat debulking may be a viable and therapeutic option.[64]

Survival of patients with malignancy and/or metastatic disease is disappointing. The average survival is approximately 1 year. There are few well documented chemotherapeutic agents for the treatment of the VIPoma syndrome. The combination of streptozotocin and 5-fluorouracil was effective in 65% of patients studied in the Eastern Cooperative Oncology Group.[65] DTIC, human leukocyte interferon and adriamycin in combination with streptozotocin have been used in small numbers of patients with variable success.[65,66] Octreotide provides symptomatic relief for most patients with metastatic disease.[67]

Somatostatinoma

Somatostatinomas are among the rarest of the functional endocrine tumors. There have been 41 males and 42 females reported with somatostatinomas. These patients have an average age of 54 years with a range of 24–84 years.[64] The most common location for somatostatinomas was within the pancreas (68%); 19% occur in the duodenum and 3% each in the ampulla of Vater and the small bowel (Table 23.1).[68] Most commonly, pancreatic tumors are found in the head and body of the gland.[13]

The classic somatostatinoma syndrome has been characterized by the triad of diabetes, diarrhea/steatorrhea and gallstones. Diarrhea/steatorrhea occurs in approximately one-third of patients and results from an increase in stool osmolarity secondary to malabsorption of fats, sugars and amino acids. Steatorrhea results from decreased pancreatic exocrine secretion and the associated impairment of fat absorption. Excessive somatostatin inhibits the release of cholecystokinin, which decreases gallbladder contraction and leads to malabsorption and cholelithiasis. Weight loss is one of the most common findings and is seen in about 40% of patients and may be attributable to malabsorption. Diabetes occurs in 25% of patients and may occur secondary to greater suppression of insulin secretion over glucagon release by somatostatin as well as indirectly by somatostatin suppression of gastric inhibitory peptide.[13,14,68]

Somatostatinomas are often large tumors at the time of presentation and imaging studies are associated with a high degree of accuracy. CT scanning correctly localized the somatostatinoma in 34 of 37 patients with pancreatic tumors. Angiography has also been used to localize difficult neoplasms.[68] The diagnosis can be established by measuring an elevated fasting somatostatin level (normal, <100 pg/ml). When evaluated preoperatively, 34 of 35 patients had elevated levels of circulating somatostatin. Plasma somatostatin measurements may also be useful in evaluating the success of treatment and to follow patients for possible recurrence.

Surgical resection is the preferred treatment for patients with somatostatinomas. Unfortunately, successful surgical management is difficult because of the high rate of metastases present at exploration (Table 23.1). Most tumors are large and enucleation is usually not possible. Pancreatic resection including a pancreaticoduodenectomy or distal pancreatectomy are often necessary. Debulking a large tumor or hepatic metastases may effectively palliate symptoms, often for prolonged periods of time.

As with other islet cell cancer, somatostatinomas may have an indolent tumor biology and long-term survival can occur. However, due to the frequent malignant behavior of this tumor, aggressive treatment is warranted and outcome is frequently poor. In one review, survival rates for these patients were 48% at 1 year and 13% at 5 years.[68] The experience with chemotherapy in this tumor is limited but streptozotocin and 5-FU has caused tumor regression and symptomatic remission in some patients and is therefore a reasonable consideration in the symptomatic patient with recurrent and/or metastatic disease.[69]

Unusual functional islet cell tumors

Other functional islet cell tumors are exceedingly rare and include growth hormone releasing factor secreting tumors, adrenocorticotropic hormone secreting tumors, parathyroid hormone like secreting tumors and neurotensinomas. The treatment of choice for these rare tumors is uncertain but appears to be primarily surgical resection. Palliative resection (debulking) of metastatic disease is also frequently indicated since it may provide symptom benefit. Octreotide acetate may prove to be useful in the symptomatic treatment of many of these tumors.[13]

Non-functional islet cell tumors

Non-functioning tumors are slow growing and occur most commonly in the head of the pancreas.[4,70] In surgical series, 38–80% of lesions are found in the pancreatic head. They tend to be relatively large, symptomatic and often present with metastatic disease. In a similar fashion to adenocarcinoma of the pancreas, the clinical presentation of these tumors is related to either local invasion or metastatic spread. Jaundice, abdominal pain, weight loss, or the appearance of an abdominal mass are the predominant signs and symptoms (Table 23.6). Many authors report the presence, in a small number of patients, of multiple non-functioning tumors scattered throughout the pancreas (Table 23.7).

Lesions in the pancreatic head may induce back pain but much less commonly than with ductal adenocarcinoma, which displays a characteristic ability to infiltrate retroperitoneal nerves. Often non-functional islet cell neoplasms in the body and tail of the pancreas do not present with many symptoms but may have a palpable mass on examination. In addition to these findings, patients may complain of nausea, vomiting, diarrhea or lethargy.[71] In contrast to adenocarcinoma of the pancreas where systemic effects are seen quite early in the presentation of the disease, patients with non-functioning islet cell tumors can present with advanced metastatic disease and relatively few systemic symptoms. An incidental presentation is not uncommon. Kent and colleagues from the Mayo Clinic noted that 4 (16%) of 25 non-functional tumors presented as an incidental finding.[4] Rarely, these tumors may present with massive hemorrhage as a result of either penetration into the gastrointestinal tract or erosion of vessels in the retroperitoneum.[72]

It is not clear whether the interval from onset of symptoms to diagnosis differs in patients with non-functioning neoplasms and those with functional

Table 23.6 Signs and symptoms of non-functional tumors at presentation

Author	N	Study years	Jaundice (%)	Abdominal pain (%)	Weight loss (%)	Mass (%)
Cheslyn-Curtis et al.[80]	20	1982–91	40	35	30	40
Broughan et al.[73]	21	1948–84	24	48	24	24
Kent et al.[4]	25	1960–78	28	36	—	8
Phan et al.[10]	58	1949–96	35	56	46	—

Table 23.7 Location of non-functional islet cell tumors in the pancreas

Author	N	Study years	Head No. (%)	Body and tail No. (%)	Multiple No. (%)
Kent et al.[4]	25	1960–78	14 (56)	5 (20)	6 (24)
Dial et al.[111]	11	1963–83	7 (64)	4 (36)	—
Broughan et al.[73]	19	1948–84	9 (47)	7 (37)	3 (16)
Eckhauser et al.[112]	10	1973–85	8 (80)	2 (20)	—
Yeo et al.[113]	13	1985–90	5 (38)	8 (62)	—
Cheslyn-Curtis et al.[80]	20	1982–91	14 (70)	5 (25)	1 (5)
Evans et al.[84]	73	1953–92	43 (59)	30 (41)	—
Madura et al.[81]	14	1972–96	11 (79)	1 (14)	1 (7)
Lo et al.[7]	34	1985–96	16 (47)	16 (47)	2 (6)

neoplasms. It has been suggested that as many small functional islet cell neoplasms cause symptoms related to hormone excess without the development of biliary or gastrointestinal obstruction due to the primary tumor, that they present earlier.[14] The duration of symptoms related to the tumor may be at least as long or longer in patients with functioning tumors as in non-functioning tumors. In a review of 64 patients with islet cell carcinomas (34 non-functional, 30 functional) treated at the Mayo Clinic, the duration of symptoms prior to diagnosis for all patients ranged from less than 1 month to 120 months (median 10 months). For functional neoplasms the median duration of symptoms was 11 months versus 8 months for non-functional neoplasms ($P > 0.1$).[7] Others have also found that the median duration of symptoms was significantly longer for functional tumors (insulinomas: 22 months, gastrinomas: 36 months) as compared to non-functional neoplasms (6 months).[73] It appears that most patients with islet cell tumors undergoing surgical treatment have a lengthy duration of symptoms. A high index of suspicion is necessary in attempting to make the diagnosis of an islet cell tumor of the pancreas.

Diagnosis

Since the clinical presentation of non-functioning islet cell tumors is similar to other pancreatic neoplasms, the major challenge is to distinguish this tumor from other forms of pancreatic neoplasia, especially from the much more common ductal adenocarcinoma. Non-functioning islet cell tumors tend to be larger than ordinary pancreatic adenocarcinomas at the time of diagnosis. Viable portions of islet cell tumors are typically well vascularized and often hypervascular relative to the unaffected portion of the pancreas. As a result this neoplastic tissue usually undergoes an appreciable degree of enhancement on images made with appropriate techniques of intravenous contrast enhancement.[74] Other morphologic features that distinguish islet cell tumors include the lack of vascular encasement and lack of obstruction of the pancreatic duct as compared to adenocarcinoma of the pancreas.

For non-functioning islet cell neoplasms, CT is the radiologic imaging modality of choice. Like other large, hypervascular neoplasms, islet cell carcinomas may have internal necrotic areas. These appear on CT as hypodense zones of low attenuation, sometimes with features of cystic degeneration or necrosis (Fig 23.4). Dystrophic calcification may develop within a tumor and is observed on CT in 20% of non-functioning islet cell tumors.[75] The characteristic features on CT of non-functioning islet cell carcinomas, including large tumor mass, hyper-enhancement, cystic degeneration and calcification, help distinguish them from ductal adenocarcinoma. Similar features are present and identified by CT in the metastatic lesions from these tumors. Metastases are found most often in the liver and in regional lymph nodes. Whereas metastases from ductal adenocarcinoma tend to be small, those from islet cell carcinoma are often large.[74]

Pancreatic tumors other than ductal adenocarcinomas can be difficult to distinguish from non-functioning islet cell tumors. In a study of 45 patients with 50 non-functioning islet cell tumors, 36 of the tumors had heterogeneous areas and over half (N = 27) had cystic degeneration visualized on CT or MRI. Only 14 of the 50 non-functioning tumors were solid homogeneous masses.[76] Therefore, an islet cell carcinoma could resemble atypical forms of serous or mucinous cystic neoplasms. More likely, a partially necrotic tumor, such as solid and papillary epithelial neoplasm, might resemble an islet cell neoplasm with similar structure. Unlike solid and papillary epithelial neoplasms, however, non-functioning islet cell tumors are often associated with large metastases and they do not typically have visible capsules. Moreover, they tend to occur in older age groups, and they do not have the predilection for female subjects (Table 23.8).

While MEN-1 syndrome has been associated with functioning endocrine tumors of the pancreas, small clinically silent endocrine tumors are often numerous in the pancreas of patients with this syndrome. Non-functioning microadenomatoses of MEN-1 patients have been found mainly to be composed of glucagon and pancreatic polypeptide producing cells. In addition to the microadenomatosis, larger,

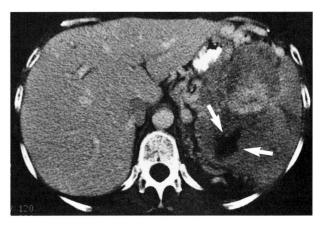

Figure 23.4 Computed tomography of patient with large non-functioning tumor of tail of pancreas. Note area of cystic degeneration and hypodense areas of necrosis (arrows). This patient underwent a potentially curative resection of the tumor.

discrete adenomas, mainly composed of pancreatic polypeptide producing cells, have been found.[77] Although increased blood levels of glucagon and pancreatic polypeptide have been frequently detected in such patients, as a rule related clinical syndromes have not been observed. Most clinically non-functioning pancreatic tumors in patients with MEN-1 syndrome have benign histologic patterns and behavior.[2]

Metastatic tumors to the pancreas such as those from renal cell carcinoma are particularly likely to have appearances indistinguishable from those of islet cell carcinoma. In these cases, clinical correlation should predict the nature of the lesion.

In addition to characteristic clinical presentations and radiologic findings, serum markers have been utilized in the diagnosis of non-functional endocrine tumors. To be able to detect a tumor by its secretion(s) implies that the tumor is no longer biochemically silent. Nonetheless, such neoplasms are not associated with any distinct clinical symptoms. Pancreatic polypeptideoma (PPoma) is one such

Table 23.8 CT characteristics of pancreatic neoplasms

Tumor type	Sex (M:F)	Vascularity	Degree of necrosis	Size	Enhancing capsule	Calcification
Adenocarcinoma	1.3:1.0	Hypovascular	Little	Small	No	No
Acinar cell	1.0:1.0	Hypovascular	Much	Large	Variable	No
Solid and papillary	1.0:9.0	Hypovascular	Much	Large	Yes	Yes—peripheral
Islet cell	1.0:1.0	Hypervascular	Variable	Mod-large	No	Yes (25%)—internal
Serous cystadenoma	1.0:2.0	Hypovascular	None	Large	Yes	Yes—central

tumor and amongst the most common of the non-functional islet cell tumors. Human pancreatic polypeptide is frequently associated with other hormones in pancreatic endocrine tumors and pancreatic polypeptide cells are most often found in glucagonomas and in non-secreting tumors.[11] In a series of eight patients with isolated pancreatic polypeptide producing islet cell tumors, clinical features included abdominal pain (N = 4), weight loss (N = 4), diarrhea (n = 2), gastrointestinal bleeding (N = 2) and jaundice in one patient. Serum basal pancreatic polypeptide was elevated in most patients with a marked response to secretin. Six of eight patients underwent tumor resection with two patients not surgical candidates due to hepatic metastases.[77] After curative resection, elevated serum pancreatic polypeptide levels fell to normal. Contrary to most reported non-functioning tumors, PPomas seem to have a benign course even when of large size and producing local symptoms, as found in six of eight cases reported above and in 10 of 10 cases reported elsewhere.[11] Other markers which have been evaluated in non-functioning islet cell tumors include neuron-specific enolase.[78] Its role in monitoring patient course or response to therapy is not known at present.

The presence of hormones in tumor cells at immunochemical staining provides useful information for the diagnosis of non-functioning islet cell tumors. Multiple hormones can be produced by these neoplasms. In a series of 61 non-functioning tumors, pancreatic polypeptide immunoreactivity was detected in 35% of cases, with a mean of 33% of all tumor cells; glucagon was found in 30% of cases and 30% of cells; somatostatin in 15% of cases and 20% of cells; serotonin in 20% of cases and 36% of cells; calcitonin in 20% of cases and 10% of cells; neurotensin in 8% of cases and 8% of cells; and insulin in 15% of cases and 2% of cells. No gastrin or VIP immunoreactivity was detected.[79] It seems clear that tumors producing pancreatic polypeptide, glucagon, somatostatin, calcitonin, and serotonin are more likely to be without an associated syndrome than are those producing clinically powerful hormones such as insulin, gastrin or VIP.

Localization and extent of disease

There are sparse data on the accuracy of non-invasive and invasive radiologic imaging in tumor localization and predicting resectability of non-functioning islet cell tumors. With improvements in CT scanning, angiography is no longer necessary in their diagnostic work-up. In a series of 20 patients studied between 1982 and 1991, dynamic CT localized the tumor in 17 of 20 patient (85%). No pancreatic lesion was seen in three patients who had obstructive jaundice. In two, the lesions were seen with angiography and the third was found at operation.[80] In another series, dynamic CT demonstrated a mass in nine of 13 patients (69%) while three of the patients had no mass seen but dilated common and/or pancreatic ducts were present.[81] In a study which evaluated both functioning and non-functioning islet cell tumors from 1949 to 1996, dynamic CT successfully localized the tumor 76% of the time. Angiography localized the tumor in 58% of patients and CT plus angiography did no better at tumor localization (79%) as compared to CT alone (76%).[10] Usually when CT shows a pancreatic mass presumed to be a non-functional islet cell neoplasm, arteriography is not warranted unless there is a question of invasion of a major vascular structure. Even then, non-invasive MR angiography has been shown to be accurate in predicting tumor vascular involvement.[82] Due to the relatively good prognosis with islet cell neoplasms, many surgeons would attempt en bloc resection with vascular reconstruction if there was vascular involvement at the time of surgery.[83] At present, the yield of new generation helical CT scanning in localizing non-functioning islet cell tumors is not known.

Although a study suggests that MR imaging is superior to CT in identification of pancreatic endocrine tumors, this study can be faulted since dynamic CT was utilized for comparison.[19] To our knowledge, no studies that compared state-of-the-art helical CT with MR imaging have been reported in the literature.

The role of laparoscopy in the management of patients with non-functioning islet cell tumors is unknown. With the goal of ruling out metastatic disease, laparoscopy would spare patients from undergoing an unnecessary laparotomy. In multiple series, evidence of metastatic disease has been found at the time of surgery in more than 50% of patients and resectability rates are low.[8,73,84] Unfortunately, most of these series have spanned long time frames and it is unknown whether metastatic disease was visible on quality preoperative imaging studies. A number of studies have demonstrated improved accuracy of laparoscopy in predicting extent of disease for pancreatic adenocarcinoma.[85] No study has specifically evaluated the use of laparoscopy in patients with islet cell tumors of the pancreas. Extrapolating from data obtained with pancreatic adenocarcinoma, it would appear that laparoscopy could spare asymptomatic patients with metastatic disease from undergoing unnecessary laparotomy (Fig. 23.5).

High-affinity somatostatin receptors have been identified in the pancreatic islet cells.[86] With this in mind, somatostatin receptor scintigraphy (SRS) has

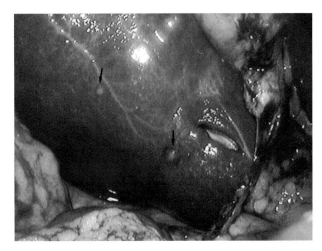

Figure 23.5 Photograph of liver metastases of a non-functioning islet cell tumor (arrows) detected at laparoscopy. The primary tumor was in the head of the pancreas. The preoperative CT scan did not reveal metastatic disease.

been developed for in vivo imaging of somatostatin receptor-positive tumors (Fig. 23.6 A–C). Studies with small numbers of patients have shown accurate localization of non-functioning islet cell tumors with SRS.[22,87] In a collective review of results from 15 centers in Europe with SRS, 82% of non-functioning tumors (N = 60) were visualized at scintigraphy.[23] Investigations in patients with non-functioning pancreatic tumors, which have compared SRS with CT scanning and MRI, have shown a similar sensitivity (60%) for both SRS and conventional imaging in detecting tumors. Somatostatin receptor scintigraphy was superior in detecting intra-abdominal and bony metastases. Conversely, tumor masses shown by conventional scanning techniques were missed by SRS in several patients. Since large tumor masses were missed by SRS in some cases, it is felt that the low density of somatostatin receptors on some tumors may be the

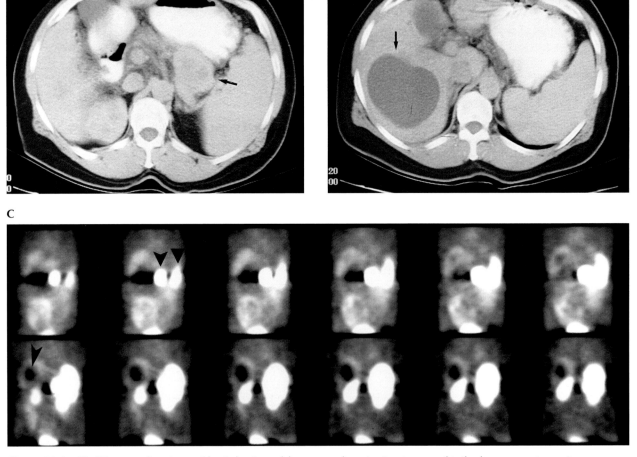

Figure 23.6 (A) CT scan of patient with cirrhosis and large non-functioning tumor of tail of pancreas (arrow). (B) Another image of the liver of the same patient shows a cystic lesion in the liver (arrrow), which was suspicious for metastatic disease. (C) Octreotide scan of the same patient. Top panel demonstrates two intense areas of uptake in the left abdomen corresponding with the tumor and the spleen (arrowheads). In the bottom panel, the large cyst in the liver is visualized and there is no uptake within this cyst in the liver (arrowhead). At operation, these findings were confirmed, no liver metastases were identified and the patient underwent a distal pancreatectomy with splenectomy.

major factor causing false negative results.[88] Since somatostatin receptors appear to be present in similar concentrations in non-functioning and functioning tumors, SRS should be of equal accuracy in detecting both types of tumors. The advantage of radionuclide scintigraphy is that adenocarcinoma of the pancreas does not take up the tracer and therefore false positive rates are low.[23] The disadvantage of this methodology is that the absence of tracer uptake by a tumor does not rule out an islet cell tumor. With rapid improvements in conventional imaging modalities (e.g. CT and MRI) in the visualization of the pancreas, liver and other intra-abdominal organs, the benefit of SRS in islet cell tumor identification may decrease.

The capacity to take up and decarboxylate amine precursors such as 5-hydroxytryptophan (5-HTP) and L-dihydroxyphenylalanine (L-DOPA) and store their amine precursors is characteristic of neuroendocrine cells and tumors. Utilizing this concept, positron emission tomography (PET) has been evaluated in the diagnosis of pancreatic endocrine tumors. In a study utilizing L-DOPA, the ability to detect the pancreatic tumor and possible metastases was evaluated in 22 patients with islet cell tumors. In the six patients with non-functioning islet cell tumors, there was relatively lower uptake of L-DOPA and in two cases the primary tumor as well as the metastases were not identified with PET, despite the fact that they were large and clearly visible with CT.[89] At present, with few available data, it appears that for localization of non-functioning endocrine tumors and their metastases, there is no general advantage of PET compared with CT. A larger patient population

is needed to determine the usefulness of L-DOPA and 5-HTP as tracers for visualization of the various subgroups of pancreatic endocrine tumors.

Treatment: curative surgery for the primary tumor

Operative resection is the only potentially curative form of therapy for patients with pancreatic islet cell tumors. Operation can be performed to resect local disease and to prevent the development of distant metastases or local recurrence. Patients with non-functional islet cell tumors may have similar clinical symptoms to ductal adenocarcinoma of the pancreas. However, in contrast to ductal adenocarcinoma, survival rates following surgical resection are quite good, and aggressive surgical therapy is indicated for non-functional neoplasms. Even though these tumors tend to be slow growing, they often present when the tumor mass is quite large. In some studies mean tumor size is 8–10 cm at presentation.[73,80] Despite this, with surgical resection, actuarial 5-year survival rates range from 44 to 63% with a median survival of 30 months to 4.8 years (Table 23.9). Surgical therapy should not be denied to patients on the basis of tumor size alone.

While ductal adenocarcinoma tends to directly encompass and invade adjacent structures early in its disease course, non-functioning islet cell tumors more often displace structures without actual invasion. The large tumor bulk may cause near obstruction of blood vessels via a compressive effect which can be relieved by tumor resection. For instance, tumors in the tail of the pancreas can

Table 23.9 Rates of curative resection and survival in non-functional islet cell tumors

Author	N	Study years	Tumor size[a] (cm)	Curative resection (%)	Survival All[b]	Curative[c]	
Kent et al.[4]	25	1960–78	>5[d]	9 (36)	44%	—	(actuarial 5-year)
Broughan et al.[73]	21	1948–84	10	12 (57)	63%	—	(actuarial 5-year)
Thompson et al.[8]	27	1965–84	—	10 (37)	58%	—	(actuarial 3-year)
Venkatesh et al.[102]	43	1950–87	—	22 (51)	40	—	months (mean)
Cheslyn-Curtis et al.[80]	20	1982–91	8	10 (50)	30	42	months (median)
Evans et al.[84]	73	1953–92	—	19 (26)	4.8	6.8	years (median)
Legaspi and Brennan[71]	33	1983–88	—	12 (36)	76%	100%	(actuarial 3-year)
Lo et al.[7]	34	1985–96	6.2	12 (35)	—	—	
Phan et al.[10]	58	1949–96	5.1	46 (79)	52%	—	(actuarial 5-year)

[a] Mean or median tumor size.
[b] Survival in entire study group: curative and non-curative resections.
[c] Survival in curatively resected patients.
[d] 18 of 25 tumors >5 cm in size.

A

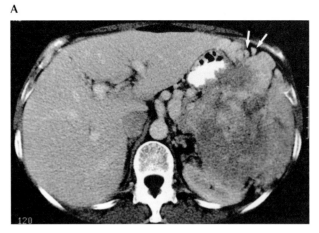

B

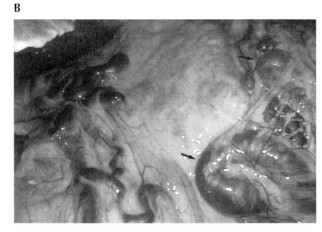

Figure 23.7 (A) Large tumor in the tail of the pancreas with splenic vein obstruction and varices (arrows). This tumor was resected with negative margins. (B) Intraoperative picture of varices encountered at the time of resection (arrows).

compress the splenic vein leading to splenomegaly and even varices (Fig. 23.7A,B). Nevertheless, these tumors can be frequently resected with negative margins. Similarly, tumors in the head of the pancreas can compress the superior mesenteric vein. Again, in the absence of known metastatic disease, every attempt should be made at tumor resection.

Tumors in the head of the pancreas should usually be treated by pancreaticoduodenectomy, while tumors in the body and tail should be treated with distal pancreatectomy. Extension of tumor from the pancreas into surrounding organs such as the stomach and colon should be resected en bloc. If the tumor is small (<2 cm) and located in the tail of the pancreas consideration should be given to distal pancreatectomy with splenic preservation. In patients with significant co-morbid conditions or for small lesions in the head of the pancreas, enucleation can be entertained.

With endocrine tumors, some authors have advocated that surgical removal of involved lymph nodes should be performed as it may improve survival. Patients with malignant endocrine tumors whose disease is confined to regional lymph nodes have a greater chance of benefit by removal of tumor than patients who have distant metastases. Therefore, regional nodes which are involved with tumor should be resected as completely as possible in an attempt to eliminate all disease and decrease the probability of distant metastases.[90] With non-functioning islet cell tumors, in the absence of metastases, it is controversial whether nodal disease outside the field of dissection should be resected. However, utilizing the data from neuroendocrine tumors of the small bowel in which extensive lymphadenectomy is recommended, it can be concluded that for non-functional islet cell neoplasms reasonable attempts should be made to remove all nodal disease.

Treatment: curative surgery for metastatic disease

There are few data available on the role for attempted curative resections of metastatic non-functional islet cell tumors. Since these tumors may follow a relatively indolent clinical course, a case to resect anatomically localized and surgically resectable metastases within the liver can be made. Of course, for this to be in the best interest of the patient, the primary disease and metastases must be completely resected. No data exist to validate this approach. It should only be considered if the metastatic lesion can be resected with acceptable morbidity and mortality.

Patients with unresected hepatic metastases from gastrointestinal neuroendocrine tumors have been reported to have 5-year survival rates of between 13% and 43%.[64] In an effort to improve survival and even cure patients who have failed other forms of therapy, liver transplantation has been applied in these patients. Reports of liver transplantation for metastatic neuroendocrine tumors have been confined to small numbers of patients and short follow-up, typically less than 3 years from the time of transplantation.[91] In the best results published to date, 12 patients (five pancreatic islet cell tumors) received transplants at a single center. Long-term survival was achieved in most patients with a median survival of 55 months.[92] However, in a multicenter report from France of 16 cases of liver transplantation for metastatic pancreatic islet cell tumors, the 4-year survival was 8%. The authors concluded that liver transplantation was not indicated for metastatic pancreatic islet cell tumors.[93] Despite some encouraging results from

Table 23.10 Surgical palliation and survival in non-functional islet cell tumors

Author	N	Palliative procedure No. (%)	Type	Survival
Kent et al.[4]	25	3 (12)	Biliary bypass (N = 2) Unknown (N = 1)	7 years (mean)
Prinz et al.[96]	8	4 (50)	Double bypass (N = 3)[a] Biliary bypass (N = 1)	4.5 years (mean)
Dial et al.[111]	11	2 (18)	Biliary bypass (N = 2)	1.5 years (AWD) 8 years (AWD)
Eckhauser et al.[112]	11	2 (18)	Double bypass (N = 2)	13 months (AWD) 26 months (DOD)
Evans et al.[84]	73	12 (16)	Distal pancreatectomy (N = 9) Pancreaticoduodenectomy (N = 3)	4.5 years (median)
Cheslyn-Curtis et al.[80]	20	7 (35)	Distal pancreatectomy (N = 2) Biliary bypass (N = 3) Pancreaticoduodenectomy (N = 2)	16 months (median)

[a] Biliary and gastric bypass.
AWD, alive with disease; DOD, dead of disease.

individual groups, until larger numbers of patients and longer follow-up are accumulated, or until the supply of donor livers increases, liver transplantation for metastatic pancreatic islet cell carcinomas should be applied with great caution.

Treatment: palliative surgery

Palliative resections of the primary tumor in the presence of metastatic disease have been performed in non-functioning islet cell tumors. In the series from M.D. Anderson, nine distal pancreatectomies and three pancreaticoduodenectomies were performed in the presence of liver metastases.[84] One perioperative death occurred in a patient who underwent distal pancreatectomy. Five of the 12 patients died of disease at a median of 3.7 years. Uncontrolled local tumor recurrence contributed to the cause of death in only one of the five patients. Overall, the median survival was 4.5 years (Table 23.10). These results can be compared to 22 patients who had metastatic disease at diagnosis and did not undergo resection of the primary tumor. Sixteen of the 22 died of disease at a median of 3.2 years. The cause of death in one patient was gastrointestinal hemorrhage caused by progression of the primary tumor in the pancreatic head. The other 15 patients died of liver metastases. The authors determined that the trend towards improved median survival in patients undergoing resection of their primary tumor in the presence of metastases could probably be explained by the smaller tumor volume in this group at the time of surgery.

In a second study, resection for palliation of local tumor symptoms was performed in two patients with non-functioning tumors. Complete relief of symptoms was achieved in both patients. One patient died 76 months after palliative resection and the other patient was still alive with disease at 10 months.[94] In the asymptomatic patient who has metastases from non-functioning islet cell tumor, due to prolonged survival regardless of primary tumor resection, it is difficult to justify primary tumor resection. In our opinion, in the absence of compelling data, resection of the primary tumor in the presence of liver metastases should be considered only in the presence of debilitating symptoms (e.g. pain) or in the presence of complications (e.g. bleeding).

Resection of metastases for palliation of symptoms has been reported more often in functioning than in non-functional islet cell carcinomas. It may play a more important role in alleviating the effects of excess production of endocrine hormones in functioning tumors. For non-functioning tumors it is rarely indicated, especially when other less invasive modalities can be utilized for treatment of symptoms due to metastatic tumor growth.

Hepatic artery embolization has been performed to palliate symptoms from metastatic disease. In a study of 22 patients with metastatic functional or non-functioning neoplasms, sequential hepatic artery embolization was performed. Patients underwent a median of four embolizations. Partial remission was achieved in 12 patients. Hormonal syndromes were frequently relieved. Moderately toxic reactions were incurred after each embolization, but they were brief. Median survival was 33.7 months.[95] Sequential hepatic artery occlusion with microembolic material may provide prolonged palliation for selected symptomatic patients with islet cell carcinoma metastatic to the liver.

Palliative biliary and/or enteric bypasses for patients presenting with unresectable disease and biliary or gastric outlet obstruction have been performed (Table 23.10). Prinz et al.[96] reported four of eight patients with unresectable tumors who underwent either a biliary bypass and gastrojejunostomy or a biliary bypass alone. The mean survival in these four patients was 4.5 years. For patients with obstructive jaundice secondary to a locally unresectable non-functioning islet cell neoplasm, operative biliary bypass should be strongly considered. The superiority of operative biliary bypass for long-term management of malignant biliary obstruction justifies this approach in patients who have islet cell tumors and potential for prolonged survival. Duodenal bypass via a gastrojejunostomy for lesions in the head of the pancreas should also be considered in these patients.

Treatment: chemotherapy

Recommended chemotherapy for advanced islet cell tumors is based on the results of a multicenter randomized trial. In this trial, 105 patients were randomized to receive one of three regimens: streptozotocin plus fluorouracil, streptozotocin plus doxorubicin, or chlorozotocin alone. Patients with either non-functioning or functioning islet cell tumors were included in this study. Streptozotocin plus doxorubicin was superior to streptozotocin plus fluorouracil in terms of the rate of tumor regression, measured objectively (69% versus 45%, $P = 0.05$, respectively), and the median length of time to tumor progression (20 versus 6.9 months, $P = 0.001$, respectively). Streptozotocin plus doxorubicin also had a significant advantage in terms of survival (median 2.2 versus 1.4 years, $P = 0.004$).[97] This regimen is now considered the standard treatment for advanced islet cell tumors, but should be considered in the context of each individual patient, as some may have prolonged survival untreated, and response to treatment is greater than the effect on overall survival.

Treatment: radiation therapy

The reported experience with radiation therapy in patients with islet cell carcinoma has been scarce. Torrisi et al.[98] treated three patients with locally advanced islet cell carcinoma. Objective responses were seen in two patients, whereas the third patient had a prolonged stabilization of the tumor. In addition, case reports of locally advanced islet cell tumors that have had complete responses to radiation therapy exist.[99] It would appear that selected patients may be palliated by radiotherapy. Radiation has, however, been reserved in the main for the treatment of pain from localized bone metastases.

Treatment: octreotide

Octreotide is a synthetic octapeptide with structure and activities similar to those of the native hormone somatostatin, but with significantly longer half-life and duration of action that the native substance. Octreotide has been reported to be effective in controlling the hormone-induced symptoms of patients with functional islet cell tumors.[100] Although rare reports of tumor regression to octreotide have been published, the drug has been primarily utilized to ameliorate the symptoms from hormonal excess in patients with functional islet cell tumors. In a study which included 13 patients with advanced, incurable non-functional islet cell tumors, octreotide was administered via subcutaneous injection. No patient experienced a major objective response. Of the 21 patients with functional tumors, 15 demonstrated either symptomatic improvement or an objective decrease in hormone level. Octreotide is useful in controlling symptoms due to hormonal excess in functional islet cell tumors. There is no evidence that octreotide would benefit patients with non-functional islet cell tumors.

Prognosis

Evans et al.[84] found that patients who underwent curative resection of their primary tumor in the absence of metastases had a 72% 5-year survival with a median survival of 6.8 years. This was in sharp contrast to patients who presented with distant metastases and who did not undergo resection. These patients had a 38% 5-year survival with a median survival of 3.3 years. In addition, amongst patients with localized disease at presentation, the survival was significantly better in patients who were able to undergo tumor resection as compared to those who did not. Therefore, important predictors of survival are the ability to undergo curative resection and the degree of local spread.

It is unclear whether non-functional tumors have a worse prognosis than functional islet cell tumors. Several studies have shown that the survival of patients with non-functional tumors is poorer than for those with functional tumors. In a report from the Cleveland Clinic, actuarial 10-year survival was 55% for non-functioning tumors while it was 92% for insulinomas and 68% for gastrinomas.[73] In a study from Johns Hopkins, median survival was 121 months in functional tumors while it was 96 months in non-functional neoplasms ($P < 0.025$).[10] In an early report from the Mayo Clinic, survival was statistically better at 3 years in those patients with gastrinomas compared with patients with non-functioning tumors, 91% versus 58%.[8] However, in a later report from the same institution, there was no survival difference between functional and non-functional neoplasms.[7] Other studies have found no difference in survival between functioning and non-functioning tumors.[101,102]

Size of the primary tumor rather than functional status may be a more important prognostic variable. In the study by Phan et al.[10] the median tumor size in the non-functional tumors was 4.0 cm as compared to 1.9 cm in the functional neoplasms. In addition, the malignancy rates were correspondingly lower in the functional tumors (47%) as compared to the non-functional ones (60%). It may be that non-functional tumors are detected at larger tumor burdens because of the absence of an endocrine syndrome. This may account for poorer survival with non-functioning neoplasms seen in some studies.

Efforts have been made to develop more sophisticated markers to determine prognosis in patients with non-functioning islet cell neoplasms. In a preliminary study of 61 non-functioning tumors, vascular or perineural microinvasion and Ki67 proliferative index were the most sensitive and specific variables that were predictive of malignancy. These variables were utilized in tumors lacking evidence of malignancy at the time of surgery, to separate cases with increased risk of malignancy from cases with limited risk, and were found to be somewhat predictive of survival.[79] Rigorous studies in larger numbers of patients with islet cell neoplasms, which examine different immunohistochemical markers, may help identify prognostic variables in these tumors.

Conclusions

Clinically, there are similarities and differences between the various functional endocrine tumors of the pancreas. These tumors vary with regard to size, location, age distribution, sex distribution, propensity for malignancy, and metastatic potential in accordance with the individual tumor type. The clinical morbidity and mortality associated with the

tumor are due to peptide hypersecretion and not to tumor mass. In addition, there is no correlation between tumor size and the severity of functional manifestations.

Non-functioning islet cell tumors are pancreatic tumors with endocrine differentiation in the absence of a clinical syndrome of hormone hyperfunction. These tumors are hormonally silent because either the principal hormone secreted by the tumor may cause no specific clinical signs although it is released in excess, the amount of hormone produced may be too small to cause symptoms, or the tumor may secrete a precursor hormone that is functionally inert, or the hormonal product of the tumor may not yet be identified.

Non-functioning islet cell tumors are slow growing and occur most commonly in the head of the pancreas. Imaging modalities such as CT scanning or MR imaging are accurate in the localization of these tumors within the pancreas. While false negative rates for tumor detection are high, octreotide scintigraphy may provide additional useful information in the evaluation for suspected metastases.

Operative resection is the only potentially curative form of therapy for patients with functioning and non-functioning islet cell neoplasms. In contrast to ductal adenocarcinoma of the pancreas, survival rates following surgical resection are quite good. Since metastatic functional and non-functional islet cell carcinomas may follow a relatively indolent course, anatomically localized and surgical resectable metastases within the liver should be considered for resection. The primary site of disease must be controlled if this is to be considered.

The survival of patients with non-functional tumors may be similar to those with functional neoplasms. Patients with non-functional tumors often present with larger tumor size, which may account for the decreased survival seen with these neoplasms in some series. Prognostic variables in islet cell tumors are limited and further work evaluating immunohistochemical markers in this disease is needed.

Key points

- Clinically silent endocrine tumors have been found in up to 10% of detailed autopsy examinations.
- Functional islet cell tumors include:
    Insulinoma
    Gastrinoma

Glucagonoma
VIPoma
Somatostatinoma.
- Localization of pancreatic endocrine tumors:
  Helical CT: sensitivity 85%
  MRI: sensitivity not known
  Angiography: sensitivity 58%

Somatostatin receptor scintigraphy: 82%
PET scan: sensitivity not known.
- Surgical excision, usually with curative intent, is the major objective of treatment.
- Surgical debulking of primary and metastatic functional islet cell tumors often achieves good palliation of symptoms.

REFERENCES

1. Kimura W, Kuroda A, Morioka Y. Clinical pathology of endocrine tumors of the pancreas. Dig Dis Sci 1991; 36: 933–42

2. Solcia E, Sessa F, Rindi G, Bonato M, Capella C. Pancreatic endocrine tumors: general concepts; nonfunctioning tumors and tumors with uncommon function. In: Dayal Y, ed. Endocrine pathology of the gut and pancreas. Boca Raton: CRC Press, 1991: 105–31

3. Solcia E, Capella C, Kloppel G. Tumors of the endocrine pancreas. In: Anonymous atlas of tumor pathology. Washington: AFIP, 1997: 145–209

4. Kent RB, Van Heerden JA, Weiland LH. Nonfunctioning islet cell tumors. Ann Surg 1981; 193: 185–90

5. Kloppel G, Heitz PU. Pancreatic endocrine tumors. Pathol Res Pract 1988; 183: 155–68

6. Howard JN, Moss NH, Rhoads JE. Collective review: hyperinsulinism and islet cell tumors of the pancreas. Int Abstr Surg 1950; 90: 417–55

7. Lo CY, Van Heerden JA, Thompson GB, Grant CS, Soreide JA, Harmsen WS. Islet cell carcinoma of the pancreas. World J Surg 1996; 20: 878–84

8. Thompson GB, Van Heerden JA, Grant CS, Carney A, Ilstrup DM. Islet cell carcinomas of the pancreas: a twenty-year experience. Surgery 1988; 104: 1011–7

9. Grant CS. Surgical management of malignant islet cell tumors. World J Surg 1993; 17: 498–503

10. Phan GQ, Yeo CJ, Hruban RH, Lillemoe KD, Pitt HA, Cameron JL. Surgical experience with pancreatic and peripancreatic neuroendocrine tumors: review of 125 patients. J Gastrointest Surg 1998; 2: 473–82

11. Heitz PU, Kasper M, Polak JM, Kloppel G. Pancreatic endocrine tumors: immunocytochemical analysis of 125 tumors. Hum Pathol 1982; 13: 263–71

12. Alpert S, Hanahan D, Teitelman G. Hybrid insulin genes reveal a development lineage for pancreatic endocrine cells and imply a relationship with neurons. Cell 1988; 53: 295

13. Mozzell E, Stenzel P, Woltering EA, Rosch J, O'Dorisio TM. Functional endocrine tumors of the pancreas: clinical presentation, diagnosis, and treatment. Curr Probl Surg 1990; 27: 303–86

14. Bieligk S, Jaffe BM. Islet cell tumors of the pancreas. Surg Clin N Am 1995; 75: 1025–40

15. Friesen SR. Tumors of the endocrine pancreas. N Engl J Med 1982; 306: 580–90

16. Norton JA. Neuroendocrine tumors of the pancreas and duodenum. Curr Probl Surg 1994; 31: 77–164

17. Grant CS. Insulinoma. Surg Oncol Clin N Am 1998; 7: 819–44

18. Van Hoe L, Gryspeerdt S, Marchal G, Baert AL, Mertens L. Helical CT for the preoperative localization of islet cell tumors of the pancreas. AJR 1995; 165: 1437–9

19. Smelka RC, Cumming MJ, Shoenut JP et al. Islet cell tumors: comparison of dynamic contrast-enhanced CT and MR imaging with dynamic gadolinium enhancement and fat suppression. Radiology 1993; 186: 799–802

20. Muller MF, Meyenberger C, Bertschinger P, Schaer R, Marincek B. Pancreatic tumors: evaluation with endoscopic US, CT and MR imaging. Radiology 1994; 190: 745–51

21. Van Byck CHJ, Bruining HA, Reubi JC, Bakker HY, Krenning EP, Lamberts SWJ. Use of isotope-labeled somatostatin analogs for visualization of islet cell tumors. World J Surg 1993; 17: 444–7

22. Krenning EP, Kwekkeboom DJ, Reubi J et al. 111In-octreotide scintigraphy in oncology. Metabolism 1992; 41: 83–6

23. Krenning EP, Kwekkeboom DJ, Oei HY et al. Somatostatin-receptor scintigraphy in gastroenteropancreatic tumors. Ann NY Acad Sci 1994; 733: 416–24

24. Thompson NW, Czako PF, Fritts LL et al. Role of endoscopic ultrasound in the localization of insulinomas and gastrinomas. Surgery 1994; 116: 1131–8

25. Pasieka JL, MeLeod MK, Thompson NW et al. Surgical approach to insulinomas: assessing the need for preoperative localization. Arch Surg 1992; 127: 442–7

26. Doppman JL, Miller DL, Chang R et al. Intraarterial calcium stimulation test for insulinomas. World J Surg 1993; 17: 439–43

27. Danforth DN, Gordon P, Brennan MF et al. Metastatic insulin secreting carcinoma of the pancreas: clinical course and role of surgery. Surgery 1984; 96: 1027–37

28. Delcore R Jr, Cheung LY, Friesen SR. Characteristics of duodenal wall gastrinomas. Am J Surg 1990; 160: 621–4

29. Ellison EH, Wilson SD. The Zollinger–Ellison syndrome: reappraisal and evaluation of 260 registered cases. Ann Surg 1964; 160: 512–30

30. Zollinger RM, Ellison EH. Primary peptic ulceration of the jejunum associated with islet cell tumors of the pancreas. Ann Surg 1955; 142: 709–23

31. Meko JB, Norton JA. Management of patients with Zollinger–Ellison syndrome. Ann Rev Med 1995; 46: 395–411

32. Waxsman I, Gardner JD, Jensen RT, Maton PN. Peptic ulcer perforation as the presentation of Zollinger–Ellison syndrome. Dig Dis Sci 1991; 36: 19–24

33. Norton JA, Doppman JL, Jensen RT. Curative resection in Zollinger–Ellison syndrome: results of a 10 year prospective study. Ann Surg 1992; 215: 8–18

34. Wolfe MM, Jensen RT. Zollinger–Ellison syndrome, current concepts in diagnosis and management. New Engl J Med 1987; 317: 1200–9

35. Bondeson AG, Bondeson L, Thompson NW. Stricture and perforation of the esophagus: overlooked threats in the Zollinger-Ellison syndrome. World J Surg 1990; 14: 361–4

36. Pisegna J, Norton JA, Slimak GG et al. Effects of curative gastrinoma resection on gastric secretory function and antisecretory drug requirements in the Zollinger–Ellison syndrome. Gastroenterology 1992; 102: 767–78

37. Norton JA. Gastrinoma: advances in localization and treatment. Surg Oncol Clin N Am 1998; 7: 845–61

38. Larsson H, Caisson E, Matsson H. Plasma gastrin and gastric enterochromaffin cell (activation and proliferation-studies with omeprazole and ranitidine in intact and adrenalectomized rats. Gastroenterology 1986; 90: 391–9

39. Stabile BE, Morrow DJ, Passaro E Jr. The gastrinoma triangle: operative implications. Am J Surg 1984; 147: 25–31

40. Farley DR, Van Heereden JA, Grant CS, Miller JL, Ilstrup DM. The Zollinger–Ellison syndrome. A collective surgical experience. Ann Surg 1992; 215: 561–9

41. Fraker DL, Norton JA, Alexander R, Venzon DJ, Jensen RT. Surgery in Zollinger–Ellison syndrome alters the natural history of gastrinoma. Ann Surg 1994; 220: 320–30

42. Ellison EC. Forty year appraisal of gastrinoma. Back to the future. Ann Surg 1995; 222: 511–24

43. Miller DL, Norton JA, Jensen RT. Prospective assessment of abdominal ultrasound in patients with Zollinger–Ellison syndrome. Radiology 1991; 178: 763–7

44. Pisegna JR, Doppman JL, Norton JA, Metz DC, Jensen RT. Prospective comparative study of ability of MR imaging and other imaging modalities to localize tumors in patients with Zollinger–Ellison syndrome. Dig Dis Sci 1993; 38: 1318–28

45. Alexander HR, Fraker DL, Norton JA et al. Prospective study of somatostatin receptor scintigraphy and its effect on operative outcome in patients with Zollinger–Ellison syndrome. Ann Surg 1998; 228: 228–38

46. Ruszniewski P, Amouyal P, Amouyal G et al. Localization of gastrinomas by endoscopic ultrasonography in patients with Zollinger–Ellison syndrome. Surgery 1995; 117: 629–35

47. Thorn AK, Norton JA, Axiotis CA, Jensen RT. Location, incidence and malignant potential of duodenal gastrinomas. Surgery 1991; 110: 1086–93

48. Howard TJ, Zinner MJ, Stabile BE et al. Gastrinoma excision for cure. Ann Surg 1990; 211: 9–14

49. Thompson NW, Vinik AI, Eckhauser FE. Microgastrinomas of the duodenum: a cause for failed operations of the Zollinger–Ellison syndrome. Ann Surg 1989; 209: 396–404

50. Carty SE, Jensen RT, Norton JA. Prospective study of aggressive resection of metastatic pancreatic endocrine tumors. Surgery 1992; 112: 1024–32

51. Norton JA, Sugarbaker PH, Doppman JL et al. Aggressive resection of metastatic disease in selected patients with malignant gastrinoma. Ann Surg 1986; 203: 352–9

52. Veldhius JD, Norton JA, Wells SAJ et al. Therapeutic controversy; surgical versus medical management of multiple endocrine neoplasia (MEN) type 1. J Clin Endocrinol 1997; 82: 357–64

53. MacFarlane MP, Fraker DL, Alexander HR et al. Prospective study of surgical resection of duodenal and pancreatic gastrinomas in multiple endocrine neoplasia type 1. Surgery 1995; 118: 973–80

54. Thompson NW. Management of pancreatic endocrine tumors in patients with multiple endocrine neoplasia type 1. Surg Oncol Clin N Am 1998; 7: 881–91

55. Modlin IM, Lewis JJ, Ahiman H, Bilchik AJ, Kumar RR Management of unresectable malignant endocrine tumors of the pancreas. Surg Gynecol Obstet 1993; 176: 507–18

56. Rothmund M, Stinner B, Arnold R. Endocrine pancreatic tumors. Eur J Surg Oncol J 1991; 17: 191–9

57. Broder LE, Carter SK. Pancreatic islet cell carcinoma: results of therapy with streptozotocin in 52 patients. Ann Intern Med 1973; 79: 101–7

58. Boden G, Ryan IG, Eisenschmid BL et al. Treatment of inoperable glucagonoma with the long acting somatostatin analogue SMS 201995. N Engl J Med 1986; 314: 1686–9

59. Verner JV, Morrison AB. Islet cell tumor and a syndrome of refractory watery diarrhea and hypokalemia. Am J Med 1958; 25: 374–80

60. Said SI, Mutt V. Isolation from porcine-intestinal wall of a vasoactive octacosapeptide related to secretin and glucagon. Eur J Biochem 1972; 28: 199–204

61. Friesen SR. Update on the diagnosis and treatment of rare neuroendocrine tumors. Surg Clin N Am 1987; 67: 379–93

62. Mekhjian HS, O'Dorisio TM. VIPoma syndrome. Semin Oncol 1987; 14: 282–91

63. Inamoto K, Yoshino F, Nakao N et al. Angiographic diagnosis of a pancreatic islet tumor in a patient with the WDHA syndrome. Gastrointest Radiol 1980; 5: 259–61

64. Delcore R, Friesen SR. Gastrointestinal neuroendocrine tumors. J Am Coll Surg 1994; 178: 188–211

65. Moertel CG, Hanley JA, Johnson LA. Streptozocin alone compared with streptozocin plus fluorouracil in the treatment of advanced islet-cell carcinoma. N Engl J Med 1980; 303: 1189–94

66. O'Dorisio TM, Mekhjian HS, Gaginella TS. Medical therapy of VIPomas. Endocrinol Metab Clin N Am 1989; 18: 545–56

67. Maton PN. Use of octreotide for control of symptoms in patients with islet cell tumors. World J Surg 1993; 17: 504–10

68. Harris GJ, Tio F, Cruz AB. Somatostatinoma of the duodenum: case report and review of the literature. J Surg Oncol 1987; 36: 8–16

69. Konomi K, Chijiiwa K, Katsuta T et al. Pancreatic somatostatinoma: case report and review of the literature. J Surg Oncol 1990; 43: 259–69

70. Thompson NW, Eckhauser FE. Malignant islet cell tumors of the pancreas. World J Surg 1984; 8: 940–51

71. Legaspi A, Brennan ME. Management of islet cell carcinoma. Surgery 1988; 104: 1018–23

72. Debas HT, Mulvihill SJ. Neuroendocrine gut neoplasms. Arch Surg 1994; 129: 965–72

73. Broughan TA, Leslie JD, Soto JM, Hermann RE. Pancreatic islet cell tumors. Surgery 1986; 99: 671–8

74. Stephens DH. CT of pancreatic neoplasms. Curr Probl Daign Radiol 1997; 26: 53–108

75. Eelkema EA, Stephens DH, Ward EM, Sheedy PF. CT features of nonfunctioning cell carcinoma. AJR 1984; 143: 943–8

76. Buetow PC, Parrino TV, Buck JL et al. Islet cell tumors of the pancreas: pathologic-imaging correlation among size, necrosis and cysts, calcification, malignant behavior, and function. AJR 1995; 165: 1175–9

77. Strodel WE, Vinik AI, Lloyd RV et al. Pancreatic polypeptide-producing tumors. Arch Surg 1984; 119: 508–14

78. Prinz RA, Marangos PJ. Serum neuron-specific enolase: a serum marker for nonfunctioning pancreatic islet cell carcinoma. Am J Surg 1983; 145: 77–81

79. La Rosa S, Sessa F, Capella C et al. Prognostic criteria in nonfunctioning pancreatic endocrine tumors. Virchows Arch 1996; 429: 323–33

80. Cheslyn-Curtis S, Sitaram V, Williamson RCN. Management of non-functioning neuroendocrine tumors of the pancreas. Br J Surg 1993; 80: 625–7

81. Madura JA, Cummings OW, Wiebke EA, Broadie TA, Goulet RL, Howard TJ. Nonfunctioning islet cell tumors of the pancreas: a difficult diagnosis but one worth the effort. Am Surg 1997; 63: 573–8

82. McFarland EG, Kaufman JA, Saini S et al. Preoperative staging of cancer of the pancreas: value of MR angiography versus conventional angiography in detecting portal venous invasion. AJR 1996; 166: 37–43

83. Harrison LE, Klimstra D, Brennan MF. Portal vein resection for adenocarcinoma of the pancreas: a contraindication for resection. Ann Surg 1996; 224: 342–9

84. Evans DB, Skibber JM, Lee JE et al. Nonfunctioning islet cell carcinoma of the pancreas. Surgery 1993; 114: 1175–82

85. Conlon KC, Dougherty E, Klimstra DS, Coit DG, Turnbull ADM, Brennan MF. The value of minimal access surgery in the staging of patients with potentially resectable peripancreatic malignancy. Ann Surg 1996; 223: 134–40

86. Patel YC, Amherdt M, Orci L. Somatostatin-receptor scintigraphy in gastroenteropancreatic tumors. Science 1982; 217: 1155–6

87. Van Eijck CHJ, Lamberts SWJ, Lemaire LCJM et al. The use of somatostatin receptor scintigraphy in the differential diagnosis of pancreatic duct cancers and islet cell tumors. Ann Surg 1996; 224: 119–24

88. Scherubl H, Bader M, Fett U et al. Somatostatin-receptor imaging of neuroendocrine gastroenteropancreatic tumors. Gastroenterology 1993; 105: 1705–9

89. Ahlstrom H, Eriksson B, Bergstrom M, Biurling P. Langstrom B, Oberg K. Pancreatic neuroendocrine tumors: diagnosis with PET. Radiology 1995; 195: 333–7

90. Zogakis TG, Norton JA. Palliative operations for patients with unresectable endocrine neoplasia. Surg Clin N Am 1995; 75: 525–38

91. Makowka L, Tzakis AG, Mazzaferro V et al. Transplantation of the liver for metastatic endocrine tumors of the intestine and pancreas. Surg Gynecol Obstet 1989; 168: 107–11

92. Lang H, Oldhafer KJ, Weimann A et al. Liver transplantation for metastatic neuroendocrine tumors. Ann Surg 1997; 225: 347–54

93. Le Treut YP, Delpero JR. Dousset B et al. Results of liver transplantation in the treatment of metastatic neuroendocrine tumors. Ann Surg 1997; 225: 355–64

94. McEntee GP, Nagorney DM, Kvols LK, Moertel CG, Grant CS. Cytoreductive hepatic surgery for neuroendocrine tumors. Surgery 1990; 108: 1091–6

95. Ajani JA, Carrasco CH, Chamsangavej C, Samaan NA, Levin B, Wallace S. Islet cell tumors metastatic to the liver: effective palliation by sequential hepatic artery embolization. Ann Int Med 1988; 108: 340–4

96. Prinz RA, Badrinath K, Chejfec G, Freeark RJ, Greenlee HB. 'Nonfunctioning' islet cell carcinoma of the pancreas. Am Surg 1983; 49: 345–9

97. Moertel CG, Lefkopoulo M, Lipsitz S, Hahn RG, Klaassen D. Streptozocin-doxorubicin, streptozocin-fluorouracil, or chlorozotocin in the treatment of advanced islet-cell carcinoma. N Engl J Med 1992; 326: 519–23

98. Torrisi JR, Treat J, Zeman R, Dritschilo A. Radiotherapy in the management of pancreatic islet cell tumors. Cancer 1987; 60: 1226–31

99. Tennvall J, Ljungberg 0, Ahren B, Gustavsson A, Nillson LO. Radiotherapy for unresectable endocrine pancreatic carcinoma. Eur J Surg Oncol 1992; 18: 73–6

100. Saltz L, Trochanowski B, Buckley M et al. Octreotide as an antineoplastic agent in the treatment of functional and nonfunctional neuroendocrine tumors. Cancer 1993; 72: 244–8

101. White TJ, Edney JA, Thompson JS, Karrer FW, Moor BJ. Is there a prognostic difference between functional and nonfunctional islet cell tumors. Am J Surg 1994; 168: 627–30

102. Venkatesh S, Ordonez NG, Ajani J et al. Islet cell carcinoma of the pancreas. Cancer 1990; 65: 354–7

103. Doherty GM, Doppman JL, Shawker TH et al. Results of a prospective strategy to diagnose, localize, and resect insulinomas. Surgery 1991; 110: 989–97

104. Grama D, Eriksson B, Martensson H et al. Clinical characteristics, treatment and survival in patients with pancreatic tumors causing hormonal syndromes. World J Surg 1992; 16: 632–9

105. Menegaux F, Schmitt G, Mercadier M, Chigot JP. Pancreatic insulinomas. Am J Surg 1992; 165: 243–8

106. Angelini L, Bezzi M, Tucci GJ et al. The ultrasonic detection of insulinomas during surgical exploration of the pancreas. World J Surg 1987; 11: 642–7

107. Grant CS, Van Heerden JA, Charboneau JW et al. Insulinoma: the value of intraoperative ultrasonography. Arch Surg 1988; 123: 843–8

108. McArthur KE, Richardson CT, Barnett CC et al. Laparotomy and proximal gastric vagotomy in Zollinger–Ellison syndrome: results of a 16-year prospective study. Am J Gastroenterol 1996; 91: 1104–11

109. Melvin WS, Johnson JA, Sparks J et al. Long-term prognosis of Zollinger–Ellison syndrome in multiple endocrine neoplasia. Surgery 1993; 114: 1183–8

110. Jaskowiak NT, Fraker DL, Alexander HR et al. Is reoperation for gastrinoma excision indicated in Zollinger–Ellison syndrome. Surgery 1996; 120: 1055–63

111. Dial PF, Braasch JW, Rossi RL, Lee AK, Jin G. Management of nonfunctioning islet cell tumors of the pancreas. Surg Clin N Am 1985; 65: 291–9

112. Eckhauser FE, Cheung PS, Vinik Al, Strodel WE, Lloyd RV, Thompson NW. Nonfunctioning malignant neuroendocrine tumors of the pancreas. Surgery 1986; 100: 978–87

113. Yeo CJ, Wang BH, Anthone GJ, Cameron JL. Surgical experience with pancreatic islet cell tumors. Arch Surg 1993; 128: 1143–8

24 Management of severe acute pancreatitis

Clement W Imrie

Approximately 20–25% of patients developing acute pancreatitis (AP), have the severe form of the disease in which respiratory insufficiency or failure is the clinical entity which is most responsible for determining outcome.[1-4] Renal compromise or failure is the next most important clinical effect, while cardiac insufficiency or failure is also very important.[2-5] Less frequently major coagulation problems, often manifest by thrombocytopenia and major neurological disturbances, may occur. It is the development of organ failure which is the most important factor determining outcome[6-9] and while much attention has been made to focus on the volume of ischaemic or necrotic pancreas detected by modern imaging techniques,[10-12] the early development of organ failure is of paramount importance.

Death and major morbidity are rare in the group of patients with mild AP, while mortality ranging from 15 to 40% and a morbidity of 50 to 60% are to be anticipated within the severe AP group.

Early identification of severe AP

Following the pioneering work of John Ranson in devising a prognostic score in the early 1970s[1,2] a similar, less complex system for use in European patients was devised in Glasgow.[3] The original 11 factor Ranson system and 9 factor Glasgow system are useful in identifying the 25% of patients at 48 hours after admission with an approximately 80% probability of being in the clinically severe AP group. Both systems were devised to identify the patients who had a maximal upset early in the disease and neither were anticipated to predict the onset of late complications such as pancreatic pseudocyst and abscess. Indeed, the main drawback of the two systems relates to the delay in grading severity requiring 2 days after admission and the

limited ability to anticipate the late complications. However, the most ill patient can usually be identified with the presence of at least three adverse prognostic factors in each system. It is most common for the Ranson system to be employed in its original description, which applies specifically to a predominantly alcohol aetiology, but is poor at accurate identification of the gallstone AP group. Ranson recognized this early on and advised the use of an alternative grading system[12] for this aetiology, but the clinician is not often aware of the aetiology at the time of admission of the patient. The Glasgow system was also modified both to simplify it and to tighten up on the too ready inclusion of patients by the original criteria with inappropriate grading into the severe group.[5] The system was reduced to eight factors with a doubling of the AST level such that in a large prospective study it was shown to perform equally well for the two major aetiologies of AP[6] (Table 24.1).

Table 24.1 **The modified Glasgow criteria for severity prediction in acute pancreatitis: a severe attack is predicted by the presence of three or more positive criteria (Corfield et al.[6])**

During the first 48 hours:	
Arterial PO$_2$	< 8.0 kPa
Serum albumin	< 32 g/l
Serum calcium	< 2.0 mmol/l
White cell count	> 15 × 10^9/l
AST	> 200 u/l
LDH	> 600 iu/l
Blood glucose	> 10 mmol/l (in the absence of diabetes mellitus)
Plasma urea	> 16 mmol/l

APACHE II

This system, which was originally devised in 1984 by Knaus et al. in Philadelphia[7] and has been applied extensively to intensive care patient assessment, has now also been applied to the grading of severe AP at an earlier stage than is possible by either of the two multifactorial systems already mentioned. In the 1980s various groups showed that this system could be valuable in the assessment of severity of AP within a few hours of admission.[8,9] The major advantage of the early grading of severity has resulted in the employment of APACHE II as the main early marker in those patients with a clinically appropriate presentation of severe upper abdominal pain and vomiting with associated hypovolaemia and appropriate raised amylase or lipase to enrol patients into therapeutic trials.[13–17] It has also considerable limitations, especially due to the heavy weighting given to age and chronic health evaluation in respect of its use in such clinical trials of severe AP therapy. This results in many older patients with clinically milder forms of AP being inappropriately graded as 'severe AP'.

An additional problem with the APACHE II system for grading severity of AP is that it was devised over 17 years ago and, with increasing longevity and fitness of older patients in the Western world, the age grading criterion is less appropriate. This means that a considerable proportion of patients who have clinically mild AP are graded in the severe category largely because of the 'chronic health evaluation and age factor' and entered into clinical trials with little prospect of them developing major systemic or local complications. A re-examination of the application of this grading system is necessary to improve its clinical efficacy. Its major advantage is the rapidity with which it can be applied compared to the Ranson and Glasgow systems.

Obesity

Lankisch and Schirren in 1990, showed that the obese patients were at greater risk of developing severe AP, particularly those manifesting respiratory complications.[18] An analysis of the role of obesity by the Cape Town group confirmed this original suggestion (as well as the bias of many surgeons who had managed such patients over many years).[19] They showed a much higher morbidity and mortality in a smaller group of patients who had a body mass index (BMI) of >30 kg/m^2. While this degree of obesity does not reach the criterion for morbid obesity (40 kg/m^2), it is a marker which others have proved valuable, particularly when combined with the APACHE II system.[20] Johnson's group in Southampton showed that the combination of obesity with the APACHE grading system resulted in a greater accuracy of diagnosis and obviously the information from height and weight can be quickly obtained at the time of admission.[20] This combination system is described as APACHE-0.

C-reactive protein

C-reactive protein (CRP) is an acute phase reactant which derives from the liver and is stimulated by the release of interleukin-6; it takes 36–48 hours to rise to a maximum significant value. The normal value is <10 mg/l and patients with an appropriate clinical course of AP and a CRP level in excess of 150 mg/l tend to have the severe form of the disease. The likelihood of clinical severity is even greater when CRP levels rise above 200 mg/l, but there is a skewed distribution of results of CRP so that, as well as having the drawback of the delay in response, CRP has a degree of non-specificity as well.

Newer methods of grading single blood sample analysis for interleukin-6[21,22] and leucocyte elastase[23] as well as urinary trypsinogen activation peptide (TAP)[24] have all shown promise when batches of blood or urine samples are assayed at a later time. None of them can be recommended for clinical use at this stage because the purchase and utilization of single assay kits has not become a reality at the present. Trials of a promising practical test for urinary TAP have now been completed.[25,26] Serum amyloid A may yet prove a better test.

Clinical assessment

While initial clinical assessment by an inexperienced doctor in the emergency admission situation has been shown to be around 30% accurate, the clinical assessment by an expert at 24 and 48 hours is probably as accurate as any of the objective grading systems which have yet been devised.[27,28] The problem with employing this approach in clinical studies is the lack of objective standards, but it is crucial to remember that the experienced clinician's assessment is a practical approach which must be utilized in scheduling treatment in the future, although it cannot be employed in prospective studies of new potential therapies.

CT scanning

Although experts believe that routine CT scanning to grade severity of AP is unreasonable in both

		Score	Necrosis (%)	Score
Normal	A	0	0	0
Focal, diffuse enlargement; contour irregularity; inhomogeneous attenuation	B	1	<30	2
B + peripancreatic haziness/steady densities	C	2	50	4
B, C + ill-defined peripancreatic fluid collection	D	3	>50	6
B, C + ill-defined pancreatic fluid collections	E	4		

Table 24.2 CT grading of acute pancreatitis (Balthazar et al.[35,36])

Score range 0–10.

practical and economic terms, it has been effectively employed to gain strong objective evidence of severe AP in several antibiotic studies. Contrast enhanced scans (CECT) can identify the volume of pancreas which is either poorly perfused or non-perfused. Where this exceeds 30% of the pancreatic volume, good evidence of a more severe clinical course exists.[10,29–31]

CECT will confirm the diagnosis of AP where doubt exists, and may be used to determine probable permanent loss of blood supply to areas of pancreas and the dynamic progress of the disease—or otherwise. It has the facility to demarcate ischaemic and infarcting tissue with considerable accuracy. CECT is also indispensable in the identification of safe fine needle aspiration (FNA) sites when peripancreatic sepsis is a diagnostic probability.[29–34] A numerical (1–10) grading system based on CECT evidence is an improvement on the poorer initial (A–E) system employed—both described by Balthazar et al.[35,36] (Table 24.2). With the increasing accuracy of magnetic resonance imaging this may well be a valuable alternative means of grading severity without the use of IV contrast agents. Experimental AP studies suggest that IV contrast employed in CECT may be harmful, but clinical evidence to support this view is lacking.

Use of organ dysfunction score

There have been several attempts to stratify ill patients with a variety of conditions and modification of the Bernard scoring system,[37] as shown in Table 24.3 has been used in the clinical studies of lexipafant in

which almost 2000 patients with a high admission APACHE II score have been studied. The initial assumption was that significant markers of organ dysfunction would develop in the disease process, but it was found that 44% of patients had scores of at least 2 at admission.[16,17] Patients who fare badly have either a non-improving organ dysfunction score or one that deteriorates. Some patients even come in with a score of 0 and develop signs of multiple organ dysfunction score (MODS) between 24 and 72 hours after admission. Our group of clinical researchers in Glasgow has already presented data suggesting that there are different patterns of behaviour in respect of organ dysfunction scores which can be categorized such that those who have a deteriorating or non-improving Bernard score can be shown to have a very high mortality.[38] It is therefore possible that in future this type of scoring system may become increasingly important, to the exclusion of others.

Treatment of severe AP

The most important aspects of treatment are:

1. Morphine is probably the best analgesic, while other opiates such as pethidine (Demerol; USA) may be used.
2. The rapid restoration of circulating volume in a manner akin to that of a patient with severe burns.
3. Satisfactory oxygen therapy.

In the most severe forms of AP it may be necessary to give between 6 and 10 litres of intravenous fluids in the first 24 hours and simple electrolyte replacement is usually adequate. Even today, more patients

Table 24.3 **Modified Bernard organ failure scoring system (excluding hepatic index)**

| Score | 0—Normal | 1—Mild | Clinically significant organ dysfunction | | |
			2—Moderate	3—Severe	4—Extreme
Cardiovascular					
SBP (mmHg)	>90	<90 Fluid responsive	<90 Not fluid responsive	<90 pH >7.3	<90 pH <7.2
Pulmonary					
PaO$_2$/F$_1$O$_2$ (mmHg)	>400	400–301	300–201 Acute lung injury	200–101 ARDS	<100 Severe ARDS
CNS					
Glasgow coma score	15	14–13	12–10	9–6	<5
Coagulation					
Platelets × 10^9/l	>120	120–81	80–50	50–20	<20
Renal creatinine:					
mol/l	<133	>133–<169	>160–<310	>310–<440	440
mg/100 ml	<1.5	1.5–1.9	2.0–3.4	3.5–4.0	>4.0

SBP, systolic blood pressure; PaO$_2$, arterial oxygen tension; F$_1$O$_2$, inspired oxygen concentration (fraction); ARDS, adult respiratory distress syndrome; CNS, central nervous system.

possibly succumb from inadequate or delayed fluid replacement than are saved by all the efforts of the most experienced clinicians utilizing a full battery of intensive care resources. After 40 years of striving to improve the management of severe AP, a 10-year study in Scotland (5.2 million people) shows that half of the patients who die do so within a week of admission to hospital.[39] We also found that for each decade of life examined, approximately 50% of the deaths occurred early. This contradicts the opinion of certain experts who have their focus primarily on data from single tertiary referral hospitals and find almost no early deaths. The implication is that such referral patterns 'select out' or filter certain patients who are not cross-referred, although it is clearly possible that geographical variations are important.

The clinical appearance of the patient often belies the degree of respiratory insufficiency and it is crucial to measure arterial blood gas levels and to correct any hypoxaemia. The provision of humidified oxygen seems such a simple measure but is often overlooked or provided at an inadequate rate without checking to see whether there has been a correction of the hypoxaemia, either by the use of oximetry or, preferably, by blood gas analysis.[40]

The simple and important first steps in the management are provision of adequate analgesia, efficient restoration of hypovolaemia and correction of hypoxaemia (Fig. 24.1). The monitoring of hourly urine output is crucial as it has already been stated that respiratory insufficiency or failure is followed in frequency by renal insufficiency or failure as the most important systemic effect of the severe variety of AP. The most common reason for inadequate urine output is a failure of satisfactory restoration of circulating blood volume and the use of a Swann Ganz or similar catheter may be necessary to determine adequate fluid resuscitation, particularly in the elderly patient. This necessitates admission to a high dependency unit, and occasionally a respiratory intensive care unit. Failure/major compromise of more than one system is now usually designated multiple organ dysfunction syndrome (MODS) rather than multiple organ failure (MOF).

The lack of a satisfactory drug therapy for the conservative management of severe AP has contributed to the reluctance of the medical profession to employ objective measures quickly and accurately in order to identify the group of patients with severe AP. It is clear from a number of audits that many patients are not graded at an early enough stage following admission to hospital and many hospital clinicians fail to utilize objective grading systems in the management of this common emergency surgical admission. This is a major topic in the national UK guidelines on the management of AP.[41] Occasionally the patients with AP are admitted under the care of physicians with what is labelled an atypical myocardial ischaemic episode or infarct. Any patient having lower left chest pain without classical ECG and/or enzyme pointers to the presence of a myocardial episode should be screened for possible AP by means of a blood amylase or lipase measurement. The fluid requirements for a patient with myocardial compromise and severe AP could scarcely be more different.

An algorithm for the management of severe AP is shown in Fig. 24.1, and it is recommended that while initial resuscitative measures are being carried out, arrangements are made for an immediate ultrasound scan to determine whether or not stones are present in the gallbladder and/or bile ducts. This is important because the presence of ultrasonic and/or biochemical evidence of stones calls for an experienced exponent of endoscopic retrograde pancreatography (ERCP) to carry out an endoscopic sphincterotomy and stone clearance of the bile duct. This is the first of three major therapeutic changes in the approach to such patients at the present time.

Evidence for the efficacy of early endoscopic sphincterotomy

In 1984 it was considered unwise to carry out even a diagnostic ERCP but now, following the original study in Leicester by Neoptolemos,[42] there is a reasonable body of evidence that an early endoscopic sphincterotomy (ES) is both practical and helpful. Randomized controlled studies carried out in Leicester[42] and Hong Kong[43] showed a statistically significant improvement in morbidity and a reduction in mortality which was not statistically significant. However, the approach was not manifestly deleterious. In addition, the uncontrolled clinical study of Nowak in Poland also claims benefit from this early approach in which his group recommended the procedure be carried out in the first 24 hours,[44] and this is my own recommendation as well, based on many years of experience.

One multicentre study which took 4 years to conduct in 22 centres in Germany suggests that caution with the employment of ERCP be advised. This is good advice, but it is important to appreciate that the German study[45] specifically recognized that patients with signs of jaundice and/or cholangitis accompanying AP required ES to the extent that they excluded them from their randomized study. Of the remaining patients only 20% had severe AP and it has previously been shown that those with mild AP do not benefit from early ES.[42] The German study, having identified patients with gallstone AP, only carried out sphincterotomy in the treatment group when stones were present in the bile ducts, but withheld ES even

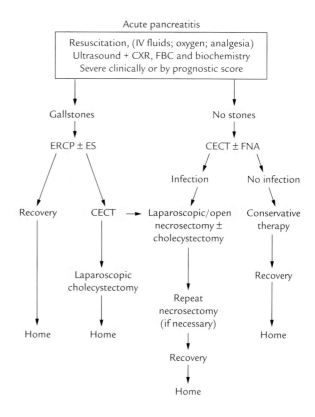

CECT = contrast enhanced CT scan
FNA = fine needle aspiration

Figure 24.1 Algorithm for treatment of AP (death may occur at any stage).

when an ERCP was carried out while stones were (at that instant confined) in the gallbladder or blocking the cystic duct.[45] This resulted in less than 50% of patients in the active treatment group receiving an ES. Our own experience of a consecutive group of 32 patients with severe AP undergoing ES within 24–36 hours of admission is that only two died. This is a low mortality, similar to the Leicester experience, so that we advocate early ES if there is any clinical evidence of a gallstone origin. As most of the patients with idiopathic AP are probably in the gallstone aetiological group (having such small stones or sand that this escapes detection on initial ultrasound) the case for carrying out an ERCP on anyone with abnormal LFTs is strong and, if indicated, a sphincterotomy. It has to be remembered that delay in the application of this technique makes it less practical day by day because of the presence of duodenal oedema causing increasing difficulty in identifying the ampulla. In addition, the longer stones are present in the tapering lower biliary tree, the greater the likelihood of an exacerbation of cholangitis and/or pancreatitis. This 'second hit' with infection or a further stone leaving the gallbladder may push a mild or resolving systemic inflammatory response syndrome (SIRS) towards MODS.

Table 24.4 **Randomized trials of early ERCP therapy**				
	Entry	**Patients**	**High bilirubin**	**Therapeutic benefit**
Neoptolemos (UK)	<72 h A	121[a]	Yes	Yes
Fan (HK)	<24 h (A)	195	Yes	Yes
Folsch (Germany)	<72 h (O)	238	No	No

[a] Separate randomization of mild and severe AP.
A, from admission; O, from onset.
Bilirubin >90 µmol/l—patients excluded in German study.

Before leaving the subject, it appears that a larger multicentre randomized study with all stone patients having ES in the treatment group is now necessary (Table 24.4).

Enteral feeding

For over 40 years in the management of AP it has been believed that a paralytic ileus accompanied the most severe forms of the disease. The recommendation to starve patients and to employ total parenteral nutrition (TPN) by feeding through an intravenous longline into the great vessels has been part and parcel of the classical approach to therapy. However, with increasing realization of the negative aspects of TPN and the potentially positive aspects of even small volumes of low fat, high peptide enteral feeding there has been a cautious reassessment of early enteral feeding, particularly in patients with the severe form of the disease.

Three important and revolutionary papers have been published which encourage the advocacy of early placement of a nasojejunal tube and the inflow of an initial small volume (20 ml per hour) of a standard low fat feed. An encouraging Greek study was published by Kalferentzos et al., in which 38 patients (all with objective evidence of severe AP) were randomized to receive an early enteral feed or TPN.[46] Although this study did not show any lowering of mortality or morbidity (in terms of days in intensive care or total hospital stay) it was shown that the enteral feeding group was treated in a more physiological and less expensive way than those receiving TPN (Table 24.5A and B).

A group of 34 patients studied in the UK by Windsor et al. contained only 13 with objective evidence of severe AP but, within this group, evidence was provided of a reduction in the systemic inflammatory response syndrome (SIRS) by means of lowered

Table 24.5A **Demographic details and prognostic scores in the study by Kalferentzos et al.**[46]		
	Enteral feed (n = 18)	**IV feed (n = 20)**
Male:female	8:10	7:13
Age (years)	63.0	67.3
Gallstones	14	16
Alcohol as cause of AP	3	2
APACHE score	12.7	11.8
Glasgow score	4.2	4.6
CRP (mg/l)	290	335

Table 24.5B **Complications and nutrition costs per day in the same study**		
	Enteral feed (n=18)	**IV Feed (n=20)**
Catheter sepsis	0	2
Glucose >10 mmol/l	4	9
Infected necrosis	1	4
Major sepsis	5	10
Cost (£ sterling)	30	100

CRP and APACHE II levels and an enhancement in antioxidant capacity within the severe AP group.[46] There was indirect evidence of greater exposure to endotoxin in the IV fed patients. Furthermore, there were two deaths in the patients who received TPN and no deaths in those fed enterally.

An uncontrolled 21 patient study utilizing endoscopically placed nasojejunal tubes found no deaths in a group with an average Ranson (original 1974) score of 3.6. The Belgian authors concluded that it was safe to utilize such an enteral feeding approach within 60 hours of admission in most patients with severe AP.[48] Thus these three pilot studies have provided encouragement that the previous recommendation to use longline intravenous feeding with total parenteral nutrition should not now be followed, but a fine bore nasojejunal tube with an increasing volume from 20 ml per hour upward should be employed. The small bowel is apparently able to cope with this and in many patients a full inflow of enteral feeding can be achieved in 48 hours. There is the practical consideration of the accurate placement and fixing of a nasojejunal tube, which is best done endoscopically. Some have used a weighted tube with a mercury filled compartment at the tip and checked the position radiologically.[48] The Belgian study[48] used an endoscopic guidewire placement, while we currently prefer to use a 7FG nasobiliary catheter (Wilson Cook, Winston, USA) for nasojejunal feeding.

In our experience nasogastric feeding may be both safe and practical as a pilot study of an initial group of 26 patients, all with severe AP[49] showed that this was possible in 22, with some technical problems in only four of the patients (three large volume aspirates, one pulled out feeding tube × 7). Compared to the nasojejunal feed, there are obvious practical advantages in using the nasogastric feed, if this proves safe. At present we are carrying out a randomized study to determine whether there are differences of practical note in the two approaches of nasogastric and nasojejunal feeding in severe AP. Whatever the outcome, it certainly appears that nasojejunal feeding can be recommended and nasogastric feeding employed cautiously. One might then wonder why not simply ask the patient to sip small volumes of appropriate enteral feed? In practical terms the patients are often too ill to do this and there is a danger that, by taking too much at one time, vomiting and clinical deterioration may be precipitated.

The place of antibiotic therapy

Prior to 1993 very few clinicians employed intravenous antibiotics at all in the management of severe AP, but increasingly since then it has become customary to provide antibiotics intravenously, usually cephalosporin with or without metronidazole, but other more expensive agents such as imipenem or ciprofloxacin and meropenem have also been recommended. A recent postal survey of clinicians with a major interest in the management of severe AP in the UK revealed that between 85 and 90% were routinely utilizing such a policy.[50]

Table 24.6A **IV antibiotic studies in severe AP**		
Author	**Patients**	**Antibiotics**
Pederzoli et al.[29] (Italy)	74	Imipenem
Sainio et al.[30] (Finland)	60	Cefuroxime
Delcenserie et al.[51] (France)	23	Ceftazidime, amikacin + metronidazole
Schwarz et al.[32] (Germany)	26	Ofloxacin + metronidazole

Table 24.6B **Aetiology and outcome in IV antibiotic studies**			
		Deaths	
Author	**Patient aetiology**	**Controls**	**Antibiotics**
Pederzoli et al.[29]	Mixed	4/33	3/41
Sainio et al.[30]	Alcohol mainly	7/30	1/30
Delcenserie et al.[50]	Alcohol only	3/12	1/11
Schwarz et al.[32]	Mixed	2/13	0/13
	Total	16/88	5/95

There have been four small controlled clinical trials of intravenous antibiotic therapy in the management of severe AP and all have tended to show benefit, but the size of the studies is such that statistical evidence in favour of the use of antibiotics is not strong (Table 24.6A and B).

In the first study, by Pederzoli et al.[29] IV imipenem was used in a dose of 500 mg three times daily in a multicentre randomized Italian study. There were 74 patients in this study, with 41 in the placebo group and 33 in the treatment group. No clear advantage in either mortality or morbidity was found, but a reduction in the incidence of infected pancreatic necrosis was claimed. It was this paper which led to the fairly widespread use of the expensive, broad spectrum imipenem, but a Finnish study of 60 young patients with a median age of 40, in which 30 were randomized to receive IV cefuroxime in a dose of 4.5 g/day, showed a reduction from 1.8 infections per patient in the placebo group to 1.0 in the treatment group.[30] Most of this reduction in infection was in terms of chest and urinary infection, but there was a reduction in mortality which was statistically significant, as there was one death in the treatment group and seven in the placebo group.[30] However, a considerable number of patients in the placebo group received a variety of antibiotics at some time late in the first week of admission and it is to be noted that this was an atypical population in the experience of the bulk of clinicians. Almost 90% of the patients were young men with alcohol induced AP, but the plea from this experience in Helsinki is reasonable for the use of this less expensive antibiotic, as a routine therapy in severe AP linked to alcohol abuse.

Two smaller studies by Delcenserie et al. from France confined to patients with alcohol as aetiology[51] and by Schwarz et al. in Germany[32] have also recommended the use of antibiotics, however there were fewer than 30 patients in each of these two studies (Table 24.6A). A meta-analysis of the four studies comes down in favour of the use of antibiotics as a routine in the early management of severe AP, but little is made of the problem of resistant organisms and fungal overinfection, which represent a considerable concern.

Before leaving the subject of antibiotic therapy it is important to consider the study by Luiten et al.[31] in which selective gut decontamination was achieved by means of 6-hourly gastric and rectal colistin sulphate, amphotericin and norfloxacin combined with intravenous cefotaxime therapy and compared with a group of intensive care patients with severe AP who did not receive such therapy.[31] This approach was associated with a statistically significant reduction in mortality from Gram-negative septicaemia but no improvement in Gram-positive septicaemia, or death from multiple organ failure. These features are reflected in a lower incidence of later deaths (Table 24.7). However, the success in virtual eradication of Gram-negative infection commends the use of this less popular gut decontamination approach plus intravenous antibiotics.

It is possible that the provision of even limited enteral nutrition reverses or slows the adverse changes in jejunal permeability and may the reduce the need for intravenous antibiotics. Our own practice has been beset by considerable problems with fungal superinfection found in the fine needle aspiration before first operation for infected necrosis, such that the safest possible policy at the present time may be to use intravenous cephalosporin plus fluconazole as an antifungal agent. A valid alternative is to withhold antibiotics until a specific event such as ERCP occurs or a specific organism and sensitivity is identified. This was certainly the policy followed in the latter part of the Belgian pilot study of nasojejunal feeding[48] and throughout our own study of 26 patients with severe AP in whom nasogastric feeding was employed.[49] While the consensus of opinion may favour routine IV antibiotic therapy in severe AP, the case has still to be proved.

Our group of clinical investigators[52] is not alone in being concerned about the dangers of fungal infection, as Grewe et al.[53] have reported similar concerns from the Mayo Clinic. They found that the patients

Table 24.7 **Deaths in the severe AP study of Luiten et al.**[31]

	Deaths <14 days	Late deaths	Total
Control (52)	8 (15%)	10 (23%)	18 (35%)
SD group (50)	8 (16%)	3 (7%)	11 (22%)

Difference in late deaths: $P = 0.07$

with fungal infection had been treated with a mean of four different antibiotics for a period of 23 days and that there was a longer stay in intensive care, a longer total hospital stay and higher mortality in those patients with fungal infection. They reported a mortality of three of seven patients (43%), which is similar to our own experience, with eight of 14 patients (57%) ultimately dying when they were found to have *Candida* peripancreatic sepsis at the primary operation. It is therefore clear that the use of antibiotics is distinctly a two-edged sword in the management of severe AP.

Potential use of platelet activating factor antagonist therapy

With the failure of many potential treatments of the severe form of AP, such as those based on antiprotease drugs, Rindernecht[54] postulated that the key to the understanding of the systemic inflammatory response syndrome (SIRS) in this disease was the appreciation of the cytokine response primarily from leucocytes. He proposed that the identification of such substances could lead to rational and effective therapy. With the passage of time it has become clear that there are a large number of interleukins and those described as IL1, IL2, IL6 and IL8 have major pro-inflammatory roles, while IL10 has an anti-inflammatory function.[55–59] Tumour necrosis factor alpha (TNF alpha) and platelet activating factor (PAF) are also very important in the pro-inflammatory response.[60–63] Various experimental animals have been utilized in the laboratory research which has led to a fuller understanding of this situation, with genetically modified 'knock-out' mice and more standard laboratory animals such as rats, rabbits and the opossum having been studied.[60–64] A whole series of cytokines, chemokines and leukotrienes are involved in different cascade systems, so that it seems very unlikely that any single agent, even given at an early stage of severe AP, could affect the disease pathway beneficially.

However, initial phase II clinical trials of lexipafant (British Biotech) in severe AP have shown encouraging results in Liverpool, UK,[13] and Glasgow.[16] These both showed a failure to develop new organ failure scores in the treatment group. Thereafter, a multicentre UK study of 290 patients with initial APACHE II scores >6 found potential benefit from early lexipafant therapy, while a delay of >50 hours was counterproductive.[17] In this phase III study new organ failures were documented in the treatment group and this was a failure of the prime objective of the study. Mortality was lower in the treatment group, but not statistically significantly so,[17] although a subgroup analysis of those given lexipafant less than 48 hours after onset of pain indicated a probable significant benefit. Hopes were accordingly raised that a new and valuable therapeutic approach was unfolding.

Disappointingly, the early assessment of an even larger multinational study of 1500 patients is not encouraging in terms of a likely drug licence for lexipafant.[65] Nevertheless, the future may still lie along the route of more than one such agent being utilized in the therapy of a more carefully selected group of patients with severe AP.

The role of surgery

As in other aspects in the management of AP, some changes are taking place in this area as well. In the milder forms of the disease it is now strongly recommended that patients who are likely or proved to have gallstones should have the risk of further similar attacks of AP minimized by definitive surgery in the same admission. Only a few older patients who are considered unfit for surgery may legitimately be treated by endoscopic sphincterotomy as an alternative. The majority should have a laparoscopic cholecystectomy in the same admission, an approach strongly endorsed by the UK national guidelines.[41]

Where sterile necrosis is present the clear recommendation is to avoid surgery and to continue conservative management unless the unusual complication of bleeding into the necrotic tissue should occur.

Where infection develops in or adjacent to the necrotic process, then surgical therapy to remove the infected necrotic material is the recommended approach and the longer the delay from the onset of the disease to the requirement for surgery, the more likely it is that a good delineation between viable and non-viable infected tissue will have taken place. The classic approach has been an anterior one, either through an upper abdominal transverse or longitudinal incision via the gastrocolic omentum (Fig. 24.2). This type of surgery invariably means that the patient requires to go to the intensive care unit after the surgery and that approximately 25–33% of patients will require further operations. Mortality for this type of surgical approach ranges from 10 to 35%. Alternative approaches exist after the removal of the necrotic tissue with the most frequently utilized method being that popularized by Beger and his disciples from Ulm,[10,66,67] with

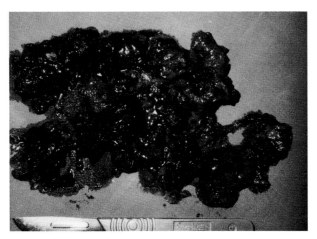

Figure 24.2 Operative specimen following necrosectomy for acute necrotizing pancreatitis.

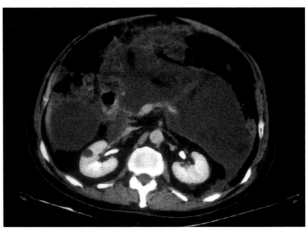

Figure 24.3 CT scan of acute necrotizing pancreatitis.

postoperative large lavage catheters being employed for approximately 25 days at flow rates of 500 ml to 1 litre per hour. Only when the fluid effluent is clear is the lavage procedure initially slowed and then stopped. A continuation of murky fluid on restarting lavage means that the procedure must be continued for longer. Repeat operations are often required for further infection, this being in approximately 30% of all patients, and those with gallstones should have their biliary tree cleared at the same operation together with cholecystectomy.

Should bleeding occur at the time of removal of necrotic tissue and debridement then intra-abdominal packing with large cotton packs enclosed in paraffin gauze will be necessary and as many as 12 or more of these packs may be needed to control venous ooze. After 2–4 days these packs can be removed and, if there is no bleeding, a lavage system established. Repeat packing is more labour intensive and often results in longer periods of time in intensive care with the consequent risks of additional complications and greater health care expense.

We have been striving to carry out surgical debridement of infected necrosis by means of a minimally invasive approach, mainly from the left flank, and now have experience in almost 50 patients, with only six being tackled from a right anterior approach. Initially the radiologist leaves a guidewire or drain down the line of the fine needle aspirate.[33] The patient is then taken to the operating theatre where the track is dilated to 1 cm diameter using the urological equipment initially advocated for the percutaneous removal of renal calculi.[68] The Amplatz graded dilator system is particularly useful and, although the procedure is time-consuming, it is usually possible at the first approach to remove all the pus and a proportion of the necrotic material with grasping forceps and the nephroscope introduced through the 1 cm

diameter port. Most of our recent patients have not required to go to intensive care, but an average of four procedures taking between 90 and 120 minutes each has proved an interesting new approach to an old problem.[69] Two other UK teams in Liverpool and Newcastle have verified the potential of this.

Pancreatic pseudocyst

It is now well established that approximately 50% of pancreatic pseudocysts which follow an attack of acute pancreatitis will resolve spontaneously with conservative management. Those which persist can often be demonstrated to have a direct link to the main pancreatic duct system and are, in effect, a localized fistula collection from the duct system. Traditional management for this problem has been an internal surgical drainage operation, either directly into the adjacent stomach or into a Roux loop. At the time of such pseudocyst drainage a cholecystectomy would usually be performed and the results of surgery tended to be good, with a low recurrence rate of pseudocyst development.

In the previous decade percutaneous drainage methods were shown to be unsatisfactory with a high recurrence rate and the potential for infection of a sterile collection.[68] Internal drainage systems by means of endoscopic cystgastrostomy or stent placement along the main pancreatic duct system and into the pseudocyst have been gaining in popularity, but no comparisons with the older standard surgical internal drainage systems have been performed. Indeed, most of the series of patients treated with the newer methods have been small and uncontrolled. There is a great need for careful audit of the data that are being collected from these more modern approaches with theoretically less risk to the patient. If the newer methods are associated with the same low recurrence rates then they will become established, but if the recurrence rates are higher then the more standard approaches may yet return to be accepted once again as the gold standard.

Key points

- Approximately one in five patients who develop acute pancreatitis suffer the severe form of the disease with respiratory compromise/failure.

- Complications of severe acute pancreatitis include:
  Respiratory failure
  Renal failure
  Coagulopathy
  Cardiac failure.
- Early ERCP and endoscopic sphincterotomy probably lead to reduced morbidity and mortality.
- Early enteral feeding may improve outcome.
- The role of antibiotic prophylaxis remains controversial.
- Patients with gallstone pancreatitis should undergo cholecystectomy during the same admission to hospital.

REFERENCES

1. Ranson HJC, Rifkind KM, Roses DF, Fink SD, Eng K, Spencer FC. Prognostic signs and the role of operative management in acute pancreatitis. Surg Gynecol Obstet 1974; 139: 69–81

2. Ranson JHC, Rifkind KM, Turner JW. Prognostic signs and non-operative peritoneal lavage in acute pancreatitis. Surg Gynecol Obstet 1976; 143: 209–19

3. Imrie CW, Benjamin IS, McKay AJ, MacKenzie I, O'Neill J, Blumgart LH. A single centre double blind trial of Trasylol therapy in primary acute pancreatitis. Br J Surg 1978; 65: 337–41

4. Renner IG, Savage WT, Pantoja JL, Renner VJ. Death due to acute pancreatitis: a retrospective analysis of 405 autopsy cases. Dig Dis Sci 1985; 30: 1005–18

5. Bradley EL, Hall JR, Lutz J. Hemodynamic consequences of severe pancreatitis. Ann Surg 1983; 198: 130–3

6. Corfield AP, Cooper MJ, Williamson RCN et al. Prediction of severity in acute pancreatitis: a prospective comparison of three prognostic indices. Lancet 1985; II: 403–6

7. Knaus WA, Wagner DP, Draper EA, Zimmerman JE. APACHE II final form and national validation results of a severity of disease classification system. Crit Care Med 1984; 12: 213

8. Larvin M, McMahon MJ. APACHE II score for assessment and monitoring of acute pancreatitis. Lancet 1989; II: 201–5

9. Wilson C, Heath DI, Imrie CW. Prediction of outcome in acute pancreatitis: a comparative study of APACHE II, clinical assessment and multiple factor scoring systems. Br J Surg 1990; 77: 1260–4

10. Beger HG, Bittner R, Block S, Buchler M. Bacterial contamination of pancreatic necrosis – a prospective clinical study. Gastroenterology 1986; 91: 433–40

11. Puolakkainen P A. Early assessment of acute pancreatitis: a comparative study of computed tomography and laboratory tests. Eur J Surg 1989; 155: 25–30

12. Ranson HJC. The timing of biliary surgery in acute pancreatitis. Ann Surg 1979; 189: 654–62

13. Kingsnorth AN, Galloway SW, Formela LJ. Randomised, double-blind phase II trial of lexipafant, a platelet-activating factor antagonist, in human acute pancreatitis. Br J Surg 1995; 82: 1414–20

14. McKay CJ, Baxter J, Imrie CW. A randomised controlled trial of octreotide in the management of patients with acute pancreatitis. Int J Pancreatol 1997; 21: 13–9

15. Uhl W, Buchler MW, Malfertheiner P, Beger HG, Adler G, Gauz W and the German Pancreatitis Study Group. A randomised, double blind, multicenter trial of octreotide in moderate to severe acute pancreatitis. Gut 1999; 45: 97–104

16. McKay CJ, Curran F, Sharples C et al. Prospective placebo-controlled randomised trial of lexipafant in predicted severe acute pancreatitis. Br J Surg 1997; 84: 1239–43

17. Johnson CD, Kingsnorth AN, Imrie CW et al. Double blind randomised, placebo controlled study of a platelet factor antagonist, lexipatant, in the treatment and prevention of organ failure in severe acute pancreatitis. Gut 2001; 48: 62–9

18. Lankisch PG, Schirren CA. Increased body weight as a prognostic parameter for complications in the course of acute pancreatitis. Pancreas 1990; 5: 626–9

19. Funnell IC, Bornmann PC, Weakley SP et al. Obesity: an important factor in acute pancreatitis. Br J Surg 1993; 80: 484–6

20. Johnson CD, Toh SKC. The APACHE II prognostic system combined with obesity, an improved method of grading severity of acute pancreatitis. In: Johnson CD, ed. Recent advances in surgery, Vol 21. Edinburgh: Churchill Livingstone, 1998

21. Viedma JA, Perez-Mateo M, Dominguez-Munoz JE, Carballo F. Role of interleukin-6 in acute pancreatitis. Comparison with CRP and phospholipase A. Gut 1992; 33: 1264–7

22. Heath DI, Cruikshank A, Gudgeon M et al. Role of interleukin-6 in mediating the acute phase protein response and potential as an early means of severity assessment in acute pancreatitis. Gut 1993; 34: 41–5

23. Dominguez-Munoz JE, Carballo F, Garcia MJ et al. Clinical usefulness of polymorph leukocyte elastase in predicting the severity of acute pancreatitis: results of a multi-centre study. Br J Surg 1991; 78: 1230–4

24. Gudgeon M, Heath DI, Hurley P et al. Trypsinogen activation peptides assay in early severity prediction of acute pancreatitis. Lancet 1990; 335: 4–8

25. Neoptolemos JP, Kemppainen EA, Mayer JM et al. Early prediction of severity in acute pancreatitis by urinary trypsinogen activation peptide: a multicentre study. Lancet 2000; 355: 1955–60

26. Kemppainen E, Mayer J, Puolakkainen P et al. Plasma trypsinogen activation peptide in patients with acute pancreatitis. Br J Surg 2001; 88: 679–80

27. Larvin M, Wilson C, Heath DI, Alexander D, Imrie CW, McMahon MJ. Intraperitoneal aprotinin therapy and the clinical course of acute pancreatitis. Br J Surg 1992; 71: 456–7

28. Heath DI, Imrie CW. The Hong Kong criteria and severity prediction in acute pancreatitis. Int J Pancreatol 1994; 15: 179–85

29. Pederzoli P, Bassi C, Vesentini S, Campedelli A. A randomised multi center clinical trial of antibiotic prophylaxis of septic complications in acute necrotizing pancreatitis with imipenem. Surg Gynecol Obstet 1993; 176: 480–3

30. Sainio V, Kemppainen E, Puolakkainen P et al. Early antibiotic treatment in acute necrotising pancreatitis. Lancet 1995; 346: 663–7

31. Luiten EJT, Hop WCJ, Lange JF et al. Controlled clinical trial of selective decontamination for the treatment of severe acute pancreatitis. Ann Surg 1995; 222: 57–65

32. Schwarz M, Isenmann R, Meyer H, Beger HG. Antibiotika bei nekrotisierender pankreatitis. Dtsch Med Wochenschr 1997; 122: 356–61

33. Gerzof SG, Banks PA, Robbins AH et al. Early diagnosis of pancreatic infection by computed tomography guided aspiration. Gastroenterology 1987; 93: 1315–21

34. Farkas G, Morton J, Mondi Y, Szederkenyi E. Surgical strategy and management of infected pancreatic necrosis. Br J Surg 1996; 83: 930–3

35. Balthazar EJ, Ranson JH, Naidich DP, Megibow AJ, Caccavale R, Cooper MM. Acute pancreatitis: prognostic value of CT. Radiology 1985; 156: 767–72

36. Balthazar EJ, Robinson DL, Megibow AJ, Ranson JH. Acute pancreatitis: value of CT in establishing prognosis. Radiology 1990; 174: 331–6

37. Bernard GR, Dorg G, Hudson LD et al. Quantification of organ failure for clinical trials and clinical practice. Am J Resp Crit Care Med 1995; 151: A32

38. Buter A, Imrie CW, Carter CR et al. Dynamic nature of early organ dysfunction determines outcome in acute pancreatitis. Br J Surg 2002; 89: 298–302

39. McKay CJ, Sinclair M, Evans S, Carter CR, Imrie CW. High early mortality from AP in Scotland 1984–1995. Br J Surg 1999; 86: 1302–5

40. Imrie CW, Ferguson JC, Murphy D, Blumgart LH. Arterial hypoxia in acute pancreatitis. Br J Surg 1977; 64: 185–8

41. Glazer G, Mann DU, Imrie CW for the British Society of Gastroenterology Study Group. UK guidelines for the management of acute pancreatitis. Gut 1998; 42 (Suppl): S1–13

42. Neoptolemos JP, Carr-Locke D, London NJM. Controlled trial of urgent ERCP and endoscopic sphincterotomy versus conservative treatment for acute pancreatitis due to gallstones. Lancet 1988; ii: 989–93

43. Fan ST, Lai ECS, Mok FPT et al. Early treatment of acute biliary pancreatitis by endoscopic papillotomy. N Engl J Med 1993; 328: 228–32

44. Nowak A, Nowakowska-Dulawa E, Marek TA, Rybicka J. Final results of the prospective, randomized, controlled study on endoscopic sphincterotomy versus conventional management in acute biliary pancreatitis. Gastroenterology 1995; 108 (Suppl): A380 (abstract)

45. Folsch UR, Nitsche R, Ludtke et al. Early ERCP and papillotomy compared with conservative treatment for acute biliary pancreatitis. N Engl J Med 1997; 336: 237–42

46. Kalfarentzos F, Kehagias J, Mead N, Kokkinis K, Gogos CA. Enteral nutrition is superior to parenteral nutrition in severe acute pancreatitis: results of a randomized prospective trial. Br J Surg 1997; 84: 1665–9

47. Windsor AC, Kanwar S, Li AG et al. Compared with parenteral nutrition, enteral feeding attenuates the acute phase response and improves disease severity in acute pancreatitis. Gut 1998; 42: 431–5

48. Nakad A, Piessevaux H, Marot JC et al. Is early enteral nutrition in acute pancreatitis dangerous? About 20 patients fed by an endoscopically placed nasogastrojejunal tube. Pancreas 1998; 17: 187–93

49. Eatock FC, Brombacher GD, Steven A, Imrie CW, McKay CJ, Carter R. Nasogastric feeding in severe acute pancreatitis may be practical and safe. Int J Pancreatol 2000; 28: 25–31

50. Powell JJ, Campbell E, Johnson CD, Siriwardena AK. Survey of antibiotic prophylaxis in acute pancreatitis in UK and Ireland. Br J Surg 1999; 86: 320–2

51. Delcenserie R, Yzet T, Ducruix JP. Prophylactic antibiotics in treatment of severe acute alcoholic pancreatitis. Pancreas 1996; 13: 198–201

52. Eatock FC, Brombacher GD, Hood J, Carter CR, Imrie CW. Fungal infection of pancreatic necrosis is associated with increased mortality. Br J Surg 1999; 86: 87A

53. Grewe M, Tsiotos GG, de Leon EL, Sarr ME. Fungal infection in acute necrotising pancreatitis. J Am Coll Surg 1999; 188: 408–14

54. Rinderknecht H. Fatal pancreatitis, a consequence of excessive leukocyte stimulation? Int J Pancreatol 1988; 3: 105–12

55. Tenaka N, Murata A, Uda K et al. Interleukin-1 receptor antagonist modifies the changes in vital organs induced by acute necrotizing pancreatitis in a rat experimental model. Crit Care Med 1995; 23: 901–8

56. Curley P J McMahon M J Lancaster F. Reduction in circulation levels of CD4-positive lymphocytes in acute

pancreatitis: relationship to endotoxin, interleukin-6 and disease severity. Br J Surg 1993; 80: 1312–5

57. Curley P, Nestor M, Collins K et al. Decreased interleukin–2 production in murine acute pancreatitis: potential for immunomodulation. Gastroenterology 1996; 110: 585–8

58. Osman MO, Kristensen JU, Jacobsen NO et al. A monoclonal anti-interleukin 8 antibody (WS-4) inhibits cytokine response and acute lung injury in experimental severe acute necrotising pancreatitis in rabbits. Gut.1998; 43: 232–9

59. Norman J. The role of cytokines in the pathogenesis of acute pancreatitis. Am J Surg 1998; 175: 76–83

60. Grewal HP, Mohey el D in A, Gaber L et al. Amelioration of the physiologic and biochemical changes of acute pancreatitis using an anti-TNF-alpha polyclonal antibody. Am J Surg 1994; 167: 214–9

61. Zhou W, Levine BA, Olson MS. Platelet-activating factor: a mediator of pancreatic inflammation during cerulein hyperstimulation. Am J Pathol 1993; 142: 1404–12

62. Emmanuelli G, Montrucchio G, Gaia E et al. Experimental acute pancreatitis induced by platelet activating factor in rabbits. Am J Pathol 1989; 134: 315–25

63. Formela LJ, Wood LM, Whittaker M, Kingsnorth AN. Amelioration of experimental acute pancreatitis with a potent platelet-activating factor antagonist. Br J Surg 1994; 81: 1783–5

64. Hofbauer B, Saluja A, Bhatia M et al . Effect of recombinant platelet-activating factor acetylhydrolase on two models of experimental acute pancreatitis. Gastroenterology 1998; 115: 1238–47

65. Larvin M, Ammori B, McMahon MJ et al. A double blind randomised, placebo controlled multi centre trial to evaluate efficacy and safety of Z doses of lexipafant in AP therapy. Pancreatology 2001; 1: 279–80

66. Beger HE, Bittner R, Buchler M et al. Necrosectomy and post operative lavage in necrotising pancreatitis. Br J Surg 1988; 75: 207–12

67. Uhl W, Buchler MW. Surgical treatment of necrotising pancreatitis. Yale J Biol Med 1997; 70: 109–17

68. Carter CR, McKay CJ, Imrie CW. Percutaneous necrosectomy and sinus tract endoscopy in the management of infected pancreatic necrosis: an initial experience. Ann Surg 2000; 232: 175–80

25 Management of pain in chronic pancreatitis

Åke Andrén-Sandberg, Asgaut Viste, Arild Horn, Dag Hoem and Hjörtur Gislason

Pain is the cardinal symptom of chronic pancreatitis[1] and is, together with the often ongoing alcoholism, the most difficult symptom to treat. For some patients with chronic pancreatitis the pain is so severe that all the waking hours are devoted to pain control and quality of life is low in every respect. Although much has been done to improve our understanding of the pathophysiology of chronic pancreatitis, there is still no therapy that counteracts the inflammatory process of the disease. As patients with chronic pancreatitis at best can be symptom-free, but never cured, treatment should be directed against symptoms and complications, of which pain is the most important, and the management of symptoms should be of prime concern in most patients with chronic pancreatitis.

Type of pain and its evolution

Several pain patterns have been described in chronic pancreatitis. The pain is most often localized to the upper part of the abdomen and is widespread. It sometimes radiates to the back, and is frequently nocturnal. Patients often present with intermittent pain that ranges from mild to moderate to severe. It is often described as deep, penetrating, and debilitating, and it may increase after a meal. Postprandial pain may contribute to weight loss by fasting.[2] Moreover, the pattern of pain changes with time, being recurrent and intermittent in the initial stages of the typical disease. Later it usually becomes persistent, but the characteristics of the pain may vary not only between patients but also in the same person from time to time.[3]

Eighty-five per cent of patients with chronic pancreatitis will develop pain at some time during the course of their disease.[4,5] The frequency, severity and other characteristics of pain in chronic pancreatitis

have a major impact or whether or not to treat and which medical and/or surgical interventions to consider. The etiology of chronic pancreatitis cannot be determined from the pain profile, but a painless course is rare in alcoholic chronic pancreatitis (<10% of cases), whereas pain-free periods are more frequent in the late-onset type of idiopathic chronic pancreatitis and in tropical chronic pancreatitis. In these cases, the disease is often only diagnosed when exocrine or endocrine insufficiency has become symptomatic by steattorhea or overt diabetes.[6–10]

In the late stages of chronic pancreatitis patients usually present with steattorhea, diabetes and pancreatic calcifications, but only moderate or miminal pain. If pain occurs it is usually due to local complications. In the early stage exocrine and endocrine function are usually normal, and there is no pancreatic calcification. Even so, the course may be uncomplicated with short episodes of recurrent pain and long pain-free intervals. There may also be a complicated course with constant pain or frequent attacks of pain without longer pain-free intervals, and there may be local complications.

Therefore in chronic pancreatitis, pain tends to precede the symptoms of diabetes and malabsorption by many years.[11] In addition to debilitation, pain often contributes to weight loss because patients voluntarily decrease their food intake in an attempt to avoid unpleasant postprandial abdominal discomfort. When pancreatic exocrine insufficiency becomes symptomatic, the discomfort associated with fat and carbohydrate malabsorption may further limit food intake. Therefore, pain should be treated aggressively, not only to improve the quality of life in these patients, but also to prevent excessive weight loss.[12]

However, there are no proven associations between imaging findings or pancreatic function test results and the presence or intensity of pancreatic pain.[9,13] Therefore assessment of pain in chronic pancreatitis has to be based primarily on clinical grounds, that is the patient's description of pain and the consumption of analgesics, and the information obtained from imaging and function tests must be correlated with great care.

The pain pattern and its treatment has also been correlated to the histological picture of the pancreatic parenchyma. Although surgical approaches to 'large duct' chronic pancreatitis have been quite successful,[4,5] patients with persisting pain from 'small duct' chronic pancreatitis have historically been a difficult group to manage. Medical therapy in this latter group has often been either inconclusive or ineffectual, and narcotic addiction is common. Surgical approaches have fared little better, with extensive ablation of pancreatic parenchyma either failing to relieve pain or leading to brittle diabetes, marginal ulceration, and serious malnutrition. Therefore the histologic picture, and the size of the ducts on morphological examinations, for example ER(C)P and CT scan, is of importance when treating the pain in patients with chronic pancreatitis.

Several additional factors interfere with the multifactorial definition of pancreatic pain and mechanisms of pain. Firstly, the pain is difficult to interpret due to psychological factors including addiction to alcohol and narcotics.[2,14] Therefore, the large number of conflicting studies on pain in chronic pancreatitis are difficult to interpret. Furthermore, symptoms have often been assessed in rather vague categories, such as mild, moderate, or severe. For example, after duct drainage combined with distal pancreatectomy, Morrow et al.[15] reported patients as asymptomatic, having occasional pain, or having no improvement. Mannell et al.[16] used a four-tiered system for pain assessment: excellent (no pain), good (better), fair (nil, better), or poor (same pain or worse), to assess the results of a variety of operations. Narcotic intake was not mentioned as part of the assessment. Russell[17] also used a four-tiered system to assess pain—none, minimal, moderate, or severe—in studying the results of preservation of the duodenum in total pancreatectomy compared with those of standard pancreaticoduodenectomy. However, he used a separate scale for assessing use of analgesics: no, minor, and moderate use of narcotics. He found no difference in pain relief between the results of the two operations. He noted that 13 (34%) of 32 patients still had severe pain after duodenum-preserving total pancreatectomy, and that six required major analgesics.

A thorough evaluation of the multidimensional construct of 'quality of life' is missing in most studies. To draw valid conclusions, it will be necessary for future studies to relate the pain pattern and profile to all important variables like etiology, onset of diagnostic criteria, stage of chronic pancreatitis, morphologic alterations, pancreatic function, possible alcohol abuse and use of narcotics.

In clinical practice the description and definitions of the pain determine the therapy for the individual patient with chronic pancreatitis. However, the strategy of treatment in each individual patient is usually established without a preoperative histologic specimen and often with limited radiologic information. Therefore, the decision making between pharmacologic treatment, resection or decompression, or other options for the treatment of pain in chronic pancreatitis must be based mostly on the history of each patient. It is then important for the physician to determine which concept of pathogenesis of pain is favored.

Pain in alcohol-related pancreatitis

In up to 30% of patients no distinct etiology of pancreatitis can be demonstrated in the Western countries.[18] However, most patients presenting with chronic pancreatitis in Europe, the United States, and South Africa will have alcohol-related disease,[19] and there are indications that this type of disease is increasing.[20]

At the present time, the most valid data on the natural course of pain in alcoholic chronic pancreatitis (ACP) are derived from the Zürich series.[6–8] Pain is the most prominent clinical feature in approximately 90% of patients with alcoholic chronic pancreatitis, and its natural cause has had a major impact on a proposed clinically based staging system.[21] Patients with early onset idiopathic chronic pancreatitis usually live through a long period of severe pain but slowly develop morphologic and functional pancreatic damage, whereas patients with late onset idiopathic chronic pancreatitis have a mild and painless course.[7,10] The most severe pain episodes are observed in early stages of alcoholic chronic pancreatitis, often before the disease has been documented clinically.

In advanced alcoholic chronic pancreatitis, pain might vanish spontaneously due to lack of functional parenchyma in patients without local complications, whereas severe pain in advanced stages is often associated with local complications. However, this pattern has been challenged by others,[9] who found few patients with deceasing pain with time. Also, pain of extrapancreatic origin must also be taken into account (gallbladder disease, peptic ulcer, and so forth), as these diseases are common in a population prone to drinking and smoking and usually eating a diet high in fat and low in protein.

In alcoholic chronic pancreatitis, cessation of alcohol abuse is said to have an impact on the natural course of the disease. Although impairment of pancreatic function progresses also after cessation in most patients, the progress is slower and less severe,[6,22,23] It has been repeatedly shown that pain relief is more frequent in those who have stopped drinking or abstain from alcohol for long periods.[23–26] Most often it can be calculated that in about 50% of patients, cessation of alcohol abuse is accompanied by a decreased severity of pain.[24,25] Therefore, doctors treating patients with chronic pancreatitis should spend considerable time convincing them of the importance of total alcohol abstinence. However, it has to be admitted that there are also studies showing no beneficial effects of abstinence.[27,28] This discrepancy may, at least partly, reflect a failure to differentiate alcohol-induced and idiopathic pancreatitis. Contrary to what has been shown about alcohol intake,[23–26] not in one trial has a relevant correlation between dietary measures and the occurrence of pain been demonstrated.

Pain mechanisms

Upper abdominal pain is the most common symptom in the clinical course of chronic pancreatitis. Although several different concepts of pain generation in chronic pancreatitis have been postulated during the last decades, the mechanisms underlying the generation and perpetuation of chronic pain are insufficiently understood and none of them can completely explain the pain in this disease. Present hypotheses include acute inflammation of the pancreas, increased pressure within the pancreatic ductal system and parenchyma, neuritis, recurrent ischemia of the parenchyma and intrapancreatic causes such as acute pseudocysts and extrapancreatic causes such as common bile duct or duodenal stenosis.[29–31] The relative contribution of inflammation, obstruction, neuritis, and scarring, etc. to the pathogenesis of pain is still unclear and may vary from patient to patient.

If the cause of pain in chronic pancreatitis is acute focal inflammation, necrosis, and scar formation, this may explain transitory attacks of pain of several days' duration. If we accept this hypothesis, it also means that the pain reflects dynamic events within the gland rather than static situations—that is, it is the formation of a scar that hurts and not the scar tissue itself; it is the expansion/dilatation of the duct or a pseudocyst that hurts and not the dilated duct or cyst itself.

Pain in chronic pancreatitis may also be caused by complications of chronic pancreatitis such as pancreatic duct strictures (obstruction), pancreatic duct stones (obstruction), pseudocysts with vascular involvement leading to hemosuccus pancreaticus (obstruction), pancreatic abscesses, ascites, bile duct stenosis with cholestasis, duodenal stenosis and malabsorption (bacterial overgrowth, meteorism). The increased pressure on the pancreas from pseudocysts and other masses may contribute as well. Especially in middle Europe, where inflammatory tumors of the pancreatic head are not unusual, masses cause local displacement of other organs, stenosis of the pancreatic and common bile duct, with alterations and occlusions of neighboring arterial and venous blood vessels. It is probable that these processes may also contribute to pain.

Increased ductal and interstitial pressure

Postinflammatory scarring of the main and side pancreatic ducts may cause strictures, calculi, or increased viscosity of pancreatic juice, all resulting in increased ductal and interstitial pressure with local ischemia and acidosis, which generates pain. Obstruction of the pancreatic duct system was for a long time seen as the major factor in the pathogenesis of chronic pancreatitis. However, the relationship between morphological changes, ductal pressures and pain has repeatedly been shown to be very variable, and other factors must be implicated.[32] An increased intracystic pressure may be assumed when a pseudocyst communicates with a stenotic duct. On the other hand, painless courses of the same anatomic abnormalities are also seen.[33,34]

One of the first to document the intrapancreatic pressure were Ebbehöl et al.[35] who recorded pancreatic tissue pressure during surgery. They found higher values in patients with pancreatitis than in control subjects. After surgical drainage of the pancreatic duct a significant drop in tissue pressure was seen.[35] It is interesting to note that they were able to follow the patients' postoperative pancreatic tissue pressures, after having developed a technique for percutaneous measurements guided by ultrasonography. In patients with recurrent pain after one year, the pressure was again increased, whereas those who remained pain-free continued to have normal values.[36] Further support for tissue hypertension was recently given by Jalleh et al.,[37] who hypothesized that pain could be associated with a situation similar to that seen in compartment syndromes in other sites, in that they found different pressures in different parts of the gland. Bradley showed increased ductal pain in painful pancreatitis compared to a control group.[30] The findings were supported by Sato et al.,[38] who in an intraoperative study found elevation of ductal perfusion and residual pressure in patients with chronic pancreatitis, compared with observations in control subjects who had had surgery for gastric cancer. Similarly, Madsen and Winkler reported high ductal pressure, measured intraoperatively in patients with chronic pancreatitis.[39]

In an endoscopic study, Okazaki et al.[40] confirmed these findings and demonstrated a statistically significant increase of the ductal pressure in chronic pancreatitis patients with pain, compared with that seen in a group of patients with painless disease. Intraductal pressure as assessed at ERCP ranged between 10 and 16 mmHg in patients without pancreatic disease and between 18 and 48 mmHg in patients with a dilated pancreatic duct. However, pain patterns and profiles were not assessed in detail in these studies.[30,39–41] Pancreatic parenchymal pressure assessed at surgery ranged between 3 and 11 mmHg in control subjects and between 17 and 21 mmHg in patients with chronic pancreatitis. Following pancreaticojejunostomy or pseudocystojejunostomy, increased pancreatic pressure fell to control values, which was associated with the relief of pain in 12 out of 14 patients.[42,43] Although these data indicate that increased intraductal or parenchymal pressure is associated with pain in chronic pancreatitis, the mechanism by which increased pressure causes pain is not clear.

With this theoretical background it is not surprising that the treatment of pain in chronic pancreatitis was for a long time largely directed at surgical decompression of the duct and more recently an endoscopic alternative.

Pancreatic neuritis

The most recent pain concept in chronic pancreatitis concerns direct alterations of pancreatic nerves as one of the major pathophysiological events of pain generation.[44–47] It has been reported that phenotypic modification of primary sensory neurones may play a role in the production of persisting pain.[48] Autodigestion with tissue necrosis and both pancreatic and peripancreatic inflammation in the earlier stages change the focal

release and uptake of mediators in the peptidergic nerves and could be an important cause of pain. Previous studies in chronic pancreatitis revealed that pancreatic nerves are preferentially retained while the exocrine pancreatic parenchyma atrophies and degenerates to be replaced by fibrosis. Moreover, in chronic pancreatitis compared with normal pancreas, the number and diameter of pancreatic nerves are significantly increased according to Bockman and analysis of neuroplasticity markers gives evidence that they actively grow.[44,46] Büchler et al.[45] found that the pattern of intrinsic and possibly extrinsic innervation of the pancreas is changed in chronic pancreatitis. This leads to a differential expression of neuropeptides such as substance P and vasoactive intestinal peptide in the chronically inflamed pancreas. Moreover, Nelson et al.[49] have shown that changes in levels of methionine-enkephalin correlates with pain, and recently it was found that immune cell infiltration and expression of growth-associated protein 43 (GAP-43), a marker of neuroplasticity in enlarged pancreatic nerves and pancreatic neurones, correlate with pain in chronic pancreatitis.[46] In addition, electron microscope examination revealed that the perineurium of these nerves is partially destroyed to a different extent, indicating a loss of the barrier between nerve fibers and bioactive material in the perineural space.[13] Bockman et al. have put forward a concept of 'pancreatitis-associated neuritis',[13,18] which implies a comparative increase in the number of sensory nerves in inflammatory pancreatic tissue together with round cell infiltration and a striking disintegration of the perineurium. The loss of function of the perineural barrier may allow an influx of inflammatory mediators or active pancreatic enzymes that could act directly on the nerve cells. In fact, they have found that the neuropeptides substance P and calcitonin gene-related peptide, CGRP, within sensory nerves in pancreatitic tissue are associated with damage of the perineural sheath.[44,47]

Based on the hypothesis that this neural inflammation is an important mechanism of pain, resection of inflammatory tissue is advocated as the treatment of choice. It can be speculated that these two mechanisms—increased pancreatic tissue pressure and neuritis—could work together. High tissue fluid pressure would facilitate influx of pain mediators into the nerves and result in more long-standing pain.

Pancreatic ischemia

There is evidence that pancreatic ischemia may occur in an experimental model of chronic pancreatitis,[50] giving decreased pancreatic blood flow, ischemia and local changes in parenchymal pH. During ischemia, xanthine oxidase becomes activated leading to the generation of toxic oxygen metabolites which may contribute to pain in chronic pancreatitis. However, a xanthine oxidase inhibiting substance, allopurinal, did not reduce pain in a randomized, double-blind cross-over clinical trial.[51]

The evidence that free radical production is increased in patients with chronic pancreatitis is derived from the observations that pancreatitics have early induction of hepatic and pancreatic mono-oxygenases and that their bile contains high levels of free radical oxidation products. The cytochrome P450 system of mono-oxygenases is intimately involved in the metabolism of lipophilic substrates such as hydrocarbons.[52] The enzymes generate oxygen-free radicals from molecular oxygen and use them to metabolize their substrates by controlled release of superoxide, and its dismutation product hydrogen peroxide. Upon exposure to exogenous agents, the activities of cytochrome P450 increase as part of a protective mechanism. This defence mechanism can be detrimental if antioxidant stores are depleted, and if agents that undergo P450 metabolism (e.g. hydrocarbons) are given concomitantly.

A case–control study[53] of patients with chronic pancreatitis has shown that they have increased exposure to hydrocarbons, in particular diesel exhaust fumes, compared to controls. These environmental chemicals would act in a manner similar to alcohol and induce cytochrome P450. Several studies have shown that the cytochrome P450 enzyme system is induced in patients suffering from chronic pancreatitis.[54–57] Foster et al.[54] employed immunohistochemistry using antibodies raised against four phase I enzymes (metabolism) and one phase II enzyme (conjugation). They found both hepatic and pancreatic biopsy specimens from patients with chronic pancreatitis and pancreatic carcinoma showed enhanced staining for cytochrome P450 compared to the staining observed in the control biopsies. Of note was the observation of cytochrome P450 induction in the islets of Langerhans. Interference of cytochrome P450 enzyme family induction is derived from theophylline clearance studies in patients with chronic pancreatitis. In one study[55] it was found that the theophylline clearance was significantly higher in patients with idiopathic and alcohol-related chronic pancreatitis compared to controls. In another study,[56] it was found that patients taking long-term anticonvulsants, known inducers of the cytochrome P450 enzyme system, had levels of enzyme induction similar to those with chronic pancreatitis but without epilepsy.

Comparison of the composition of secretin-stimulated bile from patients with pancreatic disease to controls revealed that patients with pancreatic disease had higher levels of free radical oxidation products.[58] It was also found[59] that patients with chronic pancreatitis had significantly greater bile concentrations of 9cis, 11translinoleic acid, conjugated dienes and ultraviolet fluorescence products compared to controls. Despite all indications of a beneficial role of antioxidants in chronic pancreatitis the potential reduction in morbidity and the financial savings of administering global antioxidant therapy to all patients with chronic pancreatitis. An audit of 103 patients treated with antioxidant therapy revealed that at follow-up of up to 9 years, 75 patients were pain-free and that 27 patients had substantial reduction in their pain and only seven patients required surgery (psuedocyst drainage in six).[60]

Pharmacological treatment

Analgesic drugs are still the most commonly adopted method for pain relief, such as paracetamol, dextropropoxiphene, prednisolone, non-steroidal anti-inflammatory drugs, tricyclic antidepressants or narcotic analgesic drugs given orally or rectally; opioids also may be given subcutaneously or intrathecally.[61] A problem is that due to the chronic nature of the pain many patients subsequently become addicted to powerful narcotics. A major strategy in prescribing is to therefore divide the analgesic treatment into three stages,[3,21,28,62] the principle drug in each stage being paracetamol, dextropropoxiphene and morphine, and never to proceed to the next step without very careful consideration of the short- and long-term effects of the escalation. However, the use of the dextropropoxiphene step has recently been questioned due to the sometimes fatal side effects of the drug.

Although the use of analgesic drugs is necessary in the majority of patients with chronic pancreatitis, there are no controlled trials assessing this treatment modality. However, most patients with chronic pancreatitis do not seek the help of a doctor until they have pain that requires strong analgesics. The pain-relieving drugs preferably should be taken before meals to prevent the postprandial exacerbation of pain. Initially, non-narcotic agents like paracetamol should be used and their effects maximized by increasing dose strength or frequency before switching to stronger alternatives. Time intervals and doses of drug application must be adapted to the individual pattern of pain, but it is important that analgesics are always prescribed on a time-contingent basis, because round-the-clock medications are more effective and may decrease the total daily amount of drug required. Although reluctance to use narcotic agents is advisable, such treatment should not be withheld if the treatment would otherwise not lead to adequate pain control,[3,28] despite the risk that alcohol addiction changes to narcotic addiction. Adjuvant analgesic drugs like antidepressants are often helpful in contributing to an overall dose reduction of analgesics.

There are four studies supporting the pain-relieving effect of oral enzyme preparations in a proportion of patients with chronic pancreatitis,[63–66] but further studies question the role of a negative feedback in the proximal small bowel which inhibits pancreatic secretion.[67] However, it might be worthwhile to give patients a therapeutic trial of enzyme supplements for 1 or 2 months, provided that a preparation known to increase intraduodenal trypsin activity is used.[68] Probably the use of pancreatic enzymes for the treatment of pain is also reasonable at the onset of malabsorption with flatulence, meteorism, and bowel movement, which can be rather painful. The pain should be re-evaluated after 1 or 2 months, and enzyme supplementation stopped in the case of treatment failure. Sometimes H_2 blockers or omeprazole are effective as a further adjunct, especially since patients with chronic pancreatitis have increased duodenal acidity and risk of ulcer formation.[27]

Endoscopic procedures

If decompression of the pancreatic duct is all that is needed in a majority of patients with chronic pancreatitis, it is tempting to try less invasive endoscopic procedures before resorting to surgery. However, it should be remembered that surgical sphincterotomy and sphincteroplasty have already been proved to be less efficient than formal drainage,[69,70] and that these procedures are hardly ever used nowadays. This might be due to the fact that it is unusual to find uniform dilatation of the pancreatic duct system resulting from localized obstruction at the orifice of the main duct.[61,71] More recently, however, a number of endoscopic series have been presented that suggest the complication rate is acceptable, particularly if undertaken in conjunction with stent replacement or stone extraction.

Endocscopic stone extraction has been tried with and without mechanical lithotripsy, extracorporeal shockwave lithotripsy (ESWL), laser lithotripsy and with or without stenting through the pancreatic duct orifice. Only the placement of an endoprosthesis in the pancreatic duct is reported to give pain reduction in obstructive chronic pancreatitis, but stent occlusion and migration appear to be relatively common. With all modalities taken together it is usual to find a report of 80–90% complete stone clearances and good immediate pain relief.[72] However, the long-term results in larger series are not that impressive. In a Belgian study of 123 patients only 60% experienced complete or partial pain relief during 14 months follow-up.[73] Whether this is a good result—with 60% pain-free after a cheap procedure with few complications compared to open surgery—or a bad result—with only 60% of the patients pain-free compared to the usual 80–90% after pylorus-preserving pancreaticoduodectomy (PPPD)[74] or a duodenum-preserving operation according to Beger[75]—is worth discussion. So far there has not been a randomized trial between endoscopic and surgical procedures, and as long as the endoscopic technique is still regarded as experimental it may not be fair to undertake such a trial at this time.

At present the endoscopic approach to patients with chronic pancreatitis is still no more than promising. It seems to be more useful in preventing relapsing attacks of pancreatitis as opposed to helping those with chronic pain,[76] and may better considered as an adjuvant in selection of the right patients for lateral pancreaticojejunostomy. If the patient is doing well with a stent that has to be removed and changed at certain intervals, he will probably also do well with open surgery. Pancreatic duct stents may be inserted in patients with proximal pancreatic duct stenosis and pain, with good short-term but with still variable long-term results. Within a follow-up period of up to 5 years, uncontrolled studies have reported symptom relief in 74–96% of patients and complete cessation of pain in 45–96% of patients.[77,78] Extracorporeal shock wave lithotripsy of pancreatic calculi is applied in patients with pancreatic duct stones and intermittent pain. The procedure may be combined with endoscopic sphincterotomy and extraction of calculi after one or several shock wave lithotripsy treatments. The results are still variable, ranging between symptomatic improvement in 37–83% of patients and complete pain relief in 41–79% of patients.[76,79,80] However, it must be remembered that chronic pancreatitis is not the same as simply stones in the pancreatic duct, to be compared with bile duct stones or uretherolithiasis, but is a disease primarily of the pancreatic parenchyma. Therefore it is unlikely that endoscopy could be a good alternative for more than a minority of these patients. But if this subset of patients can be well defined, important progress will have been made in the management of chronic pancreatitis.

In patients with pancreas divisum, a lesser papillotomy with intermittent stenting is an option when recurrent attacks of pancreatitis or signs of chronic obstructive pancreatitis are documented in the dorsal pancreas. Studies comparing resectional or operative drainage procedures to lesser papillotomy and stenting in pancreas divisum have not been performed to date.

Endoscopically placed biliary stents are also inserted for the acute treatment of extrahepatic cholestasis secondary to common bile duct obstruction in chronic pancreatitis. In cases of acute cholangitis, at least the sphincterotomy is mandatory. The early results of endoscopic stenting of the strictured bile duct in chronic pancreatitis are convincing, whereas long-term results in patients with significant stenosis of the common bile duct are probably better when an operative procedure is subsequently performed.

In pancreatic pseudocysts, percutaneous punctures are performed for diagnostic purposes and in large pseudocysts also for therapeutic purposes, but long-term results are unfavorable. Internal drainage may be performed by endoscopic sphincterotomy and pancreatic duct stenting when a communication between the pseudocysts and the main duct exists; otherwise, an endoscopic pseudocystogastrostomy or pseudocystoduodenostomy is being increasingly performed.[81,82] The results with regard to pain relief seem to be equal—open surgery, endoscopic stenting or percutaneous procedures—which means that the safest and easiest way for the individual patient should be favored.

Decompression procedures

Surgical decompression of the obstructed main pancreatic duct was the gold standard for a long time against which other therapies were measured.[83] Drainage operations today are most often carried out as a side-to-side pancreaticojejunostomy as this preserves pancreatic parenchyma. Longitudinal pancreaticojejunostomy according to Puestow or Partington–Rochelle, that is the duct of Wirsung opened from the tail of the pancreas to the duodenum and anastomosed to the side of the jejunum, has been one of the techniques that has been used most often.[5] The procedure is based on the concept that ductal obstruction leads to distension and that this in turn gives rise to pain and should thus be favored only if the duct is widened. Theoretically, any measure which improves drainage, either by improving flow into the duodenum or by allowing flow into the jejunum or stomach, might be expected to relieve pain. Pancreatic decompression results in immediate and lasting pain relief in a high proportion (80–90%) of patients with non-alcoholic chronic pancreatitis, which is higher than that reported in patients with alcoholic pancreatitis,

where pain relief averaged 60%.[16] This result is similar to that reported by Sato et al. who found that over a mean period of 9 years only 56% of patients with alcoholic pancreatitis had good results after surgery compared to 83% of those who had non-alcoholic pancreatitis. Although good early results have also been reported after a lateral pancreaticojejunostomy in patients with alcoholic pancreatitis, when these patients are followed for 5 years only 38–60% of them continue to be pain-free. On the other hand, Brinton et al. in a study of 39 patients who underwent lateral pancreaticojejunostomy, did not find any correlation between the pain relief seen in alcoholic patients and those who were not alcoholic; but the mean duration of follow-up was not specified in their paper. Amman et al.[6] in a study of 145 patients with chronic calcific pancreatitis, found that 85% had spontaneous and lasting relief of pain at a mean duration of 5 years after onset and Nealon and Thompson, after a well designed study, reported that pain relief was achieved in 74 of 87 patients after standard longitudinal pancreaticojejunostomy in an average follow-up of 48 months.

Prinz and Greenlee separated patients according to pain relief into three categories: complete, substantial, and none, but did not include narcotic intake in the assessment. Eighty per cent of their patients had complete or substantial pain relief after lateral pancreaticojejunostomy, with an average follow-up of 8 years. There was no explanation of how the pain assessment was performed (e.g. patient interview or questionnaire). Neither a pain scale, nor a quality of life assessment was used. During follow-up of patients after a longitudinal pancreaticojejunostomy, Bradley categorized patients' status as good, fair, or poor on the basis of communication with the patient, or referring physician, or by questionnaire. Fair was defined as decreased pain 'not requiring narcotics'; poor was defined as 'continuing to require narcotics'. Bradley's results, perhaps as a consequence of including use of narcotics as a criterion in pain assessment, gave a less optimistic picture of patient outcome than those of Prinz and Greenlee: only 28% of patients had a good result, 38% had fair, and 34% had poor results after an average follow-up of 6 years.

Using a technique for intraoperative as well as percutaneous measurement of pancreatic fluid pressure a group of Danish investigators found a close correlation between tissue pressure and pain in patients who underwent drainage operations for chronic pancreatitis. Postoperative reduction in pressure was followed by relief of pain, whereas in patients with recurrent pain the pressure rose again.[36] However, there are also a number of studies which cast doubt on the relationship between pain in chronic pancreatitis and intrapancreatic pressure. One problem in evaluating the results of the operations is the different definitions of pain relief and the different follow-ups,[14] but in spite of this it is obvious that not all patients will be pain-free after technically well performed drainage operations. It is widely accepted that the prospects for pain relief are poor if the pancreatic duct is not dilated, but even so, not all patients will experience pain relief.[14,61] About 30% of patients with chronic pancreatitis fail to obtain long-lasting relief of pain. The current opinion is that if obstructed parts of the pancreatic duct are left undrained then the operation will fail to relieve pain, but provided this is not the case there is little evidence to favor one operative procedure rather than another.

Although it has been shown that operative drainage of the pancreatic duct delays both endocrine and exocrine functional impairment in patients with chronic pancreatitis,[84] insulin requirements seem to be unchanged for a long period.

It should also be mentioned that there are numerous variations of the previously mentioned operations, the most interesting described by Frey in 1978.[85] He combined a coring out of the pancreatic head with a lateral pancreaticojejunostomy. In his own series of patients pain relief after 5 years' follow-up was complete or improved in 87% of cases, which is at least as good as any other procedure described so far. There is also one randomized series of patients comparing the techniques of Beger and Frey,[86] where no difference in decrease of pain was found but there was less postoperative morbidity after the Frey method. However, long follow-up of a more substantial series of patients operated upon by independent surgeons is still lacking.

Resection

The therapeutic principle of resection is based on the assumption that pain in chronic pancreatitis is predominantly caused by inflammation with qualitative and quantitative changes of nerve fibers. In the German literature pancreatic resections have been proposed over the last decade for pain relief in chronic pancreatitis, especially in patients with normal-sized ducts and masses involving the head of the pancreas. According to these authors, nearly 30% of patients with chronic pancreatitis develop inflammatory enlargement of the pancreatic head with subsequent obstruction of the pancreatic duct, and sometimes also of the common bile duct and duodenum. In these situations a pancreaticoduodenectomy, the 'Whipple procedure', has been the procedure of choice for many years as it provides reasonably effective pain relief. These resections, however, have a significant immediate postoperative and long-term morbidity from insulin-dependent diabetes mellitus, with an increase in the incidence of diabetes from about 20% preoperatively to about 60% in the years that follow.[84] Also postgastrectomy sequelae detract significantly from the overall quality of life. However, the long-term mortality rate and quality of life after this procedure in patients with chronic pancreatitis has not always been encouraging, and in some studies is disappointing.[83]

To counter these problems, the original Whipple procedure has been replaced by the pylorus-preserving pancreaticoduodenectomy (PPPD) and the 'Beger procedure'. The techniques of standard Whipple and PPPD are basically the same, except for the treatment of the antrum, pylorus and duodenum. The latter procedure, made popular by Traverso and Longmire,[74] attempted to preserve normal gastric function and give unimpaired nutrition and prevent bile reflux gastritis. The more conservative procedure of Beger[75] resects the pancreatic head pathology but preserves all extrapancreatic organs including the duodenum. There has been one randomized trial comparing these two procedures,[84,87] showing after 6 months' follow-up that patients undergoing the Beger procedure suffered less pain. Moreover, they had better preservation of insulin secretion and glucose tolerance, and more stable weight. These good results were confirmed in a prospective study of 298 patients with chronic pancreatitis undergoing the same procedure.[87] Furthermore, in-hospital mortality in this series was only 1%. These data suggest that in chronic pancreatitis as little as possible of extrapancreatic tissue should be removed, which seems logical. However, the limited number of patients and lack of long-term follow-up as yet preclude any definite conclusions concerning the exact method to be recommended.

The duodenum-preserving resection of the head of the pancreas has been shown to be associated with a 5-year interval of pain relief of up to 85%[84,87–89] in a selected subgroup of patients. Izbicki et al.[86] compared the results of duodenum-preserving resection of the head of the pancreas with those of local resection of the head of the pancreas using a visual analog pain scale. They noted the frequency of pain attacks, narcotic usage, and ability to work. These elements were combined into a pain score defined as the sum of the rank values of the four criteria divided by four. No details of the narcotic assessment or what was meant by 'frequency of attacks of pain' were provided, but in summary the duodenum-preserving procedure was recommended.

Morel et al.[90] reported on 20 patients with chronic pancreatitis treated with pancreaticoduodenectomy.

Of eight patients observed for follow-up for an average of 8 years, four had recurrent, moderate, intermittent abdominal pain, but no mention was made of narcotic usage. Traverso and Kozarek[91] reported on the results of the pylorus-preserving Whipple procedure for complications of chronic pancreatitis in 28 patients with a mean follow-up of 27 months. All patients were interviewed for follow-up, and 88% were said to be pain-free. No patient required reoperation for chronic pancreatitis. Narcotic usage was not described in the postoperative follow-up, although 12% of the patients continued to have enough pain to require ongoing medication.

An alternative to pancreaticoduodenectomy is Etibloc occlusion of the duct system of the preserved distal remnant and this was compared in 289 patients.[92] Slightly more than half of the patients were completely pain-free, and 35% had occasional complications. 'Minor complaints', which occurred frequently but significantly less often than they did before surgery, were reported by 11% of the patients. Two patients continued to have pain as severe as that experienced before surgery. The follow-up period averaged 6 years. The pain relief induced by pancreaticoduodenectomy was said to be constant and permanent.

Russell[17] studied the results of preservation of the duodenum in total pancreatectomy compared to standard pancreaticoduodenectomy and found no difference in pain relief between the two operations. He noted that 13 (34%) of the 32 still had severe pain after duodenum-preserving total pancreatectomy, and six had ongoing major analgesic requirements.

Distal pancreatectomy has a very limited role in management of pain. A good outcome is only seen in patients with non-dilated pancreatic ducts and pseudocyst involving the tail of the pancreas.[93] Keith et al.[94] analyzed the outcome of 80% distal pancreatectomy and pancreaticoduodenectomy and total pancreatectomy, and documented the codeine equivalent required after an average follow-up of 5 years, 6 years, and 9 years, respectively. Four of five patients, after pancreaticoduodenectomy, required ongoing narcotics, whereas 13 of 32 patients had complete pain relief after 80% distal pancreatectomy. No mention was made of the method of pain assessment.

In conclusion we believe that patients with non-dilated ducts with severe pain due to chronic pancreatitis should be considered for resection. The Beger procedure is advocated, but if the surgeon is not familiar with that technique a pylorus-preserving pancreaticoduodenectomy is a possible alternative.

Sympathectomy

The nerves in the pancreas include sympathetic, parasympathetic, sensory and motor fibers.[95] The sensory fibers mediating pain are conducted towards the central nervous system, without synapse through the celiac plexus, and the splanchnic nerves, to enter the thoracic spinal cord.[95] The cell bodies of these neurones are located in the dorsal root. The sympathetic innervation of the pancreas, including the nerves mediating pain, leaves from cells in the tractus intermediolateralis in the spinal cord from T5 to T11. The sympathetic fibers are led to the sympathetic chain and onwards by the nervus splanchnicus major (from T5 to T10) and one or more nervi splanchnici minor (from T9 to T11) to synapses in the prevertebral abdominal plexi, initially in the celiac ganglion. The postganglionic fibers pass along the arteries of the liver and spleen and the superior mesenteric artery into pancreatic tissue. Some sympathetic axons run directly to the pancreas without intra-abdominal synapses, mainly from the lower portion of the sympathetic chain (which may partly explain the limitation of pain control after surgical celiacectomy). From a theoretical point of view the pain can be inhibited by cutting the nerve fibers anywhere along these paths. The procedure most often tried is chemical ablation of the celiac ganglion, and a newer alternative is thoracoscopic sympathectomy.

The celiac block can be performed during laparotomy or percutaneously, usually from the back. The placement of the needle uses anatomical landmarks with the position checked by fluoroscopy, scout radiographic films, ultrasonography, CT, or at angiography. A nerve block with 25 ml of 50% alcohol on each side should be preceded by a positive diagnostic block with long-acting local anesthesia, carried out at least one day earlier. The method aims to block the splanchnic nerves before they reach the celiac plexus rather than block part of the celiac plexus itself. There are several different ways to ascertain that the needle tip and the fluid injected, respectively, are in the right place. The site of the needle can be documented with scout films.[96] Theoretically more appealing, is to guide the injection of local anesthetics (and later neurolytics) with fluoroscopy and contrast media in the injected fluid.[97–99]

In a critical review Sharfman and Walsh[100] analyzed data on 480 patients from 15 series (published 1964–83) celiac plexus blockade in pancreatic patients. A satisfactory response to the procedure was reported in 87% of the patients. The authors claimed, however, that there were major deficiencies in the reporting of the results. The results of celiac block have been rather unpredictable, and as the pain tended to recur after about 3 months,[61] the indication for this procedure is at present limited.

As the pain fibers run in the sympathetic chain, pain stimuli can be overcome from within the thoracic cavity where the chain lies immediately subpleural over the ribs in the posterior mediastinum. A variety of approaches to sympathectomy has been used in the past. Mallet-Guy was the first person to attempt any form of denervation of the pancreas in patients with chronic pancreatitis. Using a retroperitoneal approach, he performed unilateral left splanchnicectomy in 1942 with successful relief of pain. By 1950 he reported successful results in 84% of 37 patients followed for 1 year or more,[101] and in 1983 he reported on his expanded series of 215 patients with chronic pancreatitis who had undergone left splanchnicectomy and celiac ganglionectomy.[102] In 217 patients who had been followed for 5 years or more, relief of pain was observed in 88%. Despite this, in 1983 White reported only a 20% success rate in relieving chronic pancreatic pain with left splanchnicectomy and celiac ganglionectomy with the same technique.[103]

These nerves are easily identified at thoracoscopy. Thoracoscopic splanchnicectomy may be performed bilaterally under general anesthesia using double-lumen endotracheal intubation. In a series of 30 patients treated in Lund, only two ports were used on each side: one optical cannula (10.0 mm) and another 5.5 mm operating cannula. A small hole in the pleura on each side of a splanchnic nerve, 10 mm from the sympathetic chain, was burnt with the diathermy hook and the nerves were then cut completely so that the ends were seen to be well retracted from each other. In uncomplicated cases the patients were discharged from the hospital the day after the operation. Satisfactory stable pain relief was obtained from the first week after surgery to a median follow-up time of 18 months. All but one patient reported clearly reduced pain, but only about 20% of individuals reported immediate complete pain relief. One may conclude that thoracoscopic splanchnicectomy appears promising as a relatively simple treatment for severe chronic pancreatic pain.[62]

A different approach to pancreatic denervation was suggested by Yoshioka and Wakabayashi in 1958.[104] After studying the neuroanatomy of postganglionic nerve fibers traveling from the celiac ganglion to pancreatic parenchyma they recommended a selective bilateral neurectomy of the fibers entering the pancreas from the right and left ganglia. These authors reported that 35 of 36 patients with chronic pancreatitis experienced 'excellent' results from this challenging technique. Little or no additional information concerning these patients was provided. In a modification of this selective parenchymal sympathectomy, Hiraoka et al.[105] extended the Yoshioka procedure to include more extensive denervation of the body and tail by completely freeing the pancreas from its retroperitoneal attachments. Successful relief of pain was achieved in both patients undergoing this modified procedure.

Since the splanchnic nerves are thought to carry most if not all of the afferent sympathetic pain from the pancreatic parenchyma,[106] it is not surprising that splanchnicectomy relieves pain in patients with chronic pancreatitis. Rather, it is the failure of splanchnicectomy to completely relieve pain that is remarkable. A plausible explanation for suboptimal pain response from splanchnicectomy might be that some elements of pain in chronic pancreatitis are mediated by somatic nerve pathways. As all surgeons dealing with chronic pancreatitis know, the disease process often extends beyond the boundaries of the gland to involve the posterior abdominal wall. Pain arising from chronic inflammation of the parietal tissues is true somatic exteroceptive pain, whose pathway is through the spinal nerves to the dorsal root ganglion, and then to the lateral spinothalamic tract. In support of this theory of mixed sympathetic and somatic involvement in some patients with chronic pancreatitis was the observation of Bradley[4] that during testing with epidural analgesia in some patients with chronic pancreatitis there was some decrease of pain after sympathetic blockade, but total anesthesia required a full somatic block.

Moreover, the well-recognized failure of even total pancreatectomy to provide pain relief to some patients might be explained by somatic nerve involvement superimposed on sympathetic pain. If combined sympathetic and somatic nerve involvement is common in patients with chronic pancreatitis, an operation could be designed to add appropriate somatic denervation to the splanchnicectomy. Another explanation for the frequent absence of total analgesia after splanchnicectomy might be that pancreatic pain afferent fibers are present in mixed nerves, thereby bypassing the celiac ganglia and the splanchnic nerves. Although it is known that such fibers exist,[4] their relative importance in the neurophysiology of pancreatic pain is unknown.

Pain in pancreatic cancer in chronic pancreatitis

Sharma et al.[86] reported that 7% of patients with chronic pancreatitis died from disseminated cancer. In all forms of pancreatitis there appears to be cellular dysfunction, glandular destruction, and presumably increased cellular turnover, which has been suggested as a potential precursor of cancer in many organs. The excessive risk of pancreatic cancer that has been documented in epidemiological studies in patients with various types of pancreatitis (also in 'tropical pancreatitis') is consistent with this hypothesis. Notwithstanding, the uncertainties in epidemiological studies, the existence of a clear association between pancreatitis and the subsequent risk of pancreatic cancer is too often only random.[107]

However, in all cases of chronic pancreatitis undergoing surgery pancreatic cancer must always be considered.

Summary and options for the future

Patients with established chronic pancreatitis do not present with a uniform pattern of symptoms for the stage of the disease (early or late), the extrapancreatic, secondary symptomatology or the morphological features. This also influences the pattern of pain and the outcome of the attempts to manage not only the symptoms but the patient as a whole. The major goal of new treatment modalities in chronic pancreatitis must be an improvement of the patient's quality of life, which is a multidimensional approach. There are various studies in which pain and even quality of life have been assessed before and after surgical treatment of chronic pancreatitis.[84,86,89,108–111] Some of the studies have compared the outcome of two different operative procedures.[84,86]

A growing number of options are now available to manage pain in chronic pancreatitis, including pharmacologic, endoscopic, and surgical methods. To compare the efficacy of different treatments, it is necessary to have a baseline inventory of the patient's general health status. It should be determined specifically whether the patient's pancreatitis is caused by use of alcohol or some non-alcohol-related cause, whether the patient is addicted to narcotics, and whether the patient has exocrine and endocrine insufficiency, weight loss, pain and the grade of pain, and a record of emergency department visits and hospital admissions should be obtained. It should be noted that alcohol and narcotic addiction has an unfavorable impact on longevity and pain relief, especially if their use is continued after treatment.[112] Pain in chronic pancreatitis must always be adapted to the individual situation, and this refers especially to specific complications of the disease. At present, decision making often depends not only the individual case, but also on the local availability of methods.

Even in the most recent literature on chronic pancreatitis, there is an absence of consensus on a standard method for assessing pain relief and improved quality of life.[85,86,91–94,113,114] In the absence of a consistent, reproducible standard of assessing pain status and quality of life, it is not possible to reliably compare the result of one surgical procedure with another, nor is it possible to compare results of pharmacologic, endoscopic, and other treatments with those of operative procedures. Lankisch Andrén-Sandberg have given guidelines about which items should be assessed in the follow-up of patients treated for chronic pancreatitis.[14] Another suggestion is to use the EORTC QLQ-30, which has been used in patients suffering from chronic pancreatitis.[115] This questionnaire consists of a core of 30 generally applicable items and includes a functional scale; a working ability scale; a general symptom scale; scales on cognitive, emotional and social functioning; a financial strain scale; and a global quality-of-life scale.[115,116]

Frey et al.[85] categorized 50 patients after local resection of the head of the pancreas and lateral pancreaticojejunostomy on the basis of pain relief. Pain was quantified on a visual analog scale, VAS (graded 0–10, with VAS = 0 denoting no pain). Thirty-four per cent of the patients used no narcotics and had no pain at follow-up. Together with those with VAS <2 ('minimal pain') or taking narcotics on fewer than 3 days per month, 75% were classified as having excellent results. The patients with small improvements in pain relief (<2 on VAS) and the patients whose pain was reduced but still less than VAS 5 or who were taking minimal narcotics were considered improved (13%).

Compared with the published data from large series of patients with chronic pancreatitis both from Germany and the US, the Scandinavian results of surgical intervention are small. Even though the rate of major operations is comparatively very low, it seems that their patients are doing no worse than those in other reviewed series.[117] This may be due to differences in the disease, but should nonetheless contribute to discussions on the indications for surgery.

The principal prerequisite is to keep the frequency low and to have good personal contact with the patient on a regular basis. This may be difficult if the patient is addicted to drugs or has severe alcoholic problems, but in such cases we believe it makes no difference which medical or surgical management method is chosen, as the end result will be equally bad. However, if the patient has confidence in the doctor's overall management he or she will be able to withstand more pain without escalating analgesic requirements, and the treatment can be viewed from a long-term perspective. Therefore, the continuity in the patient–doctor relationship is of the utmost importance in these patients. An established relationship between the patient and the surgeon—not only with the general practitioner or gastroenterologist—for a long time before surgery is considered is also of importance. The knowledge that the patient can have a pain-relieving operation quickly if really needed may actually postpone the operation.

However, there are also patients who need surgical intervention. A borderline is crossed when the patient needs morphine on a regular basis. After a renewed work-up of the patient to avoid missing a pancreatic pseudocyst, a duodenal ulcer, gallbladder disease, or other extrapancreatic pathological processes, a thoracoscopic splanchnicectomy should be considered an an alternative to resective procedures as the results are equally good for pain relief and the procedure does not preclude other later interventions if needed. If pain relief is not achieved open surgery would be considered, where, if the right prerequisites are present, a longitudinal pancreaticojejunostomy would be the first choice. Surgery in patients with severe pain due to chronic pancreatitis should be performed with low morbidity and without mortality. However, the indications for resection versus drainage operations are not yet defined and therefore this type of surgery should, if possible, be performed only in centers dedicated to the scientific follow-up of all patients—operated and not operated upon—for at least 5 years.[14]

The problem of assessing pain relief in patients with chronic pancreatitis is compounded by a number of additional factors. The natural history of the disease may be characterized by spontaneous exacerbations and remissions, so there can be great variations in the course of the pain. The use of additive narcotics before and after surgery may obscure the severity of the pain and confuse attempts at comparison. Furthermore, the classification of patients undergoing surgery or other interventions for pain control into groups according to 'success' and 'failure' is clearly inadequate and fails to provide reproducible data. The need for a standard method of pain assessment to evaluate the efficacy of any therapy in chronic pancreatitis is more pressing than ever, because there are now a growing number of options for the treatment of these patients. This is especially true with surgical procedures, in that several operations with similar indications are available for ameliorating the pain of chronic pancreatitis. The surgeon must select one of these options, all of which purport to provide some degree of pain relief. In the absence of a standardized system of assessing pain relief and quality of life, it is virtually impossible to compare these operative procedures with other types of management. It is only by having a common yardstick that we can determine which is the most efficacious way of providing pain relief and maintaining a reasonable quality of life in patients with intractable pain from chronic pancreatitis. It is obvious that long-term results in chronic pancreatitis come from an appraisal of the individual's situation and that the treatment must be tailored to the patient as well as to the disease. The prognosis also depends on the attitude of the patient and may depend more on drinking habits than on the medical and surgical management!

Key points

- Pain is the cardinal symptom of chronic pancreatitis (affects 85% of sufferers) and precedes other effects (diabetes and malabsorption).
- Types of pain experienced in chronic pancreatitis:
      Constant upper abdominal radiating to back
      Intermittent, nocturnal and penetrating
      Postprandial, causing loss of appetite.
- Painless course is rare in alcoholic chronic pancreatitis.
- 'Large duct' chronic pancreatitis may be amenable to surgical drainage procedures.
- 'Small duct' chronic pancreatitis pain may be managed by:
      Cessation of alcohol (some effect)
      Analgesia and steroids (some effect)
      Endoscopic stone extraction
      Pancreatic resection
      Sympathectomy (thoracic)
      Celiac plexus block.

REFERENCES

1. Lankisch PG. Natural course in chronic pancreatitis. Pain, exocrine and endocrine pancreatic insufficiency and prognosis of the disease. Digestion 1993; 54:148–55

2. Glasbrenner B, Adler G. Evaluating pain and the quality of life in chronic pancreatitis. Int J Pancreatol 1997; 22: 163–70

3. Andrén-Sandberg Å. Pain relief in pancreatic disease. Br J Surg 1997; 84: 1041–2

4. Bradley EL. Long term results of pancreaticojejunostomy in chronic pancreatitis. Am Surg 1987; 153: 207–211

5. Andrén-Sandberg Å, Hafström A. Partington–Rochelle: when to drain the pancreatic duct and why. Dig Surg 1996; 13: 109–12

6. Amman RW, Akovbiantz A, Largiader F, Schueler G. Course and outcome of chronic pancreatitis. Longitudinal study of a mixed medical-surgical series of 245 patients. Gastroenterology 1984; 86: 820–8

7. Amman RW, Buehler H, Muench R, Freiburghaus A, Siegenthaler W. Differences in the natural history of idiopathic (nonalcoholic) and alcoholic chronic pancreatitis. A comparative study of 287 patients. Pancreas 1987; 2: 368–77

8. Amman RW, Heitz PU, Klöppel G. Course of alcoholic chronic pancreatitis: a prospective clinicomorphological long-term study. Gastroenterology 1996; 111: 224–31

9. Lankisch PG, Löhr-Happe A, Otto J, Creutzfeld W. Natural course in chronic pancreatitis. Pain, exocrine and endocrine pancreatic insufficiency and prognosis of the disease. Digestion 1993; 54: 148–55

10. Layer P, Yamamoto H, Kalthoff L, Chain JE, Bakken J, DiMagno EP. The different courses of early- and late-onset idiopathic and alcoholic chronic pancreatitis. Gastroenterology 1994; 107: 1481–7

11. Grendell JH, Cello JP. Chronic pancreatitis. In: Steisenger MH, Fordtran JS, eds. Gastrointestinal disease pathophysiology, diagnosis, management. Philadelphia: WB Saunders, 1989: 1842–72

12. Liu KJM, Atten MJ. Nutritional management in chronic pancreatitis. Probl Gen Surg 1998; 15: 17–30

13. Maifertheiner P, Pieramico O, Buchier M, Ditschuneit H. Relationships between pancreatic function and pain in chronic pancreatitis. Acta Chir Scand 1990; 156: 267–71

14. Lankisch PG, Andrén-Sandberg Å. Standards for the diagnosis of chronic pancreatitis for the evaluation of treatment. Int J Pancreatol 1993; 14: 205–12

15. Morrow CE, Cohen JL, Sutherland ER, Najanan JS. Chronic pancreatitis: long-term surgical results of pancreatic duct drainage, pancreatic resection, and near-total pancreatectomy and islet autotransplantation. Surgery 1984; 608–16

16. Mannell A, Adson MA, McIllrath DC, Ilstrup DM. Surgical management of chronic pancreatitis: long term results in 141 patients. Br J Surg 1988; 75: 467–72

17. Russell RCG. Indications for surgical treatment in chronic pancreatitis. In: Beger HG, Büchler M, Malfertheiner P, eds. Standards in pancreatic surgery. Berlin: Springer-Verlag, 1983: 350–7

18. DiMagno E, Layer P, Claim JE. Chronic pancreatitis. In: Go VLW, DiMagno EP, Gardner JD, Lebenthal E, Reber HA, Scheele GA eds. The pancreas. Biology, pathobiology, and disease. New York: Raven Press, 1993: 665–706

19. Steer ML, Waxman I, Freedman S. Chronic pancreatitis. N Engl J Med 1995; 332: 1482–4

20. Mössner J. Epidemiology of chronic pancreatitis. In: Beger HG, Büchler M, Malfertheiner P, eds. Standards in pancreatic surgery. Berlin: Springer-Verlag, 1993: 263–71

21. Amman RW. A clinically based classification system for alcoholic chronic pancreatitis: summary of an international workshop on chronic pancreatitis. Pancreas 1997; 14: 215–21

22. Sarles H. Chronic calcifying pancreatitis. Scand J Gastroenterol 1985; 20: 651–9

23. Guilo L, Barbara L, Labo G. Effect of cessation of alcohol use on the course of pancreatic dysfunction in alcoholic pancreatitis. Gastroenterology 1988; 95: 1063–8

24. Hayakawa T, Kondo T, Shibata T, Sugimoto Y, Kitagawa M. Chronic alcoholism and evolution of pain and prognosis in chronic pancreatitis. Dig Dis Sci 1989; 34: 33–8

25. Little JM. Alcohol abuse and chronic pancreatitis. Surgery 1987; 101: 357–60

26. Miyake H, Harada H, Kunichuka K, Ochi K, Kimura I. Clinical course and prognosis of chronic pancreatitis. Pancreas 1987; 2: 378–85

27. Gullo L, Corinaldesi R, Casadio R et al. Gastric acid secretion in chronic pancreatitis. Hepatogastroenterology 1983; 30: 60–2

28. Ihse I, Andersson R. The medical management of chronic pancreatitis. Probl Gen Surg 1998; 15: 31–7

29. Klöppel G. Pathology of chronic pancreatitis and pancreatic pain. Acta Chir Scand 1990; 156: 261–5

30. Bradley EL. Pancreatic duct pressure in chronic pancreatitis. Am J Surg 1982; 144: 313–6

31. Makrauer FL, Antonioli DA, Banks PA. Duodenal stenosis in chronic pancreatitis: clinicopathological correlations. Dig Dis Sci 1982; 27: 525–32

32. Leahy AL, Carter DC. Pain and chronic pancreatitis. Eur J Gastroenterol Hepatol 1991; 3: 425–33

33. Jensen AR, Matzen P, Malchow-Möller A, Christoffersen I (The Copenhagen Pancreatitis Study Group). Pattern of pain, duct morphology and pancreatic function in chronic pancreatitis. Scand J Gastroenterol 1984; 19: 334–8.

34. Malfertheiner P, Büchler M, Stanescu A, Ditschuneit H. Pancreatic morphology and function in relationship to pain in chronic pancreatitis. Int J Pancreatol 1987; 1: 59–66

35. Ebbehöj N, Borly L, Madsen P. Pancreatic tissue pressure. Technique and aspects. Scand J Gastroenterol 1984; 19: 1066–8

36. Ebbehöj N, Borly L, Bülow J, Rasmussen SG, Madsen P. Evaluation of pancreatic tissue fluid pressure and pain in chronic pancreatitis. A longitudinal study. Scand J Gastroenterol 1990; 25: 462–6

37. Jalleh RP, Aslam M, Williamson RCN. Pancreatic tissue and ductal pressures in chronic pancreatitis. Br J Surg 1991; 78: 1235–7

38. Sato T, Miyashita E, Yamauchi H, Matsuno S. The role of surgical treatment for chronic pancreatitis. Ann Surg 1986; 203: 266–71

39. Madsen P, Winkler K. The intraductal pancreatic pressure in chronic obstructive pancreatitis. Scand J Gastroenterol 1982; 17: 553–4

40. Okazaki K, Yamamoto Y, Kagiyama S et al. Pressure of papillary sphincter zone and pancreatic main duct in patients with alcoholic and idiopathic chronic pancreatitis. Int J Pancreatol 1988; 3: 457–68

41. Staritz M, Meyer zum Büschenfelde KH. Elevated pressure in the dorsal part of pancreas divisum: the cause of chronic pancreatitis? Pancreas 1988; 3: 108–10

42. Ebbehöj N, Svensen LB, Madsen P. Pancreatic tissue pressure: techniques and pathophysiological aspects. Scand J Gastroenterol 1984; 19: 1066–8

43. Ebbehöj N, Borly L, Madsen P, Svendsen LB. Pancreatic tissue pressure and pain in chronic pancreatitis. Pancreas 1986; 1: 556–8

44. Bockman DE, Büchler M, Malfertheiner P, Beger H. Analysis of nerves in chronic pancreatitis. Gastroenterology 1988; 94: 1459–69

45. Büchler M, Weihe E, Friess H et al. Changes in peptidergic innervation in chronic pancreatitis. Pancreas 1992; 7: 183–92

46. Di Sebastiano P, Fink T, Weihe E et al. Immune cell infiltration and growth-associated protein 43 expression correlate with pain in chronic pancreatitis. Gastroenterology 1997; 112: 1648–55

47. Weihe E, Büchler MW, Müller S, Friess H, Zentel HJ, Yanihara N. Peptidergic innervation in chronic pancreatitis. In: Beger HG, Büchler MW, Ditschuneit H, Malfertheiner P, eds. Chronic pancreatitis. Berlin: Springer-Verlag, 1990: 83–105

48. Woolf CJ. Phenotypic modification of primary sensory neurons: the role of nerve growth factor in the production of persisting pain. Phil Trans R Soc Lond B Biol Sci 1996; 351: 441–8

49. Nelson DK, Gress TM, Lucas DL et al. Gene expression and posttranslational processing of intrapancreatic proenkephalin: a link to pancreatic pain in chronic pancreatitis? (abstract). Gastroenterology 1993; 104: A323

50. Karanjia ND, Widdison AL, Leung F, Alvarez C, Lutrin J, Reber HA. Compartment syndrome in experimental chronic obstructive pancreatitis: effect of decompression on the main pancreatic duct. Br J Surg 1994; 81: 259–64

51. Banks PA, Hughes M, Ferrante M, Noordhoek EC, Ramagopal V, Slivka A. Does allopurinol reduce pain in chronic pancreatitis? Int J Pancreatol 1997; 22: 171–6

52. Koop DR. Oxidative and reductive metabolism by cytochrome P450 2E1. FASEBJ 1992; 6: 724–30

53. McNamee R, Braganza JM, Hogg J, Leck I, Rose P, Cherry NM. Occupational exposure to hydrocarbons and chronic pancreatitis: a case-referent study. Occupational Environ Med 1994; 51: 631–7

54. Foster JR, Idle JR, Hardwick JR Bars R, Scott P, Braganza JM. Induction of drug-metabolizing enzymes in human pancreatic cancer and chronic pancreatitis. J Pathol 1993; 169: 457–63

55. Achson DWK, Hunt LP, Rose P, Houston JB, Braganza JM. Factors contributing to the accelerated clearance of theophylline and antipyrine in adults with exocrine pancreatic disease. Clin Sci 1989; 76: 377–85

56. Uden S, Acheson DWK, Reeves J et al. Antioxidants, enzyme induction, and chronic pancreatitis: a reappraisal following studies in patients on anticonvulsants. Eur J Clin Nutr 1988; 42: 561–9

57. Sandilands D, Jeffrey IJM, Haboubi NY, MacLennan IAM, Braganza JM. Abnormal drug metabolism in chronic pancreatitis: treatment with antioxidants. Gastroenterology 1990; 98: 766–72

58. Braganza JM, Wickens DL, Cawood P, Dormandy TL. Lipid peroxidation (free-radical-oxidation) production in bile from patients with pancreatic disease. Lancet 1983; ii: 375–8

59. Guyan PM, Uden S, Braganza JM. Heightened free radical activity in pancreatitis. Free Radical Biol Med 1990; 8: 347–54

60. Whiteley GSW, Kienle APB, McCloy RF, Braganza JM. Long-term pain relief without surgery in chronic pancreatitis: value of antioxidant therapy. Gastroenterology 1993; 104(Suppl): A343

61. lhse I, Larsson J. Chronic pancreatitis: results of operations for relief of pain. World J Surg 1990; 14: 53–8

62. Andrén-Sandberg Å, Zoucas E, Lillo-Gil R, Gyllstedt E, lhse I. Thoracoscopic splanchnicectomy for chronic, severe pancreatic pain. Sem Laparscopic Surg 1996; 3: 29–33

63. Hollender LF, Laugner B. Pain-relieving procedures in chronic pancreatitis. In: Trede M, Carter DC eds. Surgery of the pancreas. Edinburgh: Churchill Livingstone, 1993: 349–57

64. lsaksson G, lhse I. Pain reduction by an oral pancreatic enzyme preparation in chronic pancreatitis. Dig Dis Sci 1983; 28: 97–102

65. Slaff J, Jacobson D, Tillman CR, Curington C, Toskes P. Protease-specific suppression of pancreatic secretion. Gastroenterology 1984; 87: 45–52

66. Rämö OJ, Poulakkainen PA, Seppälä K, Schröder TM. Self-administration of enzyme substitution in the treatment of exocrine pancreatic insufficiency. Scand J Gastroenterol 1989; 24: 688–92

67. Mössner J, Wresky HP, Kestel W, Zeeh J, Regner U, Fischbach W. Influence of treatment with pancreatic enzymes on pancreatic enzyme secretion. Gut 1989; 30: 1143–59

68. Malesci A, Gala E, Fioretta A et al. No effect of long-term treatment with pancreatic extracts on recurrent abdominal pain in patients with chronic pancreatitis. Scand J Gastroenterol 1995; 30: 392–8

69. Dreiling DA, Greenstein RJ. State of the art: the sphincter of Oddi, sphincterotomy and biliopancreatic disease. Am J Gastroenterol 1979; 72: 665–70

70. Bagley FH, Brasch JW, Taylor RH, Warren KW. Sphincterotomy or sphincteroplasty in the treatment of pathologically mild chronic pancreatitis. Am J Surg 1981; 141: 418–21

71. Moossa AR. Surgical treatment of chronic pancreatitis: an overview. Br J Surg 1987; 74: 661–7

72. Burdick JS, Hogan WJ. Chronic pancreatitis: selection of patients for endoscopic therapy. Endoscopy 1991; 23: 155–9

73. Martin RE, Hanson BL, Bosco JJ et al. Combined modality treatment of symptomatic pancreatic duct lithiasis. Arch Surg 1995; 130: 375–80

74. Traverso LW, Longmire WP. Preserving of the pylorus in pancreaticoduodenectomy. Surg Gynecol Obstet 1978; 146: 959–62

75. Beger HG, Krautzberger W, Bittner R, Büchler M. Duodenum-preserving resection of the head of the pancreas in severe pancreatitis. Surg Gynecol Obstet 1989; 209: 273–6

76. Delhaye M, Vandermeeren A, Baize M, Cremer M. Extracorporeal shock-wave lithotripsy of pancreatic calculi. Gastroenterology 1992; 102: 610–20

77. Cremer M, Devière J, Delhaye M, Baizer M, Vandermeeren A. Stenting in severe chronic pancreatitis: result of medium-term follow-up in seventy-six patients. Endoscopy 1991; 23: 171–6

78. Binmoeller KE, Jue P, Seifert H, Nam WC, lzbicki J, Soehendra N. Endoscopic pancreatic stent drainage in chronic pancreatitis and a dominant stricture: long-term results. Endoscopy 1995; 27: 638–44

79. Sauerbruch T, Holl J, Sackmann M, Paumgartner G. Extracorporeal lithotripsy of pancreatic stones in patients with chronic pancreatitis and pain: a prospective follow-up study. Gut 1992; 33: 969–72

80. Schneider HT, Andrea M, Benninger J et al. Piezoelectric shock-wave lithotripsy of pancreatic duct stones. Am J Gastroenterol 1994; 89: 2042–8

81. Barthet M, Sahel J, Bodiou-Bertei C, Bernard JP. Endoscopic transpapillary drainage of pancreatic pseudocysts. Gastrointest Endosc 1995; 42: 208–13

82. Binmoeller KE, Seifer H, Walter A, Soehendra N. Transpapillary and transmural drainage of pancreatic pseudocysts. Gastrointest Endosc 1995; 42: 219–24

83. Eckhauser FE, Knol JA, Mulholland MW, Colletti LM. Pancreatic surgery. Curr Opin Gastroenterol 1996; 12: 448–56

84. Büchler MW, Friess H, Müller MW, Wheatley AM, Beger HG. Randomized trial of duodenum-preserving pancreatic head resection versus pylorus-preserving Whipple procedure in chronic pancreatitis. Am J Surg 1995; 169: 65–70

85. Frey CE, Amikura K. Local resection of the head of the pancreas combined with longitudinal pancreaticojejunostomy in the management of patients with chronic pancreatitis. Ann Surg 1994; 220: 492–507

86. lzbicki JR, Bloechle C, Knoefel WT, Kuechler T, Binmoeller KE, Broelsch CE. Duodenum-preserving resection of the head of the pancreas in chronic pancreatitis: a prospective, randomized trial. Ann Surg 1995; 221: 350–458

87. Büchler MW, Friess H, Bittner R et al. Duodenum-preserving pancreatic head resection: long-term results. J Gastrointest Surg 1997; 1: 13–9

88. Beger HG, Krautzberger W, Bittner R, Büchler M, Limmer J. Duodenum-preserving resection in the head of the pancreas in patients with severe chronic pancreatitis. Surgery 1985; 97: 467–73

89. Beger HG, Büchler M. Duodenum-preserving reaction of the head of the pancreas in chronic pancreatitis with inflammatory mass in the head. World J Surg 1990; 14: 83–7

90. Morel P, Mathey P, Corboud H et al. Pylorus-preserving duodeno-pancreatectomy: long term complications and comparisons with the Whipple procedure. World J Surg 1990; 14: 642–7

91. Traverso LW, Kozarek RA. The Whipple procedure for severe complications of chronic pancreatitis. Arch Surg 1993; 128: 1047–53

92. Gall FP, Gebhardt C, Mesiter R, Zirngibl H, Schneider MU. Severe chronic cephalic pancreatitis: use of partial duodenopancreatectomy with occlusion of the pancreatic duct in 289 patients. World J Surg 1989; 13: 809–17

93. Rattner DW, del-Castillo F, Warshaw AL. Pitfalls of distal pancreatectomy for relief of pain in chronic pancreatitis. Am J Surg 1996; 171: 142–6

94. Keith RG, Saibil EG, Sheppard RH. Treatment of chronic alcoholic pancreatitis by pancreatic resection. Am J Surg 1989; 157: 156–62

95. Alvarado F. Distribution of nerves within the pancreas. J Int Coll Surg 1955; 23: 675–99

96. Ischia S, Ischia A, Polati E, Finco G. Three posterior percutaneous celiac plexus block techniques. A prospective, randomised study in 61 patients with pancreatic cancer pain. Anaesthesiology 1992; 76: 534–40

97. Bengtsson M, Löfström JB. Nerve block in pancreatic pain. Acta Chir Scand 1990; 156: 285–91

98. Hegedüs V. Relief of pancreatic pain by radiography-guided block. AJR 1979;133: 1101–3

99. Jackson SH, Jacobs JB. A radiographic approach to celiac ganglion block. Radiology 1969; 92: 1372–3

100. Sharfman WH, Walsh TD. Has the analgesic efficacy of neurolytic celiac plexus block been demonstrated in pancreatic cancer pain? Pain 1990; 41: 267–71

101. Mallet-Guy P, de Beaujeu MJ. Treatment of chronic pancreatitis by unilateral splanchnicectomy. Arch Surg 1950; 60: 233–41

102. Mallet-Guy P. Late and very late results of resection of the nervous system in the treatment of chronic relapsing pancreatitis. Am J Surg 1983; 145: 234–8

103. Whire TT. Pain relieving procedures in chronic pancreatitis. Contemp Surg 1983; 22: 43–8

104. Yoshioka H, Wakabayashi T. Therapeutic neurotomy on head of pancreas for relief of pain due to chronic pancreatitis. Arch Surg 1958; 76: 546–54

105. Hiraoka T, Watanabe E, Katoh T et al. A new surgical approach for control of pain in chronic pancreatitis: complete denervation of the pancreas. Am J Surg 1986; 152: 549–51

106. Ray BS, Neill CL. Abdominal visceral sensation in man. Ann Surg 1947; 126: 709–24

107. Andrén-Sandberg Å, Dervenis C, Lowenfels A. Etiological links between chronic pancreatitis and pancreatic cancer. Scand J Gastroenterol 1997; 32: 97–103

108. Imrie CW. Management of recurrent pain following previous surgery for chronic pancreatitis. World J Surg 1990; 14: 88–93

109. Stone HH, Chauvin EJ. Pancreatic denervation for pain relief in chronic alcohol associated pancreatitis. Br J Surg 1990; 77: 303–5

110. Petrin P, Andreoli A, Antoiutti M et al. Surgery for chronic pancreatitis: what quality of life ahead? World J Surg 1995; 19: 398–402

111. Broome AH, Eisen GM, Harland RC, Collins BH, Meyers WC, Pappas TN. Quality of life after treatment for pancreatitis. Ann Surg 1996; 223: 665–72

112. Frey CF. Standards for assessing outcome in chronic pancreatitis. Probl Gen Surg 1998; 15: 1–6

113. Pain JA, Knight MJ. Pancreaticogastrostomy: the preferred operation for pain relief for chronic pancreatitis. Br J Surg 1988; 75: 220–2

114. Flemming WR, Williamson RCN. Role of total pancreatectomy in the treatment of patients with end stage chronic pancreatitis. Br J Surg 1995; 82: 1409–12

115. Bloeche C, Izbicki R, Knoefel WT, Keuchler T, Broelsch CE. Quality of life in chronic pancreatitis – results after duodenum-preserving resection of the head of the pancreas. Pancreas 1995; 11: 77–85

116. Aaronson NK, Ahmedzai S, Berman B et al. The European Organization for Research and Treatment of Cancer QLQ-30: a quality-of-life instrument for use in international clinical trials in oncology. J Natl Cancer Inst 1993; 85: 365–76

117. Ihse I, Permert J. Enzyme therapy and pancreatic pain. Acta Chir Scand 1990; 156: 281–3

26 Management of localized chronic pancreatitis

ME Martignoni, H Friess and Markus W Büchler

Introduction

Definition

Chronic pancreatitis can be defined as a benign, inflammatory disorder of the pancreas which leads to permanent damage to the structure of the pancreas and impairment of pancreatic function to a varying degree, depending on the loss of pancreatic parenchyma. The evolution of the disease may be static, with some preservation of pancreatic function, or may be progressive, with the development of pancreatic insufficiency and steatorrhoea in the advanced clinical expression of the disease.

Aetiology

The most common aetiological factor (80% of the patients) for chronic pancreatitis in industrialized countries is probably long-term alcohol abuse. Recently, hereditary chronic pancreatitis was characterized by a gene mutation of the cationic trypsinogen, leading to insufficient deactivation of intracellular trypsinogen with subsequent auto-digestion. However, there is also an idiopathic form of chronic pancreatitis, with a juvenile onset (<35 years) and a late onset (>65 years), as well as an obstructive type of chronic pancreatitis. In some geographic areas chronic pancreatitis is caused by nutritional factors, such as low protein intake and cassava intake. Because this form occurs mainly in tropical regions it is called tropical pancreatitis.[1]

Symptoms

In some cases (5.8–20%) there may be only exocrine and endocrine insufficiency of pancreatic function, but for the majority of patients pain is the predominant symptom, causing much discomfort in their daily life.[2,3]

Exocrine pancreas insufficiency

Exocrine pancreas insufficiency does not play a major prognostic role in chronic pancreatitis. Occasionally, massive steatorrhoea and malabsorption leading to cachexia and susceptibility to infection has prognostic significance. However, these symptoms will not occur as long as lipase output is more than 10% of the normal lipase output, and studies have shown that it may take more than 10–20 years for the inflammatory process to destroy the pancreatic parenchyma.[4]

Endocrine pancreas insufficiency

Although almost all patients with chronic pancreatitis have some degree of exocrine pancreatic insufficiency at the time of diagnosis, this is not true for endocrine pancreatic insufficiency. In a study by Lankisch et al.,[5] only 8% of patients with chronic pancreatitis showed moderate or severe endocrine pancreatic insufficiency at the clinical onset of disease, whereas 78% of the patients had endocrine insufficiency 10 years later (Table 26.1).

Pain and its aetiology

In chronic pancreatitis pain is one of the predominant symptoms. In the natural course of the disease over 85% of patients will be affected.[6] Pain in chronic pancreatitis can be continuous or intermittent, sharp or dull, and might be exacerbated by food intake, so in some cases it mimics peptic ulcer disease. It is usually located in the epigastrium or the right or left hypochondria, and it radiates, penetrating to the back and occasionally to the left shoulder. It can last from a few hours to several days or weeks. Therapeutic attempts to manage pain in chronic pancreatitis

Table 26.1 Endocrine pancreatic insufficiency in 335 patients with chronic pancreatitis, including 24 patients with painless chronic pancreatitis[5]

Endocrine pancreatic insufficiency	At onset of disease	At end of observation (after 10 years)
Absent	307 (92%)	75 (22%)
Moderate	13 (4%)	127(38%)
Severe	15 (4%)	133(40%)
Moderate + severe	28 (8%)	260 (78%)

conservatively have been rather disappointing. Therefore the most common indication for surgical treatment of chronic pancreatitis is intractable pain, mostly in combination with complications in organs neighbouring the pancreas.[7,8]

The mechanisms which contribute to the generation of pain and the best method to manage pain in chronic pancreatitis are still controversial. The hypotheses that the pain is generated by an increase of intraductal and intraparenchymal pressure, or because of postprandial pancreatic hyperstimulation caused by the decrease of pancreatic enzyme secretion into the duodenum (with subsequent insufficient function of the so-called 'negative feedback mechanism') are now questionable as reliable explanations of abdominal pain in patients with chronic pancreatitis.[9] Studies using octreotide, a somatostatin analogue which inhibits pancreatic secretion and therefore should interrupt some of the postulated pain cycle described above, failed to reduce the pain syndrome in many patients with chronic pancreatitis.[9,10]

Published reports suggest another interesting model of pain generation describing damage of pancreatic nerves and an interaction of pancreatic nerves with inflammatory cells. In electron-microscopic analysis, foci of inflammatory cells are located close to nerves which exhibit a damaged perineurium with invasion by eosinophilic granulocytes.[11,12] Furthermore, a significantly greater diameter and density of nerves have been described in chronic pancreatitis in comparison with the normal pancreas. In addition to these morphological alterations, increased levels of growth-associated protein 43 (GAP 43) and of the pain transmitting neuropeptides substance P and calcitonin-gene-related peptide (CGRP) have been reported and proposed to be mediators of pain in chronic pancreatitis.[12,13] This new concept of pain in chronic pancreatitis is supported by recent studies, which could demonstrate that the substrates of pain-generating neuropeptides (NGF, BDNF) and the corresponding receptors (NK-1) are overexpressed in chronic pancreatitis.[14–17]

Molecular alterations in chronic pancreatitis

Molecular analysis has added continuously to our understanding of the histopathology of chronic pancreatitis in recent years. With the use of Northern blot analysis and in situ hybridization, enhanced expression of growth factors and growth factor receptors has been reported. For example, overexpression of the epidermal growth factor receptors (EGF-R) in chronic pancreatitis is frequently associated with overexpression of one of its ligands, transforming growth factor alpha (TGF-α).[18] The observation that transgenic mice, overexpressing TGF-α in their pancreas, develop pancreatic fibrosis, parenchymal degeneration and dedifferentiation of acinar cells into duct-like structures, gave the first hints that activation of the EGF-R pathway is of relevance for the progression of the disease.[19] In addition, the c-erbB-2 proto-oncogene, which is a transmembrane tyrosine kinase receptor closely related to EGF-R, is frequently enhanced in patients with chronic pancreatitis.[20] Interestingly, the levels of c-erbB-2 mRNA are positively correlated with the inflammatory enlargement of the pancreatic head, underlining the pathophysiological importance of tyrosine kinase receptor activation.[20] In addition to activation of growth factor receptors, chronic pancreatitis also features activation of acidic and basic fibroblast growth factors (aFGF, bFGF), which are strongly angio- and fibrogenic, cripto, TGF-β and platelet-derived growth factor (PDGF) and its type beta receptor.[21–23] In a recent study, connective tissue growth factor (CTGF), which is regulated by transforming growth factor beta (TGF-β), and its signaling receptors TGF-β receptor I, subtype ALK5 and TGF-β receptor II as well as collagen type I, was found to be concomitantly overexpressed in the pancreatic tissue.[24] This upregulation of profibrotic mediators is coupled with the activation of the plasminogen activating cascade, a proteolytic pathway, which allows tissue remodelling, repair and replacement of pancreatic parenchyma by fibrosis.[25] Furthermore, accumulation of fibrosis and the upregulation of extracellular matrix synthesis-promoting cascades is associated with activation of

Table 26.2 **Preoperative morbidity in chronic pancreatitis patients with and without pancreatic head enlargement**[28]

Clinical parameters	With head enlargement	Without head enlargement
Severe daily pain	67%	40%
Common bile duct obstruction	64/138 (46%)	16/141 (11%)
Pancreatic duct stenosis	72/135 (53%)	45/141 (32%)
Duodenal obstruction	37/122 (30%)	9/121 (7%)
Cysts	77/127 (61%)	43/85 (51%)
Vascular involvement	18/122 (15%)	6/73 (8%)
Diabetes mellitus	25/138 (18%)	42/141 (30%)

perforin-producing cytotoxic lymphocytes and phospholipase A type II and type IV, indicating that a variety of different pathophysiological events are of importance in the course of chronic pancreatitis.[26,27]

Inflammatory mass in chronic pancreatitis

The most frequent location of an inflammatory mass in chronic pancreatitis is the pancreatic head.[28] Because many patients are referred to a gastroenterological or surgical centre by general practitioners, outpatient gastroenterologists and smaller community hospitals, a selection bias is highly probable. Therefore, the exact prevalence of inflammatory pancreatic head enlargement in patients with chronic pancreatitis is not known.[28] Furthermore, it is not known why enlargement of the pancreas occurs predominantly in the pancreatic head region and rarely in the body or tail. However, analysis of growth factors and growth factor receptors in resected pancreatic head tissue samples has revealed that the expression of the growth factor receptor c-erbB-2, which belongs to the EGF receptor family, is positively correlated to the size of the pancreatic head.[20,28]

To evaluate the clinical consequences of inflammatory head enlargement, the prevalence and the clinical consequences of inflammatory head enlargement in patients with chronic pancreatitis were studied.[28] Out of 279 patients with chronic pancreatitis, 49% (138 patients) had pancreatic head enlargement of more than 4 cm in diameter, as shown by ultrasonography, contrast-enhanced computed tomography (CT) scan and/or intraoperative findings. There were no differences in sex, age and length of alcohol abuse in patients with and without pancreatic head enlargement. However, patients with pancreatic head enlargement showed a higher pain score and more typical complications of chronic pancreatitis, such as

common bile duct obstruction and duodenal stenosis, vascular compression and main pancreatic duct obstruction, at the time of clinical presentation. Interestingly, they also had a better preserved pancreatic exocrine and endocrine function than patients with no pancreatic head enlargement. These findings suggest that an inflammatory mass of the head of the pancreas is found early in the development of chronic pancreatitis and might lead to more morbidity of neighbouring organs (Table 26.2).

Indications for surgical treatment in localized chronic pancreatitis

When should an operation be considered?

The primary therapy for chronic pancreatitis is conservative, symptom-related treatment.[10] If complaints are not relieved, or if there are complications in the course of the disease such as pancreatic head enlargement, distal common bile duct stenosis, segmental duodenal obstruction, main pancreatic duct stenosis, vascular obstruction or pancreatic pseudocysts, surgical treatment should be considered (Fig. 26.1).[29–32] In the aim for a better understanding of the course of chronic pancreatitis, and to decide when and which operation should be performed, several classification attempts have been made. But the two classifications of the chronic pancreatitis meetings in Marseilles and the Cambridge classification (based mainly on ERCP findings) did not have the expected clinical impact.[33,34] In order to more appropriately use the clinical experience in the field of chronic pancreatitis, and to make better use of the progress in diagnostic methods, a classification of chronic pancreatitis is crucial and could possibly help the surgeon decide whether or not to operate. Therefore a new classification of chronic pancreatitis based on the combination of clinical and radiological findings was proposed by Büchler and Malfertheiner at the Chronic Pancreatitis 2000 meeting in Bern (Table 26.3).

A

B

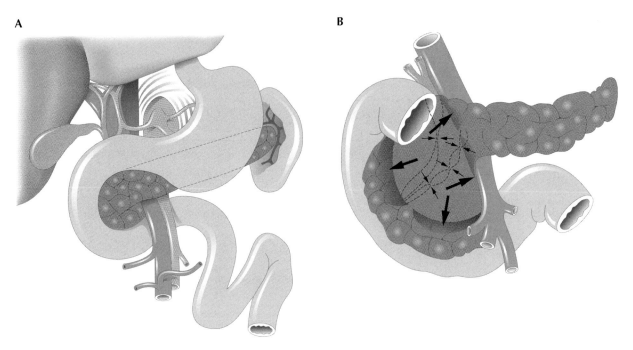

Figure 26.1 (A) Anatomy of the upper abdomen. (B) Local complications in chronic pancreatitis which require surgery; inflammatory enlargement of the pancreatic head, single or multiple obstruction of the common bile duct (medium-sized arrows), single or multiple pancreatic duct stenosis (large arrows), obstruction of retropancreatic intestinal vessels (large arrows).

Table 26.3 **Local complications in chronic pancreatitis which require surgery**[28]
1. Bile duct stenosis
2. Splenic vein thrombosis and segmental portal hypertension
3. Duodenal stenosis
4. Single or multiple pancreatic duct stenosis
5. Colonic stenosis
6. Pancreatic abscess: infected pseudocyst
7. Pancreatic fistula leading to an extrapancreatic pseudocyst or to pancreatic ascites
8. Bleeding from pseudocyst-related false aneurysm

Which operation should be performed?

Two different surgical approaches are possible. The surgeon must decide whether to perform a drainage or a resection procedure.

Drainage procedures

To preserve the exocrine and endocrine function of the pancreas, a drainage procedure should be considered first. Only a few indications for drainage lead to good long-term results; however, a strong indication for a drainage procedure must be present. Pseudocysts and dilatation of the pancreatic duct are the most common indications for an

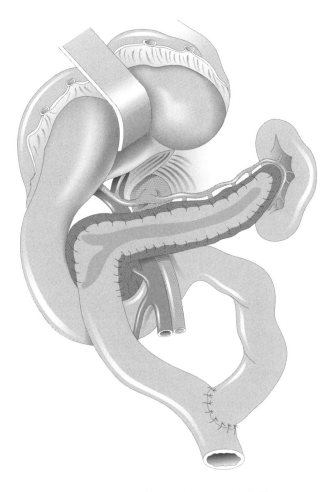

Figure 26.2 Outcome of the Partington–Rochelle operation.

operative drainage strategy. It has been shown that pseudocysts which are bigger than 6 cm in diameter need operative treatment within 1 year of presentation. The incidence for drainage procedures in pseudocysts smaller than 6 cm is about 40%.[35]

Sphincterotomy, caudal pancreaticojejunostomy and longitudinal pancreaticojejunostomy (Partington–Rochelle) are the most common operative drainage techniques. Only the last provides satisfactory results in long-term follow-up.[36,37] In patients with dilatation of the pancreatic duct, the Partington–Rochelle is a particularly suitable option (Fig. 26.2).[38] There is a lack of consensus over the extent to which the pancreatic duct must be dilated for successful drainage, with recommendations ranging from at least 3 mm to 8 mm. The procedure described by Partington and Rochelle in 1960 is a modification of the Puestow drainage.[39] Construction of the longitudinal pancreaticojejunostomy anastomosis is followed by complete drainage of the Wirsung and Santorini ducts along the whole pancreas.[39]

Although the Partington–Rochelle operation is a safe technique (with postoperative mortality between 0% and 5% and an operative morbidity of 20% to 25%), the main problem of the longitudinal pancreaticojejunostomy is that the pancreatic head is frequently enlarged and this may impair adequate drainage of the pancreatic head. Therefore, if localized pancreatitis is accompanied by pancreatic head enlargement, pancreatic head resection should be considered.

Pancreatic resection

The most common indications for resection of the pancreas are intractable pain, suspicion of carcinoma and complications involving neighbouring structures, including common bile duct stenosis, duodenal obstruction, vascular obstruction and single or multiple main pancreatic duct stenosis (Table 26.4).

The Whipple operation

During and since the last decade there has been increased willingness to perform a Whipple operation for both benign and malignant diseases. This is because most pancreatic operations are now performed in specialized centres by surgeons with considerable experience, and operative mortalities are <5%, with morbidity in an equally acceptable range, and because of improvements in postoperative care.[40,41] The indications for performing such an extensive operation in localized pancreatitis are not seen very often, but in case of suspicion of a malignant tumour this operation is still the operation of choice (Fig. 26.3).

Table 26.4 **Indications for DPPHR in 298 patients with chronic pancreatitis**

Pancreatic head enlargement	248	(83%)
Common bile duct stenosis	144	(48%)
Duodenal stenosis	95	(32%)
Vascular compression	52	(17%)
Pain	279	(94%)

A

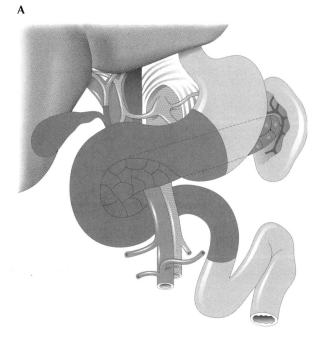

B

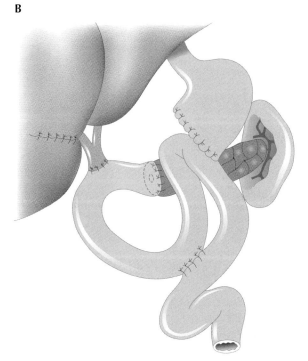

Figure 26.3 (A) Tissue removed with resection margins in classical Whipple resection. (B) Reconstruction after classical Whipple resection.

A

B

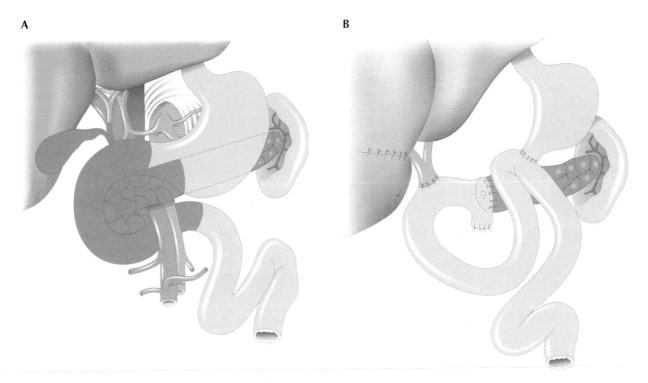

Figure 26.4 (A) Tissue removed with resection margins in PP-Whipple resection. (B) Reconstruction after PP-Whipple resection.

The distinction between chronic pancreatitis and early pancreatic cancer can sometimes be difficult. In a review by Trede et al.,[42] 15 of 100 patients (15%) who underwent Whipple resection for chronic pancreatitis were found to have pancreatic cancer. Conversely, 43 of 311 patients operated on for pancreatic carcinoma were shown by histology to have chronic pancreatitis.[42] As a result, careful evaluation with ERCP and CT and/or MRI scan is necessary preoperatively in all patients with suspected chronic pancreatitis to exclude pancreatic cancer.

Although the early postoperative results of a classical Whipple resection for chronic pancreatitis are acceptable, quality control studies have shown that the operation's long-term results are unsatisfactory.[43] These results are especially disappointing with regard to quality of life: there is often poor postoperative digestive function, including dumping, diarrhoea, peptic ulcer and dyspeptic complaints.[44]

The Whipple operation was designed for radical resection of a malignant tumour, but has subsequently been used to treat benign pancreatic disorders such as chronic pancreatitis. Today, newer organ-preserving operative techniques have been introduced which offer the same or even better results with less extensive resection. The classical procedure is now only indicated to treat localized chronic pancreatitis when there is suspicion of malignancy and intraoperative frozen section cannot exclude a malignant tumour.

The pylorus-preserving Whipple resection
The pylorus-preserving Whipple resection is a modification of the classical Whipple operation which was introduced by Kenneth Watson in 1946 as an organ-preserving operation to provide better postoperative long-term results.[45] This resection technique provides good results in pain relief and long-term follow-up. By preserving the stomach, the pylorus and the first part of the duodenum, the pylorus-preserving pancreaticoduodenectomy (PPPD) allows normal digestion of food by maintaining the volume and the mixing function of the stomach (Fig. 26.4). Furthermore, by preserving the pylorus, it prevents bile and pancreatic juice reflux into the stomach, which can lead to alkaline gastritis and eventually to gastric ulcerations.

According to recent studies, the perioperative mortality with a PPPD ranges from 0% to 4%.[46,47] The most common postoperative complication in PPPD is a subsequent problem with gastric emptying, reported in about 30% of patients.[48] However, this seems to be only a temporary problem.[49] In comparison with the classical Whipple operation, the results regarding quality of life are better, especially in long-term survivors of malignancies and in patients operated on for benign pancreatic disease. In chronic pancreatitis, 90% of patients gain weight and the operation leads to pain relief in 85–95%, even 5 years after surgery.[50] However, more than one-third of patients need oral enzyme supplementation, and about 50% develop insulin-dependent

A

B

C

D

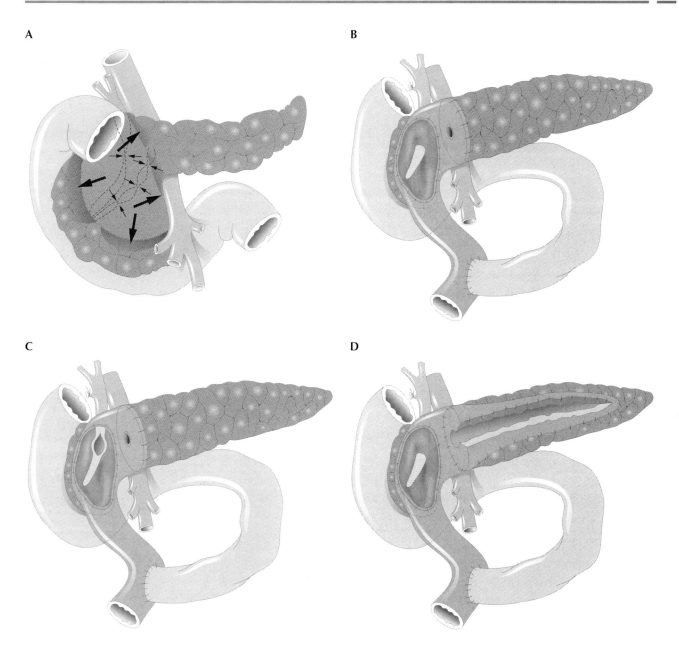

Figure 26.5 (A) Local complications in chronic pancreatitis which require surgery; single or multiple obstruction of the common bile duct (medium-sized arrows), pancreatic duct (large arrows) and retropancreatic intestinal vessels (large arrows). (B) Standard reconstruction after duodenum-preserving pancreatic head resection: 1. partial resection of the pancreatic head; 2. end-to-end anastomosis with the left pancreas and a side-to-side anastomosis with the remaining pancreatic head. (C) Reconstruction after standard duodenum-preserving pancreatic head resection creating an inner anastomosis of the common bile duct with an interposed jejunal loop for additional decompression of the common bile duct. (D) Puestow modification of the duodenum-preserving pancreatic head resection with a side-to-side anastomosis between the left pancreas and the interposed jejunal loop.

diabetes mellitus (IDDM) within 5 years of their operation.[51]

Therefore, in localized chronic pancreatitis this operation might be considered when a large inflammatory mass in the pancreatic head is found.

Duodenum-preserving pancreatic head resection (DPPHR)
In 1972 Hans Beger and co-workers introduced a new technique especially for treating pancreatic

head-related complications of chronic pancreatitis.[52,53] In this procedure the pancreatic head is resected subtotally, with the body and tail of the pancreas, the pylorus, the duodenum and the extrapancreatic bile duct being preserved. With this operation only the 'pacemaker' of chronic pancreatitis—the pancreatic head—is resected, and the normal anatomy of the upper gut is preserved (Fig. 26.5). Because of this and the preservation of the body and tail of the pancreas, there is generally no

Table 26.5 Postoperative complications after DPPHR in 298 patients[55]

Complications	No.	Percentage	Number of relaparotomies
Intestinal bleeding	17	5.7	3
Intraabdominal abcess	9	3.0	3
Anastomosis leakage	6	2.0	5
Pancreatic fistula	8	2.7	–
Sepsis	4	1.3	1
Small bowel obstruction	3	1.0	2
Duodenal wall ischemia	1	0.3	1
Common bile duct stenosis	1	0.3	1
Ulcer perforation	1	0.3	1
Total	50	16.8	17 (5.7%)

restriction of exocrine and endocrine function of the pancreas. Furthermore, patients have normal digestion, and this increases quality of life in addition to providing excellent pain relief.[54]

The duodenum-preserving pancreatic head resection is generally indicated in patients with continual abdominal pain, or if the inflammatory pancreatic head tumour starts to compromise adjacent organs, with complications such as common bile duct obstruction or duodenal stenosis (Table 26.4).

Adequate preoperative investigation needs both ERCP and CT. In the case of any clinical or ultrasonographic signs of obstruction of the retro- or peripancreatic vessels, angiography or Duplex scan of the coeliac trunk is necessary. The operative technique consists of three phases: first, exploration and full exposure of the pancreas; second, subtotal resection of the pancreatic head; and third, reconstruction by interposition of a jejunal loop and pancreaticojejunal anastomosis (Fig. 26.5).[55,56] Past experience has shown that this operation provides an excellent postoperative outcome and low mortality and morbidity rates.

In a series of 298 patients, 17 (5.7%) underwent reoperation for early postoperative complications such as bleeding or leakage of the pancreaticointestinal anastomosis (Table 26.5). One patient died because of pulmonary embolism and two died due to sepsis after anastomotic leakage, corresponding to a hospital mortality rate of 1.01% (3/298). Postoperative outcome was excellent and the long-term results are promising. In 1997 we carried out a long-term follow-up of the 298 patients operated on to date. At final evaluation 232 patients (87%) were available for long-term follow-up and the results are shown in Table 26.6.

Table 26.6 Late results of a long-term follow-up of 232 patients who underwent DPPHR. Median follow-up period: 6 years (range 1–22 years)[55]

Pain:		
none	143	(62%)
seldom	61	(26%)
frequent	28	(12%)
Professional rehabilitation:		
complete	147	(63%)
unemployed	11	(5%)
retired	74	(32%)
Body weight increase	187	(81%)
Late mortality	23	(10%)

With regard to endocrine pancreatic function, only 6 patients (2%) developed insulin-dependent diabetes mellitus in the early postoperative period.[57] A recent study of the long-term effects of DPPHS demonstrated that an excellent quality of life was being enjoyed by patients 26 years after surgery (Table 26.7).[58]

These data demonstrate the clear advantage of the duodenum-preserving pancreatic head resection over the Whipple procedures. By preserving the extrapancreatic organs, especially the stomach and duodenum, this procedure leads to normal digestion and preserves a normal glucose metabolism after surgical intervention. By resecting only the pancreatic head and preserving the other organs, which are only secondarily involved in the inflammation process, it is possible to obtain excellent results without losing normal digestion.

Table 26.7 Six months' follow-up after duodenum-preserving pancreatic head resection and pylorus-preserving Whipple resection

	Duodenum-preserving pancreatic head resection (19 patients)	Pylorus-preserving Whipple resection (17 patients)
Pain:		
none	14/19	8/17
rare	3/19	4/17
frequent	2/19	5/17
Professional rehabilitation	14/17	9/14
Hospital readmission	2/19	5/17
Weight:		
increase	16/19	12/17
loss	0/19	4/17
average increase (kg)	+4.4 ± 1.0	+2.1 ± 1.2
Exocrine pancreatic function (PLT) mean (maximum; minimum):		
preoperative	2.70 (0;8.25)	2.05 (0.48;6.6)
postoperative	1.40 (0;4.41)	1.13 (0;4.87)

The Frey procedure

In past years, especially in the United States, the duodenum-preserving pancreatic head resection was not well accepted by surgeons. In 1987 Frey and Smith introduced a modification of Beger's duodenum-preserving pancreatic head resection.[59] A local resection of the pancreatic head without dividing the pancreas was followed by a longitudinal pancreatico-jejunostomy. In this way, two principles of surgery were combined in chronic pancreatitis: partial resection and drainage.[60] In a follow-up period of 37 months Frey and Amikura found that 75% of the patients were pain-free and they reported no postoperative mortality.[60] Meanwhile Izbicki et al.[61] demonstrated comparable results in a prospective, randomized study (mean follow-up 18 months) comparing the Frey procedure with the DPPHR. The only difference was a significantly lower postoperative morbidity after the Frey procedure (11% versus 21% after DPPHR). These data show that both the duodenum-preserving pancreatic head resection and its modification, the Frey procedure, are safe and effective resection techniques in the management of pain and complications in chronic pancreatitis. However, because the Frey operation is too new for reliable long-term follow-up study, no long-term results are available.

Left pancreatic resection

This operation should be performed when the inflammatory mass of localized pancreatitis is located in the tail or the body of the pancreas. However, this situation is clinically rare in patients suffering from chronic pancreatitis. The resection can be done in two ways, either by removing about half of the pancreas, or with subtotal pancreatectomy, which includes resection of 95% of the pancreas. Twenty years ago this technique was the standard surgical treatment in localized chronic pancreatitis, but as the pathophysiology of chronic pancreatitis has become better understood (and we have learned that the pancreatic head is the cause of pain in chronic pancreatitis) left pancreatic resection has lost its clinical importance.[62] Furthermore, resection of most of the pancreatic islet cells (which are located in the tail of the pancreas) leads frequently to insulin-dependent diabetes mellitus (IDDM). This may be the reason for the high mortality and morbidity rate in the long-term follow-up of these patients, Therefore, the use of left pancreatic resection in patients with chronic pancreatitis is becoming more and more questioned.[63] There remain only a few indications for pancreatic left resection, such as persistent or bleeding pseudocysts and chronic pancreatitis with splenic vein thrombosis. A careful preoperative evaluation, including CT, ERCP and/or angio MRCP, is necessary to select the patients who will benefit from this operation.

Which operation should be the gold standard in the management of localized chronic pancreatitis? Comparison of the different types of operations

Duodenum-preserving pancreatic head resection versus classical Whipple operation

Studies have compared the duodenum-preserving pancreatic head resection and the old gold standard for resection in chronic pancreatitis, the classical Whipple operation.[64] According to their results, patients who had undergone duodenum-preserving pancreatic head resection had a significantly more rapid convalescence than patients who underwent a Whipple operation (average hospital stay 16.5 days versus 21.7 days in the Whipple group). In addition, with regard to endocrine and exocrine function of the pancreas, the DPPHR showed a clear advantage over the Whipple resection. Only 2/20 patients in the DPPHR group required pancreatic enzyme substitution, compared to all 20 patients in the classical Whipple group.[64] These data demonstrate the clear advantage of duodenum-preserving pancreatic head resection in the management of localized chronic pancreatitis.

Duodenum-preserving pancreatic head resection versus classical PP-Whipple resection

In most of the studies of patients undergoing a pylorus-preserving Whipple (PP-Whipple) operation or DPPHR, a general postoperative improvement is reported. To evaluate the advantages and disadvantages of these two techniques a unicentre, randomized study comparing the two procedures was performed.[54,65] The patients were investigated preoperatively, as well as 10 days and 6 months postoperatively, with regard to glucose tolerance, pain relief, weight gain, hospital readmission, professional rehabilitation and postoperative complications. In the 6-month follow-up, patients who underwent the duodenum-preserving pancreatic head resection had less pain, greater weight gain, a better glucose tolerance and a higher insulin secretion capacity than patients who underwent the pylorus-preserving Whipple resection (Table 26.7).

The postoperative mortality was zero and the early postoperative morbidity was comparable in both groups (DPPHR: 3/20 patients, 15%; pylorus-preserving Whipple: 4/20 patients, 20%). Of the three patients with complications who underwent duodenum-preserving pancreatic head resection, two suffered bleeding and one developed a pulmonary complication. Of the four patients with complications who underwent the pylorus-preserving Whipple operation, one suffered a stroke, one developed a fistula, and two had pulmonary complications. At the 6-month follow-up the results of the duodenum-preserving pancreatic resection were clearly superior to the pylorus-preserving Whipple operation with regard to endocrine and exocrine pancreatic function, professional rehabilitation and weight increase. Therefore we believe the duodenum-preserving pancreatic head resection should be considered as the standard operation in localized chronic pancreatitis of the pancreatic head.

Conclusion

In the 1960s and 1970s the classical Whipple operation and the pylorus-preserving Whipple resection were the two techniques generally used in the management of chronic pancreatitis. Due to increased knowledge of the pathophysiology of chronic pancreatitis and of the mechanisms which promote the inflammatory process, new operations have been developed to resect only the main source of pain in chronic pancreatitis—the pancreatic head. The effectiveness of duodenum-preserving pancreatic head resection has been evaluated in several studies. With regard to pain relief, complication rate, mortality and morbidity, and preservation of endocrine and exocrine pancreatic function, the DPPHR demonstrates a clear advantage over the classical Whipple operation or pylorus-preserving Whipple resection.

A modification of the duodenum-preserving pancreatic head resection—the Frey procedure—provides postoperative results comparable to those of DPPHR. Long-term follow-up studies with greater numbers of patients are still needed to determine whether this operation is as useful as the duodenum-preserving pancreatic head resection in the management of localized chronic pancreatitis.

For the above-mentioned reasons, and because the duodenum-preserving pancreatic head resection is the operation which tackles the current thinking on the pathophysiology of chronic pancreatitis, we believe that the duodenum-preserving pancreatic head resection should be considered as the standard operation in the management of localized chronic pancreatitis.

Key points

- Most frequent location of an inflammatory mass in chronic pancreatitis is the head of the pancreas.
- Indications for surgical treatment in localized chronic pancreatitis:
    Symptoms of pancreatic head enlargement
    Duodenal obstruction
    Distal common bile duct obstruction
    Main pancreatic duct stenosis
    Vascular obstruction
    Symptomatic pancreatic cyst and/or pseudocyst.
- Drainage procedures should aim to maintain exocrine and endocrine function.
- Indications for resection of the pancreatic head in chronic pancreatitis:
    Intractible pain
    Suspicion of carcinoma
    Duodenal obstruction
    Vascular obstruction
    Single or multiple stenoses of proximal main pancreatic duct.

REFERENCES

1. Arvanitakis C. Is chronic pancreatitis a disease of the same type? In: Dervenis CG ed. Advances in pancreatic disease. Stuttgart: Georg Thieme Verlag, 1996: 210

2. Ammann RW, Akovbiantz A, Largiadèr F, Schueler G. Course and outcome of chronic pancreatitis. Longitudinal study of a mixed medical–surgical series of 245 patients. Gastroenterology 1984; 86: 820–8

3. Miyake H, Harada H, Kunichika K, Ochi K, Kimura I. Clinical course and prognosis of chronic pancreatitis. Pancreas 1987; 2: 378–85

4. Layer P, Yamamoto H, Kalthoff L, Clain JE, Bakken LJ, DiMagno EP. The different courses of early- and late-onset idiopathic and alcoholic chronic pancreatitis. Gastroenterology 1994; 107: 1481–7

5. Lankisch PG, Lohr-Happe A, Otto J, Creutzfeldt W. Natural course in chronic pancreatitis. Pain, exocrine and endocrine pancreatic insufficiency and prognosis of the disease. Digestion 1993; 54: 148–55

6. Forell MM. Diagnostic procedure in chronic pancreatitis in relation to the values of individual technics. Internist (Berl) 1979; 20: 360–6

7. Tzias B. Chronic pancreatitis: pain aetiology and management. In: Dervenis CG ed. Advances in pancreatic disease. Stuttgart: Georg Thieme Verlag, 1996: 213

8. Evans JD, Wilson PG, Carver C et al. Outcome of surgery for chronic pancreatitis. Br J Surg 1997; 84: 624–9

9. Di Magno EP, Layer P, Clain JE. Chronic pancreatitis. In: Go VLW, DiMagno EP, Gardner JD, Lebenthal E, Reber HA, Scheele GA, eds. The pancreas. New York: Raven Press, 1993: 707

10. Di Magno EP. Conservative management of chronic pancreatitis. In: Beger HG, Büchler MW, Malfertheiner P eds. Standards in pancreatic surgery. New York: Springer Verlag, 1993: 325

11. Bockman DE, Büchler MW, Malfertheiner P, Beger HG. Analysis of nerves in chronic pancreatitis. Gastroenterology 1988; 94: 1459–69

12. Büchler MW, Weihe E, Friess H et al. Changes in peptidergic innervation in chronic pancreatitis. Pancreas 1992; 7: 83–192

13. Weihe E, Nohr D, Muller S, Büchler MW, Friess H, Zentel HJ. The tachykinin neuroimmune connection in inflammatory pain. Ann NY Acad Sci 1991; 632: 283–95

14. Di Sebastiano P, di Mola FF, Di Febbo C et al. Expression of interleukin 8 (IL-8) and substance P in human chronic pancreatitis. Gut 2000; 47: 423–8

15. Friess H, Zhu ZW, di Mola FF et al. Nerve growth factor and its high-affinity receptor in chronic pancreatitis. Ann Surg 1999; 230: 615–24

16. Shrikhande SV, Friess H, di Mola FF et al. NK-1 receptor gene expression is related to pain in chronic pancreatitis. Pain 2001; 91: 209–17

17. Zhu ZW, Friess H, Wang L et al. Brain-derived neurotrophic factor (BDNF) is upregulated and associated with pain in chronic pancreatitis. Dig Dis Sci 2001; 46: 1633–9

18. Korc M, Friess H, Yamanaka Y, Kobrin MS, Büchler MW, Beger HG. Chronic pancreatitis is associated with increased concentrations of epidermal growth factor receptor, transforming growth factor alpha, and phospholipase C gamma. Gut 1994; 35: 1468–73

19. Bockman DE, Merlino G. Cytological changes in the pancreas of transgenic mice overexpressing transforming growth factor alpha. Gastroenterology 1992; 103: 1883–92

20. Friess H, Yamanaka Y, Büchler MW et al. A subgroup of patients with chronic pancreatitis overexpress the c-erb B-2 protooncogene. Ann Surg 1994; 220; 183–92

21. Friess H, Yamanaka Y, Büchler MW et al. Increased expression of acidic and basic fibroblast growth factors in chronic pancreatitis. Am J Pathol 1994; 144: 117–28

22. Friess H, Yamanaka Y, Büchler MW, Kobrin MS, Tahara E, Korc M. Cripto, a member of the epidermal growth factor family, is over-expressed in human pancreatic cancer and chronic pancreatitis. Int J Cancer 1994; 56; 668–74

23. Ebert M, Kasper HU, Hernberg S et al. Overexpression of platelet-derived growth factor (PDGF) B chain and type beta PDGF receptor in human chronic pancreatitis. Dig Dis Sci 1998; 43: 567–74

24. di Mola FF, Friess H, Martignoni ME et al. Connective tissue growth factor is a regulator for fibrosis in human chronic pancreatitis. Ann Surg 1999; 230: 63–71

25. Friess H, Cantero D, Graber H et al. Enhanced urokinase plasminogen activation in chronic pancreatitis suggests a role in its pathogenesis. Gastroenterology 1997; 113: 904–13

26. Hunger RE, Mueller C, Z'graggen K, Friess H, Büchler MW. Cytotoxic cells are activated in cellular infiltrates of alcoholic chronic pancreatitis [see comments]. Gastroenterology 1997; 112: 1656–63

27. Kashiwagi M, Friess H, Uhl W et al. Phospholipase A2 isoforms are altered in chronic pancreatitis. Ann Surg 1998; 227: 220–8

28. Büchler MW, Malfertheiner P, Friess H, Senn T, Beger HG. Chronic pancreatitis with inflammatory mass in the head of the pancreas: a special entity. In: Beger HG, Büchler MW, Malfertheiner P, eds. Standards in surgery. New York: Springer Verlag, 1993: 41

29. Beger HG, Büchler MW, Biffner. R. The duodenum preserving resection of the head of the pancreas (DPRHP) in patients with chronic pancreatitis and an inflammatory mass in the head. An alternative surgical technique to the Whipple operation. Acta Chir Scand 1990; 156: 309–15

30. Beger HG, Büchler MW. Chronic pancreatitis: indications and successes of surgical therapy. Z Gastroenterol Verh 1989; 24: 107–10

31. Beger HG, Büchler MW, Malfertheiner P. Standards in pancreatic surgery. New York: Springer-Verlag, 1993

32. Largiadèr F. Chronic pancreatitis: indications for surgery. Dig Surg 1994; 11: 304–7

33. Chari ST, Singer MV. The problem of classification and staging of chronic pancreatitis. Proposals based on current knowledge of its natural history [see comments]. Scand J Gastroenterol 1994; 29: 949–60

34. Axon AT. Endoscopic retrograde choliangiopancreatography in chronic pancreatitis. Cambridge classification. Radiol Clin North Am 1989; 27: 39–50

35. Yeo CJ, Bastidas JA, Lynch-Nyhan A. The natural history of pancreatic pseudocysts: a unified concept of management. Surg Gynecol Obstet 1990; 170: 411–7

36. Ebbehöj N, Borly U, Madsen P. Svendsen LB. Pancreatic tissue pressure and pain in chronic pancreatitis. Pancreas 1986; 1: 556–8

37. Andrén-Sandberg A, Hafstöm A. Partington–Rochelle: when to drain the pancreatic duct and why. Dis Surg 1996; 13: 109–12

38. Lankisch PG, Andrén-Sandberg A. Standards for the diagnosis of chronic pancreatitis and for the evaluation of treatment. Int J Pancreatol 1993; 14: 205–12

39. Partington PF, Rochelle REL. Modified Puestow procedure for retrograde drainage of the pancreatic duct. Ann Surg 1960; 152: 1037–43

40. Stone WM, Starr MG, Nagorney DM, McIlrath DC. Chronic pancreatitis: results of Whipple's resection and total pancreatectomy. Arch Surg 1988; 23: 815–9

41. Rossi RL, Rothschild J, Braasch JW, Munson JL, ReMine SG. Pancreaticoduodenectomy in the management of chronic pancreatitis. Arch Surg 1987; 122: 416–21

42. Trede M, Schwall G, Saeger H. Survival after pancreaticoduodenectomy. Ann Surg 1990; 211: 447–58

43. Traverso LW, Kozarek RA. The Whipple procedure for severe complications of chronic pancreatitis. Arch Surg 1993; 128: 1047–53

44. Ammann RW. Quality control following surgery for chronic pancreatitis. In: Beger HG, Malfertheiner P, eds. Standards in pancreatic surgery. New York: Springer Verlag, 1993: 496

45. Watson K. Carcinoma of the ampulla of Vater: successful radical resection. Br J Surg 1946; 31: 368–73

46. Traverso LW, Longmire WP. Preservation of the pylorus in pancreatico-duodenectomy. Surg Gynecol Obstet 1978; 146: 959–62

47. Grace PA, Pitt HA, Longmire WP. Pylorus-preserving pancreatoduodenectomy: an overview. Br J Surg 1990; 77: 968–74

48. Sadowski S, Uhl W, Baer HU, Reber P, Seiler C, Büchler MW. Delayed gastric emptying after classic and pylorus-preserving Whipple procedure: a prospective study. Dis Surg 1997; 14: 159–64

49. Morel P, Rohner A. Pylorus-preserving technique in duodenopancreatectomy. Surg Ann 1992; 24: 89–105

50. Martin RF, Rossi RL, Leslie KA. Long-term results of pylorus-preserving pancreatoduodenectomy for chronic pancreatitis. 1995. San Diego, 19th annual meeting of the Pancreas Club.

51. Hunt DR, McLean R. Pylorus-preserving pancreatectomy: functional results. Br J Surg 1989; 76: 173–6

52. Beger HG, Büchler MW, Bittner R, Oettinger W, Roscher R. Duodenum-preserving resection of the head of the pancreas in servere chronic pancreatitis. Ann Surg 1989; 209: 273–8

53. Beger HG, Büchler MW, Bittner R, Uhi W. Duodenum-preserving resection of the head of the pancreas: an alternative procedure to the Whipple operation in chronic pancreatitis. Hepatogastroenterology 1990; 37: 283–9

54. Büchler MW, Friess H, Muller MW, Wheatley AM, Beger HG. Randomized trial of duodenum-preserving pancreatic head resection versus pylorus-preserving Whipple in chronic pancreatitis. Am J Surg 1995; 169: 65–9

55. Beger HG, Krautzberger W, Bittner R, Limmer J, Büchler MW. Duodenum-preserving resection of the head of the pancreas in patients with severe chronic pancreatitis. Surgery 1985; 97: 467–73

56. Friess H, Muller M, Ebert M, Büchler MW. [Chronic pancreatitis with inflammatory enlargement of the pancreatic head]. Zentralbl Chir 1995; 120: 292–7

57. Büchler MW, Friess H, Bittner R et al. Duodenum-preserving pancreatic head resection: long-term results. J Gastrointest Surg 1997; 1: 13–19

58. Beger HG, Schlosser W, Friess HM, Buchler MW. Duodenum-preserving head resection in chronic pancreatitis changes the natural course of the disease: a single-center 26-year experience. Ann Surg 1999; 230: 513–19

59. Frey CF. Smith GJ. Description and rationale of a new operation for chronic pancreatitis. Pancreas 1987; 2: 701–7

60. Frey CF, Amikura K. Local resection of the head of the pancreas combined with longitudinal pancreaticojejunostomy. Dig Surg 1994; 11: 325–30

61. Izbicki RJ, Boechle C, Knoefel WT, Wilker DK, Dornschneider G, Broelsch CE. Comparison of two techniques of duodenum-preserving resection of the head of the pancreas in chronic pancreatitis. Dig Surg 1994; 11: 331–7

62. Frey CF. Subtotal pancreatectomy and pancreaticojejunostomy in surgery in chronic pancreatitis. J Surg Res 1981; 31: 361–70

63. Sawyer R, Frey CF. Is there still a role for distal pancreatectomy in surgery for chronic pancreatitis? Am J Surg 1994; 168: 6–9

64. Klempa J, Spatny M, Menzel J et al. Pankreasfunktion und Lebensqualität nach pankreaskopfresektion bei der chronischen Pankreatitis. Der Chirurg 1995; 66: 350–9

65. Friess H, Müller WH, Büchler MW. Duodenum-preserving resection of the head of the pancreas: the future. Dis Surg 1994; 11: 318–24

27 Management of chronic pancreatitis without endocrine failure

Marco Siech, Wolfgang Schlosser, Andreas Schwarz and Hans G Beger

Natural course of chronic pancreatitis

The incidence of chronic pancreatitis varies between countries from 1.9 to 10 per 100 000 (mean values are 6.7 for men and 3.2 for women).[1–3] The increasing incidence of chronic pancreatitis in women might be explained by increasing alcohol consumption and a more rapid absorption of alcohol by women.[1,4] Thus, the risk of chronic pancreatitis in women could rise more rapidly than in men because they require less alcohol over a shorter time than men to be at significant risk for the development of chronic pancreatitis.

Treatment of chronic pancreatitis has improved over the past decades, with the result that 50% of patients with chronic inflammation of the pancreas live for more than 20 years.[5] Amman found that approximately half of his patients with chronic pancreatitis required operative intervention for complications of the disease.[5] Of the 50% of his patients not requiring surgery, none of them ever experienced severe persistent pain. Spontaneous and long-lasting pain relief was associated with severe exocrine dysfunction ('pancreas burnout'). Among Amman's patients, maximum pain relief occurred at a median of 4–5 years from the onset of symptoms. According to Levy et al.,[6] about 58% to 67% of chronic pancreatitis patients need surgery during the course of pancreatitis. As shown in Table 27.1, 93% of surgical patients suffered from severe intractable pain. Patients with an inflammatory mass of the head of the pancreas prevail in most surgical series (Table 27.1).

Bockman et al.[7] demonstrated that patients with an inflammatory mass of the head of the pancreas had

Table 27.1 **Chronic pancreatitis with inflammatory mass of the pancreatic head. Morbidity leading to surgical intervention in 380 patients (November 1972 to April 1992, Department of General Surgery, University of Ulm)**

	N[a]	%
Pain	302	93
Tumour of the pancreatic head >4 cm	187	79
Stenosis of the common bile duct	65	47
Stenosis of the superior mesenteric vein, portal vein	23	17
Symptomatic duodenal stenosis	23	6
Small pseudocysts in the head	212	56

[a] N = 380 patients for DPPHR.

an increased diameter of nerves in this area. Additionally, the perineurial sheath was damaged by inflammatory cells. In addition to the increase in diameter of the nerves, the mean area served per nerve was diminished.[7] These mechanisms might be responsible for the attack of severe pain seen in patients with inflammatory mass of the head of the pancreas due to chronic pancreatitis. In 79% of patients, the inflammatory mass within the head of the pancreas was larger than 4 cm.[8]

Büchler et al.[9] demonstrated by immunostaining of neuropeptides within the head of the pancreas in patients with chronic pancreatitis, there was increased neuropeptide Y, substance P and calcitonin gene-related peptide when compared to organ donors. Ductal hypertension is another condition that received attention with regard to a possible relationship to development of pain during the disease process. Okazaki et al.[10] cannulated the pancreatic duct during ERCP and measured the pressure of the main pancreatic duct in 20 control subjects and 38 patients with chronic pancreatitis. They found elevated main duct pressures which averaged 44.9 mmHg in patients with 'minimum change pancreatitis'. Ebbehoj et al.[11] performed fine needle puncture in 39 patients with chronic pancreatitis to measure pancreatic parenchymal fluid pressure. The pressures were significantly higher in those patients suffering pain.[12]

Patients with chronic pancreatitis have a much shorter life expectancy than others. Thorsgaard-Pedersen et al.[13] found that once patients develop chronic pancreatitis they have a 5-year survival of 65%, a 10-year survival of 43% and a 20-year survival of 20%. In 19% of cases, the mortality was related to the patient's disease; however, in the other 81%, the causes of death were related to factors other than chronic pancreatitis, such as malignancies, alcoholic hepatitis and cirrhosis and severe infections[13] (Table 27.2). Lankisch et al.[14] found a 13% mortality related to chronic pancreatitis within 15 years of the diagnosis. Chronic pancreatitis may also cause pancreatic cancer in 3% of the patients who suffer from chronic pancreatitis for longer than 10 years.[15] This finding was confirmed by our own data,[16] where pancreatic cancer developed in 3.8% of our chronic pancreatitis patients.

Forty-seven per cent of patients with chronic pancreatitis in our own series additionally suffered from common bile duct stenosis within the lower third of the common bile duct (Table 27.1). The duct usually passes through the substance of the pancreas, where it is vulnerable to stricture, should the pancreas be inflamed and fibrotic, or compression by a pseudocyst. The common bile duct is the peripancreatic structure most frequently obstructed in chronic pancreatitis, and this is the most common complication of chronic pancreatitis after a pseudocyst formation. Strictures most frequently involve the entire intrapancreatic course of the common bile duct and occur in 3.1–47% of patients with chronic pancreatitis. The incidence of common bile duct stricture varies from 3.5% to 9.9% among hospitalized patients with chronic pancreatitis.[17] The incidence of duodenal obstruction is less common than bile duct obstruction, although they often occur together. Five of 878 (0.6%) hospitalized patients with chronic pancreatitis had evidence of duodenal obstruction.[18] Prinz noted that 8 of 55 patients (14.6%) had duodenal obstruction.[19,20] In our own series, 10.5% of all patients had duodenal obstruction. Most of those

Table 27.2 Co-morbidity in chronic pancreatitis

Diseases of heart and circulation	19%[5]
Malignancies	Extrahepatic 4%,[14] 19%[5]
Alcoholic hepatopathy	8%[5]
Severe infections	14%[5]

obstructions, however, were asymptomatic and only appeared radiologically, although 6% of all those patients had symptomatic duodenal stenosis (Table 27.1). Both of these mechanical problems are caused by an enlargement of the head of the pancreas. Seventeen per cent of these patients also had vascular stenoses, which were mainly caused by infiltration of the superior mesenteric vein and portal vein (Table 27.1). Lemaitre et al.[21] found vascular anomalies in as many as 60% of all patients with chronic pancreatitis undergoing operations. These findings included splenic vein thrombosis, left-sided portal hypertension, bleeding from gastric varices and pseudoaneurysms with or without bleeding. Pseudoaneurysms of the splenic artery are often associated with splenic vein thromboses.[22] Left-sided portal hypertension and bleeding gastric varices may occur in 10 to 20% of patients with splenic vein thrombosis.[22]

It has been shown that endocrine and exocrine function interfere with each other in vivo; insulin acts as a trophic factor to maintain the tissue level of amylase in the acini of diabetic animals[23] and also potentiates the action of CCK on pancreatic enzyme secretion.[24] The influence of islet hormones on surrounding acinar tissue can be either direct (paracrine) or indirect (endocrine). Endocrine and exocrine cells may exert a direct influence on each other, since there is direct contact of their cell membranes in areas where the thin capsule which separates them is deficient. Studies in rats showed that the amylase content of the pancreas was reduced in the diabetic state and that in vivo administration of insulin resulted in the increased synthesis of pancreatic amylase.[25,26]

Because diabetes mellitus has a large impact on the quality of life of patients, the surgeon should preserve endocrine function whenever possible. In man, pancreatic enzymes in the duodenum stimulate release of pancreatic polypeptide. Thus, there is a feedback whereby pancreaticobiliary secretions release pancreatic polypeptide which internally inhibits pancreatic secretion. Physiologically, postprandial release of pancreatic polypeptide may be important in modulating pancreatic secretion after digestion is complete and all the chyme has passed into the jejunum. This enteropancreatic islet axis therefore provides an important autoregulatory mechanism for proper function of the pancreas in digestion and regulation of metabolism of nutrients. Therefore, the duodenum should be preserved whenever possible. Newer techniques like the duodenum-preserving pancreatic head resection and the Frey procedure were developed to suit this purpose (see below).

Gullo and Lankisch have shown that the natural progression of chronic pancreatitis may be slowed down but not stopped by abstinence from alcohol.[14,27] In contrast, Nealon et al.[28] found that abstinence from alcohol did not influence the deterioration of endocrine function during the period of observation.[28] Chronic pancreatitis remains within the domain of conservative treatment and the indication for surgery remain intractable pain, mechanical organ complications (Table 27.1) or the suspicion of the development of malignant change. There are different surgical options in the treatment of chronic pancreatitis. These options need to be judged by both their efficacy to treat the problems which indicate an operation and their own specific postoperative morbidity.

Surgical options in chronic pancreatitis

The opportunities to treat chronic pancreatitis surgically are outlined in Table 27.3. Procedures like Puestow operation combining a drainage procedure

and a small left-sided pancreatic resection are no longer used and therefore not discussed further in this chapter. Also, other procedures, like Kausch–Whipple operation and total pancreatectomy are nowadays only rarely used and have been replaced by other procedures. Therefore, these procedures are discussed only briefly (see below). The classic procedures are discussed together with new procedures in order to weigh the advantages of one procedure compared to another. Nowadays, the most frequently used procedures for chronic pancreatitis worldwide are pylorus-preserving partial duodenopancreatectomy and duodenum-preserving pancreatic head resection. Therefore, both these procedures are compared below.

Technique and results of Partington–Rochelle drainage

Regarding the Partington and Rochelle procedure,[29] instead of small left resection (as performed in the Puestow procedure), the authors proposed an incision of the main pancreatic duct longitudinally throughout the whole pancreas and then performed a Roux-en-Y reconstruction with side-to-side pancreaticojejunostomy (Fig. 27.1). Because this procedure does not include any resection, the perioperative mortality and morbidity is much lower than in other techniques which include resection of the pancreas. Therefore, for many years, the lateral pancreaticojejunostomy was favoured in treatment of chronic pancreatitis. Table 27.4 shows a meta-analysis of 205

Table 27.3 **Surgical options in chronic pancreatitis**		
	Resection	**Drainage**
Historical	• Partial duodenopancreatectomy (Kausch–Whipple)	• Puestow procedure
Classic	• Pylorus-preserving partial duodenopancreatectomy	• Partington–Rochelle procedure
Standard today	• Duodenum-preserving pancreatic head resection	• Frey procedure
	• Spleen-preserving pancreatic left resection	

Table 27.4 **Pain relief after pancreaticojejunostomy >5 years follow-up. Meta-analysis of 290 patients.**

Reference	N	Complete pain relief (%)	Pain but improved (%)	Failure (%)
Leger et al. 1974[30]	205	44	31	25
White and Hart 1979[31]				
Prinz and Greenlee 1981[20]				
Morrow et al.1984[32]				
Bradley 1987[18]				
Adams et al.1994[33]	85	24	31	45

A

B

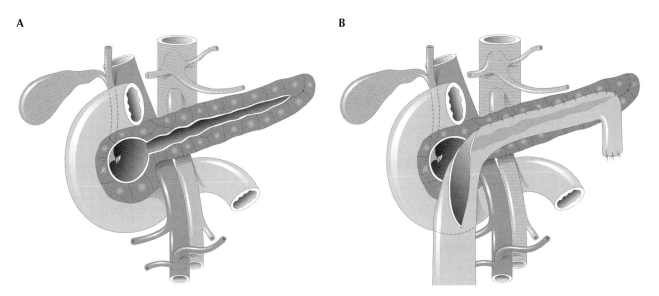

Figure 27.1 Technique of the Frey procedure. (A) The main pancreatic head is opened longitudinally and the head is cored out. (B) A Roux-en-Y limb is used for reconstruction. (With permission of the publisher.)

patients treated by lateral pancreaticojejunostomy in the 1970s and 1980s.

This meta-analysis, shows that, despite good early postoperative results, there is complete pain relief in only 44%, while another 31% continue to suffer pain; however, the overall situation was regarded as improved. Twenty-five per cent of all patients had complete failure of pain control 5 years after the operation. Adams et al.[33] in 1994, published their results in 85 patients observed for a median of 5 years after surgery (Table 27.4). In their study, a good result was recorded in 24%, fair results in 31% and poor results in 45% (Table 27.4). These authors regarded the reasons for failure of Partington–Rochelle as follows: recurrent chronic pancreatitis, further complications of chronic pancreatitis and finally further alcohol abuse. In 1994, Markowitz and co-workers reported on 15 patients who were transferred on to their hospital after failure of primary Partington–Rochelle operations at other centres, with a median of 5 months after primary operation.[34] Fourteen of these 15 patients required further surgery. Thirteen underwent pancreatic head resection and one required a left-sided pancreatic resection. Their median follow-up time after reoperation was 39 months. After the second operation, there was one death from pancreatic cancer, while ten patients were pain-free. The authors concluded that the reasons for failure of the Partington–Rochelle procedure at the first operation were: pancreatic cancer (N = 2), inadequate duct decompression (N = 2), biliary stenosis (N = 2), inflammation of the head of the pancreas (N = 10).[34] These ten patients clearly demonstrate that, in most cases, the major problem faced by the drainage procedures is enlargement of the pancreatic head. Furthermore,

pancreatic cancer cannot always be excluded by the Partington–Rochelle procedure. In our own series, the vast majority of patients with chronic pancreatitis, transferred to our hospital for surgery, suffered with an inflammatory mass of the head of the pancreas. The last two studies[33,34] show that this inflammatory mass of the head of the pancreas cannot be sufficiently treated by a simple drainage procedure. Consequently, we feel that the Partington–Rochelle procedure is only indicated when either the main pancreatic duct is larger than 6 to 8 mm or a chain of lakes occurs without inflammatory mass of the head of the pancreas. In our own series, these criteria were met in only 12 out of 644 patients (2% of all patients).

Technique and results of the Frey modification of Partington–Rochelle drainage

This relatively new technique was first described by Frey et al. in 1987.[35] In this procedure, the main pancreatic duct is opened throughout its length in the head, body and tail of the pancreas, as far as possible to the duodenum. This step is similar to the Partington–Rochelle drainage. After location of the superior mesenteric vein and portal vein (to avoid injuries to these structures), the head of the pancreas is cored out to remove retention of cysts, areas of necrosis and impacted calculi (Fig. 27.1A). Then, a Roux-en-Y limb is used to drain the main pancreatic duct in the head, body and tail of the pancreas by means of a two layer side-to-side pancreaticojejunostomy (Fig. 27.1B). Because only a small portion of the pancreatic head is cored out (approximately 5 g according to Frey), biliary and duodenal stenosis cannot be treated by this method in patients with inflammatory mass in the head of the pancreas.

Izbicki et al. performed a prospective study comparing Frey's procedure and duodenum-preserving pancreatic head resection in 40 patients.[36] These authors found similar good early results with both procedures. However, in this prospective trial there were no patients with duodenal stenosis or obstruction of the common bile duct.[36] Since common bile duct stenosis and duodenal stenosis can be easily treated by DPPHR but not by the Frey procedure, the latter can only be used in cases without damage to these structures. The coring-out technique of pancreatic head tissue advocated by Frey results in an operative tissue specimen of 5 g and is considered a modification of the Partington–Rochelle duct drainage procedure.[35] There have not been any published scribes of long-term results of the Frey procedure so far. Therefore, this method still needs to be evaluated.

Duodenum-preserving pancreatic head resection

The duodenum-preserving resection of the head of the pancreas is a surgical procedure which was especially developed for patients with chronic pancreatitis. It was described by Beger in 1980 for treatment of inflammatory mass of the head of the pancreas.[37] In our own institution, more than 400 patients have been operated upon so far using this procedure, and this approach is now widely accepted.

There are three major steps during resection: exposure of the head of the pancreas, subtotal resection of the head and reconstruction using an upper jejunal loop for interposition. The head of the pancreas is exposed as described by Kocher, and the ligaments are divided. The resection starts with a transection of the pancreas ventrally to the portal vein at the level of the duodenoportal vein wall (Fig. 27.2). After transection of the pancreatic neck, the head of the pancreas is rotated to the ventral dorsal level (Fig. 27.3). Subtotal resection of the pancreatic head is carried out from the dorsal surface of the pancreatic head toward the intrapancreatic common bile duct (Fig. 27.4). In most patients it is not difficult to dissect the pancreatic tissue along the wall of the intrapancreatic common bile duct toward and up to the uncinate process. A 5 to 8 mm shell-like piece of the pancreatic head along the the duodenal wall is preserved to maintain the blood supply of the third part of the duodenum (Fig. 27.2).

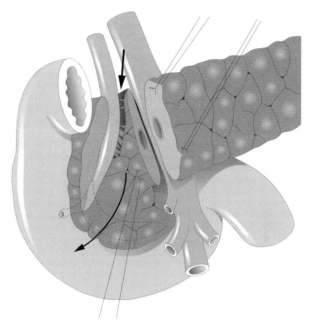

Figure 27.3 After transection of the pancreas, the pancreatic head is rotated to a ventrodorsal position.

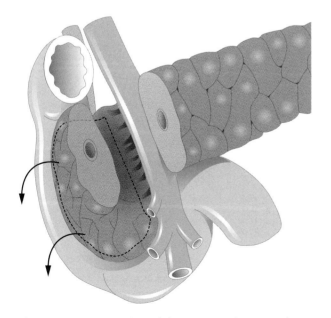

Figure 27.2 Transection of the pancreas between the head and body along the duodenal border of the portal vein.

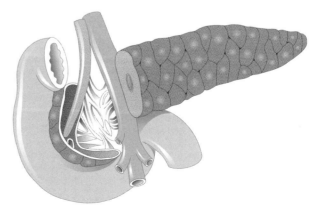

Figure 27.4 A subtotal resection of the head of the pancreas results in a decompression of the intrapancreatic segment of the common bile duct.

Preservation of the gastroduodenal artery is not necessary. Restoration of the pancreatic secretory flow from the body and tail to the upper gastrointestinal tract is maintained by interposition of the first jejunal loop (Fig. 27.5); two pancreatic anastomoses must be carried out (Fig. 27.5). In most patients, subtotal excision of the inflammatory mass in the head leads to a decompression of the pancreatic segment of the common bile duct. Patients in whom cholestasis is caused by narrowing of the prepapillary common bile duct segment because of intraductal wall inflammation, a biliary anastomosis

with the jejunal loop is necessary (Fig. 27.6A and B). In cases with multiple stenoses and dilatations of the main pancreatic duct, a Partington–Rochelle modification using the side-to-side anastomosis must be performed (Fig. 27.7). To restore upper gastrointestinal tract continuity, a Roux-en-Y jejunal anastomosis must be carried out. The medium wet weight of dissected pancreatic tissue using the duodenum-preserving subtotal head resection in our series was 28 g (range 18–52 g). In 380 patients in whom the duodenum-preserving head resection was employed, the following pathological findings were noted: a single pancreatic main duct stenosis in the prepapillary segment of the pancreatic head in 39%, pseudocystic cavities in 51%, small focal necrosis in 9%, common bile duct stenosis in 48%, severe duodenal stenosis in 7% and portal vein compression caused by pancreatic head enlargement in 13%. An additional common bile duct anastomosis had to be carried out in 23% and a drainage procedure of the left pancreas in 7%. Portal vein thrombosis necessitated an additional recanalization procedure in six patients, and an additional decompression procedure of the narrowed duodenum was performed in 4% (Table 27.5).

Early results after duodenum-preserving head resection are shown in Table 27.6. The median postoperative hospitalization time was 13.9 days; 5.3% of the patients had to undergo reoperation for complications. The hospital mortality was 0.8%. Subtotal pancreatic head resection resulted in improved glucose metabolism (of preoperatively latent or insulin-dependent diabetes) in 96%; only 2% of the patients showed deterioration with newly developed diabetes mellitus in the early postoperative phase.[39]

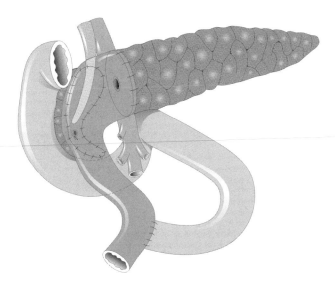

Figure 27.5 Restitution of pancreatic secretory flow is accomplished by interposition of the upper jejunal loop between the left pancreas and the pancreatic shell along the duodenum. Two pancreatic anastomoses are carried out.

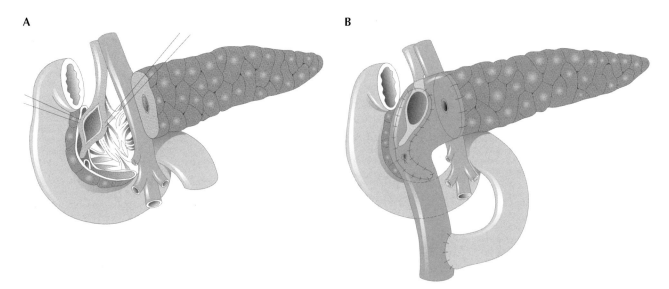

A

B

Figure 27.6A and B In patients with chronic pancreatitis and inflammatory mass, who suffer from a severe stricture of the common bile duct in the prepapillary intrapancreatic segment, an additional common bile duct anastomosis with the jejunal loop has to be carried out to restore the bile flow into the upper intestine.

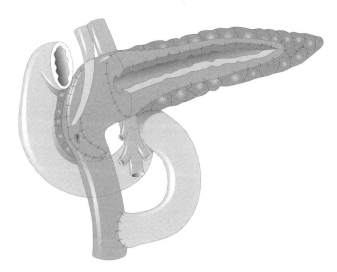

Figure 27.7 In patients with multiple stenoses of the pancreatic main duct in the left pancreas, a side-to-side anastomosis like the Partington–Rochelle procedure is performed.

Table 27.5 Duodenum-preserving head resection in chronic pancreatitis: additional surgical procedures for 380 patients.[a] (From Beger et al.[38] with permission of the publisher)

Procedure	No. of patients (%)
CBD anastomosis	86 (23)
Duct drainage	26 (7)
Decompression of duodenum	16 (4)
Cholecystectomy	102 (27)
Portal vein recanalization	6 (2)
Drainage of pseudocysts	4 (1)
Left resection	2 (1)
Splenectomy	3 (1)
Other	15 (4)

[a] 11/1972–4/1982, Department of Surgery, FU Berlin. 5/1982–9/1995 Department of General Surgery, University of Ulm.

During the follow-up period (from 6 months to 23 years), it was demonstrated that late morbidity and mortality after duodenum-preserving head resection are surprisingly low. In 1983, 1987 and 1993, re-evaluations of all patients after duodenum-preserving head resection were carried out; the follow-up response was 92%, 96% and 88%, respectively.[8,40,41] In terms of relief of abdominal complaints, 75–82% of all patients were absolutely pain-free, and an additional 7–11% did not need analgesic medication in spite of occasional upper abdominal pain sensations. With regard to recurrence of pain, 8–11% suffered further pain with a need for analgesic treatment at the re-evaluation. As to working status, more than 60% of all patients were in professional employment. Body weight increase occurred in more than 80% in the first postoperative months. After surgical treatment, only one-third of the patients were still on a full dose of enzyme supplementation; 50% of the patients had only an occasional enzyme supplementation. Late mortality after duodenum-preserving head resection was 7.7%, at a median 6 years.[41] Only 10% of patients had to be rehospitalized because of further attacks of pancreatitis.[41] This low postoperative hospitalization rate in chronic pancreatitis deserves special mention, because on the basis of our knowledge of the natural course of chronic pancreatitis, at least 50% of patients should experience further severe attacks of pancreatitis. The low late morbidity in spite of progression of chronic pancreatitis provides evidence that the surgical excision of the inflammatory process in the head of the pancreas promotes the transformation of clinically manifest chronic pancreatitis into a resolution of the disease (Table 27.7).

Subtotal resection of the head of the pancreas preserving the duodenum in chronic pancreatitis does not lead to a deterioration of glucose metabolism as an early consequence of surgical resection of pancreatic tissue. Compared to preoperative endocrine function, glucose metabolism was

---

Table 27.6 Duodenum-preserving head resection in chronic pancreatitis: early postoperative results in 380 patients[a] (From Beger et al.,[18] with permission of the publisher)

Relaparotomy	20 patients (5.3%)
Postoperative newly developed DM	8 patients (2.0%)
Postoperative improved glucose metabolism	33 patients (9.0%)
Postoperative hospitalization	13.9 days (median)
Hospital mortality	3 patients (0.8%)

[a]11/1972–4/1982, Department of Surgery, FU Berlin. 5/1982–9/1995, Department of General Surgery, University of Ulm.

Table 27.7 Duodenum-preserving head resection in chronic pancreatitis: early and late outcome after DPPHR in 298 patients[a] (From Büchler et al.[41] and Beger et al.,[43] with permission of the publisher)

Early:	Hospital mortality	1.01%
	Relaparotomy	5.7%
	Postoperative newly developed diabetes mellitus	2%
	Postoperative hospitalization	13.9 days (median)
Late outcome after 6-year	Late mortality	7.7%
follow-up (median) in 232 patients:	Pain: none/rare	88%
	Professionally rehabilitated	63%
	Rehospitalization	10%

[a]11/1972–12/1994, Department of General Surgery, University of Ulm

unchanged in 82% of patients, improved in 9% and deteriorated in only 2%. Glucose tolerance tests in a small group of patients early and late after duodenum-preserving head resection showed an improvement of glucose tolerance in the first 6–12 months after surgical treatment. Preoperative and late postoperative insulin secretion was almost identical. The basal levels of glucagon, pancreatic polypeptide and somatostatin were postoperatively significantly reduced compared to the preoperative levels, contributing to the postoperative improvement of glucose metabolism.[42]

The rationale behind the use of the duodenum-preserving pancreatic head resection in patients with chronic pancreatitis and an inflammatory mass in the pancreatic head is based on our present knowledge of chronic pancreatitis. The inflammatory process as the pacemaker of the disease develops in a subgroup of patients in the head of the pancreas; pain is generated by the inflammatory process, which leads to a specific pancreatitis-associated neuritis and a liberation of pain hormones in the head of the pancreas. The preservation of the stomach, duodenum and extrahepatic biliary tree offers the major advantage when using the duodenum-preserving head resection in chronic pancreatitis deriving from the conservation of the endocrine capacity of the pancreas and duodenum in the early and late postoperative course. In contrast to the Whipple procedure, the duodenum-preserving pancreatic head resection means preservation of stomach, biliary tract and duodenum. Early and late morbidity after Whipple's procedure are related to the reduction in insulin secretion, the occurrence of early and late dumping complaints, and attacks of cholangitis.[30,44–49] The results of two prospective clinical trials comparing the duodenum-preserving pancreatic head resection with the pylorus-preserving Whipple procedure in chronic pancreatitis have been published. After 6 months,

patients who had undergone the duodenum-preserving resection had significantly less frequent pain, a greater weight gain, a significantly better glucose tolerance and a higher insulin secretory capacity than patients after pylorus-preserving Whipple resection.[40] Duodenum-preserving head resection does not lead to a complete restoration of the reduced exocrine and endocrine function of the pancreas, because the impairment resulting from chronic pancreatitis cannot be compensated for by any surgical intervention.

Duodenum-preserving pancreas resection for chronic pancreatitis results in a subtotal resection of the pancreatic head, leading on average to a removal of 28 g of tissue. Of 380 patients suffering from chronic pancreatitis who did not respond to medical pain treatment, 79% had an inflammatory mass in the pancreatic head, 49% had a common bile duct stenosis, 6% a severe duodenum stenosis and 13% a portal vein obstruction. Hospital mortality after duodenum-preserving head resection was 0.8%, late mortality after a follow-up of 6 years on average (range, 3 months to 23 years) was 8.9%. In the late follow-up, 88% of patients were pain-free or had rare minor pain; 63% were professionally rehabilitated. The incidence of early postoperative diabetes mellitus amounted to 2%, and in the late follow-up an additional 10% developed insulin-dependent diabetes mellitus; 9% of patients had a postoperative improvement in their glucose metabolism. In patients after duodenum-preserving head resection, early and late postoperative glucose metabolism and insulin secretion are significantly better than in patients after pylorus-preserving pancreatic head resection for chronic pancreatitis. Duodenum-preserving head resection should be the standard surgical procedure in chronic pancreatitis because of the low early and late postoperative morbidity and mortality and a favourable maintenance of glucose metabolism and upper gastrointestinal tract physiology.

Pylorus-preserving pancreatic head resection

Pylorus-preserving pancreatic head resection was first applied for small periampullary carcinomas by Watson.[50] Later, it was introduced into routine clinical use by Traverso et al.[51] This technique allows a sufficient distance between the tumour and the pylorus of the stomach in small carcinomas. Compared to the classic Whipple operation,[52] it avoids the problems of gastric dumping. More recently, this technique has been used for patients with chronic pancreatitis, since there is no need to remove a part of the stomach. In this setting, operating mortality (1.7%) is lower than that seen in patients undergoing the classic Whipple operation. The long-term postoperative results were better than in the classic Whipple operation, but not, however, as good as in the duodenum-preserving pancreatic head resection (see Table 27.14, later). After pylorus-preserving pancreatic head resection there was complete pain relief in 82%, compared to 72% in classic Whipple and 89% after duodenum-preserving pancreatic head resection of our patients. In Büchler's prospective randomized trial only 40% of patients were completely pain-free after pylorus-preserving pancreatic head resection, compared to 75% after duodenum-preserving pancreatic head resection (Table 27.8).[40] Similarly, in Klempa's randomized trial, after a median follow-up of 5.5 years, 30% of patients needed analgetics after a classic Whipple operation, compared to none of the patients after duodenum-preserving pancreatic head resection.[53] It is not completely clear why patients after duodenum-preserving pancreatic head resection have less pain than after classic or pylorus-preserving Whipple procedure. Possibly, one of the reasons is less operative trauma and a lower postoperative rate of cholangitis.

In 50% of patients after the classic Whipple procedure, there is a median weight gain of 4 kg (Table 27.9). However, in pylorus-preserving pancreatic head resection and also in duodenum-preserving pancreatic head resection, 80 to 90% of all patients had a median weight gain of 7 kg. In our own randomized trial, patients with duodenum-preserving pancreatic head resection had a significantly higher weight gain compared to patients with pylorus-preserving pancreatic head resection. This concurs with the results seen by Klempa, showing a significantly high rate of underweight patients in classic Whipple operation after 5 years.[53]

The short-term results of pylorus-preserving pancreatic head resection are much better than after a classic Whipple resection. The morbidity and mortality of pylorus-preserving pancreatic head resection is much better than in the classic Whipple procedure. However, morbidity and mortalitiy have improved in all procedures during the last 10 years. Ten years ago the classic Whipple procedure carried mortality rates higher than 10% whereas at the time of writing the mortality rate of classic Whipple procedures is in the region of 3.2%. A meta-analysis of 1180 patients showed early postoperative mortality in classic Whipple at 3.2%, in pylorus-preserving pancreatic head resection 2.1%, and the best mortality rate in duodenum-preserving pancreatic head resection with 0.8%. Also the long-term mortality in pylorus-preserving pancreatic head resection is better (10.1%) than after a classic Whipple (22%); however, both are not as good as that seen in patients after duodenum-preserving pancreatic head resection (8.4%).

The preservation of exocrine and endocrine pancreatic function seems to be of importance for long-term

---

Table 27.8 Results of the Ulm prospective randomized trial DPPHR versus PPDP; 6-month follow-up. (From Büchler et al.,[40] with permission of the publisher)

	DPPHR N = 20	PPDP N = 20	
Pain-free (%)	75	40	P <0.05
Weight gain (kg)	4.1 + 0.9	1.9 + 1.2	P <0.05
New hospital stays (%)	13	27	NS
Ability to work (%)	80	65	NS
Oral glucose tolerance (mg/dl/min)	20.5	25.3	P <0.05
Insulin secretion capacity (µU/ml/min)	32.1	24.5	P <0.05

DPPHR, duodenum-preserving pancreatic head resection; PPDP, pylorus-preserving partial duodenopancreatectomy.

Table 27.9 Results of the Ulm prospective randomized trial. Follow-up 36 months to 5.5 years. (From Büchler et al.,[40] with permission of the publisher)

	DPPHR (N = 20)	PPDP (N = 20)	Significance
Use of analgesics (%)	0	30	$P < 0.05$
Weight gain (kg)	6.4	4.9	NS
Normal weight or overweight (%)	80	30	$P < 0.05$
Underweight (%)	20	70	$P < 0.05$
Median hospital stay (days)	16.5	21.7	$P < 0.05$
Endocrine function: newly-detected, insulin-dependent diabetes mellitus (%)	2/17=11.8%	6/16=37.5%	NS
Exocrine function: steatorrhoea (%)	15	100	$P < 0.05$
CCK[a] (pg/h)	190 ± 63	60 ± 17	$P < 0.05$
Gastrin[a] (pg/h)	1805 ± 1378	0	$P < 0.05$
Neurotensin[a] (pg/h)	1194 ± 499	812 ± 358	NS
C-Peptide[a] (ng/h)	16 + 3.7	13 + 5.7	NS

DPPHR, duodenum-preserving pancreatic head resection; PPDP, pylorus-preserving partial duodenopancreatectomy.
NS = not significant.
[a] Integrated total secretion after stimulation.

survival. Early postoperative delayed gastric emptying is a specific postoperative problem after pylorus-preserving pancreatic head resection occurring in 17% of patients (range 4 to 32%). Additionally, 8.4% (range 5 to 11%) of all patients develop late postoperative anastomotic ulcerations.

In a prospective randomized trial, comparing the gastric emptying after pylorus-preserving pancreatic head resection and duodenum-preserving pancreatic head resection,[54] 10 days postoperatively, the median velocity of gastric emptying was delayed after pylorus-preserving pancreatic head resection, compared to a normal gastric emptying after duodenum-preserving pancreatic head resection. However, 6 months postoperatively, all patients (both pylorus-preserving and duodenum-preserving pancreatic head resection) had normal gastric emptying, compared to their preoperative status. There is little information available on postoperative exocrine function in the literature, however, several authors have compared postoperative endocrine function after several types of procedures (see Tables 27.9 and 27.13 later), and this is discussed below (see preservation of endocrine functions).

Pancreatic duct stenting: an experimental approach

Stricture of the main pancreatic duct leads to increasing intraduct pressure and consequently to attacks of pain.[11] In contrast, after restoring pancreatic duct drainage, exocrine pancreatic function is to some degree reversible.[55] This was demonstrated in a prospective clinical trial in patients with operative drainage of the pancreatic duct.[28] Consequently, pancreatic drainage using endoscopically placed stents, without pancreatic surgical exploration has been tried in a number of patients with chronic pancreatitis. The first of these studies reported on 75 patients with prepapillary stenosis who were stented by plastic stents of major or minor papillae.[56] Early pain relief was achieved in as many as 94% of these patients.[56] However, during the subsequent follow-up of 37 months, 15% of patients nevertheless needed an operation. An additional 29% of these patients came to replacement of their plastic stents by metal stents and the median stent replacement in these patients was once a year.[56] Also, in other studies a poor rate of pain improvement was found, despite good technical success (Table 27.10).

From the experimental background, pancreatic stenting leads to induction of chronic pancreatitis.[57]

Similar to work in animals models Kozarek et al.[59] showed that 72% of their patients developed new areas of fibrosis within the pancreas, induced by the stents. This finding was confirmed by Sherman et al.[57] (over 50%) and Smith et al.[62] in 80% of their patients. Additionally, it has been shown by Ikenberry et al.[63] that the function period of a plastic pancreatic duct stent was a median of 6 weeks. After that, the stent had either to be unblocked or replaced

Table 27.10 **Effect of stent placement within the pancreatic duct in relieving pain in chronic pancreatitis**

Reference	No. of patients	Technical success	Pain improvement
Huibregtse et al. 1988[58]	11	8 (73%)	6 (54%)
Kozarek et al. 1989[59]	6	5 (83%)	5 (83%)
Smits et al. 1995[60]	51	49 (96%)	40 (82%)
Treacy and Worthley 1996[61]	9	7 (78%)	7 (78%)
Total	77	69 (89%)	58 (75%)

Table 27.11 **Pancreatic stents in patients with chronic pancreatitis and inflammatory mass of the head of the pancreas: Ulm experience in 35 patients**

Indication for surgery	Pain despite stenting	35/35 patients	100%
Patients with stents	Recurrent acute pancreatitis	27/35 patients	77%
	Necrotizing pancreatitis	5/35 patients	14%
	Closure of the stent	11/35 patients	31%

6/1992–4/1997, Department of General Surgery, University of Ulm.

by another stent. These complications concur with our own results (Table 27.11). Besides blockage of stents in approximately 55% of cases,[60] other complications include recurrent and necrotizing pancreatitis. Even gastroenterological units with a large experience of the use of stents state that the use of pancreatic stents should remain largely experimental.[62] Stenting of intrapancreatic common bile duct strictures may play a role as an adjunct in the management of patients with cholangitis. However, up to now, this approach is unsatisfactory for long-term treatment in patients with chronic pancreatitis.

Outdated surgical procedures: Whipple, total pancreatectomy

The Kausch–Whipple procedure was first described by Kausch in 1912,[64] and then by Whipple in 1935[52] and was introduced for treatment of periampullary carcinomas. Because of the wide safety margin, the lower part of the common bile duct and a part of the stomach is also removed in this procedure. Chronic pancreatitis, however, is a benign disease and a radical resection is not necessary. Tailoring the operation to clinical and morphological characteristics remains the basic principle in the management of chronic pancreatitis. Following this principle, the removal of the antrum and pylorus does not appear to be necessary. On the other hand, the 'Whipple' is a standard procedure familiar to all gastrointestinal surgeons. Standard procedures are usually employed by preference in as many patients as possible, unless there are significant reasons for a change. Many authors have studied the perioperative mortality and morbidity of Whipple procedure in chronic pancreatitis.[65–68] (Tables 27.12–27.14). The early and late mortality of the classic Whipple operation compared to pylorus-preserving duodenopancreatectomy and duodenum-preserving pancreatic head resection is shown in Table 27.12. Compared to others, the Whipple procedure yielded the highest hospital mortality (3.2% versus 0.6 and 2.1%). Also, the late mortality was significantly higher in this procedure when compared to pylorus-preserving pancreatic head resection and duodenum-preserving pancreatic head resection (22% versus 10.1 and 8.4%, respectively, Table 27.12).

Consequently, the higher postoperative mortality is a significant reason to change to other techniques. Moreover, postoperative morbidity is also highest following the classic Whipple procedure. Postoperative 'surgical' diabetes is 17.6% compared to 12.5% in pylorus-preserving pancreatic head resection and 2% in duodenum-preserving pancreatic

Table 27.12 **Meta-analysis of early and long-term mortality after three different methods of pancreatic head resection (≥4 years)**

	Reference	Total N	DPPHR N	DPPHR %	PPDP N	PPDP %	pDP N	pDP %
Mortality: early postoperative	Gall et al. 1981,[45] Frick et al. 1987,[66] Horn and Hohenberger 1987,[73] Köhler et al. 1987,[69] Stone et al. 1988,[67] Beger and Büchler 1990,[8] Braasch 1990,[70] Howard and Zhang 1990,[65] Morel et al. 1990,[68] Izbicki et al. 1994,[36] Büchler et al. 1995,[40] Martin et al. 1996,[71] Traverso and Kozarek 1996,[72] Eddes et al. 1997[74]	1180	3/501	0.6	3/140	2.1	19/602	3.2
Long-term mortality	Gall et al. 1981,[45] Frick et al. 1987,[66] Köhler et al. 1987,[69] Stone et al. 1988,[67] Beger and Büchler 1990,[8] Braasch 1990,[70] Howard and Zhang 1990,[65] Morel et al. 1990,[68] Izbicki et al. 1994,[36] Martin et al. 1996,[71] Traverso and Kozarek 1996[72]	983	25/296	8.4	11/109	10.1	127/578	22

DPPHR, duodenum-preserving pancreatic head resection; PPDP, pylorus-preserving partial duodenopancreatectomy; pDP, partial duodenopancreatectomy.

Table 27.13 **Meta-analysis of postoperative endocrine function, new diabetes mellitus**

	Reference	No. of patients	DPPHR N	DPPHR %	PPDP N	PPDP %	pDP N	pDP %
Early postoperative	Gall et al. 1981,[45] Braasch 1990,[70] Izbicki et al. 1994,[36] Büchler et al. 1995,[40] Martin et al. 1996,[71] Schlosser et al. 1996,[16] Traverso and Kozarek 1996,[72] Eddes et al. 1997[74]	950	10/511	2	10/80	12.5	60/340	17.6
In long-term follow-up	Gall et al. 1981,[45] Frick et al. 1987,[66] Stone et al. 1988,[67] Beger and Büchler 1990,[8] Braasch 1990,[70] Howard and Zhang 1990,[65] Morel et al. 1990,[68] Izbicki et al. 1994,[36] Martin et al. 1996,[71] Traverso and Kozarek 1996[72]	691	8/147	6	30/99	30.3	107/445	24

DPPHR, duodenum-preserving pancreatic head resection; PPDP, pylorus-preserving partial duodenopancreatectomy; pDP, partial duodenopancreatectomy.

head resection (Table 24.13). This also holds true during the long-term follow-up (Tables 27.13 and 27.14) showing 24% develop diabetes after the classic Whipple operation compared to 6% for the duodenum-preserving pancreatic head resection. This increased postoperative morbidity and mortality has to outweigh the expected benefits of this operation. Long-term results are not as good as other techniques involving resection of the head of the pancreas (Tables 27.12–27.14). With regard to long-term follow-up in 11 studies between 4 and 10 years after operation (Table 27.14), only 72% of patients are pain-free compared to 82% after pylorus-preserving duodenopancreatectomy and 89% after duodenum-preserving pancreatic head resection.

Table 27.14 **Pain-free patients in long-term follow-up after three different methods of head resection of the pancreas (≥4 years)**

Reference	No. of patients	DPPHR		PPDP		pDP		Follow-up (median) (years)
		N	%	N	%	N	%	
Köhler et al. 1987[69]	18					12/18	67	10
Frick et al. 1987[66]	62					28/68	45	6
Stone et al. 1988[67]	15					8/15	53	6
Gall et al. 1990[45]	201					170/201	88	8
Morel et al. 1990[68]	38			17/20	85	14/18	78	5
Howard and Zhang 1990[65]	16					15/16	94	5
Braasch 1990[70]	33					20/33	61	5
Izbicki et al. 1994[36]	38	35/38	92					4
Martin et al. 1996[71]	45			43/45	95			5
Traverso and Kozarek 1996[72]	35			30/35	86			4
Beger et al. 1997[43]	258	227/258	88					6
All	774	262/296	89	141/173	82	267/369	72	

DPPHR, duodenum-preserving pancreatic head resection; PPDP, pylorus-preserving partial duodenopancreatectomy; pDP, partial duodenopancreatectomy.

It has been proposed that the Whipple procedure may serve as a procedure of choice for severe complications in chronic pancreatitis.[75] In the series of Traverso et al. a total pancreatectomy was found to be necessary in 9 patients out of 28 (32%).[75] These authors reasoned that the necessity for total pancreatectomy was due to anatomic problems which would not allow the surgeon to leave a remnant of pancreatic tissue. Eight of these nine patients were diabetic preoperatively. In our own experience of 517 patients, there were only 11 (2.1%) in which the classic Whipple procedure was regarded preoperatively to be necessary because malignancy was suspected. We have not found a pancreatectomy to be necessary in any of our 517 patients.

Because of the high associated morbidity and mortality, total pancreatectomy is not indicated and the general tendency is towards organ-preserving resectional procedures, yielding much better results than multivisceral resection. Apart from the experience of Traverso et al.[75] only two studies have been published during the last 10 years or so reporting total pancreatectomy. Both originated from the United Kingdom and mainly described total pancreatectomy as a second operation after the first one had failed to cure pain.[76,77] The perioperative mortality is quite high (2.4–5%).[76,77]

After 1.5 years (median), 72% of these patients were pain-free, while others still needed analgesics.[76] Because 38% of these patients had difficulties with control of endocrine function in spite of insulin,[76]

we feel that this procedure cannot outweigh the probable benefit of 72% pain-free.

Because the long-term results are worse than in other procedures, and also the postoperative morbidity and mortality is higher than in pylorus-preserving pancreatic head resection and duodenum-preserving pancreatic head resection, we feel that the classic Whipple operation as a standard procedure should be considered outdated. The few indications for the classic Whipple operation include the suspicion of malignancy in a large mass in the head of the pancreas. Also, in rare cases, there might be a limited indication for the classic Whipple operation where other surgical treatments for chronic pancreatitis have failed. However, we propose that this resection includes preservation of the pylorus.

Preservation of endocrine functions

The development of endocrine insufficiency depends on the degree of pancreatic calcification. Amman has shown that patients with diffuse calcifications had a significantly higher incidence of diabetes mellitus than patients without calcifications.[5] In another series, diabetes occurred in 30% of patients with chronic non-calcific pancreatitis, rising to 70% of patients with chronic calcifying pancreatitis.[78] Overall, 45% of patients with chronic pancreatitis had overt diabetes. It was thought that diabetes mellitus occurs more often in patients with alcoholic chronic pancreatitis than in the non-alcoholic disease.[79] It has been shown by Gullo et al.[27] that the risk and characteristics of diabetic retinopathy are similar in patients with diabetes secondary to chronic pancreatitis and patients with idiopathic diabetes mellitus. Diabetic neuropathy is probably more common because of the additive effect of alcohol abuse and malnutrition.[80] To evaluate endocrine pancreatic function, we performed a meta-analysis of data of 950 patients (Table 27.13). In the early postoperative period, 2% of patients after duodenum-preserving pancreatic head resection developed insulin-dependent diabetes mellitus. After pylorus-preserving pancreatic head resection, 12.5% of all patients developed insulin-dependent diabetes mellitus. After classic Whipple operation, this rate was highest at 17.6%. Also in our own randomized trial during the early postoperative period, there was a significantly higher insulin secretion capacity after duodenum-preserving pancreatic head resection and we also saw more physiological blood glucose regulation when compared to pylorus-preserving pancreatic head resection. In long-term follow-up for more than 4 years, the incidence of newly developed insulin-dependent diabetes mellitus was 6% after duodenum-preserving pancreatic head resection and 30.3% after pylorus-preserving pancreatic head resection (Table 27.13). After classic Whipple, this rate was 24%. In the randomized trial of Klempa,[53] after a median follow-up of 5.5 years, 11.8% of patients after duodenum-preserving pancreatic head resection developed new insulin-dependent diabetes mellitus compared to 37% after classic Whipple operation. The reasons for these different rates of postoperative diabetes mellitus are not completely clear. In duodenum-preserving pancreatic head resection, only 20 to 30% of the pancreatic parenchyma are removed when compared to 50% of the parenchyma at Whipple procedure. A possible explanation is the preservation of the passage of food through the duodenum. Contact of food with duodenal mucosa may enhance release of the insulinotrope gastrointestinal hormones such as CCK and GIP, leading to a stimulation of the enteroinsulin axis of insulin secretion, regulating the blood glucose level. Therefore, the major advantage of duodenum-preserving pancreatic head resection, compared to pylorus-preserving pancreatic head resection and classic Whipple, is mainly the preservation of endocrine function, also leading to better quality of life and long-term survival of patients (see Table 27.3).

Quality of life after surgical treatment of chronic pancreatitis

There are few data in the literature evaluating quality of life in patients with chronic pancreatitis.

During the natural course of the disease, 65% of patients live longer than 5 years, 50% more than 10 years and 43% more than 20 years.[13] A major impact on life expectancy is the co-morbidity of those patients (cardiovascular diseases, malignancies, alcoholic hepatopathy and severe infections; see also Table 27.2). However, 13 to 18% of the increased morbidity is directly due to the chronic pancreatitis.[5,6,14] Between 58 and 67% of all patients need surgery for their chronic pancreatitis during their life. Therefore, the subsequent quality of life closely depends on the success of the surgical intervention. Because different kinds of surgical interventions are employed for chronic pancreatitis, the impact of each operation for quality of life must be addressed. Lankisch et al.[14] are of the view that the natural course of chronic pancreatitis was only briefly interrupted by surgery. However, they compared operated and non-operated patients and the surgical procedures reviewed ranged between standard Whipple operation, left resection and Partington–Rochelle drainage operations. Long-term follow-up on patients after left resection resulted in 49 to 67% of all patients not becoming pain-free after operation.[81] Table 27.1 shows that 93% of all patients suffered from severe pain attacks almost daily. Severe pain is subjectively one of the most powerful arguments counting for the quality of life. Consequently, patients who do not become pain-free after surgical intervention, do not regain quality of life. A single drainage procedure yields unsatisfactory results, after a median time of 5 years in 45%.[33] The duodenum-preserving pancreatic head resection first described in 1980[37] leads to the best long-term relief of pain (89%, Table 27.14) and also preserves the duodenal passage and the common bile duct. Moreover, postoperative pancreatic endocrine function is better than in other operations.[8,42,53] For the first time, Bloechle et al. prospectively followed up 25 patients after duodenum-preserving pancreatic head resection and studied quality of life using three different quality of life indexes.[82] After 18 months the physical status improved by 44%, the working ability by 50%, the emotional and social function by 50% and the global quality of life by 67% (Tables 27.15 and 27.16). Their findings on pain development and ability to return to work are shown in Table 27.15.

It has been shown that after duodenum-preserving pancreatic head resection, during follow-up to 22 years, only 32% failed to return to work.[41] Sixty-two per cent were completely pain-free and an additional 26% of patients suffered pain only rarely.[41] Endocrine function of the pancreas has a large impact on quality of life because of insulin dependency. In long-term follow-up, 47.7% of

Table 27.15 **Preoperative and follow-up (18-month) results for the pain score after DPPHR (N = 25). (From Bloechle et al.,[82] with permission of the publisher)**

Criterion	Preoperative	Median follow-up	Significance[a]
Pain VAS	82	12	$p < 0.001$
Frequency of pain attacks	75	0	$p < 0.001$
Pain medication	17	0	$p < 0.001$
Inability to work	75	0	$p < 0.001$
Total	249	12	$p < 0.001$
Pain score	62,25	3	$p < 0.001$

[a] Wilcoxon rank test was used to estimate statistical significance.

Table 27.16 **Quality of life after duodenum-preserving pancreatic head resection; 25 patients, prospective re-evaluation after 18 months. (From Bloechle et al.,[82], with permission of the publisher)**

- Physical status   44% improvement
- Ability to work   50% improvement
- Emotional well-being   50% improvement
- Social well-being   60% improvement
- Global quality of life 67% improvement

388 patients (1982–97), 303 of them were available for follow-up; median 5.5 years.

patients after duodenum-preserving pancreatic head resection had normal endocrine function, 25.7% had impaired glucose tolerance and 26.6% had insulin-dependent diabetes mellitus.[8]

Of these patients followed long term 8.3% improved their endocrine function and 81.7% remained unchanged. However, 6% suffered deteriorating endocrine function during this period.[8]

In conclusion, patients with chronic pancreatitis suffer from an increased long-term morbidity and mortality which impacts on their lifestyle. The long-term prognosis regarding morbidity and ability to work is determined by the choice of operative procedure employed by the surgeon. It has also been shown that 50% of all patients with chronic pancreatitis coming to the surgeon are already unable to work before operative treatment. Patients who have already been retired before their operative procedure, do not return to work. In contrast, after duodenum-preserving pancreatic head resection, only 4% of patients were retired at a median of 5.5 years after operation. As a thought, maybe in the future, retirement should not be considered before all possible treatment concepts including surgery have been employed.

Key points

- 50% of patients with chronic pancreatitis live with their symptoms for more than 20 years.
- 50% of patients with chronic pancreatitis benefit from surgical intervention.
- Spontaneous and long-lasting pain relief is associated with severe exocrine dysfunction (usually after 4–5 years from onset of symptoms).
- Patients with chronic pancreatitis suffer significant co-morbidity (cardiac, hepatic, malignancy, infection, endocrine).
- Surgical options to relieve symptoms and maintain both endocrine and exocrine function include:
    Duodenum-preserving pancreatic head resection
    Spleen-preserving left pancreatic resection
    Partington–Rochelle procedure
    Frey procedure.

REFERENCES

1. Riela A, Zinsmeister AR, Melton LJ, Di Magno EP. Trends in the incidence and clinical characteristics of chronic pancreatitis. Pancreas 1990; 5: 727.

2. O'Sullivan JN, Nobrega FT, Morlock CG, Brown AL, Bartholomew LG. Acute and chronic pancreatitis in Rochester, Minnesota, 1940 to 1969. Gastroenterology 1972; 62: 373–9

3. Worning H. Incidence and prevalence of chronic pancreatitis. In: Beger HG, Büchler M, Ditschuneit R, Malfertheiner P, eds. Chronic pancreatitis. Berlin, Heidelberg: Springer, 1990: 8–14

4. Frezza M, DiPadova C, Pozzato G, Terpin M, Baraona E, Lieber CS. High blood alcohol levels in women. N Engl J Med 1990; 323: 95–9

5. Amman RW, Akovbiantz A, Largiadèr F et al. Course and outcome of chronic pancreatitis. Gastroenterology 1984; 56: 820–8

6. Levy P, Milan C, Pognon JP, Baetz A, Bernardes P. Mortality factors associated with chronic pancreatitits. Unidimensional and multidimensional analysis of a medical–surgical series of 240 patients. Gastroenterology 1989; 96: 1165–72

7. Bockman D, Büchler M, Malfertheiner P, Beger HG. Analysis of nerves in chronic pancreatitis. Gastroenterology 1988; 94: 1459–69

8. Beger HG, Büchler M. Duodenum-preserving resection of the head of the pancreas in chronic pancreatitis with inflammatory mass in the head. World J. Surg 1990; 14: 83–7

9. Büchler M, Weihe E, Friess H, Beger HG. Changes in peptidergic innervation in chronic pancreatitis. Pancreas 1992; 7: 183–92

10. Okazaki K, Yamamoto Y, Kagiyama S et al. Pressure of papillary sphincter zone and pancreatic main duct in patients with chronic pancreatitis in the early stage. Scand J Gastroenterol 1988; 23: 501–7

11. Ebbehoj N, Borly L, Madsen P, Matzen P. Pancreatic tissue fluid pressure during drainage operations for chronic pancreatitis. Scand J Gastroenterol 1990; 25: 1041–5

12. Ebbehoj N, Borly L, Bulow J et al. Pancreatic tissue fluid pressure in chronic pancreatitis. Relation to pain morphology and function. Scand J Gastroenterol 1990; 25: 1046–51

13. Thorsgaard-Pedersen N, Nyboe-Andersen B, Pedersen Worning H. Chronic pancreatitis in Copenhagen. a retrospective study of 64 consecutive patients. Scand J Gastroenterol 1982; 17: 925–31

14. Lankisch PG, Löhr-Happe A, Otto J, Creutzfeldt W. Natural course in chronic pancreatitis. Digestion 1993; 54: 148–55

15. Lowenfels AB, Maisoneuve P, Cavallini G et al. Pancreatitis and the risk of pancreatic cancer. N Engl J Med 1993; 328: 1433–7

16. Schlosser W, Schoenberg M, Rhein E, Siech M, Gansauge F, Beger HG. Pankreaskarzinom bei chronischer Pankreatitis mit entzündlichem Pankreaskopftumor. Z Gastroenterol 1996; 34: 3–8

17. Yadegar J, Williams RA, Passaro E, Wilson SE. Common duct stricture from chronic pancreatitis. Arch Surg 1980; 115: 582–6

18. Bradley EL. Long-term results of pancreaticojejunostomy in patients with chronic pancreatitis. Am J Surg 1987; 153: 207–13

19. Prinz RA, Aranha GV, Greenlee HB. Combined pancreatic duct and upper gastrointestinal and biliary tract drainage in chronic pancreatitis. Arch Surg 1985; 120: 361–6

20. Prinz RA, Greenlee HB. Pancreatic duct drainage in 100 patients with chronic pancreatitis. Ann Surg 1981; 194: 313–20

21. Lemaitre G, L'Hermine C, Maillard JP, Toison F. L'Hypertension portale segmentaire des pancreatites. Lille Med 1971; 16: 928–32

22. Hofer BO, Ryan JA Jr, Freeny PC. Surgical significance of vascular changes in chronic pancreatitis. Surg Gynecol Obstet 1987; 164: 499–505

23. Malaisse-Lagae F, Ravazzola M, Robberecht P et al. Exocrine pancreas: Evidence for topographic partition of secretory function. Science 1975; 190: 795–7

24. Kanno T, Ueda N, Saito A. Insulo–acinar axis: a possible role of insulin pontentiating the effects of pancreozymin in the pancreatic acinar cell. In: Fujita T, ed. Endocrine gut and pancreas. Amsterdam: Elsevier, 1976: 335–45

25. Soling HD, Unger KO. The role of insulin in the regulation of α-amylase synthesis in the rat pancreas. Eur J Clin Invest 1972; 2: 199–212

26. Adler G, Kern HF. Regulation of exocrine pancreatic secretory process by insulin in vivo. Horm Metab Res 1975; 7: 290–6

27. Gullo L, Parenti M, Monti L, Pezilli R, Barbara L. Diabetic retinopathy in chronic pancreatitis. Gastroenterology 1990; 98: 1577–81

28. Nealon WH, Townsend CM, Thompson JC. Operative drainage of the pancreatic duct delays functional impairment in patients with chronic pancreatitis. Ann Surg 1988; 208: 321–9

29. Partington PF, Rochelle REL. Modified Puestow procedure for retrograde drainage of the pancreatic duct. Ann Surg 1960; 152: 1037–43

30. Leger L, Lenriot JP, LeMaigre G. Five to twenty year follow-up after surgery for chronic pancreatitis in 148 patients. Ann Surg 1974; 180: 185–91

31. White TT, Hart MJ. Pancreaticojejunostomy versus resection in the treatment of chronic pancreatitis. Am J Surg 1979; 138: 129–35

32. Morrow CE, Cohen JI, Sutherland DER, Najarian JS Chronic pancreatitis: long-term surgical results of pancreatic duct drainage, pancreatic resection, and near-total pancreatectomy and islet autotransplantation. Surgery 1984; 96: 608–15

33. Adams DB, Ford MC, Anderson MC. Outcome after lateral pancreaticojejunostomy for chronic pancreatititis. Ann Surg 1994; 219: 289–93

34. Markowitz JS, Rattner DW, Warshaw AL. Failure of symptomatic relief after pancreaticojejunal decompression for chronic pancreatitis. Strategies for salvage. Arch Surg 1994; 129: 374–9

35. Frey CF, Smith GJ. Description and rationale of a new operation for chronic pancreatitis. Pancreas 1987; 2: 701–7

36. Izbicki JR, Bloechle C, Knoefel WT et al. Complications of adjacent organs in chronic pancreatitis managed by duodenum-preserving resection of the head of the pancreas. Br J Surg 1994; 81: 1351–5

37. Beger HG, Witte C, Kraas E, Bittner R. Erfahrung mit einer das Duodenum erhaltenden Pankreaskopfresektion bei chronischer Pankreatitis. Chirurg 1980; 51: 303–7

38. Beger HG, Imaizumi T, Harada N, Schlosser W, Kunz R. Duodenum-preserving head resection: a standard operation for chronic pancreatitis. In: Hanyu F, Takasaki M, eds. Pancreatoduodenectomy. Tokyo: Springer, 1997: 269–78

39. Beger HG, Büchler M, Bittner R, Oettinger W, Roscher R. Duodenum-preserving resection of the head of the pancreas in severe chronic pancreatitis. Early and late results. Ann Surg 1989; 209: 273–8

40. Büchler MW, Friess H, Müller MM, Beger HG. Randomized trial of duodenum-preserving pancreatic head resection versus pylorus-preserving Whipple in chronic pancreatitis. Am J Surg 1995; 169: 65–70

41. Büchler MW, Friess H, Bittner R et al. Duodenum-preserving pancreatic head resection: long-term results. J Gastrointest Surg 1997; 1: 13–9

42. Bittner R, Butters M, Büchler M, Nägele S, Roscher R, Beger HG. Glucose homeostasis and endocrine pancreatic secretion in patients with chronic pancreatitis before and after surgical therapy. Biomed Res 1988; 9: 28

43. Beger HG, Schoenberg MH, Link KH, Safi F, Berger D. Die duodenumerhaltende Pankreaskopfresektion – Ein Standardverfahren bei chronischer Pankreatitis. Chirurg 1997; 68: 874–80

44. Doutre LP, Perissat J, Pernot F, Houdelette P. Réflexions statistiques sur une série de 142 interventions pour pancréatite chronique primitive. Chirurgie 1977; 103: 169–76

45. Gall FP, Mühe E, Gebhardt C. Results of partial and total pancreaticoduodenectomy in 117 patients with chronic pancreatitis. World J Surg 1981; 5: 269–75

46. Guillemin G, Cuilleret J, Michael A, Berard P, Foroldi J. Chronic relapsing pancreatitis. Surgical management. Including 63 cases of pancreatico-duodenectomy. Am J Surg 1971; 122: 802–7

47. Trede M. Therapie der chronischen Pankreatitis – Schlußkommentar. Langenbeck's Arch Cir 1987; 373: 379–82

48. Proctor HJ, Mendes OC. Surgery for chronic pancreatitis. Ann Surg 1979; 189: 664–71

49. Grant CSJ, van Heerden JA. Anastomotic ulceration following subtotal and total pancreatectomy. Ann Surg 1979; 190: 1–5

50. Watson K. Carcinoma of ampulla of Vater: successful radical resection Br J Surg 1944; 31: 368–73

51. Traverso LW, Longmire WP. Preservation of the pylorus during pancreatico-duodenectomy. Surg Gynecol Obstet 1978; 146: 959–62

52. Whipple AO, Pearson WB, Mullins CR. Treatment of carcinoma of the ampulla of Vater. Ann Surg 1935; 102: 763–79

53. Klempa I, Spatny M, Menzel J et al. Pankreasfunktion und Lebensqualität nach Pankreaskopfresektion bei der chronischen Pankreatitis. Eine prospektive, randomisierte Vergleichsstudie nach duodenumerhaltender Pankreaskopfresektion versus Whipple'scher Operation. Chirurg 1995; 66: 350–9

54. Müller MW, Fress H, Beger HG et al. Gastric emptying following pylorus-preserving Whipple and duodenum-preserving pancreatic head resection in patients with chronic pancreatitis. Am J Surg 1997; 173: 257–63

55. Garcia-Pueges AM, Navarro S, Ros E et al. Reversibility of exocrine pancreatic failure in chronic pancreatitis. Gastroenterology 1986; 1991: 17–24

56. Cremer M, Deviere J, Delhaye M, Baize M, Vandermeeren A. Stenting in severe chronic pancreatitis: results of medium-term follow-up in seventy-six patients. Endoscopy 1991; 23: 171–6

57. Sherman S, Alvarez C, Robert M, Ashley SW, Reber HA, Lehman GA. Polyethylene pancreatic duct stent-induced changes in the normal dog pancreas. Gastrointest Endosc 1993; 39: 658–64

58. Huibregtse K, Schneider B, Vrij AA, Tytgat GN. Endoscopic pancreatic drainage in chronic pancreatitis. Gastrointest Endosc. 1988; 34: 9–15

59. Kozarek R, Patterson DJ, Ball TJ, Traverso LW. Endoscopic placement of pancreatic stents and drains in the management of pancreatitis. Ann Surg 1989; 209: 261–6

60. Smits ME, Badiga SM, Rauws EA, Tytgat GN, Huibregtse K. Long-term results of pancreatic stents in chronic pancreatitis. Gastrointest Endosc 1995; 42: 461–7

61. Treacy PJ, Worthley CS. Pancreatic stents in the management of chronic pancreatitis. Aust NZ J Surg 1996; 66: 210–3

62. Smith MT, Sherman S, Ikenberry SO, Hawes RH, Lehman GA. Alterations in pancreatic ductal morphology following polyethylene pancreatic stent therapy. Gastrointest Endosc 1996; 44: 268–75

63. Ikenberry SO, Sherman S, Hawes RH, Smith M, Lehman GA. The occlusion rate of pancreatic stents. Gastrointest Endosc 1994; 40: 611–3

64. Kausch W. Das Carcinom der Papilla duodeni und seine radikale Entfernung. Beitr Klin Chir 1912; 78: 439–86

65. Howard JM, Zhang Z. Pancreaticoduodenectomy (Whipple resection) in the treatment of chronic pancreatitis. World J Surg 1990; 14: 77–82

66. Frick S, Jung K, Rückert K. Chirurgie der chronischen Pankreatitis. Deut Med Wochenschr 1987; 112: 629–35

67. Stone WM, Sarr MG, Nagorney DM, Mellrath DC. Chronic pancreatitis. Results of Whipple resection and total pancreatectomy. Arch Surg 1988; 123: 815–9

68. Morel P, Mathey P, Corboud H, Huber O, Egeli RA, Rohner A. Pylorus-preserving duodenopancreatectomy: long-term complications and comparison with the Whipple procedure. World J Surg 1990; 14: 642–7

69. Köhler H, Schafmayer A, Peiper HH. Follow-up results of surgical treatment of chronic pancreatitis. Dig Surg 1987; 4: 67–75

70. Braasch JW. Pyloric-preserving pancreatectomy for chronic pancreatitis. In: Trede M, Saeger HD, eds. Aktuelle Pankreaschirurgie Berlin: Springer-Verlag, 1990: 165–9

71. Martin RF, Rossi RL, Leslie KA. Long-term results of pylorus-preserving pancreatoduodenectomy for chronic pancreatitis. Arch Surg 1996; 131: 247–52

72. Traverso LW, Kozarek RA. Long-term follow-up after pylorus-preserving pancreatoduodenectomy for severe complications of chronic pancreatitis. Dig Surg 1996; 13: 118–26

73. Horn J, Hohenberger P. Chronische Pankreatitis – Drainage und Resektionsverfahren: Standortbestimmung. Chirurg 1987; 58: 14–24

74. Eddes EH, Masclee AAM, Gooszen HG, Frölich M, Lamers CBH. Effect of duodenum-preserving resection of the head of the pancreas on endocrine and exocrine pancreatic function in patients with chronic pancreatitis. Am J Surg 1997; 174: 387–92

75. Traverso LW, Kozarek R. The Whipple procedure for severe complications of chronic pancreatitis. Arch Surg 1993; 128: 1047–53

76. Cooper MJ, Williamson RC, Benjamin IS et al. Total pancreatectomy for chronic pancreatitis. Br J Surg 1987; 74: 912–5

77. Linehan IP, Lambert MA, Brown DC, Kurtz AB, Cotton PB, Russell RC. Total pancreatectomy for chronic pancreatitis. Gut 1988; 29: 358–65

78. Marks IN, Bank S, Vinik AI. Clinical and hormonal aspects of pancreatic diabetes. Am J Gastroenterol 1975; 64: 13–22

79. Kalthoff L, Layer P, Clain JE, DiMagno EP. The course of alcoholic and nonalcoholic chronic pancreatitis. Dig Dis Sci 1984; 29: 953–7

80. Bank S, Marks IN. Alcohol-induced pancreatitits (AIP). Med S Afr 1973; 8: 577–86

81. Gebhardt C, Zirngibl H, Gossler M. Pankreaslinksresektion zu Behandlung der chronischen Pankreatitis. Langenbecks Arch Chir 1981; 354: 209–20

82. Bloechle C, Izbicki JR, Knoefel WT, Kuechler T, Broelsch CE. Quality of life in chronic pancreatitis – results after duodenum-preserving resection of the head of the pancreas. Pancreas 1995; 11: 77–85

28 Blunt trauma to the duodenum and pancreas

James A Murray and Thomas V Berne

Regional anatomy

Duodenum

The region of the duodenum and pancreas is an anatomically complex region (Fig. 28.1). A thorough understanding of this anatomy is essential due to the proximity of other organs, ducts and major vessels. The duodenum is arbitrarily divided into four portions beginning at the pylorus and ending at the ligament of Trietz. The majority of the duodenum is retroperitoneal, except for the first portion. The duodenum is fixed throughout most of its course, being adherent to the pancreas along its medial surface. The two ends of the duodenum are relatively mobile. The duodenum also lies directly over the lumbar portion of the vertebral column. A vast arcade of vessels supplies the duodenum and pancreas with multiple anastomoses.

The common bile duct passes posterior to the junction of the first and second portions of the duodenum. It enters the duodenum at the junction between the second and third portions. In 85% of individuals the common bile duct and pancreatic duct enter through a common channel, in 5% the ducts enter the ampulla of Vater through separate channels, and 10% have separate openings.[1] The superior mesenteric artery and vein pass anterior to the duodenum at the junction of the third and fourth portions.

Pancreas

The pancreas lies transversely over the lumbar vertebrae in the retroperitoneum of the upper abdomen. The splenic artery and vein are in close association with the superior border of the pancreas. The superior mesenteric artery and vein travel posterior to the body of the pancreas and are closely associated with

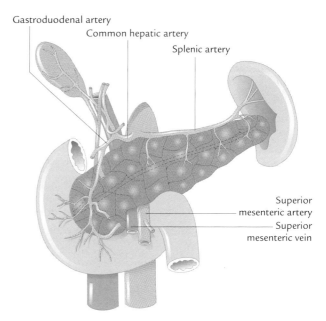

Figure 28.1 Anatomy of the pancreaticoduodenal region.

the uncinate process. The superior mesenteric vein becomes the portal vein after joining with the splenic vein. The main pancreatic duct of Wirsung travels parallel to the long axis of the pancreas just above the midline. The accessory duct of Santorini usually empties into the duodenum about 2.5 cm above the ampulla of Vater. Up to 90% of the pancreas can be resected prior to the development of endocrine insufficiency, if otherwise normal.

Preoperative evaluation

Blunt pancreatic and duodenal injuries occur from high-energy crushing forces applied to the epigastric region. Most commonly these are motor vehicle crashes, with unrestrained drivers who impact the

453

steering wheel. Children are also commonly injured after bicycle accidents that result in impacts to the handlebars. Other similar mechanisms such as assaults or abuse can result in these blunt duodenal perforations.

Due to the insidious nature of these largely retroperitoneal injuries diagnosis can be difficult. A high index of suspicion is required to ensure a timely diagnosis. Delays in diagnosis are common, but unfortunately can lead to an increase in complications.[2–4]

The appropriate evaluation and tests for diagnosing injuries to the pancreas and duodenum depend upon the physiologic status of the patient, associated injuries, and indications for operation. Patients without obvious indications for operation may require extensive assessment. In the presence of indications for laparotomy a thorough evaluation of the duodenum and pancreas can be performed intraoperatively.

Abdominal findings may lead directly to operative exploration or further evaluation. Epigastric pain out of proportion to physical exam is suggestive of a retroperitoneal injury. Patients with equivocal findings on physical exam can be evaluated with a CT scan (Fig. 28.2). This provides an excellent assessment of retroperitoneal structures as well as solid organs within the abdomen. CT scan has largely replaced other diagnostic modalities, such as plain films with or without the infusion of air through the nasogastric tube, as well as contrast studies of the upper GI tract. However, a negative CT scan does not entirely exclude the presence of a significant duodenal or pancreatic injury.

Serum amylase levels may be misleading.[5–8] Patients with an elevated serum amylase require close observation and serial measurements, or further investigation. A normal amylase does not rule out an injury to either the pancreas or duodenum.

The role of diagnostic peritoneal lavage (DPL) is also limited in evaluating the retroperitoneal structures. Obviously, if the DPL is positive an operation is mandatory. A negative lavage does not exclude a retroperitoneal injury.

Injury grading system

An injury scale was instituted by the American Association for the Surgery of Trauma (AAST) (Table 28.1), ranging from I, least severe, to V, most severe.[9] This system provides a means and structure to report and classify injuries for the evaluation of outcome and comparisons between institutions, and for stratification in clinical investigations. The best method for individual cases is for the operating surgeon to record the grade of the injury, and provide a detailed description of the size of the wound, its location, and the viability of surrounding tissue, in addition to the extent of debridement

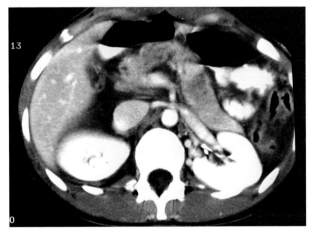

Figure 28.2 CT scan of blunt pancreatic injury showing prevertebral fracture of the pancreas slightly to the left of the spine.

Table 28.1 American Association for the Surgery of Trauma duodenal injury scale

Grade		Injury description
I	Hematoma	Involving single portion
	Laceration	Partial thickness; no perforation
II	Hematoma	Involving more than one portion
	Laceration	Disruption <50% of circumference
III	Laceration	Disruption 50–75% of circumference of second portion
		Disruption 50–100% of circumference of first, third or fourth portion
IV	Laceration	Disruption of >75% of circumference of second portion
		Involvement of the ampulla or distal common bile duct
V	Laceration	Massive disruption of duodenopancreatic complex
	Vascular	Devascularization of the duodenum

required and surgical maneuvers performed. The associated injuries as well as physiologic status of the patient often play an important role in the operative decision making, and should also be noted in the operative report.

Inspection and mobilization

Visualization of the retroperitoneum is necessary to identify clues indicating an injury to the duodenum. Obvious hematomas, bile staining, saponification, or crepitance of the tissues provide strong indications of a potential injury. The absence of such signs does not exclude an injury. Adequate mobilization of the duodenum should be performed in all blunt trauma patients to ensure the integrity of the duodenum. Since a missed injury to the duodenum can be rapidly fatal, thorough mobilization and visualization of the entire duodenum should be performed during the initial operation.

Inspection of the duodenum begins with the mobilization of the hepatic flexure of the colon to allow inspection and palpation of anterior surface of the duodenum. The duodenum is then Kocherized by incising laterally, rotating the duodenum anteriorly. This should allow visualization of the entire retroperitoneal duodenum (Fig. 28.3). Caution must be exercised near the hepaticoduodenal ligament to prevent injury to the portal structures. The head of the pancreas can also be well visualized when the maneuver is done completely.

Additional exposure to the distal duodenum can be obtained by dividing the ligament of Treitz (Fig. 28.4). This allows the distal portion of the duodenum to be freely mobile behind the superior mesenteric vessels for inspection and resection if necessary. Further exposure of the retroperitoneum and distal duodenum can be obtained through a Cattell–Braasch manuever[10] (Fig. 28.5). This involves mobilizing the cecum and ascending colon along with the small bowel mesentery and rotating these

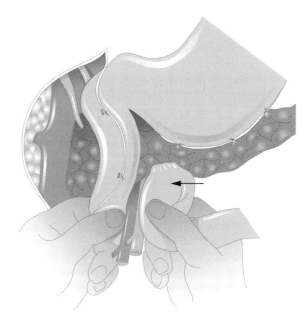

Figure 28.4 Additional exposure of distal duodenum by division of the ligament of Treitz.

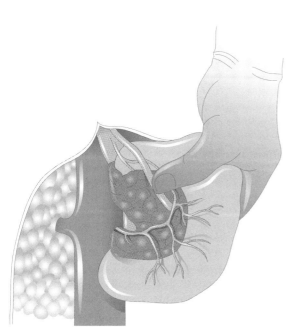

Figure 28.3 Wide Kocher maneuver of pancreatic head and duodenum.

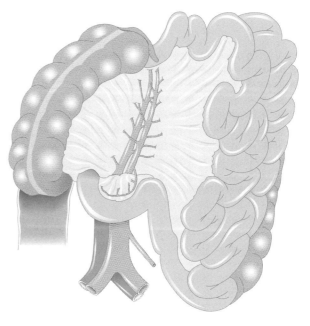

Figure 28.5 Cattell–Braasch maneuver for exposing the distal duodenum, uncinate process and superior mesenteric vessels.

structures superiorly. This allows visualization of the retroperitoneum from the pancreas and duodenum inferiorly towards the bifurcation of the aorta and inferior vena cava.

It must be emphasized that adequate exposure and mobilization are necessary to properly inspect the duodenum and assess the degree of injury. A thorough knowledge of these maneuvers, which are often performed expeditiously, is required.

Management of duodenal injuries

The majority of duodenal injuries are relatively minor, requiring repair with simple surgical procedures. Some guidelines must be remembered during these procedures. The duodenum is fixed along the medial border to the pancreas. This does not allow for generous resections. Primary repair of injuries must be performed without tension or significant narrowing. Two-layered closures are preferred, but single-layered repairs are possible, or even necessary at times to prevent additional tension on the suture line. The routine use of closed suction drains is recommended to prevent disaster in the unfortunate case of an anastomotic leak. These drains should be placed in proximity to, but not in contact with, the suture line.

A wide variety of surgical techniques have been employed for the repair of duodenal injuries. We will focus on the most commonly used techniques and the indications for their use.

Intramural hematomas

Intramural duodenal hematomas usually present with obstructive symptoms or may be seen on CT scan. Obstructive symptoms may be delayed in onset. This lesion most frequently occurs in the pediatric population. The diagnosis can be confirmed by an upper gastrointestinal study or a contrast enhanced CT scan. The appearance of the duodenum on the upper GI study is described as a 'coiled spring'. Sonography has also been used to diagnose intramural duodenal hematomas.[11] The initial management of these injuries is non-operative, with nasogastric decompression, intravenous hydration, and parenteral nutrition.[12] Operative intervention is reserved for those patients who do not resolve after 2–3 weeks.[13] If this lesion is detected during an abdominal exploration it should be opened.

Operative management of these injuries consists of a wide mobilization of the duodenum through a Kocher maneuver. An antimesenteric incision is

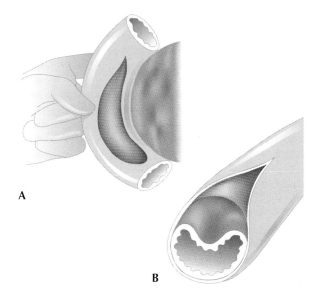

Figure 28.6 Duodenal hematoma and cross-section demonstrating compression of lumen.

made through the serosa and muscularis layers of the duodenal wall (Fig. 28.6). Care must be taken not to violate the mucosa. Opening of the wall will allow evacuation and decompression of the hematoma. It is not uncommon to perceive this portion of the duodenum as being non-viable. No resection should be performed since this is an erroneous perception.

Simple perforations

These injuries range from grade I to III, being from partial thickness disruption of the duodenal wall, to more than 50% of the circumference of the duodenum. Again, wide mobilization with a Kocher maneuver is required to fully visualize the organ and the extent of the injury. The edges of the injury should be debrided of any non-viable tissue. Primary closure should be performed either in a transverse or longitudinal fashion, whichever produces the least amount of luminal narrowing, and suture line tension (Fig. 28.7).

Complex injuries

These more advanced injuries, grade III to V, frequently require more extensive repair due to the loss of tissue. Again, the fixed nature of the duodenum with injuries requiring extensive debridement, large amounts of tissue loss, or the need for resection, does not allow for primary closure in most cases. Further challenges can be present when the injury is in association with the pancreas, pancreatic duct, biliary duct, or the ampulla of Vater.

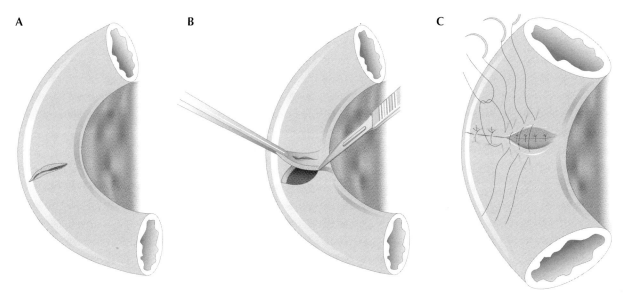

Figure 28.7 Closure of a simple duodenal injury: (A) injury, (B) debridement of edge, and (C) two-layered closure.

For large wounds that can be closed primarily, but are somewhat tenuous, an onlay jejunal patch can be performed[14] (Fig. 28.8). A loop of jejunum is brought up to the area of the repair and sutured in place to cover the defect and prevent fistulization.

For complex injuries with significant tissue loss prohibiting primary closure, or when a large segment of juxta-ampullary duodenum is involved, a Roux-en-Y duodenojejunostomy can be constructed (Fig. 28.9). The segment of jejunum is brought through the transverse colon mesentery and opened along the antimesenteric border. The opening into the jejunum must be of a length equal to that of the defect in the duodenum.

Pyloric exclusion

Pyloric exclusion should be performed for injuries of the duodenum where primary repair is possible but is felt to be at high risk for leakage.[15,16] General guidelines for such injuries are those that involve more then 50% of the circumference of the duodenum, associated with pancreatic injuries with an intact duct, associated common bile duct injuries, extensively edematous tissues, or those that were diagnosed after considerable delay.[17]

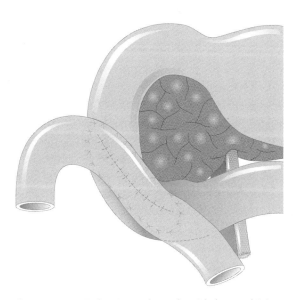

Figure 28.8 Onlay jejunal patch with loop of jejunum secured to duodenum after primary repair of duodenal injury.

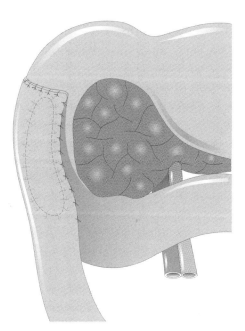

Figure 28.9 Roux-en-Y side-to-side duodenojejunostomy for large defect in duodenal wall.

Pyloric exclusion blocks the flow of gastric juice and contents away from the duodenum. This is postulated to prevent pancreatic stimulation, decrease flow of material, food particles, and digestive enzymes past the anastomosis, and prevent distention of the duodenum. In addition, if a duodenal leak occurs, the resultant fistula is easier to manage because gastric effluent is diverted into the jejunum.

Pyloric exclusion is performed by occluding the pylorus. This can be done with a row of staples placed externally across the pylorus. Alternatively, the pylorus can be sutured closed from inside the stomach (Fig. 28.10). This is done through a gastrostomy in the fundus of the stomach. The gastrostomy is then used to provide outflow through a gastrojejunostomy. The gastrojejunostomy can be performed by a handsewn or stapled anastomosis.

In the majority of cases, flow through the pylorus is restored spontaneously within 6 weeks. The advantage of a sutured closure of the pylorus is the ability to reopen the pylorus with endoscopic assistance. With the stapled closure of the pylorus, placement must be accurate to prevent excluding a portion of the antrum and creating an ulcerogenic mechanism.

Duodenal diverticulization

This procedure is reserved for injuries similar to those for which pyloric exclusion is performed, but there is devitalization of the proximal duodenum, pylorus or distal antrum.[18] An antrectomy is performed and a gastrojejunostomy created (Fig. 28.11). The injury is closed primarily with a tube duodenostomy placed into the duodenal stump to

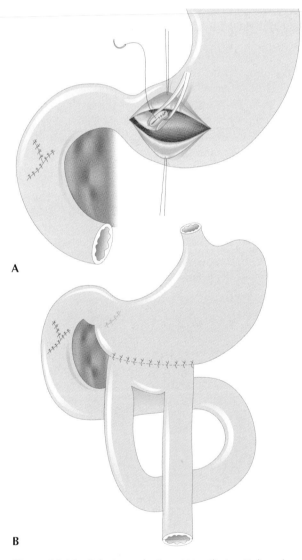

A

B

Figure 28.10 Pyloric exclusion: (A) utilizing Babcock clamp grasping pylorus to facilitate pyloric sutures and (B) restoration of continuity using gastrojejunostomy.

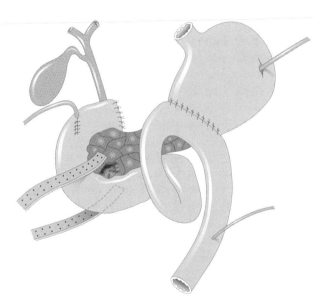

Figure 28.11 Duodenal diverticulization for severe injury of the first portion of duodenum, pylorus or distal antrum.

allow decompression. A common bile duct T-tube was advocated in the original procedure. Due to the small size of the normal common bile duct this is often omitted. This procedure antidates pyloric exclusion and its principle is similar. With this reconstruction, restoration of normal flow is no longer possible.

Adjuvant maneuvers

Duodenostomy tubes have been advocated to provide internal drainage after duodenal repairs. These can be placed antegrade, retrograde, or

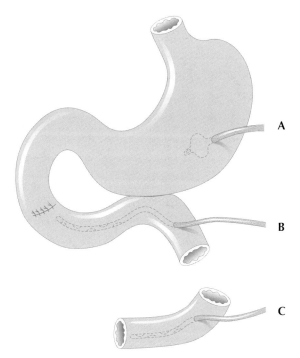

Figure 28.12 Adjuvant drainage techniques: (A) gastrostomy, (B) retrograde duodenostomy, and (C) feeding jejunostomy.

directly into the duodenum (Fig. 28.12). Direct drainage through the injury should be avoided since it is associated with a higher fistula rate. Some studies have shown a decrease in fistula rates when compared to historic controls,[19–21] while other reports find them to be of no benefit[22,23] and complications can occur due to the duodenostomy itself. We use them occasionally for complex injuries. We prefer to place them in a retrograde fashion with a Witzel technique. This provides a tunnel to prevent a leak when the catheter is removed.

Gastrostomy tubes are occasionally employed when patients have a gastrojejunostomy performed. There may be a prolonged period of gastric outlet dysfunction, requiring a long course of decompression. These are temporary and can be removed once the patient is tolerating a diet.

A feeding jejunostomy catheter is placed for many complex injuries where oral intake is unlikely to be provided during the early postoperative period. This catheter allows early enteral feeding, which can be rapidly advanced in most patients to provide full caloric needs. The complications associated with parenteral nutrition and line sepsis are avoided. In randomized control trials there seems to be a trend towards a greater intra-abdominal abscess rate associated with parenteral nutrition. The mechanism for such a finding is not clear.

Marginal ulcers at the site of the gastrojejunostomy are an infrequent problem (in approximately 10% of cases).[23] Routine vagotomy is not performed for patients requiring a gastrojejunostomy. Antiulcer therapy is administered routinely.

Outcome/postoperative complications

The mortality associated with blunt injuries to the duodenum ranges from 10 to 35%. The mortality directly attributable to the duodenal injury is 2%.[24] Associated intra- and extra-abdominal injuries account for the additional increase in mortality. Duodenal leaks can lead to profound sepsis. Factors that contribute to a higher risk for leaks are severity of injury, associated injuries, especially pancreatic injuries, and delay in operative repair.[2,25]

Management of pancreatic injuries

Intraoperative evaluation of the pancreas

Those trauma surgeons involved in research or the collection of trauma registry data will need to know the American Society for the Surgery of Trauma (AAST) pancreatic organ injury scale,[9] shown in Table 28.2. For a thin patient with little retroperitoneal fat, in whom the suspicion of injury is low, full mobilization may not be necessary. The surgeon should look carefully in the region of the pancreas for any evidence of edema, bilious staining, saponification, or hemorrhage into peripancreatic tissues. If none of these are present it is highly unlikely that

Table 28.2 **American Association for the Surgery of Trauma pancreatic injury scale**	
Grade	**Injury description**
I	Minor contusion or superficial laceration without duct injury
II	Major contusion or laceration without duct injury or tissue loss
III	Distal transection or parenchymal injury with duct injury
IV	Proximal transection[a] or parenchymal injury involving the ampulla
V	Massive disruption of pancreatic head

a To the right of the superior mesenteric vein.

injury is present. However, if there are any of these findings or if a fatty retroperitoneum precludes adequate visualization, the surgeon should further expose the organ.

Exposure of the pancreas for intra-operative examination requires several surgical maneuvers. Some of them are similar to those described earlier in this chapter on mobilization of the duodenum. These include a wide Kocher maneuver, which should extend from the portal structures to the distal duodenum as it passes behind the right colon (Fig. 28.3). Examination of the body and the tail of the pancreas requires opening of the lesser peritoneal sac through the gastrohepatic ligament. The point of entry should be on the colonic side of the gastroepiploic vascular arcade. The stomach is retracted superiorly and the colon inferiorly. Retracters are often placed under the stomach to lift it anteriorly in order to see the entire length of the pancreatic tail to the splenic hilum. Care should be taken to avoid tearing omental vessels and cause troublesome bleeding. Usually division of the developmental adhesions between the stomach and the anterior portion of the pancreas is required in order to see the entire anterior surface of the pancreas. If, during the lesser sac exposure, there are signs suggesting gland injury, the pancreas should be further explored. This is particularly important when a 'masking hematoma' over a pancreatic fracture is present as shown in Fig. 28.13. The pancreas is usually cracked over the spinal column, just to the left of the superior mesenteric vessels. To visualize this injury, an incision should be made in the peritoneum which is just inferior to the pancreas and in the region of suspicion (Fig. 28.14). The areolar avascular nature of this tissue plane allows the index finger to be slipped behind the pancreas where the fracture can often be felt and, using Army retractors, visualized. It is important to avoid the error of simply examining the anterior surface of the pancreas, because a significant parenchymal injury may occur yet be invisible while the anterior capsule remains intact.

At this time it must be determined whether or not there is a major pancreatic duct (duct of Wirsung or Santorini) disruption. Mobilization of the area with careful inspection usually detects injuries which are serious enough to have disrupted a major pancreatic duct. If there is concern about either common bile duct or pancreatic duct injury near the ampulla of Vater, a cholangiogram should be done. A cholecystocholangiogram will usually adequately assess the distal common bile duct, and the dye will often demonstrate the pancreatic duct. If disruption of the duodenum is present, then a transduodenal pancreatic ductogram can be done safely through the ampulla. If these maneuvers fail, some surgeons

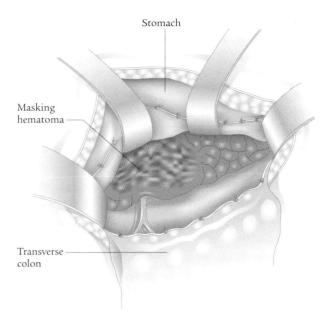

Figure 28.13 Masking hematoma demonstrated through an opening in the gastrocolic ligament.

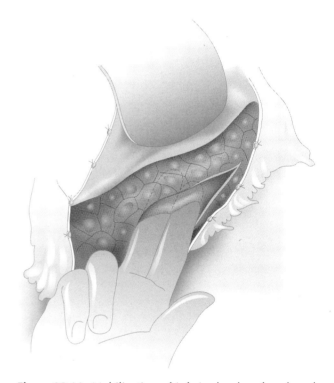

Figure 28.14 Mobilization of inferior border of neck and tail of the pancreas.

advocate obtaining a pancreaticogram by amputating the tail of the pancreas or opening the duodenum. Obtaining access in this way is rarely warranted, because the potential for breakdown of the duodenum or fistulization from the pancreatic tail is too great. We would first attempt to obtain an intraoperative ERCP when a pancreaticogram is necessary (Fig. 28.15). Careful inspection of the lacerated

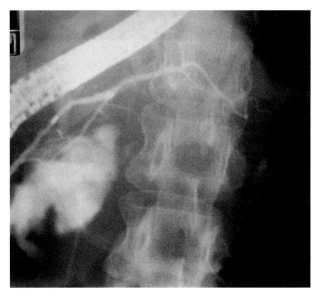

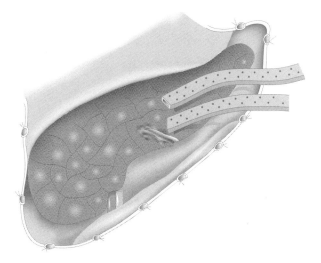

Figure 28.16 Simple drainage of pancreatic injury thought not to involve a major pancreatic duct.

Figure 28.15 Intraoperative ERCP demonstrating disruption of major pancreatic ducts.

pancreatic tissue, particularly if loupe magnification is used, often reveals the pancreatic duct. Collection of clear fluid suggests an open major duct. Intravenous secretin (1 IU per kg body weight over one minute) enhances pancreatic secretion, making ductal identification easier. In essentially all circumstances, one of these options will yield adequate information about ductal continuity.

Treatment of minor injuries to the pancreas

Pancreatic wounds which are considered to be minor, such as small lacerations or contusions of the parenchyma which do not transect a major duct, require only drainage of the closed suction type (Fig. 28.16). Some surgeons recommend suture closure of the pancreatic capsule, but this is not of proven value.

Treatment of injuries to the tail and body of the pancreas

If major disruption of the tissue indicates the likelihood of ductal transection in the region of the neck, body or tail of the pancreas, distal pancreatic resection is most often required. Re-attachment of the pancreas with anastamosis of the duct of Wirsung to itself almost invariably leads to anastomotic breakdown. Others have attempted to deal with this problem by utilizing Roux-en-Y drainage of both cut surfaces or of only the distal pancreatic segment. These maneuvers are carried out in order to preserve pancreatic tissue and maintain the endocrine function of the distal pancreas. However, in trauma

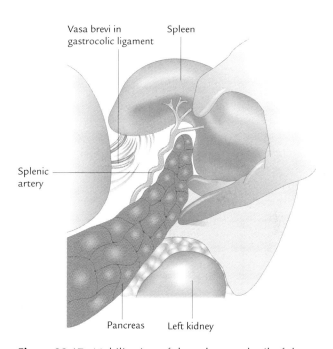

Figure 28.17 Mobilization of the spleen and tail of the pancreas by the Aird maneuver.

surgery the pancreaticojejunal anatamosis is likely to break down. It also requires significantly more time to perform such an anastamosis than a subtotal resection of the pancreas with the spleen. Fortunately, there have been no reports of diabetes mellitus in those patients with distal pancreatectomy for trauma. However, we lack follow-up on the glucose tolerance status of these patients in later life.

In the procedure for distal pancreatectomy with splenectomy (Fig. 28.17) mobilization of the spleen and the tail of the pancreas should progress from the patient's left to the right, by first dividing the peritoneal attachments of the spleen posteriorly over

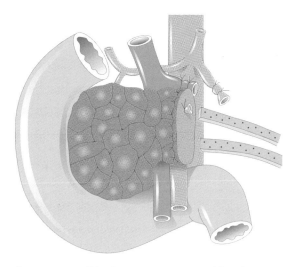

Figure 28.18 Distal pancreatectomy with splenectomy.

the renal fossa and the diaphragm. The spleen and the tail of the pancreas are then lifted anteriorly and to the right using the Aird maneuver.[26] Identification of the splenic artery and vein is most easily done from behind. They should be individually suture ligated just to the right of the proposed pancreatic resection. The site of the fracture is chosen as the point for transection and any devitalized or remaining bridging tissue is divided. Magnification is used to identify the open pancreatic duct in the retained segment, which should be ligated with a fine non-absorbable suture such as 4/0 Prolene™. Non-absorbable suture (silk or Prolene™) should be placed to close the cut end with horizontal mattress sutures (Fig. 28.18). Gastrointestinal stapling devices can also be utilized to close the proximal end. The surgical literature indicates that no matter how this transection is carried out, there is a small but significant incidence of pancreatic leak (see the next section).[27] For this reason, the transected end of the pancreas should be drained with two closed suction drains placed in close proximity.

Splenectomy, carried out as part of distal pancreatectomy, is of concern because an asplenic patient may develop the overwhelming postsplenectomy sepsis syndrome (OPSS). This problem is of greater concern in children than adults. The data regarding the incidence and lethality of OPSS were largely collected prior to the availability of vaccination for *Pneumococcus* and *Haemophilus* influenzae. Therefore, it is difficult to know what the risk of OPSS is when appropriate prophylaxis has been given. From a practical point of view, attempts to preserve the spleen when distal pancreatectomy is carried out for trauma should be limited to patients who are entirely stable hemodynamically, with few other significant injuries. In addition, the surgeon should have had experience in working around the splenic vein. This structure is very closely adherent to the pancreas, and there are many short and very fragile venous connections. These tributaries are easily torn and may lead to significant blood loss and the failure of the operation due to operative injury of the splenic vein.

Distal pancreatectomy with splenic preservation is carried out as shown in Fig. 28.19. Ideally, this operation should be performed using magnification to better identify the small venous tributaries mentioned above. The operation can proceed from right to left after division of the pancreas. As the distal pancreas is lifted anteriorly and slightly cephalad, good exposure to the area of dissection is provided. Fine silk ties may be used on the small venous tributaries and arterial branches. Small hemoclips can be applied to the pancreatic side. This procedure can also be carried out from the spleen towards the central pancreas, with the pancreas and spleen rolled forward, utilizing the Aird maneuver.[26]

If during the procedure, repair or ligation of a torn splenic vein leads to significant narrowing, splenic

Figure 28.19 Distal pancreatectomy with splenic preservation.

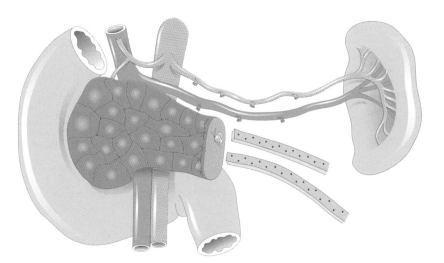

preservation should be abandoned because of the high likelihood of splenic vein thrombosis with subsequent splenic rupture.

Pancreatic head injury

If major pancreatic injury with apparent duct disruption is identified in the head of the pancreas there are several options. In recent years, major bleeding from injuries to the pancreatic head is increasingly managed by packing and rapid abdominal closure, so-called 'damage control'. This is particularly true in the blunt trauma situation because of the frequent association with hepatic injury. In other instances where there is little bleeding but worrisome fracturing of the head of the pancreas, and it is not deemed safe because of hemodynamic instability to proceed with a major resectional operation, liberal drainage around the head of the pancreas with several closed suction drains is also appropriate. Some seemingly deep pancreatic injuries will drain fluid for a number of days or weeks, but the fistula will ultimately close without significant sequelae. We discuss below what should be done if a pancreatic fistula persists. If an extensive pancreatic head injury includes involvement of the duodenum for which there is likely to be a tenuous duodenal suture line (Fig. 28.20), and if the patient is hemodynamically stable, pancreaticoduodenectomy is the best option.

The pancreaticoduodenectomy procedure is shown in Fig. 28.21. One of the important steps in the procedure is to establish a plane between the anterior wall of the portal vein and the posterior pancreatic neck. This plane is generally avascular and is best achieved by digital exploration. Care is taken to stay directly in front of the portal vein because the venous tributaries enter into the side walls of the portal vein from the pancreatic head. The common bile duct in young patients is usually of very small caliber and T-tube drainage of the common bile duct, as might be done in a Whipple procedure for malignancy, is impractical. Either no such drainage is carried out or a small 'pediatric feeding' type tube is placed through the jejunal loop into the common duct. The gallbladder can also be used for biliary decompression. However, retention of the gallbladder when the sphincter of Oddi has been resected is thought to lead to the formation of gallstones.

When a pancreatic head injury is associated with a major duodenal injury, but the duodenal injury can be closed as noted in the above section, another option is to drain the pancreatic head widely and carry out duodenal exclusion (Fig. 28.10) or diverticulization (Fig. 28.11) as discussed above for serious duodenal injury.

Postoperative complications of duodenal and pancreatic trauma

Leaks from both the duodenum and pancreas are most often detected by the presence of drainage into the closed suction drains that were placed at the time of the initial operation. Drainage of small volumes of amylase-containing fluid is quite common, but persistent high volume leaks of fluid containing bile or high levels of amylase suggest significant leak. Occasionally, the operative drains will not adequately evacuate these leaks. The patient will

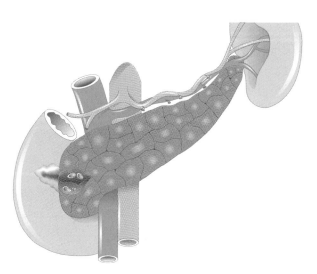

Figure 28.20 Extensive pancreatic head and duodenal injury involving ductal structures, which may require pancreaticoduodenectomy.

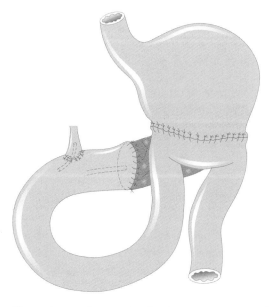

Figure 28.21 Pancreaticoduodenectomy at completion.

develop a collection or peritonitis. In the former case, abdominal discomfort, a palpable mass, fever and/or white blood cell count elevation may herald the collection. If generalized peritonitis develops it must be dealt with by operative exploration. Localized collections are usually identified by CT scan and can be effectively treated, in most instances, by the placement of percutaneous catheters. Occasionally, such patients require reoperation, either because sepsis cannot be controlled with catheter drainage or a pancreatic or duodenal fistula persists for a long period of time. If reoperation has been done for a septic picture, removal of infected devitalized tissue and debris is carried out and drains are placed. Operation for persistent fistula should only be done after several months of management utilizing somatostatin and either jejunal or parenteral feeding. It appears that somatostatin reduces the volume of both duodenal and pancreatic fistula drainage and leads to earlier closure. Studies on prophylactic use of somatostatin to prevent pancreatic fistulas after trauma surgery are yet inconclusive. If this management fails, placement of a Roux-en-Y loop over the fistula's opening can be done to control the fistula. For pancreatic fistula from the neck, body or tail, resection of the distal pancreas is sometimes possible. Suture closure alone is likely to fail. In each instance suction drains should be left in the operative area.

Delayed gastric emptying with gastric outlet obstruction due to narrowing of a gastrojejunal or duodenal suture line will occasionally occur. A water-soluble upper gastrointestinal contrast (WSUGI) study should be performed to define the problem and, in some instances, provide relief of the obstruction. Usually a partial obstruction will be identified and further non-operative management should be carried out for 2 to 3 weeks until gastrointestinal function improves. Occasionally a clearly mechanical problem will be identified on WSUGI and require early reoperation. Unrelenting duodenal obstruction will usually require creation of a gastrojejunostomy, while gastrojejunostomy dysfunction often necessitates revision of that gastrojejunostomy. When gastric atony is a contributing factor, removal of additional stomach may be necessary. Because these remedies often require some time before oral intake can be re-established, jejunostomy and gastrostomy are often included so early enteral feeding is possible.

When duodenal diverticulization or diversion is carried out the patient is at some small risk of developing gastrojejunal ulceration, particularly if vagotomy has not been done. As noted earlier, this should be a relatively infrequent occurrence, particularly if the patient is managed postoperatively with intensive antiulcer therapy. Only very rarely will patients require ulcer curative surgery.

Key points

- Blunt trauma to the pancreas and duodenum result from high-energy crushing forces applied to the epigastric region.
- Diagnosis may be difficult because of the insidious nature of largely retroperitoneal injury— therefore always suspect after blunt abdominal trauma.
- Serum amylase levels and diagnostic peritoneal lavage results are often misleading.
- Operative evaluation includes:
  Mobilization of duodenum and head of pancreas and evaluation of hematoma
  Full exposure of length of pancreas
  Exclusion of other injuries: liver, spleen, mesentery.
- Postoperative complications:
  Duodenal/pancreatic fistula/collection
  Gastric outflow obstruction
  Peptic ulceration
  Pancreatic duct stricture and localized chronic pancreatitis.

Acknowledgements

Acknowledgements to Pat Garcia and Martha Eide for typing this chapter.

REFERENCES

1. Milburn EL. On excretory ducts of pancreas in man, with special reference to their relation to each other, to common bile duct, and to duodenum: radiological and anatomical study. Acta Anat 1950; 9: 1–34

2. Lucas CE, Ledgerwood AM. Factors influencing outcome after blunt duodenal injury. J Trauma 1975; 15: 839–46

3. Leppaniemi AK, Haapiainen RK. Risk factors of delayed diagnosis of pancreatic trauma. Eur J Surg 1999; 165: 1134–7

4. Allen GS, Moore FA, Cox CS Jr, Mehall JR, Duke JH. Delayed diagnosis of blunt duodenal injury: an avoidable complication. J Am Coll Surg 1998; 187: 393–9

5. Cogbill TN, Moore EE, Kashuk JL. Changing trends in the management of pancreatic trauma. Arch Surg 1982; 117: 722–8

6. White PH, Benfield JR. Amylase in the management of pancreatic trauma. Arch Surg 1972; 105: 158–63

7. Moretz JA, Campbell DP, Parker DE et al. Significance of serum amylase level in evaluating pancreatic trauma. Am J Surg 1975; 130: 739–41

8. Olsen WR. The serum amylase in blunt abdominal trauma. J Trauma 1973; 12: 200–4

9. Moore EE, Cogbill TH, Malagoni MA et al. Organ injury scaling II. Pancreas, duodenum, small bowel, colon, rectum. J Trauma 1990; 30: 1427–9

10. Cattell RB, Braasch JW. A technique for exposure of the duodenum. Surg Gynecol Obstet 1954; 98: 376–7

11. Lorente-Ramos RM, Santiago-Hernando A, DelValle-Sanz Y, Arjonillo-Lopez A. Sonographic diagnosis of intramural duodenal hematomas. J Clinical Ultrasound 1999; 27: 213–6

12. Wooley M, Mahoor G, Sloan T. Duodenal hematoma in infancy and childhood. Am J Surg 1978; 136: 8–14

13. Touloukian R. Protocol for the nonoperative treatment of obstructing intramural duodenal hematoma. Am J Surg 1983; 145: 330–4

14. Kobold EE, Thai AP. A simple method for the management of experimental wounds of the duodenum. Surg Gynecol Obstet 1963; 116: 340–3

15. Graham JM, Mattox, KL, Vaughan GD III, Jordan GL. Combined pancreaticoduodenal injuries. J Trauma 1979; 19: 340–6

16. Kelly G, Norton L, Moore G et al. The continuing challenge of duodenal injuries. J Trauma 1987; 18: 160–5

17. Fang JF, Chen RJ, Lin BC. Surgical treatment and outcome after delayed diagnosis of blunt duodenal injury. Eur Journal Surgery 1999; 165: 133–9

18. Berne CJ, Donovan AJ, White EJ et al. Duodenal 'diverticulization' for duodenal and pancreatic injury. Am J Surg 1974; 127: 503–7

19. Corley RD, Norcross WJ, Shoemaker WC. Traumatic injuries to the duodenum. A report of 98 patients. Am Surg 1974; 181: 92–8

20. Stone HH, Fabian TC. Management of duodenal trauma. J Trauma 1979; 19: 334–9

21. Hasson JE, Stern D, Mosds GS. Penetrating duodenal trauma. J Trauma 1984; 24: 471–4

22. Ivatury RR, Guadino J, Ascer E et al. Treatment of penetrating duodenal injuries: primary repair vs repair with decompressive enterostomy/serosal patch. J Trauma 1985; 25: 337–41

23. Martin TD, Feliciano DV, Mattox KL et al. Severe duodenal injuries. Arch Surg 1983; 118: 631–5

24. Jurkovich GJ. Injuries to the duodenum and pancreas. In: Feliciano DV, Moore EE, Mattox KL, eds. Trauma, 3rd edn. Stamford, Connecticut: Appleton and Lange, 1996: 573–94

25. Tyburski JG, Dente CJ, Wilson RF, Shanti C, Steffer CP, Carlin A. Infectious complications following duodenal and/or pancreatic trauma. Am Surg 2001; 67: 227–30

26. Aird I, Helman P. Bilateral anterior transabdominal adrenalectomy. Br Med J 1955; 2: 708

27. Fitzgibbons TJ, Yellin AE, Maruyama MM et al. Management of the transected pancreas. Surg Gynecol Obstet 1982; 154: 225–31

29 Liver trauma, including caval injury

Timothy G John and Myrddin Rees

Introduction

The liver is the abdominal organ most commonly injured following both blunt and penetrating trauma. The type and severity of liver injuries vary greatly and many different approaches to their treatment have been described. While the majority of liver injuries may prove to be relatively minor and inconsequential, and it is now clear that even patients with severe liver trauma do not necessarily require operative intervention, other patients with hepatic trauma present the ultimate surgical challenge to even the most experienced trauma or hepatobiliary surgeon. Not surprisingly, a wide spectrum of outcomes has been reported, with the issue further complicated by the consequences of other organ injuries.

The management of liver trauma continues to evolve apace with dramatic advances in its management reported during and since the last decade. Consensus now exists in certain areas of treatment, and this has facilitated protocols for the management of liver trauma. Conversely, other aspects of its treatment remain the focus of controversy.

Anatomical considerations and mechanisms of injury

The major cause of death following liver trauma is haemorrhage. The liver is the largest solid abdominal organ and its dual vascular inflow, comprising the portal vein and hepatic artery, delivers up to 2 litres of blood per minute to the hepatic parenchymal mass. This fragile pulp is contained within the thin fascial investment comprising Glisson's capsule. Some protection is afforded by the lower chest wall and the liver is secured by various peritoneal reflections. However, it is the intimate connections between the liver capsule, the major

hepatic veins and the retrohepatic inferior vena cava (IVC) which are primarily responsible for anchoring the liver within the upper abdominal cavity. Most of the venous return from the lower body flows within these thin-walled veins, and injuries to these vulnerable, high volume flow 'juxtahepatic' vessels are a uniquely challenging feature of severe liver trauma.

The liver is thus susceptible to a variety of types of injury. It presents a large target for penetrating injuries to the trunk. Blunt trauma delivers compressive impacts, and deceleration or shearing forces which cause parenchymal rupture and intrahepatic or subcapsular haematoma formation. The deceleration forces inherent in motor vehicle accidents may avulse the right hepatic vein or one of its major tributaries in their short extrahepatic course. Major parenchymal lacerations along the plane between the posterior (segments VI and VII) and anterior sections (segments V and VIII) of the right hemiliver also characterize such injuries. The fundamental aims of treatment in the patient with liver trauma are to arrest bleeding, preserve hepatic function and prevent late complications, mainly infection.

Classification of liver trauma

The liver is a complex organ and the very diversity of liver trauma and its management resists generalizations. Furthermore, the reported overall mortality in various liver trauma series varies widely, and is undoubtedly influenced by the prevailing casemix.[1] This confounds superficial comparisons of overall mortality as reported outcomes often reflect the types of injury as much as any particular treatment policy. As observed by Krige and colleagues,[2] overall reported mortalities in centres experiencing mainly penetrating liver injuries (e.g. Detroit, Dallas, Houston and New Orleans) are lower than those where blunt injuries predominate (e.g. Toronto, Baltimore and Sydney).

The importance of a standardized method of classifying liver trauma is fundamental to meaningful comparisons of treatment outcomes. Several different classifications have been devised, usually based on the degree and nature of anatomical disruption, but also on the type of treatment required. A basic classification which has been adopted by several authors in the past describes liver injuries as 'simple' (grades I–II) or 'complex' (grades III–IV).[3–5] In this system, haemostasis is achieved spontaneously or by suture ligation in 'simple' liver injuries, whereas 'complex' injuries imply major life-threatening haemorrhage requiring advanced surgical and/or interventional radiological skills.

The more sophisticated classification of liver injuries described by Moore and co-workers in 1989,[6] and revised in 1994,[7] has now been adopted as the 'industry standard' by the American Association for the Surgery of Trauma (AAST) (Table 29.1). The liver injury scale of I–VI reflects the anatomical extent of liver injury defined not only at operation (or autopsy), but also from imaging studies in patients managed non-operatively. This reflects the importance of the radiologist in the modern management of liver trauma, and serves to emphasize that diagnostic and interventional radiological techniques are indispensable in the multidisciplinary approach to liver trauma management.

Validation of the AAST organ injury scale was first attempted by Croce and co-workers in which 37 patients with blunt liver trauma were studied.[8] The liver injury scale was assigned at operation in each case and correlated with preoperative CT, transfusion requirements and operative management. Good correlation was observed between operative score severity on the one hand, and transfusional requirements and methods of operative management necessitated on the other. A similar study from Toronto applied the AAST organ injury scale to a cohort of 170 liver injury patients (90% blunt trauma).[9] Again, blood transfusions, surgical interventions and liver-related morbidity and mortality all correlated well with the grade of injury.

However, the liver injury scale as determined by preoperative computed tomography (CT) was not always as accurate. Instances of both understaging and overstaging by CT were documented in the Memphis study,[8] while the need for laparotomy or the length of hospital stay could not be predicted reliably in the Canadian study.[9] Despite such anxieties regarding CT-graded liver injury scores in the non-operative management of patients with apparent minor injury,[8] the AAST classification has been widely adopted as a paradigm, and is the basis of modern protocol-guided management of liver trauma in most institutions (vide infra).

Initial assessment and diagnosis of liver trauma

Resuscitation: priorities in the initial management of liver trauma

Initial management of the patient with suspected liver trauma follows advanced trauma life support (ATLS) principles,[10] and aggressive fluid resuscitation should be instigated immediately through multiple, large-bore, upper limb peripheral venous cannulae. Nasogastric tubes and urinary catheters should be inserted as appropriate. The importance of temperature monitoring and the prevention of systemic hypothermia during resuscitation and transfer deserve emphasis.[11] Hypothermia in trauma patients exacerbates coagulopathy and the bleeding diathesis

Table 29.1 **American Association for the Surgery of Trauma liver injury scale (1994 revision)[7]**

Grade[a]		Injury description[b]
I	Haematoma	Subcapsular, non-expanding, <10% surface area
	Laceration	Capsular tear, non-bleeding, <1 cm parenchymal depth
II	Haematoma	Subcapsular, 10–50% surface area; Intraparenchymal, <10 cm in diameter
	Laceration	1–3 cm parenchymal depth, <10 cm in length
III	Haematoma	Subcapsular, >50% surface area or expanding Ruptured subcapsular or parenchymal haematoma Intraparenchymal haematoma >10 cm or expanding
	Laceration	>3 cm parenchymal depth
IV	Laceration	Parenchymal disruption involving 25–75% of hepatic lobe or 1–3 Couinaud's segments within a single lobe
V	Laceration	Parenchymal disruption involving >75% of hepatic lobe or >3 Couinaud's segments within a single lobe
	Vascular	Juxtahepatic venous injuries; i.e. retrohepatic vena cava/central major hepatic veins
VI	Vascular	Hepatic avulsion

[a] Advance one grade for multiple injuries to the same organ.
[b] Based on most accurate assessment at autopsy, laparotomy, or radiological study.

and is associated with increased mortality.[12] Rewarming measures include the use of heated and convective air blankets and a turban around the head. Active core rewarming using warm intravenous infusions and blood products (ideally using a rapid infusion pump with heat exchanger) and intraoperative body cavity lavage are simple and effective measures which should not be neglected.[12] Intensive monitoring and early treatment of abnormalities of acid–base balance, coagulation and electrolytes (including ionized calcium) are essential, with anticipation of adverse events through good communication between surgeons and anaesthesiologists.

Prompt transfer to the operating room to permit operative control of intra-abdominal bleeding is of paramount importance in the haemodynamically unstable patient. This principle was emphasized by the findings of the Western Trauma Association's study of death in the operating room following major trauma at eight North American Level I trauma centres between 1985 and 1992.[13] Of 537 patients studied, uncontrolled haemorrhage was judged to have been the primary cause of death in 82% of patients. Delays in transfer to the operating room and inadequate perioperative resuscitation were implicated in 29 out of 54 intraoperative deaths (54%) judged to have been preventable.

Investigate further or operate immediately?

The possibility of liver injury should be suspected in all cases of blunt or penetrating thoracoabdominal trauma. Its diagnosis may be readily apparent in the patient presenting in a shocked state with abdominal distension and blunt or penetrating injuries to the right thoracoabdominal region. Conversely, the diagnosis of significant liver trauma may initially prove surprisingly elusive. The development of organized and systematic algorithms for the assessment of abdominal trauma in recent years has undoubtedly improved methods for the evaluation and management of liver trauma.

The first principle of liver trauma management is that haemodynamically unstable patients (systolic blood pressure <90 mmHg) who do not respond to fluid resuscitation (2 litres of intravenous fluid) require immediate operation to arrest intra-abdominal haemorrhage. Inappropriate delays caused by the quest for diagnostic information in such cases may ultimately prove fatal (vide supra). Thus, transfer to the operating room for immediate laparotomy is indicated in the unstable patient following penetrating abdominal trauma—attention to concomitant injuries rarely demands priority. Similarly with blunt liver injuries, although it is necessary to confirm the abdominal cavity as the major site of

bleeding in patients with blunt polytrauma (vide infra). Obviously it is important first to exclude ongoing haemorrhage in the chest cavity, pelvis or long bones by thorough clinical assessment and appropriate plain radiographs.

The haemodynamically stable patient with liver trauma: operation or observation?

Opinions regarding the optimal method of establishing the diagnosis of liver trauma in the haemodynamically stable patient vary according to the prevailing experience and expertise in individual institutions. Perhaps of more importance in this scenario is the decision of whether to proceed straight to laparotomy or to pursue an expectant policy of observation. The main modalities employed in this role include diagnostic peritoneal lavage (DPL), abdominal ultrasonography, abdominal computerized tomography (CT) and laparoscopy (Table 29.2). In addition, the diagnostic and therapeutic roles of selective hepatic arteriography have assumed increased importance.

Diagnostic peritoneal lavage

Advantages of diagnostic peritoneal lavage (DPL) include its simplicity, speed and high sensitivity in detecting intraperitoneal blood. Its performance by the 'open technique' remains a fundamental tenet of trauma assessment as recommended by the American College of Surgeons Committee on Trauma.[10] Alternatively, DPL maybe performed by the 'closed technique' using a peritoneal dialysis type catheter over a percutaneously introduced trocar or flexible wire. A (non-randomized) study from Los Angeles reported that while closed DPL was found to be as sensitive and specific as the open method, it was also quicker and less likely to yield inconclusive results.[14] Closed DPL is therefore particularly useful for confirming haemoperitoneum prior to laparotomy in the haemodynamically unstable patient with suspected blunt liver trauma.

Nevertheless, DPL is fallible. Its principal drawback is its very sensitivity in detecting even small quantities of intraperitoneal blood in the effluent, and the observer is in practice liable to overestimate the degree of blood staining and its clinical significance.[15] Although decisions based on laboratory determined red and white cell counts might be expected to introduce objectivity and improve specificity, there is evidence that even this approach may fail in instances of penetrating injury.[16] This explains the consistent failure of DPL to identify those patients with minor liver (or splenic) injuries who stop bleeding spontaneously, and in whom

Table 29.2 **Summary points: investigations for suspected liver trauma**

Diagnostic peritoneal lavage
1. Rapid and sensitive method for confirmation of haemoperitoneum
2. ATLS recommended
3. Open or closed techniques

Limitations
1. Non-specific. Unnecessary laparotomies due to false positive results
2. Insensitive for diaphragmatic, retroperitoneal and hollow viscus injuries
3. Invasive. Associated risk of visceral injury

Ultrasonography
1. Rapid, accurate, repeatable, non-invasive and inexpensive
2. 'FAST' protocol. May be performed by (trained) attending surgeon
3. First-line modality for precordial wounds and blunt truncal injury
4. May have superceded DPL as a prelude to laparotomy in the unstable patient

Limitations
1. Operator-dependent. Requires aptitude and appropriate training
2. Insensitive for diaphragmatic and hollow viscus injuries
3. Imprecise anatomical delineation of hepatic parenchymal injuries
4. Not suitable for monitoring non-operative management of liver trauma

Laparoscopy
1. Highly specific. Avoids non-therapeutic laparotomy for non-bleeding liver lacerations—especially penetrating injuries and tangential gunshot wounds
2. Identifies 'occult' diaphragmatic lacerations and some hollow viscus injuries
3. Feasible as an emergency department/local anaesthetic procedure

Limitations
1. Little evidence for benefit in blunt trauma
2. Invasive and potentially time-consuming. Possible risk of tension pneumothorax and gas embolism
3. May miss retroperitoneal and hollow viscus injuries
4. Logistically difficult to perform in the busy emergency department

Computed tomography
1. Excellent definition of hepatic parenchymal injury/haemoperitoneum
2. The basis for non-operative management of liver trauma
3. Accurate evaluation of associated abdominal and retroperitoneal injuries

Limitations
1. Liable to understage or overstage grade of liver injury (AAST organ injury scale)
2. Potentially time-consuming and risks delaying operative control of haemorrhage
   Not suitable for triage of the haemodynamically unstable patient
3. May miss hollow viscus injury
4. Expensive

'non-therapeutic' laparotomy might have been avoided. Against this background, a review of liver trauma management in The Royal Infirmary, Edinburgh, in the 1980s revealed that spontaneous haemostasis was observed at laparotomy in 13 out of 24 patients with 'simple' penetrating liver injuries (54%), and in 14 out of 27 patients with 'simple' blunt liver injuries (52%).[5] The literature contains numerous other studies which reproducibly report similar data.[11]

The role of DPL has become more restricted in the evaluation of selected stable patients with liver trauma since the advent of CT-guided non-operative management (vide infra). However, it deserves emphasis that DPL remains useful for the rapid demonstration of haemoperitoneum prior to emergency laparotomy in haemodynamically unstable patients with blunt polytrauma. Even so, ultrasonography has now assumed a dominant role in this scenario (vide infra).

Ultrasonography

Emergency department ultrasonography seems destined to play an increasing role in decision making in patients with liver trauma. Its advantages include its non-invasiveness, its reported high accuracy, the rapidity of the examination, the ease with which it may be repeated and its relative inexpense. However, abdominal ultrasonography is inherently operator-dependent and much depends on the experience and enthusiasm of the sonographer. Nevertheless, there is increasing evidence testifying to the feasibility of surgeon-performed ultrasound in the setting of blunt abdominal trauma.[17,18]

The importance of a systematic and comprehensive sonographic examination is emphasized, with particular attention to the (subxiphoid) pericardial region for haemopericardium, and the left and right upper abdominal quadrants and pelvis for haemoperitoneum.[18–21] This is imbued in the concept of the 'Focused Assessment for the Sonographic examination of the Trauma patient' (FAST), which has gained acceptance in many North American trauma centres (Fig. 29.1). A landmark study of surgeon-performed FAST in 1540 patients with blunt and penetrating truncal injuries reported high sensitivity (83.3%) and specificity (99.7%) for the technique, most pronounced following blunt injury. Because of its rapidity and accuracy, it was concluded that FAST should become the initial diagnostic modality for the evaluation of patients with precordial wounds and blunt truncal injuries.[18] In particular, immediate surgical intervention was recommended on the basis of a positive ultrasound examination in the hypotensive patient with blunt truncal injury, i.e. the role previously fulfilled by DPL. The algorithm for the use of ultrasonography in blunt abdominal trauma suggested by Rozycki and Shackford[22] summarizes current opinion (Fig. 29.2).

Thus, sufficient evidence seems to have emerged to recommend ultrasonography as a rapid, non-invasive,

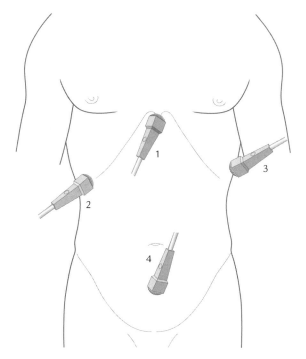

Figure 29.1 Probe positions and sequence for focused assessment for the sonographic examination of the trauma patient (FAST). (1) pericardial area, (2) right upper quadrant, (3) left upper quadrant and, (4) pelvis.

low-cost method of providing triage to patients with suspected blunt liver trauma. However, it should be appreciated that ultrasonography is limited in its ability to define hepatic parenchymal damage and is no substitute for CT in the non-operative management of the stable patient with hepatic trauma. It is also insensitive in detecting hollow viscus and diaphragmatic injuries.

Laparoscopy

The rationale for emergency laparoscopy in the evaluation of abdominal trauma is attractive—excellent views of the abdominal cavity are obtained using

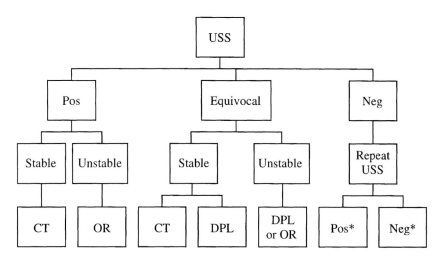

Figure 29.2 Suggested algorithm for the use of ultrasonography in the patient with blunt abdominal trauma.[22] USS, ultrasonography; OR, operating room; Pos, positive; Neg, negative; * indicates that algorithm for initial positive or negative sonogram should be followed (after Rozyck: and Shackford[22]).

modern videolaparoscopic camera systems and light sources. Minor liver injuries which stop bleeding spontaneously may be identified and unnecessary laparotomy avoided. Also, visceral and diaphragmatic injuries missed by ultrasonography or CT may be identified and repaired. Thus, enthusiasts have re-explored the role of diagnostic laparoscopy in the assessment of haemodynamically stable patients with both blunt and penetrating abdominal trauma, no doubt stimulated by recent advances and increased confidence with minimal access general surgery.

These apparent advantages were highlighted by the preliminary results of the only randomized (multi-centre) study in which 'mini-laparoscopy' (using a 4 mm laparoscope under IV sedation) was compared with DPL in 55 patients with blunt abdominal motor vehicle trauma.[23] Although both techniques were sensitive in detecting significant haemoperitoneum, mini-laparoscopy was more specific in recognizing minimal static bleeds and avoiding unnecessary laparotomy (8%, versus 27% for DPL). However, later studies have failed consistently to reproduce such findings or show an advantage for diagnostic laparoscopy over DPL in the context of blunt abdominal trauma.[24,25]

Conversely, the diagnostic yield of trauma laparoscopy seems more evident in patients with abdominal penetrating wounds. In 100 laparoscopies for penetrating injuries, Ivatury and co-workers in New York reported the avoidance of unnecessary laparotomy in 34% of stab wounds and 60% of gun shot wounds, and demonstrated diaphragmatic lacerations in 47% of those with peritoneal penetration.[26] Ditmars and Bongard even highlight the potential cost savings attributed to reduced negative laparotomy rates and early patient discharge following laparoscopy based on a study of 106 haemodynamically stable patients with penetrating abdominal injuries in Los Angeles (including 66 gunshot wounds).[27] In a systematic review of laparoscopy in trauma, Villavicensio and Aucar analysed 37 studies comprising nearly 2000 trauma patients.[28] Laparoscopy helped prevent laparotomy in 63% of patients with a variety of injuries, although the great majority of these followed penetrating trauma.

Detractors of diagnostic laparoscopy cite the (theoretical) risk of gas embolism and tension pneumothorax, its limitations and dangers in the presence of intra-abdominal adhesions, the potential fallibility of laparoscopy in overlooking significant bowel injuries and, perhaps most importantly, the risk of delaying definitive, life-saving treatment. However, the overall reported rates of missed injuries and procedure-related complications have been estimated as 1% in each case.[28]

Diagnostic laparoscopy thus remains a controversial approach in the setting of suspected liver trauma. While there is a paucity of evidence to support a prime role in the assessment of blunt abdominal injury, diagnostic laparoscopy may yet fulfil a unique role in both evaluating diaphragmatic injuries after penetrating thoracoabdominal wounds, and confirming or refuting peritoneal penetration, and eliminating unnecessary laparotomies following tangential gunshot wounds.[29]

Computed tomography

Abdominal CT has become the method of choice for the evaluation of the stable patient with suspected blunt liver trauma[30] (Fig. 29.3). Detailed cross-sectional

A

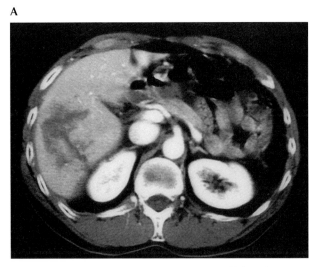

B

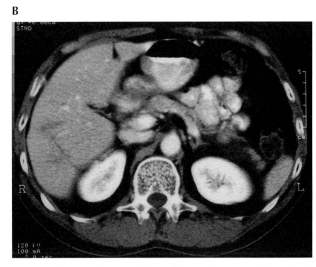

Figure 29.3 Non-operative management of blunt hepatic trauma in the haemodynamically stable patient. (A) Abdominal CT reveals grade IV parenchymal disruption of the right hemiliver. (B) Follow-up CT 5 weeks later confirmed near complete healing of the hepatic lacerations.

Table 29.3 **Estimation of volume of haemoperitoneum based on eight intraperitoneal spaces (after Knudson et al.)[31]**

Intraperitoneal
Right and left subphrenic
Right and left subhepatic
Right and left paracolic
Pelvic
Intramesenteric

Blood location	Estimate of blood volume
1–2 spaces	Small (<250 ml)
3–4 spaces	Moderate (250–500 ml)
>4 spaces	Large (>500 ml)

imaging of the abdominal organs permits precise delineation of the type and extent of the liver injury, estimation of the volume of haemoperitoneum[31] (Table 29.3) and demonstration of associated intraperitoneal and retroperitoneal injuries. The status of CT as a paradigm in the non-operative management of blunt liver trauma (vide infra) has been enhanced by technical refinements such as the development of rapid spiral CT scanners, protocols optimizing vascular contrast enhancement and CT-scanning suites adjacent to the emergency department and equipped for critical care monitoring.[30]

Hepatic parenchymal injuries may be defined in terms of:

1. Subcapsular haematoma,
2. Intrahepatic haematoma,
3. Laceration,
4. Vascular injury, and/or,
5. Active haemorrhage.[30]

Although reliable predictors of failure of non-operative management are lacking, contrast extravasation and 'pooling' merit emphasis as cardinal signs of active haemorrhage mandating prompt (angiographic and/or surgical) intervention[11,30,32-34] (Fig. 29.4). Fang et al.[34] reported contrast pooling in eight out of 150 stable patients treated non-operatively, six of whom (75%) developed haemodynamic instability requiring liver-related laparotomy.

Concerns persist regarding the reliability of CT in the detection of hollow viscus injuries.[35] However, recent evidence refutes the necessity for the administration of oral contrast solution in patients with blunt abdominal trauma. Indeed, a randomized study by Stafford and colleagues indicates that oral contrast administration was both unnecessary and a source of delay in obtaining abdominal CT.[36]

Based on their successful experience with the non-operative management of 37 selected patients with blunt hepatic trauma, Mirvis and co-workers devised an injury severity classification specific for CT-based management of blunt hepatic trauma.[37] However, the updated 1994 AAST liver injury scale also embodies such imaging information and has superseded the former (Table 29.1).[7] As discussed above, the fallibility of CT in calculating surgically determined AAST liver injury grades was highlighted in the study by Croce et al.[8] They noted understaging of injury severity in 15 out of 37 cases (41%), and overestimation of its severity in 12 (32%). Factors implicated in CT misclassifications included intrahepatic haematomas not evident at operation (Fig. 29.5), underestimation of parenchymal lacerations

A

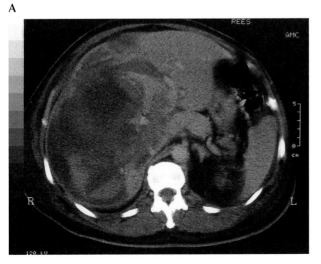

B

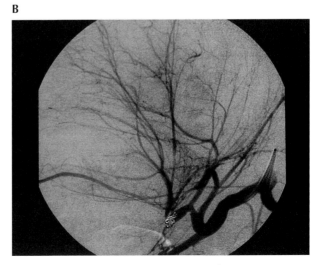

Figure 29.4 (A) Abdominal CT following penetrating trauma to the right liver showing a massive intrahepatic haematoma with contrast pooling indicative of active haemorrhage. (B) Selective hepatic arteriography defined a right sectoral artery laceration. Angioembolization was succesfully performed.

A

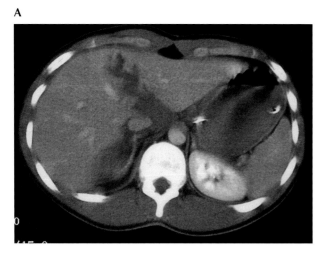

B

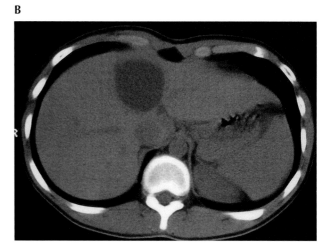

Figure 29.5 (A) Laceration through the left hemiliver in the vicinity of the ligamentum teres insertion following a motor vehicle accident. Despite haemodynamic stability, increasing peritonism secondary to a pancreatic injury mandated laparotomy. The liver appeared undamaged to external inspection and required no further intervention. (B) Follow-up CT at 6 weeks demonstrated a resolving intrahepatic biloma/haematoma.

near the falciform ligament and suboptimal quality scans. However, the majority of reported discrepancies were inexplicable.[8]

Principles of non-operative management of blunt liver trauma

The concept of 'surgical abstention' in selected patients with suspected liver injuries is now firmly established. Indeed, the advent of non-operative management may justifiably be regarded as one of the most important advances in liver trauma management in recent times. Factors which heralded this change include:

1. The recognition that as many as two-thirds of patients with blunt injuries operated on the basis of positive DPL were found to have relatively trivial injuries during non-therapeutic laparotomy (vide supra).
2. Improved imaging techniques, i.e. abdominal CT (vide supra).
3. The precedents for successful non-operative management of liver trauma documented in the paediatric literature.[38-40]
4. A better understanding of the pathophysiology of liver injury.

Reports indicate that as many as 50–82% of all adult patients with blunt liver trauma may be managed non-operatively.[11,41-43] Indeed, it now seems likely that at least 90% of patients with blunt liver trauma may be satisfactorily managed thus in future.[11,32,44] Evidence for the success of non-operative management was presented in a collective review of 16

published series comprising 609 adult patients with liver trauma managed non-operatively between 1988 and 1997.[32] 'Success rates' of 84–100%, mean hospital stays of 11.5–16.6 days and mean transfusional requirements of 1–4 units were documented.[31,37,42-55]

Having established a likely diagnosis of liver trauma in the haemodynamically stable patient, a critical decision must be made whether to embark on a surgical approach or to attempt non-operative management. Although there is no consensus defining criteria for the non-operative management of blunt liver trauma, the following principles are at least accepted:[11,32]

1. Haemodynamic stability, with CT delineation of,
2. Simple hepatic parenchymal laceration or intrahepatic haematoma,
3. Absence of active haemorrhage,
4. Haemoperitoneum of less than 500 ml, and,
5. Limited need for liver-related blood transfusions,
6. Absence of diffuse peritoneal signs in patients not neurologically impaired and,
7. Absence of other (visceral or retroperitoneal) injuries which would otherwise require operation.

However, treatment failures are difficult to predict and it is obvious that intensive care monitoring by an appropriately experienced multidisciplinary team is a prerequisite for non-operative management of the patient with liver trauma.[41]

It should be noted that increased experience and confidence with non-operative treatment has

Table 29.4 **Contraindications to non-operative management of blunt liver trauma**

1. Haemodynamic instability (after initial resuscitation)
2. Peritoneal irritation (except localized to right hypochondrium)
3. Suboptimal quality abdominal CT
4. Suspected associated abdominal injuries
5. Continued requirement for liver-related blood transfusion (>4 units)

lowered the threshold to include patients with hepatic trauma regardless of the severity of the liver injury on CT. Furthermore, the arbitrary acceptable upper limit of haemoperitoneum of 500 ml is no longer regarded as sacrosanct.[44] It has also become accepted that neurological integrity, of itself, is not a necessity for safe non-operative management in the stable patient.[33] However, it should be emphasized that careful clinical judgement must be exercised in selecting such patients for non-operative management, and delays in arresting haemorrhage by surgical means while obtaining CT scans or angiograms must be avoided if the overall success of this approach is to be maintained (vide supra). Suggested contraindications to non-operative management are summarized in Table 29.4.

There is no consensus as to the need for follow-up imaging, nor for the duration of bed rest, inpatient observation or return to physical activity such as contact sport. However, the available evidence does not support repeating CT scans as routine.[11,32]

Complications of non-operative management

Contamination of the peritoneal cavity with blood and bile is an inevitable consequence of a policy of non-operative management in patients with liver trauma, particularly those with more severe injuries. Both localized peritoneal signs and a systemic inflammatory response with persisting fever, leucocytosis and tachycardia may be expected. Furthermore, the anticipation and management of specific complications is inherent to the successful non-operative management of severe liver injuries. Typically these include arterio–venous fistulae, bile leaks, intra or perihepatic abscesses and vascular–biliary communications (bilhaemia and haemobilia). Carillo and Richardson have noted that such complications are 'virtually obligatory consequences' of non-operative management.[56] Moreover, they have redefined the philosophy of surgical abstention by emphasizing that delayed surgery

and/or interventional procedures are not only justified, but should be deemed an inherent part of the overall management plan rather than treatment failure. Although conjectural, it seems highly probable that the adoption of non-operative management rather than operative intervention has heralded a substantial reduction in mortality associated with severe blunt liver injuries.[11,33]

It has been estimated that approximately 60% of grade IV–V liver lacerations treated in this way require delayed intervention for complications.[56] However, the role of surgery for complications has declined in favour of 'alternative' interventions (e.g. angioembolization, percutaneous tube drainage, ERCP and laparoscopy). Thus, 32 patients out of 135 (24%) with blunt liver trauma managed non-operatively at the University of Louisville, Kentucky during 1995–97 developed such complications, 94% of which comprised grade IV–V injuries.[33] Strategies employed in their treatment included angioembolization (37%), CT-guided drainage of collections (31%), ERCP (25%) and laparoscopic drainage of collections (7%). The increasing tendency to attempt non-operative management of severe liver trauma further emphasizes the role of the multidisciplinary team in managing the recognized pitfalls, and close consultation between surgeon, interventional radiologist and/or endoscopist and intensive care specialist is essential.

Haemorrhage

It is increasingly recognized that selective angiography with transcatheter embolization may be effective in arresting hepatic arterial bleeding at an early stage in the course of non-operative management (Fig. 29.4). This strategy seems most appropriate in the stable patient. Moreover, it has been suggested that the role of selective hepatic arterial embolization may be extended as an alternative to surgery in the shocked patient who responds to initial resuscitative measures (Table 29.5). Ciraulo and colleagues reported an encouraging preliminary experience with 'resuscitative' angioembolization in 'bridging' operative and non-operative management.[57] Seven out of 11 patients with CT-determined grade IV–V blunt hepatic injuries and requiring continuous resuscitation were successfully managed by hepatic embolization as definitive therapy. The 'alternative' management of haemorrhage from grade V juxtahepatic venous lacerations by percutaneous hepatic venous stenting has also been reported.[58] Clearly, much depends on the timing of such intervention and the prompt availability of appropriate expertise (with an operating room on standby).[33]

The recognition and prompt treatment of ongoing or recurrent bleeding in the non-operatively managed

Table 29.5 **Summary points: the role of selective hepatic arteriography in the management of patients with liver trauma**

1. Diagnosis of active haemorrhage in subcapsular and intrahepatic haematomas, arterio–venous fistulae, false aneurysms and haemobilia
2. Resuscitative angioembolization as a bridge between operative and non-operative management
3. Salvage embolization for ongoing/recurrent bleeding in non-operative management of stable patients
4. Salvage embolization for ongoing/recurrent bleeding after perihepatic packing/conservative surgery

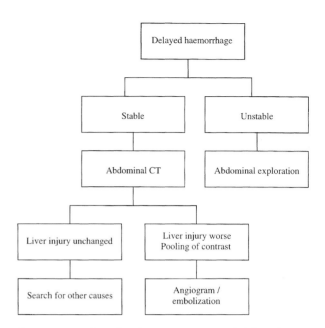

Figure 29.6 Algorithm for management of delayed haemorrhage following blunt liver injury (after Carrillo et al.[32,33]).

patient is imperative. This is usually manifest as haemodynamic instability with a gradually declining haematocrit and the requirement for repeated transfusions. Recognized pitfalls include assumptions or overestimation of associated non-hepatic bleeding, underestimation of haemoperitoneum or active bleeding (e.g. 'pooling') on CT and the expectant administration of multiple transfusions (>4 units). It should also be noted that while liver enzyme derangement is commonplace in the aftermath of severe blunt liver trauma, escalating serum transaminases reflect ongoing hepatocellular damage and should prompt further intervention such as angiography or surgery. The algorithm for management of delayed haemorrhage following blunt liver injury instituted by Carrillo and colleagues[32,33] is shown in Fig. 29.6. In their experience, angioembolization for delayed haemorrhage was successful in six out of eight instances.[33] However, it merits re-emphasis that failure to control ongoing bleeding in the unstable patient mandates surgical intervention (vide infra). Complications of angioembolization itself include gallbladder infarction and late biliary strictures, while a systemic inflammatory response with fever is common, presumably reflecting regional hepatic ischaemia.

Intrahepatic arterio–venous fistulae and hepatic artery pseudoaneurysms are less common sequelae of blunt liver trauma. Such lesions are likely to be detected by contrast-enhanced CT, and angioembolization has become the first-line treatment rather than surgery[59,60] (Table 29.5).

Biliary complications

Intrahepatic or perihepatic bile collections ('bilomas' have been documented in up to 20% of

cases through radionuclide scanning,[41] although most are insignificant and resolve spontaneously. The incidence of clinically significant bilomas detected by CT scanning seems much lower (approximately 0.5%[11,49]). Such collections are almost always amenable to percutaneous guided drainage, which may establish a controlled biliary fistula. In the absence of an infected cavity or distal biliary obstruction, disrupted intrahepatic biliary radicles may be expected to heal by fibrosis with spontaneous resolution of the fistula. However, biliary decompression by ERCP, sphincterotomy and endobiliary stent insertion may be required if a peripheral bile leak persists.[33]

A less well understood aspect of the pathophysiology of intrahepatic bile duct disruption and its healing concerns subsequent biliary stricture formation. Sugimoto and colleagues documented intrahepatic duct injuries in six out of 28 such patients (21%) with severe liver trauma and investigated by ERCP, although only one of these patients required surgery.[53] Thus, clinically significant, delayed biliary stricturing seems unlikely to be a dominant legacy of non-operative management, although further evaluation is clearly required.

Disruption of the gallbladder or extrahepatic bile ducts is uncommon and usually encountered with severe trauma and associated hepatic parenchymal or pancreatic injuries.[61] Interventional procedures are unlikely to suffice following major 'central' biliary injuries and surgery is usually required. Cholecystectomy, operative cholangiography, temporary external drainage and delayed bilio–enteric reconstruction are the mainstays of treatment.

Haemobilia and bilhaemia are uncommon consequences of traumatic vascular–biliary communication, in which interventional techniques have largely superseded the role of surgery. Haemobilia implies intrahepatic pseudoaneurysm formation and is characterized by pain, deranged liver function tests, jaundice, anaemia and/or overt gastrointestinal bleeding. Angioembolization, with or without ERCP (for evacuation of blood from the biliary tree) fulfills both diagnostic and therapeutic roles in the management of traumatic haemobilia.[33,62] Bilhaemia can occur in the aftermath of hepatic venous–biliary disruption and is characterized by jaundice with a massive rise in serum bilirubin (e.g. >2000 μmol/l), disproportionate to any abnormality of liver enzymes. Again, such fistulae may resolve successfully with endoscopic biliary decompression, hepatic venous embolization and/or occlusion of the fistula with selective endobiliary tissue glue injection.[63,64]

Intra-abdominal sepsis

Abdominal CT remains the modality of choice in the investigation of sepsis of unknown origin in the critically ill trauma patient. A recent study of CT in 85 such patients indicated that a septic focus was identified in 58%, of whom 69% experienced therapeutic benefit as a direct consequence.[65] It was emphasized that sequential CT scans may be required and that the yield was greatest in patients with penetrating trauma who had undergone emergency laparotomy. However, it should also be noted that poor specificity might be expected during the first postoperative week, and that any potential benefits must be balanced against the haemodynamic and respiratory risks inherent in patient transfer to the CT scanner.[65]

The role of CT in the diagnosis and treatment of delayed perihepatic collections following non-operative management of liver trauma is well established. CT-guided drainage procedures were successful in eight out of ten such patients in the experience of Carrillo and associates,[35] although those with infected collections proved more difficult to manage, with three out of five requiring operative drainage. The same group also reported the use of laparoscopy in selected patients with biliary peritonitis, although its role is less well defined at present.

Gunshot wounds to the liver: the role of non-operative management

Gunshot wounds involving the liver present unique problems because of the high incidence of associated organ (and vascular) injuries. Because of the attendant high risk of peritoneal violation, operative management has traditionally been regarded as mandatory in patients with gunshot wounds to the liver. Nevertheless, there have been precedents for the successful non-operative management of selected patients with abdominal gunshot wounds,[66] and the concept was supported by data from Los Angeles between 1994 and 1998.[67]

In this study, 928 patients presented with abdominal gun shot wounds, of which 152 (16%) involved the liver, and of which 52 (34%) were isolated liver injuries. Of these 52 patients with isolated liver injuries, 16 (31%) were selected for non-operative management, five of whom required delayed operation for peritonitis. Thus, out of nearly 1000 patients presenting with abdominal gun shot wounds to a busy, North American level I trauma centre, successful non-operative management of liver gun shot wounds was accomplished in 11, i.e. 7% of all liver injuries, or 21% of isolated liver injuries.[67] While this confirms the feasibility of such an approach in selected patients with isolated grade I–II wounds, it appears that candidates for observation are infrequent and this approach is potentially fraught with complications.[66]

Important prerequisites for non-operative management of liver gun shot wounds include: haemodynamic stability without blood transfusion, minimal, localized abdominal signs and the absence of associated injuries which preclude adequate serial physical examination. While CT findings should not be the sole determinant of non-operative management, the importance of corroboration with interventional radiologists is again emphasized as angioembolization may be required for treatment of false aneurysms or active bleeding.[66,67] It remains to be seen whether the role of diagnostic laparoscopy will increasingly identify the isolated non-bleeding liver gun shot wound, as suggested by some workers.[26,27,29,68]

The profoundly shocked patient: the role of 'resuscitative thoracotomy'

Haemorrhage is the prime killer in liver trauma and control of bleeding remains the absolute priority. When confronted with the severely traumatized patient with profound hypovolaemic shock and a tense haemoperitoneum, it may be tempting for the surgeon to attempt 'resuscitative thoracotomy' whereby a left anterolateral thoracotomy is performed with cross-clamping of the descending thoracic aorta. The manoeuvre is performed as a prelude to laparotomy in an attempt to pre-empt the haemodynamic collapse anticipated following the release of tamponade in such patients with severe liver injuries. However, little evidence has emerged to recommend this approach in the management of such patients. In the Houston experience of 31 cases of grade VI liver injury between 1977 and 1987, all 13 patients (42%) in whom resuscitative thoracotomy was attempted subsequently exsanguinated and died in the operating room.[69] A similar experience was described in Cape Town.[2]

This is not to decry the role of emergency room thoracotomy in patients exsanguinating from *penetrating* intrathoracic injuries where such an approach may prove lifesaving. Nevertheless, it must be emphasized that initial control of haemorrhage from the traumatized liver can usually be achieved by relatively simple manoeuvres during emergency laparotomy following rapid transfer of the patient to the operating room (vide infra).

Principles of operative management

Operative exposure

Midline laparotomy remains the standard approach in the patient with abdominal trauma, permitting expeditious access to all areas of the abdominal and pelvic cavities. A transverse/subcostal extension along the right 12th rib ('L' or 'T' incision) further improves access to the liver and right subhepatic/subphrenic space (Fig. 29.7). The importance of effective, fixed costal margin retraction using a device such as a Rochard frame (or simply improvising with retractor blades, heavy tapes and lithotomy stirrups) is worthy of emphasis. This affords excellent access such that thoracotomy or sternotomy are indicated only in exceptional circumstances. Nevertheless, the incision may be extended across the right costal margin to create right thoracoabdominal access to the liver ('Y' incision), an approach favoured by some trauma surgeons. The bilateral subcostal ('rooftop/chevron') incision preferred by some hepatobiliary surgeons also provides good access, albeit at the expense of time and access to the lower abdomen, such that many trauma surgeons would consider this unacceptable in the haemodynamically unstable patient.

Early decision making during laparotomy: strategies for the arrest of haemorrhage

Following a rapid, systematic exploratory laparotomy with evacuation, (warm) lavage and the insertion of abdominal packs as appropriate, the persistence of active bleeding from the injured liver will be obvious and local control of bleeding becomes the priority.

A

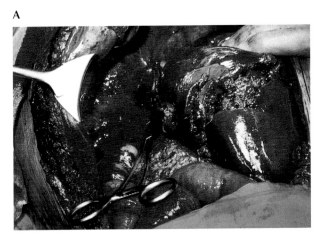

B

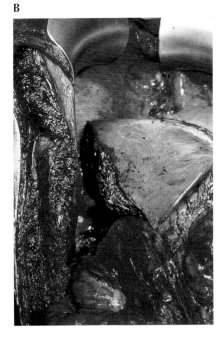

Figure 29.7 (A) Laparotomy for blunt liver trauma. Excellent access has been provided by a lateral extension to the midline incision with fixed subcostal retraction. Complete mobilization of the right hemiliver reveals extensive parenchymal disruption and an avulsion injury of the right hepatic vein (grade V injury). Control of haemorrhage was achieved by hepatic inflow and outflow occlusion (note a vascular clamp has been applied to the right hepatic vein stump immediately distal to the laceration). (B) A formal right hemihepatectomy was performed under controlled conditions.

Simple manoeuvres for simple liver injuries

In many cases where the bleeding has not already ceased, haemostasis can be achieved by simple measures such as bimanual compression of the adjacent parenchyma, diathermy (using high coagulation settings, e.g. 60–90 watts) or suture ligation of visible bleeding points. Topical haemostatic agents such as Surgical (Ethicon, Somerville, NJ, USA), collagen sheets, fibrin glue, etc., may be of use in promoting haemostasis. Careful suture with 'figure of 8' stitches (e.g. 2/0 silk) are often sufficient to stop bleeding from capsular tears and shallow grade I–II lacerations, although the surgeon should beware of overtightening the sutures and 'cheese wiring' the liver. The argon beam coagulator is especially useful for treating the raw surface oozing of decapsulating injuries.

Caution should also be exercised in the practice of blind 'suture hepatorrhaphy' of deeper lacerations or penetrating wounds. This risks formation of a bursting-type intrahepatic haematoma when deep-seated arterial bleeding is merely concealed, worsening the injury and causing large areas of parenchymal necrosis. Ongoing bleeding, which is not easily controlled by aforementioned simple manoeuvres, requires prompt consideration of temporary vascular inflow control with or without perihepatic packing as the next step.

Hepatic inflow occlusion

Pringle manoeuvre

Manual occlusion of the portal triad in the free edge of the hepatoduodenal ligament (i.e. 'the Pringle manoeuvre'[70]) is a simple and effective method of temporarily reducing active bleeding from severed parenchymal branches of the hepatic arterial and portal venous blood supply (Fig. 29.8). Extended periods of hepatic inflow occlusion are usually achieved using atraumatic soft bowel or vascular

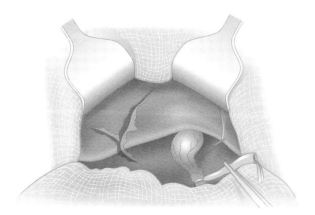

Figure 29.8 Hepatic inflow occlusion (Pringle manoeuvre) by application of an atraumatic (vascular or bowel) clamp to the hepatoduodenal ligament.

clamps. It is advisable to 'test' such clamps on one's finger as a prelude to cross-clamping to avoid inadvertent crushing trauma from faulty or inappropriately selected instruments (with the attendant risk of vascular thrombosis). Experience with elective liver resection has documented the ability of the normal liver to tolerate 1 hour of continuous warm ischaemia,[71] and this may be extended to 2 hours if 15–20 minute intermittent periods of occlusion are employed.

An effective Pringle manoeuvre with local manual compression applied to the liver injury will diminish active bleeding, facilitate anaesthetic resuscitation and rewarming, permit careful assessment of the liver injury and generally 'buys time' for the surgeon. This is reflected by its use, for a mean occlusion time of 32 minutes, in 74% of 113 surviving liver trauma patients reported by Pachter and colleagues in New York.[72]

Selective hepatic artery ligation

When local attempts to arrest parenchymal haemorrhage fail, especially when repeated Pringle manoeuvres are required to control rebleeding, ligation of the regional hepatic arterial supply remains an option. This requires a rapid, precise dissection of the appropriate extrahepatic pedicle. Mays popularized this approach in the 1960s and 1970s, citing no instance of liver failure or massive hepatic necrosis in a series of 60 patients, including nine cases of common hepatic artery ligation.[73]

Of course, similar principles to selective hepatic artery ligation are deployed during angioembolization in the patient with the closed abdomen. It may also be employed in conjunction with selective portal vein ligation as a prelude to more formal hepatic resections, and this manoeuvre should be differentiated from isolated common hepatic artery ligation. It should be noted that the need to ligate the common hepatic artery is exceptional, in which case prophylactic cholecystectomy is advised in anticipation of gallbladder necrosis. The incidence of hepatic artery ligation in series of liver trauma varies widely from 0.6 to 17%, although some commentators cite a figure of 2% as more representative of North American trauma centre practice.[74] This seems to support the contemporary authoritative opinion that hepatic artery ligation alone is 'rarely useful'.[75]

Liver mobilization

Adequate exposure of the traumatized liver is essential and it may be necessary to mobilize the liver formally from its ligamentous diaphragmatic attachments. This can be especially important for injuries of the posterior sector (segments VI and VII) of the

> **Table 29.6 Advanced surgical manoeuvres for complex hepatic trauma: the options**
>
> - Hepatic vascular inflow occlusion (Pringle manoeuvre)
> - Perihepatic packing (resuscitative or therapeutic), or mesh hepatorrhaphy
> - Hepatotomy and selective vascular ligation
> - Selective hepatic artery ligation
> - Anatomical hepatic resection
> - Total hepatic vascular isolation and direct vascular repair
> - Atriocaval shunt or veno–venous bypass
> - Total hepatectomy and liver transplantation

right hemiliver, where injudicious attempts at manual retraction can inadvertently extend and deepen the rents in the liver parenchyma. Careful division of the ligamentum teres, falciform ligament and right and left coronary ligaments through the retrohepatic 'bare area' to the IVC allows the liver to be delivered into the wound without aggravating the injury, and may facilitate the process of perihepatic packing (vide infra)[76] (Fig. 29.9).

Liver mobilization in this way may permit digital compression and control of bleeding in the region of the right hepatic vein confluence. Conversely, grade IV–V injuries with hepatic venous/caval lacerations may not respond to inflow occlusion and any attempts to mobilize the liver or inspect the retrohepatic space may be met with profuse venous bleeding. Other strategies must be considered under such circumstances (Table 29.6).

Perihepatic packing

Performed appropriately, perihepatic packing works for most surgeons most of the time and has been identified as one of the most important factors in reducing the mortality following liver trauma in recent years.[11] Perihepatic packing should be considered at an early stage by any surgeon faced with ongoing haemorrhage from a traumatized liver, irrespective of the specific injury type. In the lexicon of liver trauma management, temporary 'resuscitative' packing should be distinguished from definitive 'therapeutic' packing. The former aims to achieve haemodynamic stability, allows the surgeon to regain his composure, repair other priority vascular injuries and await more experienced surgical assistance if necessary. Most importantly, pack tamponade often pre-empts the rapid cascade of events leading to refractory hypotension, dilutional coagulopathy, hypothermia, acidosis and 'metabolic failure'.

Depending on circumstances, a decision can be taken either to attempt definitive control of bleeding or to proceed with 'therapeutic' packing with abdominal closure and staged reoperation.

The role of therapeutic packing for severe liver trauma has re-emerged as an important part of a prevalent philosophy of 'surgical restraint' and 'damage control'.[77] The accepted indications for perihepatic packing include:

1. Established coagulopathy or prolonged haemodynamic instability,
2. Transfer to a specialist institution (e.g. level I trauma centre or hepatobiliary unit),[4]
3. Severe bilobar injuries,
4. A large expanding or ruptured subcapsular haematoma, and
5. After repeated failed attempts to control haemorrhage.[74,76]

Although packing tends to be reserved for the subset of patients with severe liver injuries, proponents of packing cite a mean survival of no less than 72% in data culled from a collected series of 145 patients from 1976 to 1986.[11] While there remains some debate as to the role of therapeutic packing compared with more aggressive resectional approaches, perhaps of more importance to the surgeon facing severe bleeding from liver trauma is the timing of his decision to pack, that is the avoidance of packing as a desperate last resort when all other measures have failed.

In this regard, Garrison and associates have emphasized the potential for fatal delays in surgical judgement and identify the need to pack at an early stage in patients with severe injuries, metabolic failure and prolonged hypotension.[78] They speculate that preoperative selection of such patients for 'abbreviated laparotomy' may prevent avoidable deaths. Furthermore, a multicentre study performed by the Western Trauma Association identified the sequence of attempted resection and later hepatic packing (together with splenectomy and nephrectomy) as the most common scenario in which patients died in the operating room.[13] Fatal exsanguination following liver trauma occurred irrespective of mechanism (i.e. blunt versus penetrating), but failure to recognize the value of timely packing rather than an injudicious attempt at resection was implicated in several (potentially salvageable) instances. The authors highlight the concept of rapid haemostasis without regard to repair, but with attention to temperature and acidosis control.

It should be noted that perihepatic packing may engender a false sense of security when a 'pack and peek' sequence is allowed to develop.[79] This particular scenario consists of a 'vicious cycle' of repeated packing, resuscitation, unsuccessful attempts at definitive haemostasis and repeated rebleeding into shock.

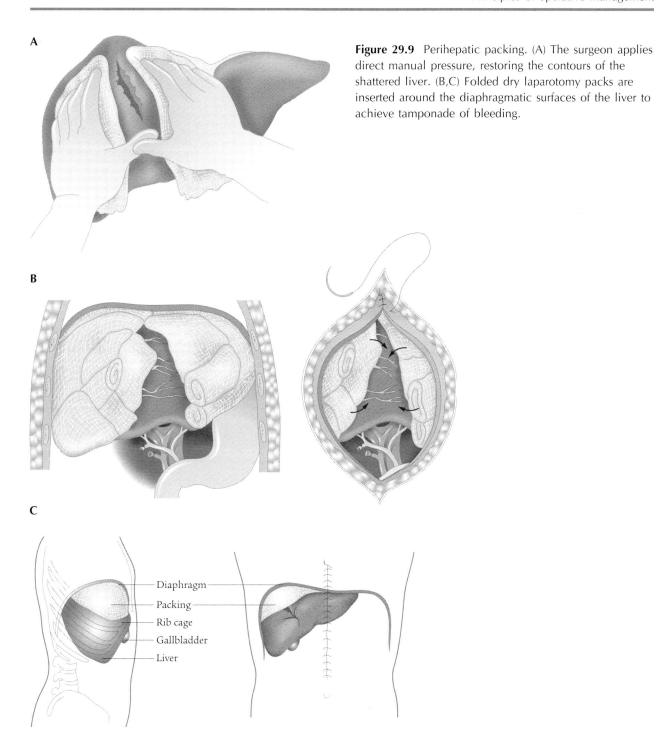

Figure 29.9 Perihepatic packing. (A) The surgeon applies direct manual pressure, restoring the contours of the shattered liver. (B,C) Folded dry laparotomy packs are inserted around the diaphragmatic surfaces of the liver to achieve tamponade of bleeding.

Diaphragm
Packing
Rib cage
Gallbladder
Liver

Meantime, a massive cumulative transfusion becomes established and metabolic failure sets in. Beal has stressed the importance of surgical–anaesthetic team dialogue in maintaining awareness of the ongoing volume of blood loss and curtailing this cycle.[79]

Several technical points deserve emphasis. Therapeutic perihepatic packing evolved from the experiences of World War II, when packs were inserted directly into liver wounds. Although packing of raw injured liver surfaces may temporarily stop bleeding, intrahepatic venous lacerations may also be extended by distractive forces and recurrent bleeding is an inevitable consequence of pack removal. Rather, perihepatic packing requires careful insertion of large, folded, dry gauze laparotomy packs around the diaphragmatic surfaces of liver and aims to restore its external contours (Fig. 29.9). Sufficient packs must be inserted to provide adequate external counterpressure to achieve tamponade, most of this external force being provided by the body wall and rib cage. In this regard, Krige and colleagues describe a 'six-pack technique'.[2] Abdominal closure completes the tamponade effect, allowing continued physiological stabilization in the intensive care unit. The patient

A

B

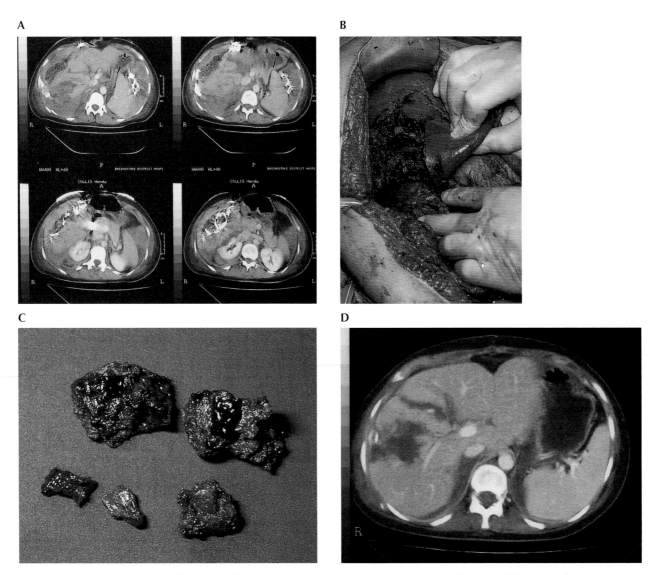

C

D

Figure 29.10 Therapeutic perihepatic packing for a major segment VI/VII injury, and repair of bowel and mesenteric injuries were performed during abbreviated laparotomy following a motor vehicle accident. (A) Postoperative (day 2) CT scan showing tamponaded peri- and intrahepatic haematomas. (B) Relaparotomy, pack removal, resectional debridement and drainage were performed following intensive care stabilization and reversal of metabolic failure. (C) Non-anatomical resection of devitalized hepatic parenchyma. (D) Follow-up CT confirms healing of the liver injury.

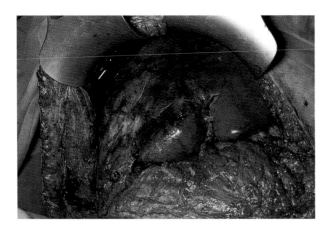

Figure 29.11 Relaparotomy on day 2 after perihepatic packing and abbreviated laparotomy for grade IV lacerations complicated by coagulopathy. Pack removal revealed contusions and patchy necrosis of the right hepatic lobe without active bleeding.

is later returned to the operating room for relaparotomy and pack removal after 24–72 hours, according to the progress of 'metabolic recovery' (Figs 29.10 and 29.11). Saturation of the gauze packs with irrigant facilitates their subsequent retrieval, together with judicious evacuation of residual blood clot with or without resectional debridement and/or drain placement.

Refinements in the technique of liver packing have been devised to facilitate delayed pack removal with reduced risk of attendant haemorrhage. Some surgeons have advocated using a mobilized, viable omental pedicle which is covered by a sterile plastic Steri-drape to protect the pack–liver interface.[76]

Perhaps the ultimate refinement in therapeutic perihepatic packing is the 'mesh hepatorrhaphy' technique which employs a synthetic (polyglycolic acid or polygalactin) mesh which is absorbable and obviates the need for relaparotomy. Originally developed for salvage of the traumatized spleen, Reed and co-workers describe a 'pita pocket' technique whereby the mobilized hepatic lobes are manually compressed and wrapped with stretched mesh sheets.[1] The edges of the mesh are sutured to the falciform ligament or anterior abdominal wall anteriorly, along the right edge of the IVC posteriorly and together elsewhere. Mesh hepatorrhaphy has been reported in several small series of patients with both blunt and penetrating grade III–V liver injuries for a combined mortality rate of nine out of 24 (37.5%).[1] The technique seems particularly well suited for extensive lobar stellate lacerations, but unsurprisingly is ineffective in instances of juxtahepatic or caval injury.

Definitive surgical procedures in complex liver trauma

A common scenario, therefore, consists of the patient with grade III–V liver injuries, in whom prompt laparotomy with the Pringle manoeuvre and 'resuscitative' packing has successfully, albeit temporarily, controlled active haemorrhage. Under such circumstances it is reasonable to assume that there is no significant juxtahepatic venous injury. The dilemma facing the surgeon is whether to take an early decision to institute 'therapeutic packing' (e.g. at the earliest sign of coagulopathy or to permit patient transfer to a specialist unit), or to attempt definitive control of parenchymal/vascular bleeding with or without debridement of devascularized parenchyma.

The latter option requires the use of one or more recognized manoeuvres. Although these techniques all have their proponents and detractors, they should not be considered mutually exclusive. No controlled trials exist to provide an 'evidence base' for the superiority of one particular method over the other and much depends on anecdote, local expertise and individual experience. As stated by Cox, 'Myriads of measures to deal with serious liver injury have been proposed, used, studied and reported. No one surgical technique has emerged

that is clearly superior and applicable to every patient. Each has proponents and when expertly applied in the correct situation will have rewarding results'.[80] Thus, a variety of techniques are available to the surgeon facing the challenge of severe liver trauma and he may select his preferred approach *a la carte* (Table 29.6).

Hepatotomy and selective vascular ligation

Rapid exposure and selective vascular suture/ligation of deep-seated, actively bleeding intrahepatic vessels by finger fracture hepatotomy under hepatic inflow control has become the mainstay of management in many centres[11] (Fig. 29.12). Of course, 'finger fracture' usually entails the use of a small artery forceps to crush the parenchyma and skeletonize the vascular and biliary radicles. Intermittent release of hepatic inflow occlusion 'declares' the site of arterial/portal venous bleeding and allows the precise application of ligatures, sutures and/or clips. Some hepatobiliary surgeons prefer a more refined approach to hepatotomy using sophisticated equipment such as an ultrasonic aspirator (e.g. CUSA) and argon beam coagulator (e.g. ValleyLab). Obviously this assumes its rapid availability and a familiarity with the use of such equipment, which tends to restrict it to specialist centres.

Although the prospect of deliberately extending the liver laceration through normal parenchyma to further 'split' the liver may seem daunting, an extensive literature testifies to the safety and efficacy of this technique. In the series of 107 patients with grade III–IV liver injuries reported from New York by Pachter and colleagues, the finger fracture hepatotomy technique was successful in controlling haemorrhage in no less than 100 cases (93.5%) for a cumulative mortality of 15%.[72] It should be noted, however, that 83% of these patients had penetrating injuries. Similarly, Beal reported the use of hepatotomy in 53 out of 121 patients (44%) with complex liver trauma, citing success in 87% of cases.[79] The popularity of the technique in large North American trauma centres during the 1980s is evidenced by its reported use in approximately 43% of nearly 3000 collected cases of complex hepatic trauma,[79,81,82] and in 28 out of 85 (33%) such cases reported from Cape Town.[2]

An important issue relates to the early recognition of the more severe (grade V) injuries where major IVC or hepatic venous bleeding following blunt hepatic trauma is unlikely to be controlled by the intrahepatic route.[72] It is also worth re-emphasizing that actively bleeding deep penetrating liver injuries (e.g. knife or gunshot wounds) should not simply be oversewn with 'liver sutures' at the point of entry.

A

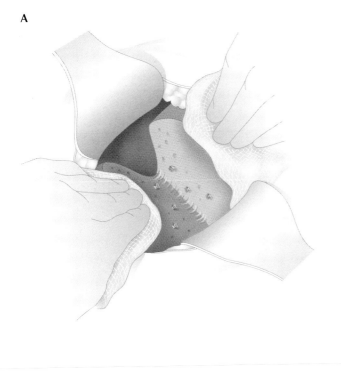

B

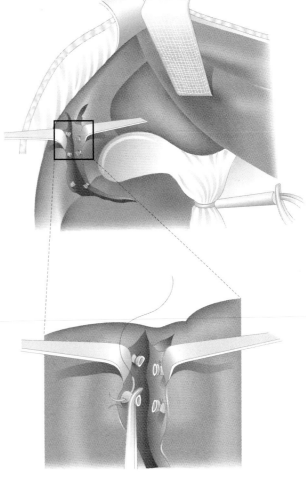

Figure 29.12 Hepatotomy and direct vascular ligation. The parenchymal laceration is extended to reveal the source of bleeding in the depths of the wound under hepatic inflow occlusion. Direct suture ligation or clipping of intrahepatic vessels and ducts is performed until haemostasis and bilistasis is achieved.

As mentioned previously, this risks creating a cavitating intrahepatic haematoma leading to delayed necrosis and rupture.

Non-anatomic resection

In the nomenclature of non-anatomic liver resection for trauma, Strong and colleagues emphasize that such procedures are appropriately defined as either 'partial resections', where devascularized liver peripheral to the fracture line is removed, or 'resectional debridement', which involves limited removal of non-viable liver bordering the injury[75] (Fig. 29.13). Such 'atypical' liver resections may be performed during the index operation after haemostasis has been achieved, or during subsequent staged reoperations following therapeutic perihepatic packing. The limited removal of non-viable tissue in this way has gained popularity as part of the concept of 'surgical restraint' in the management of severe liver trauma, as distinct from a more aggressive approach of anatomical hepatic resection. For instance, resectional debridement was

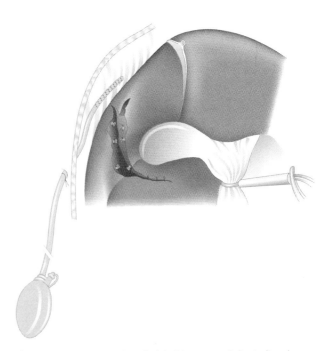

Figure 29.13 Resectional debridement of devitalized liver parenchyma, with hepatorrhaphy and direct vascular suture for control of bleeding. A closed tube drain has been inserted.

performed in this way in 31 out of 85 cases (36%) of complex liver trauma in the Cape Town series.[2]

The extent of resectional debridement is largely determined by the site and severity of the liver injury, and a haemodynamically stable patient with satisfactory coagulation is obviously a prerequisite. As with the technique of hepatotomy, 'finger fracture', 'clamp fracture', ultrasonic dissection or simple suction tip/aspiration may be used. Limited debridement of areas of peripheral liver tissue may be very straightforward, with the caveat that inappropriate pursuit of this manoeuvre to the point of uncontrolled hepatectomy is a pitfall that must be avoided.

At the other end of the spectrum, limited finger fracture may be all that is required to complete a *de facto* liver resection through a grade IV–V laceration which has already partially detached a portion of liver. This scenario is not uncommon following severe blunt trauma to the right hemiliver where a massive fracture causes avulsion of the posterior sector (i.e. segments VI and VII) from its point of fixation along the right coronary ligament (Fig. 29.7) Such injuries are often associated with a juxtahepatic venous tear (vide infra) and a rapid 'partial hepatectomy' may thus be achieved by extension of this plane of cleavage.

Anatomical hepatic resection

The decision to embark upon an anatomical liver resection for complex liver trauma must be regarded as one of the most difficult and controversial. As previously discussed, most authorities emphasize a policy of 'conservative surgery' and 'damage limitation' based on the use of inflow control, perihepatic packing, hepatotomy and selective vascular ligation and/or resectional debridement. Detractors of formal resection cite prohibitive mortalities of 40–60%,[51,79,83] and observe its dwindling usage (2–4% incidence) in the trauma centres of North America.[11] Others recommend that formal hepatic resection be restricted to a limited role in the management of the rare instance of major burst injuries with extensive lobar devitalization.[2]

The rationale for hepatic resection is nevertheless logical in fulfilling the dual role of eradicating both the site of haemorrhage and the source of necrosis (Fig. 29.7). It has therefore been suggested that conservative, non-resectional procedures are 'based on misguided principles',[84] and that condemnation of the role of anatomic resection has led to 'less than adequate surgery for the shattered liver injury' with the attendant morbidity of recurrent haemorrhage and intra-abdominal sepsis.[75]

Although there is a paucity of positive evidence for anatomical resection in this scenario, the principles of surgical restraint observed in most North American trauma centres have also been challenged by some surgeons in Japan[85] and France.[86] Kasai and Kobayashi reported emergency hepatic resection in 30 out of 37 patients with grade IV and V liver injuries, for mortalities of 5% and 33%, respectively. Also, in an 18-year retrospective study of blunt liver trauma in Paris, Menegaux and colleagues cited an apparent increase in the operative mortality of grade III–V injuries following the abandonment of the liberal use of resection in the 1980s.[86] Although careful not to attribute this entirely to changes in surgical practice, the authors nevertheless question the role of conservative treatment in this context.

Perhaps the most compelling data to support an enhanced role for anatomic resection in severe liver trauma emanates from the Princess Alexandra Hospital, Brisbane.[75] In their monograph, Strong and colleagues describe anatomical liver resection in 37 patients presenting with severe liver trauma.[75] Right hepatectomy was the most commonly performed procedure (27 cases (73%)), and grade V juxtahepatic venous injuries were encountered in 11 patients (30%). There were no on-table deaths, three postoperative deaths (due to ARDS and multiorgan failure), the overall mortality was 8.1% and re-exploration was performed in seven instances (three of which were for removal of postresection packs). However, this remarkable experience should be considered in the context of a specialist supraregional hepatobiliary team with formidable experience in elective liver resection and transplant techniques. Initial laparotomy had previously occurred at the referring hospital in two-thirds of cases, and in this regard the lifesaving role of perihepatic packing prior to transfer was emphasized.

Although an element of case selection seems inevitable in a study of this type, the majority of patients were undoubtedly extremely ill with severe liver injuries. The results seem to support the authors' contention that anatomical resection retains an important role in the armamentarium of the dedicated liver team managing blunt hepatic trauma.[75] It remains to be seen whether such results will become more widely reproduced over the next decade, or whether the role of major resections in this context will remain the preserve of the surgical virtuoso.

As previously discussed, there is currently little 'scientific' evidence on which to recommend definitively one approach over another. The debate between proponents of 'conservative' measures based on perihepatic packing,[87] and those advocating major

Table 29.7A **Rationale for 'conservative' surgical management of severe liver trauma**

1. Permits rapid resuscitation with reversal of coagulopathy and 'metabolic failure'
2. 'Buys time' for transfer to specialist unit
3. Avoids high mortality rates traditionally associated with emergency major resection
4. Rebleeding and delayed sepsis may be succesfully managed by interventional radiological techniques

Table 29.7B **Rationale for anatomical resection in the management of severe liver trauma**

1. Removes source of both bleeding and sepsis
2. Low mortality and morbidity reported in experienced hands
3. Appropriately undertaken by specialist hepatobiliary surgeon subsequent to 'pack and transfer'

hepatic resection[88] underlines this. As observed by Reed and associates, the result may be regarded as 'a draw' with overall mortalities of approximately 30% on each side.[1] Table 29.7 summarizes the main points in favour of each management philosophy. However, it should be re-emphasized that these should not necessarily be regarded as mutually exclusive approaches.

Specific manoeuvres for control of haemorrhage from juxtahepatic/caval injuries

Grade V injuries are recognized by profuse venous bleeding from the retrohepatic region which cannot be controlled by inflow occlusion. The type of venous injury can usually be estimated by inspection or palpation of the adjacent parenchymal defect. In this scenario, the surgeon has several options.

Therapeutic packing

As discussed previously, perihepatic packing may achieve tamponade of high flow, but low pressure, retrohepatic venous bleeding. In this way, Beal reported success with packing in 20 patients with grade V venous injuries.[79] Strong and colleagues observed that this manoeuvre, while not always achieving complete haemostasis and haemodynamic stability, nevertheless permitted patient transfer and avoided early death from exsanguination.[75] However, additional measures are required when the severity of haemorrhage defies control by perihepatic packing.

Total hepatic vascular isolation

Originally described in the 1960s by Heaney and colleagues,[89] this technique requires rapid mobilization of the liver with exposure, isolation and cross-clamping of both suprahepatic and infrahepatic segments of the IVC. This may seem a daunting prospect to the uninitiated in the face of heavy bleeding, but is usually managed relatively rapidly by the surgeon experienced in liver resection and transplantation techniques[90] (Fig. 29.14). Indeed, the main issue relates to the ability of the hypovolaemic patient to withstand caval occlusion without circulatory collapse. Also, reperfusion with gut endotoxins may cause tachyarrhythmias following clamp removal.

If a trial of cross-clamping is tolerated then vascular repair may be achieved in dry field. Alternatively, a drop in systolic blood pressure (e.g. <60 mmHg) may be controlled by temporary sub-diaphragmatic aortic cross-clamping, as reported by Khaneja and colleagues.[91] A modification which may control back-bleeding from the hepatic veins while preserving caval flow entails clamping of the extrahepatic hepatic veins immediately proximal to their confluence with the IVC.[92] Also, vascular stapling devices (e.g. Autosuture EndoGIA 30, USSC, Hartford, Connecticut, USA) have become increasingly popular in securing hepatic vascular inflow and outflow pedicles during elective resections,[93] and may facilitate expeditious occlusion and division of hepatic vein stumps in such cases. It should again be emphasized that adequate operative exposure for these manoeuvres is virtually always afforded by the combination of a subcostal or 12th rib extension to the midline incision combined with fixed costal margin retraction (Fig. 29.7). Thoracotomy or sternotomy is rarely required, even when access to the intrapericardial, suprahepatic IVC is require.[75,91]

Excellent results were reported for direct repair of penetrating juxtahepatic IVC injuries when total vascular isolation techniques were employed.[91] In this way, Khaneja and co-workers reported operative survival in nine out of ten such patients presenting with grade V stab and gun shot wounds between 1988 and 1996 in New York, for an overall survival of 70%.[91]

A

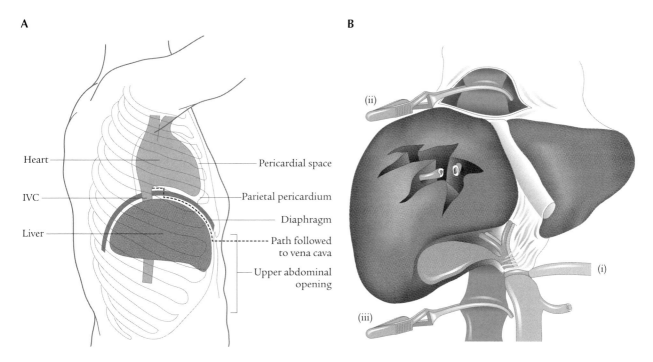

Heart — — Pericardial space
IVC — — Parietal pericardium
— Diaphragm
Liver — — Path followed to vena cava
— Upper abdominal opening

B

(ii)
(i)
(iii)

Figure 29.14 Total vascular hepatic inflow and outflow occlusion allowing direct repair and/or resection for juxtahepatic injuries. (A) Access to the suprahepatic, (i) supradiaphragmatic and (ii) infradiaphragmatic IVC by the intra-abdominal route. (B) Vascular clamps are applied to the (i) hepatoduodenal ligament, (ii) suprahepatic and (iii) infrahepatic IVC.

Hepatotomy and hepatectomy

Anecdotal evidence cites successful control of grade V haemorrhage by a combination of hepatotomy and intrahepatic hepatic vein clamping combined with packing and delayed clamp removal.[94] Nevertheless, the intrahepatic route to blunt juxtahepatic venous injuries seems unnecessarily hazardous and there is scant evidence to support such an approach otherwise (vide supra).[72]

A scenario where rapid liver resection and control of juxtahepatic haemorrhage seems of particular benefit pertains to isolated injuries of the left hepatic vein with parenchymal damage limited to the left hemiliver (i.e. segments II–IV). Such injuries seem to have a significantly better prognosis compared with isolated right-sided or combined hepatic venous injuries.[95]

Atriocaval shunts

The concept of atriocaval shunting seems logical. In reality it has remained the preserve of enthusiasts and reported results have been generally unsatisfactory.[69,95,96] Briefly, the technique involves median sternotomy, control of the intrapericardial and infrahepatic IVC and insertion of a No. 36 chest tube (with additional sidehole cut proximally) via the right atrial appendage (Fig. 29.15). Alternatively, a No. 8 endotracheal tube may be used, utilizing the distal balloon to occlude the infrahepatic cava. It is claimed that the successful diversion of systemic venous return directly to the right atrium facilitates

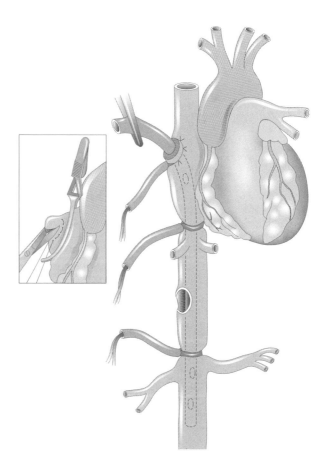

Figure 29.15 Atriocaval shunt fashioned from a chest tube and inserted via the right atrial appendage. Note the additional sidehole cut to lie above the level of suprahepatic IVC occlusion (after Burch et al.[69]).

repair of the injury in a bloodless field, and there have been reports of modest success in the management of grade V penetrating injuries.[69]

It seems likely that surgical indecision, delay and/or technical difficulty in the face of haemorrhage are likely contributors to the generally poor results.[91] In the same way that practising trauma surgeons are liable to disparage the role of hepatic isolation and anatomic hepatic resection,[74] conversely specialist hepatobiliary surgeons have come to disregard the technique of sternotomy and atriocaval shunting as 'almost obsolete'.[75] A controlled trial to address this issue seems inconceivable at the present time.

Veno–venous bypass

Extracorporeal veno–venous bypass circuits (i.e. from common femoral and inferior mesenteric veins to axillary or internal jugular veins) obviate the haemodynamic sequelae of uncompensated IVC occlusion during total hepatic vascular isolation. While a small but beneficial experience has been reported by enthusiasts,[97] the logistics of this approach in the emergency setting obviously restrict its use to specialist surgical teams with hepatobiliary and transplantation experience.

Total hepatectomy and liver transplantation

Total hepatectomy is the ultimate strategy in desperate circumstances when haemorrhage from a shattered liver cannot be controlled, or when a grade VI avulsion injury renders the liver remnant non-viable. Techniques for maintaining venous return during the anhepatic period include portosystemic veno–venous bypass, a temporary portocaval shunt or the insertion of a heparinized Gott shunt to bridge a retrohepatic caval defect. However, the logistical and ethical dilemmas presented by this scenario are obviously daunting as the future survival of the patient depends at the very least on the availability of a suitable donor organ. While an increasing number of reports have testified to the feasibility of this approach,[98,99] the grim reality of the situation was illustrated by Ringe and Pichlmayr, who described the Hannover experience with eight such patients.[100] A variety of operative manoeuvres had failed, culminating in uncontrolled haemorrhage (four patients) and hepatic necrosis (four patients), with six out of eight patients subsequently succumbing from multiorgan failure and sepsis. The authors emphasize the importance of the (early) timing of hepatectomy, but stress that this approach can only be justified in exceptional circumstances.

Deep stab/gunshot wounds

The main options for the surgeon facing an actively bleeding, deep penetrating liver wound have already been discussed. To summarize, inflow occlusion, pack tamponade, hepatotomy and selective vascular ligation and anatomic resection all have a role depending on the circumstances. Total vascular occlusion and direct repair of juxtahepatic IVC injuries following penetrating liver trauma has already been described.[91] A technique which merits endorsement in this context, and which (anecdotally) has yielded successful results, involves intrahepatic 'track tamponade' using ribbon gauze[101] or a balloon catheter.[102,103] This manoeuvre seems most appropriate for selected patients with central, bilobar gunshot wounds.

It is pertinent to note the 1989–93 experience of surgeons at the Baragwanath Hospital, Johannesburg, in dealing with 304 patients with gunshot (often high velocity) liver injuries.[101] They reported grade I–III injuries in approximately 80% of cases, most of which were treated by 'simple' surgical measures. The latter included the frequent use of 'mattress suture hepatorrhaphy' which in their experience was not associated with problems of hepatic necrosis or traumatic haemobilia. Resectional debridement and perihepatic packing were used liberally in patients with more severe grade III–V injuries, and were associated with 15% and 31.5% mortality rates, respectively (usually due to rebleeding, sepsis or associated injuries).

Abdominal wall closure

Closure of the anterior abdominal wall is notoriously difficult (or impossible) following surgery for severe liver trauma when profound midgut distension is established, especially following perihepatic packing[104] (Fig. 29.16). A variety of closure methods have been advocated, including skin-only techniques employing skin-edge towel clips or sutured plastic silos (or mesh) to retain the viscera.[77,104] While rates of definitive abdominal closure of less than 50% are commonplace, Rotondo and colleagues reported success in 12 out of 14 such patients (86%).[77] They cite the utility of temporary, continuous polypropylene skin suture without recourse to fascial closure at the conclusion of the index operation, and discourage towel clip closure for its potential interference with subsequent angiographic studies. Ultimately, healing by granulation of the open abdomen with delayed skin grafting may be the only available option.

Postoperative management following surgery for liver trauma

The principles of postoperative care are the same as for the non-operatively managed patient irrespective

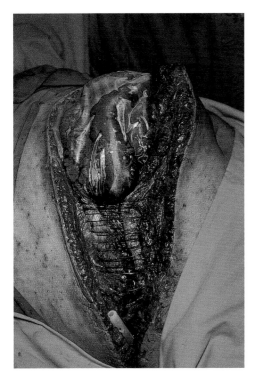

Figure 29.16 Perihepatic packing complicated by midgut oedema and congestion. Note partial fascial closure of the abdominal wall with temporary insertion of a plastic drape silo to contain the bowels.

<20 mmHg) and timely alleviation of this secondary syndrome by pack removal can therefore be critical to patient survival, but must be balanced against the degree of metabolic recovery. Inferior vena caval thrombosis is another recognized complication of packing which may mandate interventional radiological expertise.[107]

The principles of management of postoperative bile collections and biliary fistulae are also identical to those observed for the non-operatively managed patients, that is abdominal CT, percutaneous drainage, ERCP, sphincterotomy and/or endobiliary stent insertion (vide supra). In the aftermath of hepatorrhaphy for a variety of grade III–IV liver injuries in 175 patients, Howdieshell and colleagues reported an incidence of biliary complications of 6%.[108] Abdominal CT and HIDA scans were the diagnostic mainstays, and although biliary fistulae persisted for a mean of 44 days (range 5–120 days), all eventually healed spontaneously without operative intervention. Hollands and Little reported a similar experience in 13 out of 306 patients (4%), although noting the possible contribution of major duct injuries and bile peritonitis to the high incidence of systemic and respiratory complications in their experience.[109]

of the type of surgical intervention, i.e. intensive care monitoring with particular attention to rebleeding, hepatic function and intra-abdominal sepsis. As previously discussed, abdominal CT and selective hepatic arteriography with embolization retains an important role in stable patients with signs of ongoing bleeding (Table 29.5). The role of CT in the diagnosis and percutaneous drainage of septic foci in the postoperative trauma patient has also been discussed,[65] although surgical exploration will obviously be mandated on occasion. Bender and colleagues reported a 12% incidence of sepsis in patients surviving laparotomy for liver trauma, amongst whom there was a 31% mortality.[105] Not surprisingly, factors associated with abdominal abscess formation included perihepatic packing, massive transfusions, severe liver injuries and open drains.

Although perihepatic packing and abbreviated laparotomy may be an expedient, life-saving manoeuvre, specific complications can occur in its aftermath. The 'abdominal compartment syndrome' secondary to pathological intra-abdominal hypertension is responsible for both impaired abdominal organ perfusion, most notably causing acute renal failure, and significant cardiopulmonary compromise.[106] Bladder pressure monitoring (e.g.

Conclusion

Liver injuries are relatively common in victims of both blunt and penetrating abdominal trauma. The AAST hepatic injury scale has become the accepted term of reference. Ultrasonography has gained popularity in the rapid diagnosis of haemoperitoneum and CT is the mainstay of non-operative treatment. The latter has revolutionized liver trauma management for the haemodynamically stable patient, irrespective of injury grade.

A variety of surgical strategies for complex liver injuries in haemodynamically unstable patients have been advocated. A broad dichotomy of opinion has emerged with the current vogue for 'surgical restraint' and 'damage limitation' (i.e. perihepatic packing, resectional debridement and/or hepatotomy with direct vascular ligation) exemplified by practice in the trauma centres of North America. Other (specialist hepatobiliary) surgeons cautiously support a renaissance for definitive anatomical hepatic resection in selected patients.

The various heroic manoeuvres for the repair of juxtahepatic venous injuries generally require the skills of an experienced liver surgeon and may mandate a decision to 'pack and transfer'. Ultimately, optimal outcomes following liver trauma require the multidisciplinary skills of a specialist team consisting of hepatobiliary surgeons, anaesthetists/intensivists and interventional radiologists and endoscopists. The latter are indispensable to the modern management of the formidable postoperative complications which characteristic both surgical and non-operative management of liver trauma.

Key points

- Suspect major liver injury in all cases of haemodynamically unstable blunt and penetrating abdominal trauma.
- If stable: attempt conservative management.
- If unstable: proceed to surgery.
- If definitive surgery not possible then pack and transfer to regional centre.

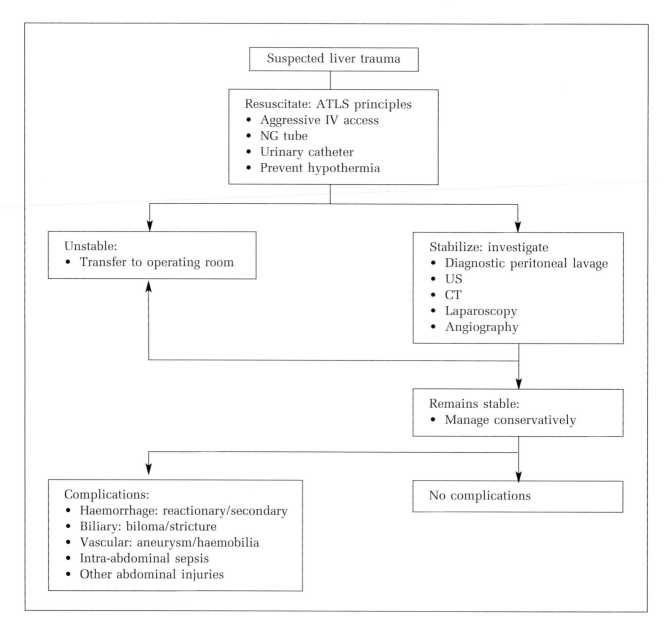

REFERENCES

1. Reed RL, Merrell RC, Meyers WC, Fischer RP. Continuing evolution in the approach to severe liver trauma. Ann Surg 1992; 216: 524–38

2. Krige JEJ, Bomman PC, Terblanche J. Liver trauma in 446 patient. S Afr J Surg 1997; 35: 10–5

3. Calne RY, Wells FC, Firty J. Twenty six cases of liver traum. Br J Surg 1982; 69: 365–8

4. Watson CJE, Calne RY, Padhani AR, Dixon AK. Surgical restraint in the management of liver trauma. Br J Surg 1991; 78: 1071–5

5. John TG, Greig JD, Johnstone AJ, Garden OJ. Liver trauma: a ten year experience. Br J Surg 1992; 79: 1352–6

6. Moore EE, Shackford SR, Pachter HL et al. Organ injury scaling: spleen, liver, and kidney. J Trauma 1989; 29: 1664–6

7. Moore EE, Cogbill TH, Jurkovich GJ, Shackford SR, Malangoni MA, Champion HR. Organ injury scaling: spleen and liver (1994 revision). J Trauma 1995; 38: 323–4

8. Croce MA, Fabian TC, Kudsk KA et al. AAST organ injury scale: correlation of CT-graded liver injuries and operative findings. J Trauma 1991; 31: 806–12

9. Rizoli SB, Brenneman FD, Hanna SS, Kahnamoui K. Classification of liver trauma. HPB Surg 1996; 9: 235–8

10. Alexander RH, Proctor HJ. Advanced trauma life support program for physicians, 5th edn. Chicago: American College of Surgeons, 1993.

11. Pachter HL, Feliciano DV. Complex hepatic injuries. Surg Clin N Am 1996; 76: 763–82

12. Peng RY, Bongard FS. Hypothermia in trauma patients. J Am Coll Surg 1999; 188: 688–96

13. Hoyt DB, Bulger EM, Knudson MM et al. Death in the operating room: an analysis of a multi-center experience. J Trauma 1994; 37: 426–32

14. Velmahos GC, Demetriades D, Stewart M et al. Open versus closed diagnostic peritoneal lavage: a comparison on safety, rapidity, efficacy. J R Coll Surg Edin 1998; 43: 235–8

15. Wyatt JP, Evans RJ, Cusack SP. Variation among trainee surgeons in interpreting diagnostic peritoneal lavage fluid in blunt abdominal trauma. J R Coll Surg Edin 1992; 37: 104–6

16. Muckart DJ, McDonald MA. Unreliability of standard quantitative criteria in diagnostic peritoneal lavage performed for suspected penetrating abdominal stab wound. Am J Surg 1991; 162: 223–7

17. Smith RS, Kern SJ, Fry WR, Helmer SD. Institutional learning curve of surgeon-performed trauma ultrasound. J Trauma 1998; 133: 530–6

18. Rozycki GS, Ballard RB, Feliciano DV, Schmidt JA, Pennington SD. Surgeon-performed ultrasound for the assessment of truncal injuries. Ann Surg 1998; 228: 557–67

19. Rozycki GS, Ochsner MG, Schmidt JA et al. A prospective study of surgeon performed ultrasound as the primary adjuvant modality for injured patient assessment. J Trauma 1995; 39: 492–500

20. Pearl WS, Todd KH. Ultrasonography for the initial evaluation of blunt abdominal trauma: a review of prospective trials. Ann Emerg Med 1996; 27: 353–61

21. McGahan JP, Richards JR. Blunt abdominal trauma: the role of emergent sonography and a review of the literature. AJR 1999; 172: 897–903

22. Rozycki GS, Shackford SR. Ultrasound, what every trauma surgeon should know. J Trauma 1996; 40: 1–4

23. Cuschieri A, Hennessy TPJ, Stephens RB, Berci G. Diagnosis of significant abdominal trauma after road traffic accidents: preliminary results of a multicentre clinical trial comparing minilaparoscopy with peritoneal lavage. Ann R Coll Surg Engl 1988; 70: 153–5

24. Fabian TC, Croce MA, Stewart RM, Pritchard FE, Minard G, Kudsk KA. A prospective analysis of diagnostic laparoscopy in trauma. Ann Surg 1993; 217: 557–65

25. Salvino CK, Esposito TJ, Marshall WJ, Dries DJ, Morris RC, Gamelli RL. The role of diagnostic laparoscopy in the management of trauma patients: a preliminary assessment. J Trauma 1993; 34: 506–15

26. Ivatury RR, Simon RJ, Stahl WM. A critical evaluation of laparoscopy in penetrating abdominal trauma. J Trauma 1993; 34: 822–8

27. Ditmars ML, Bongard F. Laparoscopy for triage of penetrating trauma: the decision to explore. J Laparoendosc Surg 1996; 6: 285–91

28. Villavicencio RT, Aucar JA. Analysis of laparoscopy in trauma. J Am Coll Surg 1999; 189: 11–20

29. Simon RJ, Ivatury RR. Current concepts in the use of cavitary endoscopy in the evaluation and treatment of blunt and penetrating truncal injuries. Surg Clin N Am 1995; 75: 157–74

30. Shanmuganathan K, Mirvis SE. CT scan evaluation of blunt hepatic trauma. Radiol Clin N Am 1998; 36: 399–411

31. Knudson MM, Lim RC, Oakes DD, Jeffrey RB. Nonoperative management of blunt liver injuries: the need for continued surveillance. J Trauma 1990; 30: 1494–500

32. Carrillo EH, Platz A, Miller FB, Richardson JD, Polk HC. Non-operative management of blunt hepatic trauma. Br J Surg 1998; 85: 461–8

33. Carrillo EH, Spain DA, Wohltmann CD et al. Interventional techniques are useful adjuncts in nonoperative management of hepatic injuries. J Trauma 1999; 46: 619–24

34. Fang JF, Chen RJ, Wong YC et al. Pooling of contrast material on computed tomography mandates aggressive management of blunt hepatic injury. Am J Surg 1998; 176: 315–9

35. Shankar KR, Lloyd DA, Kitteringham L, Carty HML. Oral contrast with computed tomography in the evaluation of blunt abdominal trauma in children. Br J Surg 1999; 86: 1073–7

36. Stafford RE, McGonigal MD, Weigelt JA, Johnson TJ. Oral contrast solution and computed tomography for blunt abdominal trauma: a randomized study. Arch Surg 1999; 134: 622–7

37. Mirvis SE, Whitley NO, Vainwright JR, Gens DR. Blunt hepatic trauma in adults: CT-based classification and correlation with prognosis and treatment. Radiology 1989; 171: 27–32

38. Karp MP, Cooney DR, Pros GA et al. The non-operative management of pediatric hepatic trauma. J Pediatr Surg 1983; 18: 512

39. Cywes S, Rode H, Miller AJ. Blunt liver trauma in children: non-operative management. J Pediatr Surg 1985; 20: 14

40. Oldham KT, Guice KS, Ryckman F, Kaufman RA, Martin LW, Noseworthy J. Blunt liver injury in childhood: evolution of therapy and current perspective. Surgery 1986; 100: 542–9

41. Croce MA, Fabian TC, Menke PG et al. Nonoperative management of blunt hepatic trauma is the treatment of choice for hemodynamically stable patients. Results of a prospective trial. Ann Surg 1995; 221: 744–55

42. Meredith JW, Young JS, Bowling J, Roboussin D. Nonoperative management of blunt hepatic trauma: the exception or the rule. J Trauma 1994; 36: 529–35

43. Sherman HF, Savage BA, Jones LM et al. Nonoperative management of blunt hepatic injuries: safe at any grade? J Trauma 1994; 37: 616–21

44. Pachter HL, Hofstetter SR. The current status of nonoperative management of adult blunt hepatic injuries. Am J Surg 1995; 169: 442–54

45. Farnell MB, Spencer MP, Thompson E, Williams HJ, Mucha P, Ilstrup DM. Nonoperative management of blunt hepatic trauma in adults. Surgery 1988; 104: 748–56

46. Hiatt JR, Harrier HD, Koenig BV, Ransom KJ. Non-operative management of major blunt liver injury with hemoperitoneum. Arch Surg 1990; 125: 101–3

47. Frederico JA, Horner WR, Clark DE, Isler RJ. Blunt hepatic trauma. Nonoperative management in adults. Arch Surg 1990; 125: 905–9

48. Pachter HL, Liang HG, Hofstetter SR. Liver and biliary tract trauma. In: Feliciano DV, Moore EE, Mattox KL, eds. Trauma, 3rd edn. Norwalk, Connecticut: Appleton and Lange, 1996: 508–9

49. Durham RM, Buckley J, Keegan M, Fravell S, Shapiro MJ, Mazuski J. Management of blunt hepatic injuries. Am J Surg 1992; 164: 477–81

50. Bynoe RP, Bell RM, Miles WS, Close TP, Ross MA, Fine JG. Complications of nonoperative management of blunt hepatic injuries. J Trauma 1992; 32: 308–15

51. Hollands MJ, Little JM. Non-operative management of blunt liver injuries. Br J Surg 1991; 78: 968–72

52. Hammond JC, Canal DF, Broadie TA. Nonoperative management of adult blunt hepatic trauma in a municipal trauma center. Am Surg 1992; 58: 551–6

53. Sugimoto K, Asari Y, Sakaguchi T, Owada T, Maekawa K. Endoscopic retrograde cholangiography in the nonsurgical management of blunt liver injury. J Trauma 1993; 35: 192–9

54. Boone DC, Federle MP, Billiar TR, Udekwu AO, Peitzman AB. Evolution of management of major hepatic trauma: identification of patterns of injury. J Trauma 1995; 39: 344–50

55. Allins A, Hartunian SL, Grossman PH, Hiatt JR. Blunt hepatic trauma in adults: evolution of a strategy for nonoperative management. Surg Rounds 1997; 20: 419–24

56. Carrillo EH, Richardson JD. Delayed surgery and interventional procedures in complex liver injuries. J Trauma 1999; 46: 978

57. Ciraulo DL, Luk S, Palter M et al. Selective hepatic arterial embolization of grade IV and V blunt hepatic injuries: an extension of resuscitation in the non-operative management of traumatic hepatic injuries. J Trauma 1998; 45: 353–9

58. Denton JR, Moore EE, Coldwell DM. Multimodality treatment for grade V hepatic injuries: perihepatic packing, arterial embolization, and venous stenting. J Trauma 1997; 42: 964–8

59. Schmidt B, Bhatt GM, Abo MN. Management of post-traumatic vascular malformations of the liver by catheter embolization. Am J Surg 1980; 1980: 332–5

60. Schwartz RA, Teitelbaum GP, Katz MD, Pentecost MJ. Effectiveness of transcatheter embolization in the control of hepatic venous injuries. J Vasc Intervent Radiol 1993; 4: 359–65

61. Burgess P, Fulton RL. Gallbladder and extrahepatic biliary duct injury following abdominal trauma. Injury 1992; 23: 413–4

62. Clancy TE, Warren RL. Endoscopic treatment of biliary colic resulting from hemobilia after nonoperative management of blunt hepatic injury: case report and review of the literature. J Trauma 1997; 43: 527–9

63. Sattawattamrong Y, Janssens AR, Alleman MJA, Huibregtse K, Rauws EAJ, Tytgat GNJ. Endoscopic treatment of bilhaemia following percutaneous liver biopsy. HPB 1999; 1: 33–5

64. Glaser K, Wetscher G, Pointner R et al. Traumatic bilhemia. Surgery 1994; 116: 24–7

65. Velmahos GC, Kamel E, Berne TV et al. Abdominal computed tomography for the diagnosis of intra-abdominal sepsis in critically injured patients. Arch Surg 1999; 134: 831–8

66. Moore EE. When is nonoperative management of a gunshot wound to the liver appropriate? J Am Coll Surg 1999; 188: 427–8

67. Demetriades D, Gomez H, Chahwan S et al. Gunshot injuries to the liver: the role of selective nonoperative management. J Am Coll Surg 1999; 188: 343–8

68. Sosa JL, Markley M, Sleeman D, Puente I, Carrillo E. Laparoscopy in abdominal gunshot wounds. Surg Laparosc Endosc 1993; 3: 417–9

69. Burch JM, Feliciano DV, Mattox KL. The atriocaval shunt. Facts and fiction. Ann Surg 1988; 207: 555–68

70. Pringle JH. Notes on the arrest of hepatic hemorrhage due to trauma. Ann Surg 1908; 48: 541–9

71. Hannoun L, Bone D, Delva E et al. Liver resection with normothermic ischaemia exceeding 1 hour. Br J Surg 1993; 80: 1161–5

72. Pachter HL, Spencer FC, Hofstetter SR, Liang HG, Coppa GF. Significant trends in the treatment of hepatic trauma. Experience with 411 injuries. Ann Surg 1992; 215: 492–502

73. Mays ET. Hepatic trauma. Curr Probl Surg 1976; 13: 6–73

74. Feliciano DV. Continuing evolution in the approach to severe liver trauma. Ann Surg 1992; 216: 521–3

75. Strong RW, Lynch SV, Wall DR, Liu C-L. Anatomic resection for severe liver trauma. Surgery 1998; 123: 251–7

76. McHenry CR, Fedele GM, Malangoni MA. A refinement in the technique of perihepatic packing. Am J Surg 1994; 168: 280–2

77. Rotondo MF, Schwab CW, McGonigal MD et al. 'Damage control': an approach for improved survival in exsanguinating penetrating abdominal injury. J Trauma 1993; 35: 375–83

78. Garrison JR, Richardson JD, Hilakos AS et al. Predicting the need to pack early for severe intra-abdominal hemorrhage. J Trauma 1996; 40: 923–9

79. Beal SL. Fatal hepatic hemorrhage: an unresolved problem in the management of complex liver injuries. J Trauma 1990; 30: 163–9

80. Cox EF, Flancbaum L, Dauterive AH, Paulson RL. Blunt trauma to the liver. Ann Surg 1988; 207: 126–34

81. Feliciano DV, Mattox KL, Jordan GL et al. Management of 1000 consecutive cases of hepatic trauma (1979–1984). Ann Surg 1986; 204: 438–42

82. Cogbill TH, Moore EE, Jurkovich GJ et al. Severe hepatic trauma: a multi-center experience with 1,335 liver injuries. J Trauma 1988; 28: 1433–8

83. Moore FA, Moore EE, Seagraves A. Nonresectional management of major hepatic trauma. An evolving concept. Am J Surg 1985; 150: 725–9

84. Balasegaram M, Joishy SK. Hepatic resection: the logical approach to surgical management of major trauma to the liver. Am J Surg 1981; 142: 580–3

85. Kasai T, Kobayashi K. Searching for the best operative modality for severe hepatic injuries. Surg Gynecol Obstet 1993; 77: 551–5

86. Menegaux F, Langlois P, Chigot J-P. Severe blunt trauma of the liver: a study of mortality factors. J Trauma 1993; 35: 865–9

87. Feliciano DV. Packing for major liver injury is a life-saving maneuver. In: Simmons RL, Udekwu AO, eds. Debates in clinical surgery, Volume 1. Chicago: Year Book Medical Publishers, 1990: 141–51

88. Peitzmann AB, Udekwu AO, Iwatsuki S. Resection: optimal therapy for major liver injury. In: Simmons RL, Udekwu AO, eds. Debates in clinical surgery, Volume 1. Chicago: Year Book Medical Publishers, 1990: 152–61

89. Heaney JP, Stanton WR, Halbert DS et al. An improved technique for vascular isolation of the liver. Ann Surg 1966; 163: 237–44

90. Bismuth H, Castaing D, Garden OJ. Major hepatic resection under total vascular exclusion. Ann Surg 1989; 210: 13–9

91. Khaneja SC, Pizzi WF, Bane PS, Ahmed N. Management of penetrating juxtahepatic inferior vena cava injuries under total vascular occlusion. J Am Coll Surg 1997; 184: 469–74

92. Elias D, Lasser P. Debaena B et al. Intermittent vascular exclusion of the liver (without vena cava clamping) during major hepatectomy. Br J Surg 1995; 82: 1535–9

93. Fong Y, Blumgart L. Useful stapling techniques in liver surgery. J Am Coll Surg 1997; 185: 93–100

94. Carrillo EH, Spain DA, Miller FB, Richardson JD. Intrahepatic vascular clamping in complex hepatic vein injuries. J Trauma 1997; 43: 131–3

95. Chen RJ, Fang JF, Lin BC, Jeng LBB, Chen MF. Surgical management of juxtahepatic venous injuries in blunt hepatic trauma. J Trauma 1995; 38: 886–90

96. Rovito PF. Atrial caval shunting in blunt hepatic vascular injury. Ann Surg 1987; 205: 318–321

97. Baumgartner F, Scudamore C, Nair C, Karusseit 0, Hemming A. Venovenous bypass. J Trauma 1995; 39: 671–3

98. Jeng LB, Hsu CH, Wang CS et al. Emergent liver transplantation to salvage a hepatic avulsion injury with a disrupted suprahepatic vena cava. Arch Surg 1993; 128: 1075–7

99. Demirbas A, Fragulidis GP, Karatzas T et al. Role of liver transplantation in the management of liver trauma. Transplant Proc 1997; 29: 2848

100. Ringe B, Pichlmayr R. Total hepatectomy and liver transplantation: a life-saving procedure in patients with severe hepatic trauma. Br J Surg 1995; 82: 837–9

101. Degiannis E, Levy RD, Velmahos GC, Mokoena T, Daponte A, Saadia R. Gunshot injuries of the liver: the Baragwanath experience. Surgery 1995; 117: 359–64

102. Poggetti RS, Moore EE, Moore FA, Mitchell MB, Read RA. Balloon tamponade for bilobar transfixing hepatic gunshot wounds. J Trauma 1992; 33: 694–7

103. Seligman JY, Egan M. Balloon tamponade: an alternative in the treatment of liver trauma. Am Surg 1997; 63: 1022–3

104. Feliciano DV, Burch JM. Towel clips, silos, and heroic forms of wound closure. In: Maull KI, Cleveland HC, Feliciano DV et al., eds. Advances in trauma and critical care. Mosby Year Book, 1991: 231–50

105. Bender JS, Geller ER, Wilson RF. Intractable sepsis following liver trauma. J Trauma 1989; 29: 1140–5

106. Meldrum DR, Moore FA, Moore EE, Haenel JB, Cosgriff N, Burch JM. Cardiopulmonary hazards of perihepatic packing for major liver injuries. Am J Surg 1995; 170: 537–42

107. John TG, Chalmers N, Redhead DN, Kumar S, Garden OJ. Inferior vena caval thrombosis following severe liver trauma and perihepatic packing – early detection by intraoperative ultrasound enabling treatment by percutaneous mechanical thrombectomy. Br J Radiol 1995; 68: 314–7

108. Howdieshell TR, Purvis J, Bates WB, Teeslink CR. Biloma and biliary fistula following hepatorrhaphy for liver trauma: incidence, natural history, and management. Am Surg 1995; 61: 165–8

109. Hollands MJ, Little JM. Post-traumatic bile fistulae. J Trauma 1991; 31: 117–20

Index